OTHER BOOKS BY STEPHEN HARROD BUHNER

Ensouling Language: On the Art of Nonfiction and the Writer's Life

The Fasting Path: The Way to Spiritual, Physical, and Emotional Enlightenment

Healing Lyme: Natural Healing and Prevention of Lyme Borreliosis and Its Coinfections

Herbs for Hepatitis C and the Liver

The Lost Language of Plants: The Ecological Importance of Plant Medicines for Life on Earth

The Natural Testosterone Plan

One Spirit, Many Peoples: A Manifesto for Earth Spirituality

Pine Pollen: Ancient Medicine for a Modern World

Sacred and Herbal Healing Beers: The Secrets of Ancient Fermentation

Sacred Plant Medicine: The Wisdom in Native American Herbalism

The Secret Teachings of Plants: The Intelligence of the Heart in the Direct Perception of Nature

The Taste of Wild Water: Poems and Stories Found While Walking in Woods

Vital Man: Natural Health Care for Men at Midlife

HERBAL
ANTIBIOTICS

NATURAL ALTERNATIVES
FOR TREATING DRUG-RESISTANT BACTERIA

STEPHEN HARROD BUHNER

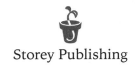

Storey Publishing

For David Hoffmann,
who began it all

The mission of Storey Publishing is to serve our customers by
publishing practical information that encourages
personal independence in harmony with the environment.

Edited by Nancy Ringer and Lisa H. Hiley
Art direction and book design by Mary Winkelman Velgos
Text production by Vicky Vaughn Shea/Ponderosa Pine Design and Jennifer Jepson Smith
Cover photography by © Eric Delmar/iStockphoto.com: mortar and pestle, © Kryczka/
    iStockphoto.com: juniper berries, and © VMJones/iStockphoto.com: tincture bottle
Indexed by Nancy D. Wood

**This publication is intended to provide educational information for the reader on the
covered subject. It is not intended to take the place of personalized medical counseling,
diagnosis, and treatment from a trained health professional.**

**Storey books are available at special discounts when purchased in bulk for premiums
and sales promotions as well as for fund-raising or educational use. Special editions or book
excerpts can also be created to specification. For details, please call 800-827-8673, or send
an email to sales@storey.com.**

Storey Publishing
210 MASS MoCA Way
North Adams, MA 01247
www.storey.com

Printed in the United States by Sheridan Books
23 22 21 20 19 18 17 16 15 14 13 12 11

Library of Congress Cataloging-in-Publication Data

Buhner, Stephen Harrod.
  Herbal antibiotics / by Stephen Harrod Buhner. — 2nd ed.
    p. ; cm.
  Includes bibliographical references and index.
  ISBN 978-1-60342-987-0 (pbk. : alk. paper)
  I. Title.
  [DNLM: 1. Herbal Medicine—methods. 2. Anti-Bacterial
  Agents—therapeutic use. 3. Bacterial Infections—drug therapy.
  4. Plant Preparations—therapeutic use. WB 925]
  616.9'201—dc23
              2012004609

CONTENTS

ACKNOWLEDGMENTS

Julie McIntyre, Robert Chartier, Nikki Darrell, Rosemary Gladstar, James Duke,
Kathleen Gilday, Don Babineau, Melanie and Jeff, William LaSassier, Michael Moore,
Ryan Drum, James Green, Matthew Wood, Susun Weed, Naava, Candace Catin Packard,
Jim McDonald, Redbird, Kevin, Eric, Erica, and of course, Buck and the boys.

FOREWORD TO THE FIRST EDITION

by James A. Duke, PhD

Stephen Buhner has arrived at (and shares with you, the reader) the frightening truth that you won't find in the *Journal of the American Medical Association:* We are running out of weapons in the war on germs. Since germs can go through a generation in 20 minutes or so, instead of the 20 years or so it takes us humans to reproduce ourselves, it's no small wonder that the germs are evolving resistance to our chemical weapons as rapidly as we develop them.

When the drug vancomycin falls completely by the wayside, as it will, we may, just as Stephen predicts here and I have predicted elsewhere, fall back on the bimillennial biblical medicinal herbs such as garlic and onion. These herbs each contain dozens of mild antibiotic compounds (some people object to using the term "antibiotic" to refer to higher plant phytochemicals, but I do not share their disdain for such terminology). It is easy for a rapidly reproducing bug or bacterial species to outwit (out-evolve) a single compound by learning to break it down or even to use it in its own metabolism, but not so easy for it to outwit the complex compounds found in herbs. Scientists are recognizing this fact and developing more complex compounds such as the AIDS cocktail and multiple chemotherapies for cancer. The same super-scientists who downplay the herbalists' claims of synergies that account for the effectiveness of particular herbs and herbal formulas are now resorting to synergies of three or four compounds in their pharmaceutical formulas.

It is certainly easier to demonstrate how two compounds can work synergistically than it is to figure out how 200 or 2,000 different compounds (and more, as are present in all herbs) can work synergistically. So the scientific community will be reluctant to consider the remarkable synergistic suites of compounds that have evolved naturally in plants. But we really cannot afford to ignore these. For nature favors synergies among beneficial, plant-protective compounds within a plant species (with antibacterial, antifeedant, antifungal, antiviral, and insecticidal properties) and selects against antagonisms.

When we borrow the antibiotic compounds from plants, we do better to borrow them all, not just the single solitary most powerful among them. We lose the synergy when we take out the solitary compound. But most important, we facilitate the enemy, the germ, in its ability to outwit the monochemical medicine. The polychemical synergistic mix, concentrating the powers already evolved in medicinal plants, may be our best hope for confronting drug-resistant bacteria.

The Evolution of "Modern" Medicine
(as imagined and adapted by Jim Duke from Internet surf castings)

8,000,000 years ago: One chimp to another: "I have a tummy ache . . ." (*in chimpanzeze, rubbing tummy*). Response: "Here, chimp, eat these bitter herbs!" (*in chimpanzeze*).

5,000,000 years ago: "Here, Hominid, eat these bitter herbs!" (*in hominidese*).

2,500,000 years ago: "Here, Homo, eat these bitter herbs and leave some for the Leakeys to find!" (*in homonoid sign language*).

2500 BCE: "Here, man, eat these bitter herbs!" (*in Arabic, Coptic, Farsi, Hebrew, etc.*).

0 CE: "The Savior is born! Faith can heal. Eat these bitter herbs (*if faith should fail!*)."

1200 CE: "Those bitter herbs aren't Christian. Say a prayer when you take those bitters!"

1850 CE: "That prayer is superstition. Here, drink this bitter potion!"

1900 CE: "That bitter potion is snake oil. Here, swallow this bitter pill!"

1950 CE: "That bitter pill is ineffective. Here, take this bitter antibiotic!"

2000 CE: "That bitter antibiotic is artificial, ineffective, and toxic; besides, all the microbes are resistant, and some even feed on it (*even vancomycin*). Here, eat these bitter herbs. And pray they will help you (*95 percent of Americans, but only 33 percent of psychologists, are reported to pray*)."

PREFACE TO THE SECOND EDITION

If you've reached the point where you don't pay attention to anything that might disturb your orthodoxy, you're not doing science, you're not even pursuing a discipline. All you're doing is perpetuating a smug, closed-minded sect.

— **Paul Krugman**

In the years since I wrote the first edition of this book, my knowledge of plant medicines and their use in healing has increased tremendously. Thus this new edition of *Herbal Antibiotics* is a great deal more comprehensive than that first, more simplistic effort. There are many more herbs included, and some of the old ones are gone or have been moved into another category of action — from an antibiotic to an immune herb, for instance (echinacea is an example). And much of the original material on bacteria and bacterial resistance has been expanded considerably.

Over the years I have received a great many questions as to why this or that herb was included in the book while such and so herb was not. It's a good question; here's why.

I've included the herbs you'll find here for either one of two reasons: 1) I, or practitioners I respect, have found them to be highly effective in practice in the treatment of antibiotic-resistant diseases, or 2) in-depth research and use in other countries has found them to be highly effective. I think when you read the expanded material on treatment strategies and the plants that I've included you will understand the reasoning more clearly; there are some fairly sophisticated understandings of resistant bacteria treatment that were not described in the first edition of the book, primarily because neither I nor the herbal community in the United States had developed enough understanding, sophistication, and experience in clinical work with them at that point.

I've excluded the plants that you won't find here for one of two reasons: either 1) I have not found them to be potently effective in clinical practice (though they might be mildly effective or effective in some circumstances), or 2) there is just not enough clinical research showing they are effective. That is why olive leaf, for example, is not described in any depth in this book. It is not that olive leaf is not antibacterial — it is; all plants contain antibacterial compounds — but rather, both clinical practice and in-depth research have not convinced me that olive leaf is as good as the rather ecstatic reports that circulate on the Internet say it is. For some people and some circumstances, it is a valuable herb to use in the treatment of disease. However, in this book I am interested in herbs that are more potent and effective in the treatment of antibiotic-resistant microorganisms — and more reliable.

In other words, if someone came to me for help and they were in serious danger of dying, the herbs in this book are the ones I would use. If I myself were at risk of death from an antibiotic-resistant disease, these are the herbs that I personally would use (and have used). Without hesitation.

Olive leaf has not, at least in my experience, shown that broad and reliable of an effect, even though in some circumstances and for some people it is highly effective.

Garlic didn't make the cut either, in spite of having been included in the older edition of this book. After observing garlic in clinical practice for over 20 years, I no longer feel it is very effective in the treatment of internal bacterial infections. The plant and its constituents are active and very widely so — in vitro, but that activity doesn't translate well to the real world. Clinical trials and in vivo research just haven't found that those in vitro studies translate to efficacy in the treatment of diseases in humans, especially of resistant bacterial organisms. For topical use, because of its broad antibacterial actions, I think garlic useful — though there are many other plants that are as good or better. And in certain, very limited situations, it can help with some systemic infections — if you use it properly. Generally, though, its effectiveness lies elsewhere. Garlic is very useful

> If I myself were at risk of death from an antibiotic-resistant disease, these are the herbs that I personally would use.

for lowering blood pressure and for helping with high cholesterol, it is excellent as a regular food additive for raising immune function (in a general, tonic sort of way), and it does help a bit in the prevention of colds and flu.

The dreaded "garlic breath" effect doesn't actually come just from eating garlic but instead from the plant's compounds being expressed through the lung tissue as they are moved out of the body. This is why the plant works to some extent for viral respiratory infections. Nevertheless, in spite of its reputation and long use as an antibacterial, I just haven't seen the kind of potency I want to see to label garlic a primary plant to use in the treatment of resistant organisms. If my life depended on it, which it may, garlic would not, even remotely, be my first choice for treatment. I can hardly then recommend it for you.

If you are familiar with the first edition of this book, you will probably notice that I have removed grapefruit seed extract (GSE) from this new edition. The grapefruit plant, *Citrus paradisi*, contains, as all citrus plants do, a great many antibacterial compounds that are effective against a wide variety of organisms (see, for instance, Z. Cvetnic and S. Vladimir-Knezevic, "Antimicrobial activity of grapefruit seed and pulp ethanolic extract," *Acta Pharm* 54 (3): 243–50). Its antibacterial potency is not in doubt, nor is its use for millennia in traditional medicine as an antibacterial, among other things. However, intensive research has found that nearly all commercial GSE products contain synthetic disinfectants such as benzethonium or benzalkonium salts. (The best article on this is N. Sugimoto et al., "Survey of synthetic disinfectants in grapefruit seed extract and its compounded products," *Shokuhin Eiseigaku Zasshi* 49 (1): 56–62.)

For those who have insisted that grapefruit is not antibacterial and that it is only the synthetic disinfectants that make GSE effective, you are, and always have been, incorrect. For those who have insisted that GSE is natural (myself among them), you (we) are, and apparently always have been, wrong. The commercial grapefruit seed extracts just aren't a natural herbal medicine; thus GSE is out. And while all parts of the grapefruit plant are antibacterial, there are nevertheless a great many antibacterial herbs that are more effective than *Citrus paradisi*; hence the plant's absence from this book.

As with my earlier effort, this new edition of *Herbal Antibiotics* is focused on the treatment of antibiotic-resistant diseases. Resistant bacteria caught my attention in 1991, and they've never let it go. The data were clear then: we had a very limited time in which to alter our behavior if we wished antibiotics to remain part of our pharmaceutical options, and many people, including scores of bacterial researchers and epidemiologists, knew it. But knowing something and intelligently acting on it are two different things; there is perhaps nothing more difficult for human beings than actually acting on what we know to be the sensible thing to do. As a species, when it comes to the overuse of antibiotics, we haven't altered our behavior to match what the researchers have been saying, and finding, for decades, that we must do — that is, stop using antibiotics except in absolutely essential circumstances, which is to say, in situations where there is a strong possibility of death or permanent disability if they aren't used.

In consequence the difficulties that face us are now dire; we cannot escape the emergence of pharmaceutically untreatable, and very serious, diseases in our countries or in our communities. These diseases will not be limited to isolated individuals here and there but will instead be widespread epidemics of tremendous virulence. And those epidemics will not come only from the organisms we currently know about; more types of resistant bacteria (and viruses) are emerging yearly.

The growth curve is inexorable, and the emergence of a resistant epidemic only a matter of time, and a very short time at that. When it comes, most, if not all, pharmaceutical antibiotics will be useless.

There are alternatives, however, to the pharmaceuticals that once seemed our saviors and are now our bane, for bacteria do not develop resistance to plant medicines. They can't. For plants have been dealing with bacteria a great deal longer than the human species has even existed, some 700 million years.

Plants have long been, and still are, humanity's primary medicines. They possess certain attributes that pharmaceuticals never will: 1) their chemistry is highly complex, too complex for resistance to occur — instead of a silver bullet (a single chemical), plants often contain hundreds to thousands of compounds; 2) plants have developed sophisticated responses to bacterial invasion over millions of years — the complex compounds within plants work in complex synergy with each other and are designed to deactivate and destroy invading pathogens through multiple mechanisms, many of which I discuss in this book; 3) plants are free; that is, for those who learn how to identify them where they grow, harvest them, and make medicine from them (even if you buy or grow them yourself, they are remarkably inexpensive); 4) anyone can use them for healing — it doesn't take 14 years of schooling to learn how to use plants for your healing; 5) they are very safe — in spite of the unending hysteria in the media, properly used herbal medicines cause very few side effects of any sort in the people who use them, especially when compared to the millions who are harmed every year by pharmaceuticals (adverse drug reactions are the fourth leading cause of death in the United States, according to the *Journal of the American Medical Association*); and 6) they are ecologically sound. Plant medicines are a naturally renewable resource, and they don't cause the severe kinds of environmental pollution that pharmaceuticals do — one of the factors that leads to resistance in microorganisms and severe diseases in people.

Plants are the people's medicine. They always have been. They have been with us since we emerged out of the ecological matrix of this planet — and they still are. And as they always have done, they bring their healing to those in need, at least to those who know about them. And make no mistake: we are going to need them.

It is naive to think we can win.

David Livermore, MD

PROLOGUE: RISE OF THE SUPERBUGS

In the late 1940s, the successes of Waksman and Schatz (streptomycin) and Duggar (tetracycline) led many to believe that bacterial infections were basically conquered. That conceit led to widespread misuse and outright abuse of antibacterial agents. Nonetheless, we still neither fully understand nor appreciate resistance to antibacterial agents. . . . Many important advances in the practice of medicine are actually at serious risk. Multi-drug resistant bacteria are compromising our ability to perform what are now considered routine surgical procedures. . . . A ubiquitous phrase encountered in obituaries is "died from complications following surgery," but what is not well understood is that these "complications" are quite frequently multi-drug resistant infections.

— **Steven Projan,** *Bacterial Resistance to Antimicrobials*

We have let our profligate use of antibiotics reshape the evolution of the microbial world and wrest any hope of safe management from us. . . . Resistance to antibiotics has spread to so many different, and such unanticipated types of bacteria, that the only fair appraisal is that we have succeeded in upsetting the balance of nature.

— **Marc Lappé,** *When Antibiotics Fail*

It's hard to escape the realization that when it comes to bacterial disease we are in trouble. Twenty years ago, when my interest was first stimulated by it, there might have been a newspaper article on antibiotic resistance or a resistant disease outbreak perhaps once a month. I come across them almost daily now. The headlines often look like this:

Hospital Continues to Limit Visitors as It Fights Superbugs
   Ottawa Citizen, December 21, 2010

Staph Bacteria: Blood-Sucking Superbug Prefers Taste of Humans
   Science Daily, December 16, 2010

Hospitals preparing for killer bug
   AsiaOne, December 2, 2010

Eight Deadly Superbugs Lurking in Hospitals
   Nikhil Hutheesing, *Health Care,* October 17, 2010

New "superbugs" raising concerns worldwide
   Rob Stein, *Washington Post,* October 11, 2010

New Drug-Resistant Superbugs Found in 3 States
   Associated Press, September 14, 2010

The Spread of Superbugs
   Nicholas Kristof, *New York Times,* March 7, 2010

Report: Superbugs killed record number
   UPI, May 23, 2008

Sometimes they take a more personal turn:

The fight for life against superbugs
   Boonsri Dickenson, *Smartplanet,* March 24, 2010

'The NHS failed my mum,' says distraught daughter
   Grantham Journal, December 14, 2010

The 'catalogue of errors' that cost this father his life
   Denis Campbell and Anushka Asthana, *The Guardian,* November 27, 2010

The first sort of article (i.e., "Superbugs on the increase in care homes," Daniel Martin, *The Mail Online,* July 16, 2007) tends to focus on numbers and statistics and rarely reflects the human face of the problem. Such articles often end with a statement from a government or medical authority mentioning how new procedures are being instituted or that new antibiotics are just down the road a ways (they aren't). Nothing to be concerned about even though it sounds a bit scary, say the experts; we have it all in hand (they don't).

The second sort of piece, growing more common every year, presents the human face of the problem. These articles are rarely so blasé. This report, from an article by Sarah White, "The empowered patient," is representative. It recounts the story of Jeanine Thomas (who later began a "survivors of MRSA support group") and the moment when all those headlines changed from the theoretical to the very personal:

> Thomas' expertise in the MRSA patient perspective comes from her life-threatening battle with bacteria. In 2001, she was in critical condition after contracting MRSA [methicillin-resistant *Staphylococcus aureus*] following ankle surgery.
>
> "You're just living a normal life — never been sick, never been unhealthy, and all of a sudden you are fighting for your life. And this is happening to individuals every day," Thomas said.
>
> The infection went to her blood stream and bone marrow and caused septic shock and organ failure. After undergoing multiple surgeries including a bone-marrow transplant and a "never-ending cycle of antibiotics," she survived the ordeal.[1]

Thomas survived relatively intact. Some don't, losing limbs in a desperate bid to stop the infection from spreading and then living permanently debilitated lives. Others aren't even that "lucky."

Denis Campbell's and Anushka Asthana's article appeared in November 2010 in the English paper *The Guardian*. It describes the last few months of Frank Collinson's life.

> Ex-docker Frank Collinson, 72, was admitted to hospital following a fall in May 2009. When he went home days later he had cracked ribs and a skin infection .... Four months later he was dead....
>
> Soon after arriving in Hull's main hospital, Collinson contracted the deadly superbug MRSA. Astonishingly, no health professional told his son, Gary. It was only by Googling the name of the drug being administered through a drip that Gary discovered that it was a strong antibiotic and that his father had the potentially fatal infection. "I went ballistic," he said.[2]

This is often how the personal face of the resistance epidemic emerges into someone's awareness. They, or a relative, go into the hospital for a minor procedure or for help after an accident but what they find in the hospital is far worse than the trouble that sent them there in the first place.

> Devastated siblings still reeling from the death of their mother several months ago continue to push for answers on how she contracted a deadly superbug.
>
> Fiona Weatherstone and her four brothers were shocked when their 73-year-old mother, Sylvia Weatherstone, died at Lincoln County Hospital after being admitted for a simple pain-killing injection....
>
> It was in January that Mrs. Weatherstone, formerly of Bristol Close, was admitted for a nerve root injection to numb pain in her back, caused by severe pressure on a nerve root.
>
> The following day, Mrs. Weatherstone's health began to deteriorate and tests were undertaken to find the source of an infection.
>
> Several days later, C. Diff [*Clostridium difficile*] was diagnosed and Mrs. Weatherstone later passed away after a month in hospital.[3]

In fact, other than factory farms, hospitals and doctors' offices are the primary breeding ground of superbugs. A simple injection or a minor surgery can now, fairly routinely, lead to months in the hospital, or loss of limb, or loss of life. It's a new world out there, or rather it's an old one that is letting us know there is a price to be paid for hubris....

1

THE END OF ANTIBIOTICS

[Once] the germ theory of contagion finally caught on, it did so with a vengeance. Different types of bacteria were implicated in anthrax, gonorrhea, typhoid, and leprosy. Microbes, once amusing little anomalies, became demonized. . . . [They] became a virulent "other" to be destroyed.
— **Lynn Margulis and Dorion Sagan, *What Is Life?***

It is worth considering that despite being smaller than one millionth of a meter long, microbes compromise fully 60 percent of the mass of life on the planet.
— **Brad Spellberg, *Rising Plague***

There is a unique smell to hospitals, composed of equal parts illness, rubbing alcohol, fear, and hope. Few of us who have been in a hospital can forget that smell or the feelings it engenders. But underneath those memory-laden smells and feelings is the belief that in this place, this hospital, an army of men and women is fighting for our lives, working to bring us back from the brink of death. We have learned, been taught, know for a fact, that this army is winning the war against disease, that antibiotics have made an end to most bacterial diseases. It is a comforting belief. Unfortunately, what we "know" couldn't be more wrong.

Late in 1993, as *Newsweek*'s Sharon Begley reported, infectious disease specialist Dr. Cynthia Gilbert entered the room of a long-term kidney patient. Her face was set in the mask that physicians have used for centuries when coming to pass sentence on their patients. The man was not fooled; he took it in in a glance. "You're coming to tell me I'm dying," he said.

She paused, then nodded curtly. "There's just nothing we can do."

They each paused then. One contemplating the end of life, the other the failure of her craft and the loss that goes with it.

Dr. Gilbert took a deep, painful breath. "I'm sorry," she said.

The man said nothing; for what he was contemplating there were no words. His physician nodded sharply as if settling her mind. Then she turned and left him, facing once again the long hall filled with the smells of illness, rubbing alcohol, fear, and hope, and the questions for which she had no answer.

Her patient was going to die of something easily curable a few years earlier — an enterococcal bacterial infection. But this particular bacteria was now resistant to antibiotics; for 9 months she had tried every antibiotic in her arsenal. The man, weakened as he was by disease, could not fight off a bacteria impervious to pharmaceuticals. Several days later he succumbed to a massive infection of the blood and heart.

This outcome, inconceivable even a few decades earlier, is growing ever more common. Millions of people are contracting resistant infections every year in the United States, and hundreds of millions more are doing so around the globe. Increasingly, as the virulence and resistance of bacteria worsen, more of them are succumbing to formerly treatable diseases. Estimates of the dead and maimed rise every year with little hope in sight for their reduction.

The toll is mounting because the number of people infected by resistant bacteria is increasing, especially in places where the ill, the young or old, or the poor congregate, such as homeless shelters, inner cities, prisons, and child care centers. And the most dangerous place of all? Well, it's your average hospital. For there is no place else on Earth where so many sick people congregate. No place else where so many pathogenic bacteria congregate. And there is no place else where the bacteria will experience such a multiplicity of antibiotics.

We face an uncertain future but it's not widely understood just how this has come to pass.

The Antibiotic Age

You probably haven't heard of Anne Miller; almost no one has. Never-theless, when she died in 1999 at the age of 90, her obituary was pub-lished in the *New York Times*. Why did "the paper of record" publish the obituary of an obscure elderly woman? Well, because she was the first person to be saved by a very new, experimental drug — a drug that altered human history.

In March of 1942 Anne Sheafe Miller was in a hospital in New Haven, Connecticut, dying from pneumonia caused by a streptococcal infection. She was delirious, slipping in and out of consciousness, with a temperature near 107°F. Her doctors had tried everything they could think of, sulfa drugs and blood transfusions, and nothing had worked. But then someone remembered reading about a new, highly experimental drug. The doctors managed to get a small amount of it from a laboratory in New Jersey. Once they injected her with it, Anne's temperature dropped to near normal overnight. The next day she was no longer delirious and within a few days she was sitting up, eating full meals, and chatting with her visitors. That moment changed our world. News of her miraculous recovery made headlines across the country. The pharmaceutical companies took note and began full pro-duction of the first "miracle" drug in existence. The drug? Penicillin.

In 1942 the world's entire supply of penicillin was a mere 32 liters (its weight? about 64 pounds). By 1949, 156,000 pounds a year of penicillin and a new antibiotic, streptomycin (isolated from common soil fungi), were being produced. By 1999 — *in the United States alone* — this figure had grown to an incredible 40 million pounds a year of scores of antibiotics for people, livestock, research, and agricultural plants. Ten years later some *60 million pounds per year of antibiotics were being used in the United States* and scores of millions of pounds more by other countries around the world. Nearly 30 mil-lion pounds were being used in the United States solely on animals raised for human consumption. And those figures? That is *per year*. Year in, year out.

Epidemiologist and veterinarian Wendy Powell, of the Canadian Food Inspection Agency, comments that "in 1991, there were more than 50 penicillins, 70 cephalosporins, 12 tetracyclines, 8 aminoglycosides, 1 monobactam, 3 carbapenems, 9 macrolides, 2 new streptogramins and 3 dihydrofolate reductase inhibitors" on the market.[1] Those numbers are even higher now.

Most people don't realize it, but — these antibiotics? They never go away.

Antibiotics, in their pure or metabolized states, form a significant part of hospital waste streams. They are excreted in their millions of pounds from the millions of patients who visit hospitals each year. Expired antibiotics (sold or unsold, in their millions of pounds) are simply thrown into the garbage. Antibacterials, as disinfectants, and antibiotic remnants from various treatments also enter the hospital waste streams. *All* of the antibiotics that hospitals buy end up, one way or another, in the environment, usually in wastewater streams. They travel to treatment plants and pass relatively unchanged into the world's water supplies.

American physicians outside of hospitals dispense an additional 260 million antibiotic prescriptions yearly, and those, too, are excreted into the environment. Adding to the antibiotic waste stream, pharmaceutical manufacturers discharge thousands of tons of spent mycelial and other antibiotic-related waste into the environment, much of it still containing antibiotic residues. Yearly, American factory farms dispense nearly 30 million pounds, or more, of antibiotics so that America's food animals — primarily pigs, cattle, and chickens — will survive overcrowding (low levels of antibiotics also stimulate weight gain, increasing revenue). The millions of gallons of their excrement is funneled into waste lagoons, from where it flows relatively unchanged into local ecosystems. Open-range farm animals (as well as millions of other domesticated animals — mostly dogs and cats), deposit their antibiotic-laden feces directly onto the ground. Ninety-seven percent of the antibiotic kanamycin passes unchanged through animal gastrointestinal (GI) tracts onto the surface of the soil.

In short, the American continent, like much of the world, is literally awash in antibiotics. And as physician and researcher Stuart Levy remarks, many of these antibiotics are not easily biodegradable. "They can remain intact in the environment unless they are destroyed by high temperatures or other physical damage such as ultraviolet light from the sun. As active antibiotics they continue to kill off susceptible bacteria with which they have contact."[2]

In an extremely short period of geologic time, the earth has been saturated with hundreds of millions of tons of nonbiodegradable, often biologically unique pharmaceuticals designed to kill bacteria. Many antibiotics (whose name literally means "against life") do not discriminate in their activity but kill broad groups of diverse bacteria whenever they are used. The worldwide environmental dumping over the past 65 years of such huge quantities of synthetic antibiotics has initiated the most pervasive impacts on the earth's bacterial underpinnings since oxygen-generating bacteria supplanted methanogens 2.5 billion years ago. It has, as Levy comments, "stimulated evolutionary changes that are unparalleled in recorded biologic history."[3] In the short run this means the emergence of unique pathogenic bacteria in human, animal, and agricultural crop populations. In the long run it means the emergence of infectious disease epidemics more deadly than *any* in human history.

> Hospital-acquired resistant infections, by conservative estimates, are now the fourth leading cause of death in the United States.

The Limits of Antibiotics

Perhaps no technological advance has been more widely advertised and capitalized upon than the development of antibiotics. It is routinely lauded as one of the primary accomplishments of the application of science and modern medicine in Western culture — the success of the scientific method over the uninformed medicine of the past.

The excitement over the discovery and successful use of antibiotics in medicine was so strong in the late 1950s and early 1960s that many physicians, including my great-uncle Lee Burney, then surgeon general of the United States, and my grandfather David Cox, president of the Kentucky Medical Association, jointly proclaimed the end for all time of epidemic disease. A 1963 comment by the Australian physician Sir F. Macfarlane Burnet, a Nobel laureate, is typical. By the end of the twentieth century, he said, humanity would see the "virtual elimination of infectious disease as a significant factor in societal life."[4]

Seven years later, one of my great-uncle's successors, Surgeon General William Stewart, testified to Congress that "it was time to close the book on infectious diseases."[5] Smallpox was being eradicated and polio vaccines were showing astonishing success in preventing infection in millions of people in the United States, Africa, and Europe. Tuberculosis and malaria, it was predicted, would be gone by the year 2000. With satisfaction David Moreau observed in an article in *Vogue* magazine that "the chemotherapeutic revolution [had] reduced nearly all non-viral disease to the significance of a bad cold."[6]

They couldn't have been more wrong.

In spite of Moreau's optimism, when his article appeared in 1976, infectious disease was already on the rise. By 1997 it had become so bad that three million people a year in the United States were being admitted to hospitals with difficult-to-treat, antibiotic-resistant, bacterial infections. The Centers for Disease Control (CDC) estimated in 2002 that another 1.7 million were becoming infected while visiting hospitals and 100,000 were estimated to be dying after contracting a resistant infection in a hospital.

"To reiterate," says Brad Spellberg of the Infectious Diseases Society of America, "these people come into the hospital for a heart attack, or cancer, or trauma after a car accident, or to have elective surgery, or with some other medical problem and then ended up dying of infection that they picked up in the hospital. . . . The number of people who die from hospital-acquired infections is unquestionably much higher now, and is almost certainly more than 100,000 per year in the United States alone."[7]

This would make hospital-acquired resistant infections, by conservative estimates, the fourth leading cause of death in the United States. And that doesn't even include the death toll from infectious diseases in general, the same infectious diseases that were going to be eradicated by the year 2000. R. L. Berkelman and J. M. Hughes commented in 1993 in the *Annals of Internal Medicine* that "the stark reality is that infectious diseases are the leading cause of death worldwide and remain the leading cause of illness and death in the United States."[8] Pathologist and researcher Marc Lappé went even further, declaring in his book *When Antibiotics Fail*, "The period once euphemistically called the Age of Miracle Drugs is dead."[9]

The End of Miracle Drugs

Though penicillin was discovered in 1929, it was only with World War II that it was commercially developed and it wasn't until after the war that its use became routine. Those were heady days. It seemed science could do anything. New antibiotics were being discovered daily; the arsenal of medicine seemed overwhelming. In the euphoria of the moment no one heeded the few voices raising concerns. Among them, ironically enough, was Alexander Fleming, the discoverer of penicillin. Dr. Fleming noted as early as 1929 in the *British Journal of Experimental Pathology* that numerous bacteria were already resistant to the drug he had discovered, and in a 1945 *New York Times* interview, he warned that improper use of penicillin would inevitably lead to the development of resistant bacteria. Fleming's observations were prescient. At the time of his interview just 14 percent of *Staphylococcus aureus* bacteria were resistant to penicillin; by 1953, as the use of penicillin became widespread, 64 percent to 80 percent of the bacteria had become resistant and resistance to tetracycline and erythromycin was also being reported. (In 1995 an incredible 95 percent of staph was resistant to penicillin.) By 1960 resistant staph

11

had become the most common source of hospital-acquired infections worldwide. So physicians began to use methicillin, a *beta*-lactam antibiotic that they found to be effective against penicillin-resistant strains. Methicillin-resistant staph (MRSA) emerged within a year. The first severe outbreak in hospitals occurred in the United States in 1968 — a mere 8 years later. Eventually MRSA strains resistant to all clinically available antibiotics except the glycopeptides (vancomycin and teicoplanin) emerged. And by 1999, 54 years after the commercial production of antibiotics, the first staph strain resistant to all clinical antibiotics had infected its first three people.

Originally limited to patients in hospitals (the primary breeding ground for such bacteria), by the 1970s resistant strains had begun appearing outside hospitals. Now they are common throughout the world's population. In 2002 I saw my first resistant staph infection outside a hospital setting. Now (2011) every month brings an e-mail or call from someone with another.

> The period once euphemistically called the Age of Miracle Drugs is dead.
> — *Marc Lappé*

This rate of resistance development was supposed to be impossible. Evolutionary biologists had insisted that evolution in bacteria (as in all species) could come only from spontaneous, usable mutations that occur with an extremely low frequency (from one out of every 10 million to one out of every 10 billion mutations) in each generation. That bacteria could generate significant resistance to antibiotics in only 35 years was considered impossible. That the human species could be facing the end of antibiotics only 60 years after their introduction was ludicrous. But in fact, bacteria are showing extremely sophisticated responses to the human "war" on disease.

The Rise of Bacterial Resistance

The thing that so many people missed, including my ancestors, is that *all* life on Earth is highly intelligent and very, very adaptable. Bacteria are the oldest forms of life on this planet and they have learned very, very well how to respond to threats to their well-being. Among those threats are the thousands if not millions of antibacterial substances that have existed as long as life itself.

One of the crucial understandings that those early researchers ignored, though tremendously obvious now (only hubris could have hidden it so long), is that the world is filled with antibacterial substances, most produced by other bacteria, as well as fungi and plants. Bacteria, to survive, learned how to respond to those substances a very long time ago. Or as Steven Projan of Wyeth Research puts it, bacteria "are the oldest of living organisms and thus have been subject to three billion years of evolution in harsh environments and therefore have been selected to withstand chemical assault."[10]

What makes the problem even more egregious is that most of the antibiotics originally developed by human beings came from fungi, fungi that bacteria had encountered a very long time ago. Given those circumstances, *of course* there were going to be problems with our

> The trend in the bacterial development of antibiotic resistance is not unlike the increasing resistance of agricultural pests to pesticides. In 1938, scientists knew of just seven insect and mite species that had acquired resistance to pesticides. By 1984 that figure had climbed to 447 and included most of the world's major pests. In response to heavier pesticide use and a wider variety of pesticides, pests have evolved sophisticated mechanisms for resisting the action of chemicals designed to kill them. Pesticides also kill the pests' natural enemies, much like antibiotics kill the natural enemies of harmful bacteria in the body.
> — *Michael Schmidt,* Beyond Antibiotics

antibiotics. Perhaps, *perhaps*, if our antibiotic use had been restrained, the problems would have been minor. But it hasn't been; the amount of pure antibiotics being dumped into the environment is unprecedented in evolutionary history. And that has had tremendous impacts on the bacterial communities of Earth, and the bacteria have set about solving the problem they face very methodically. Just like us, they want to survive, and just like us, they are very adaptable. In fact, they are much more adaptable than we ever will be.

Developing Resistance

As soon as a bacterium encounters an antibiotic, it begins to generate possible responses. This takes time, usually a number of bacterial generations. But bacteria live a lot more quickly than we do; a new generation can occur every 20 minutes for many species. This is some 500,000 times faster than us. And during that quickened time scale, bacteria have found a lot of different ways to respond to our antibiotics.

> Just like us, bacteria want to survive, and just like us, they are very adaptable.

ALTERED UPTAKE

Bacteria can decrease the amount of the antibiotic that gets inside them. Antimicrobials, in most instances, need to enter bacterial cells in order to kill them — they need to negotiate the cell envelope that surrounds the bacteria. Some do this by taking advantage of the normal influx of materials that must go into the bacterial cells daily in order for them to live. In other words, they sneak in by attaching themselves to nutrients of one sort or another or even appear to be a necessary nutrient so that the bacteria take them up.

To avoid this infiltration the bacteria alter the permeability of their cell membranes, often by altering the structure of the doorways that let outside substances into the cell. This makes it harder, or impossible, for antibiotics to sneak in — essentially keeping the level of the drug below that needed to affect the bacteria.

TARGET MODIFICATION

Bacteria can alter their internal structure so that the intended target of the antibiotic won't be affected by it. As David Hooper at the Division of Infectious Diseases at Massachusetts General Hospital puts it, "Resistance by the general mechanisms of target modification can be brought about, however, by a remarkable variety of specific means, which have been exploited by different clinically important bacteria. The modification mechanism often results in an altered structure of the original drug target structure that binds the drug poorly or not at all."[11]

In other words, they change the structure of their bodies so specifically that the parts of themselves that would be affected by the antibiotics aren't. The antibiotic enters the cell, but it just doesn't do anything.

ANTIBIOTIC MODIFICATION

Bacteria can degrade or destroy the antibiotic, even if it gets inside them, by creating antibiotic-specific inactivation or disabling compounds — often these are enzymes such as extended-spectrum beta-lactamases (ESBLs). As Harry Taber of the New York Department of Health puts it, "It is not surprising to find, then, that antibiotic inactivating enzymes are found in the [cell] envelope: β-lactamases and aminoglycoside-modifying enzymes are examples."[12]

The newest member of this group is NDM-1, New Delhi metallo-beta-lactamase. NDM-1 is a kind of ESBL but much more problematical than any known so far because it is potently active against carbapenem antibiotics, a class of beta-lactams that were previously resistant to ESBL deactivation. NDM-1 is carried on plasmids and transfers easily to a wide range of bacteria. "The frightening thing about this," says Timothy Walsh, a professor of microbiology and antibiotic resistance at Cardiff University in the UK, is that "it appears to be spreading fast."[13]

EFFLUX PUMPS

Bacteria can remove antibiotics from their cells as fast as they enter them using something called an efflux pump. Essentially they create a kind of sump pump that will pump out exactly the things they want pumped out. There are a variety of efflux pumps in all bacteria, each coded for particular substances. Some efflux pumps act on only a single substance, while others (multidrug efflux pumps) can pump out a wide range of compounds. Often the compounds have very little in common with each other; no one yet understands why one pump can act on so many different kinds of substances.

But when one of those substances is identified by a bacterium, the pump kicks in, the drug goes out. Researchers have commented that these "pumps can recognize and extrude positive-, negative-, or neutral-charged molecules, substances as hydrophobic as organic solvents and lipids, and compounds as hydrophilic as aminoglycoside antibiotics."[14]

Bacteria have, over long evolutionary time, created a wide range of pump types in order to protect themselves from the millions of antimicrobial substances that exist in the world. There are five main forms:
- The major facilitator superfamily (MFS)
- The APT-binding cassette superfamily (ABC)
- The small multidrug resistance family (SMR)
- The resistance-nodulation-cell division superfamily (RND)
- The multi-antimicrobial extrusion protein family (MATE)

Most Gram-positive bacteria use MFS as their primary efflux mechanism. Most Gram-negative bacteria use RND. These pumps have a wide variety of purposes, among them the protection of the organism from things like bile salts and stomach acids, which, in their own way, act much like antimicrobials on pathogenic bacteria.

SUPER ADAPTABILITY

Sometimes bacteria learn how to live and prosper in antimicrobial environments, such as the cleaning solutions in hospitals. As one journal article put it, "Contamination, mainly by Gram-negative bacteria, was found in 10 freshly prepared solutions and in 21 of 22 at discard."[15] Sometimes, they even learn to use the antibiotics for food.

Sharing Resistance

Once a bacterium develops a method for countering an antibiotic, it systematically begins to pass the knowledge on to other bacteria at an extremely rapid rate. Under the pressure of antibiotics, bacteria are interacting with as many other forms and numbers of bacteria as they can. In fact, bacteria are communicating across bacterial species lines, something they were never known to do before the advent of commercial antibiotics. The first thing they share is resistance information and they do this in a number of different ways.

ENCODING PLASMIDS

Bacteria encode several different kinds of plasmids, essentially chromosome-independent DNA strands, each of which contains resistance information, and they pass these on to other bacteria. Plasmids are highly mobile genetic strands and are widely exchanged throughout the bacterial world. Aminoglycosides, for example, some of the most potent antibacterials known, were originally isolated from actinomycetes, a type of bacteria. Those bacteria created and used aminoglycosides themselves to kill invading or competing bacteria, but the aminoglycosides could also kill actinomycetes, so the actinomycetes also created something to deactivate aminoglycosides and they stored that information on plasmids inside themselves. *All* resistance to aminoglycosides worldwide, including in *Pseudomonas* and *Acinetobacter* organisms, has come from those ancient plasmids created by the actinomycetes. Once aminoglycosides began to be promiscuously prescribed by the medical community, the actinomycetes released the plasmids like a puff of dandelion seeds on the wind.

USING TRANSPOSONS AND INTEGRONS

Bacteria use transposons, unique movable segments of DNA that are a normal component of their genome. Sometimes called "jumping genes," transposons easily move between chromosomes and plasmids. They are readily integrated into DNA structures, and when they are, the genetic makeup, and hence the physical form of the organism, is altered. Bacteria use transposons to transfer a significant amount of resistance information and often release them in free form into the environment to be taken up later by other bacteria.

They use integrons as well, a type of DNA sequence that integrates into the genome structure at specific sites. Integrons are especially active in the transfer of both resistance and virulence information.

USING VIRUSES

Bacterial viruses, or bacteriophages, also help transfer resistance information between different bacteria. It is now known that instead of making only copies of themselves when they reproduce, bacteriophages take up and make copies of host chromosome segments that contain resistance information, which are then transferred to newly infected bacteria. In other words, the viruses that infect bacteria (they get colds, too) teach them how to be resistant to antibiotics.

Bacteria can share resistance information directly or simply extrude it from their cells, allowing it to be picked up later by other roving bacteria. They often experiment, combining resistance information from multiple sources in unique ways that increase resistance, generate new resistance pathways, or even stimulate resistance to antibiotics that they have never encountered before. Even bacteria in hibernating or moribund states will share whatever information on resistance they have with any bacteria that encounter them. When bacteria take up any encoded information on resistance, they weave it into their own DNA, and this acquired resistance becomes a genetic trait that can be passed on to their descendants forever — distressingly Lamarckian. Researchers have noted that the rise of resistance over the past 50 years has had a one-to-one correlation to the production and use of antibiotics and that resistance mechanisms are not just passed on to other bacteria but are conserved within species.

Bacterial Learning

Antibiotics, ultimately and regrettably for us, have actions similar to pheromones; they act as chemical attractants and literally pull bacteria to them. Once in the presence of an antibiotic, a bacterium's learning rate immediately increases by several orders of magnitude. Tetracycline, in even extremely low doses — in fact, especially in low doses — stimulates from one hundred to one thousand times the transfer, mobilization, and movement of transposons and plasmids. (Treatment of acne and fattening of industrial farm animals, by the way, generally involves low doses of tetracycline, often over years.) Wendy Powell comments that "this means that in times of stress, predicated by the presence of antibiotics, the antibiotics themselves promote the exchange of plasmids, which may contain resistance genes."[16]

> Bacteria are not competing with each other for resources, but rather cooperating in the sharing of survival information.

The fairly recent discovery that *all* of the water supplies in the industrialized countries are contaminated with minute amounts of antibiotics (from their excretion into water supplies) means that bacteria everywhere are experiencing low doses of antibiotics *all the time*. This exposure is exponentially driving resistance learning; the more antibiotics that go into the water, the faster the bacteria learn.

What is more, as bacteria gain resistance, they pass that knowledge on to *all* forms of bacteria they meet. They are not competing with each other for resources, as standard evolutionary theory predicted, but rather promiscuously cooperating in the sharing of survival information. "More surprising," one research group commented, "is the apparent movement of genes, such as *tetQ* and *ermB* between members of the normal microflora of humans and animals, populations of bacteria that differ in species composition."[17] Anaerobic and aerobic, Gram-positive and Gram-negative, spirochetes and plasmodial parasites, all are exchanging resistance information — something that, prior to antibiotic usage, was never known to occur (and contributing

How Smart Are Bacteria, Anyway?

After placing a single bacterial species in a nutrient solution containing sublethal doses of a newly developed and rare antibiotic, researchers found that within a short period of time the bacteria developed resistance to that antibiotic *and* to 12 other antibiotics that they had never before encountered — some of which were structurally dissimilar to the first. Stuart Levy observes, "It's almost as if bacteria strategically anticipate the confrontation of other drugs when they resist one."[18]

In essence, bacteria are anticipating the creation of antibiotics that people haven't even thought of yet. They are also teaching themselves how to become more virulent, how to make their diseases stronger, by sharing virulence factors among themselves through the same mechanisms they use to share resistance information. In fact, they are acting in concert so well in response to the human "war on disease" that it has led Levy to remark, "One begins to see bacteria, not as individual species, but as a vast array of interacting constituents of an integrated microbial world."[19] Former FDA commissioner Donald Kennedy echoes this, stating, "The evidence indicates that enteric microorganisms in animals and man, their R plasmids, and human pathogens form a linked ecosystem of their own in which action at any one point can affect every other."[20]

And wherever antibacterial use is high, bacterial congregation and rate of learning are also high. Heavy antibiotic usage in fact causes immediate bacterial congregation, rapid learning, and a subsequent cascade of resistance information throughout the microbial membrane, where it can be accessed at any time. Researcher J. Davies notes, "This gene pool [of resistance information] is readily accessible to bacteria when they are exposed to the strong selective pressures of antibiotic usage in hospitals, for veterinary and agricultural purposes, and as growth promotants in animal and poultry husbandry."[21]

Wherever antibiotics and overcrowded or ill animal life meet in large numbers, resistance cascades occur: nursing homes, day care centers, homeless shelters, prisons, inner cities, animal hospitals, and factory farming operations. But they aren't the worst. In spite of the apparent cleanliness of hospitals, the white coats, the quiet voices, the surety of purpose, the truth is that there is no place on Earth that contains more resistant bacteria.

to a growing recognition that nature may not be red in tooth and claw but much more mutualistic and interdependently connected than formerly supposed). The recognition, long delayed by incorrect assumptions about the nature of the genome, is now widespread — genetic structures in all organisms are not static but fluid, sometimes along a wide range. Barbara McClintock, who early recognized the existence of transposons, noted in her 1983 Nobel lecture that the genome "is a highly sensitive organ of the cell, that in times of stress can initiate its own restructuring and renovation."[22] She noted as well that the instructions for how the genotype reassembled came from not only the organism but the environment itself. The greater the stress, the more fluid and specific the action of the genome in responding to it.

Research, new since the first edition of this book, has borne out McClintock's observations with a vengeance. The genome of an organism is stored in its DNA. It turns out that antibiotics often damage bacterial DNA through boosting production of free-radical oxygen molecules inside the bacteria. In other words this highly flexible organ of the cell is partially corrupted by antibiotics. Once that occurs the organism immediately begins repairing the damage. The bacteria begins to reweave the DNA, including the genomic structure encoded within it. Part of the data that informs those repair processes is the factors that caused the damage. So the bacteria literally restructure the genome in such a way as to counteract the damaging event. And since the damaging event *is* the antibiotic creation of free radicals, the bacteria develop resistance to *all* antibiotics that create free radicals.

The Spread of Resistant Disease

Resistant bacteria tend to specialize in what part of the body they infect. *Enterococcus*, *Pseudomonas*, *Staphylococcus*, and *Klebsiella* bacteria take advantage of surgical procedures to infect surgical wounds or patients' blood in hospitals.

It turns out that staph bacteria need the iron that occurs naturally in blood cells, and the organisms prefer one kind of blood — ours. Anyplace where human blood is widely available, staph organisms congregate in large numbers. *Staphylococcus* organisms are "the leading cause of pus-forming skin and soft tissue infections, the leading cause of infectious heart disease, the number one hospital acquired infection, and one of the four leading causes of food-borne illness."[23] And the organisms keep learning.

Effluent streams from cities, filled with excreted antibiotics and resistant staph organisms, flow into the seas surrounding cities. Resistant staph is endemic in all oceans abutting land masses — and the adjoining beaches. It also learned how to transmit itself from person to person during sex. Welcome to the newest STD.

Haemophilus, Pseudomonas, Staphylococcus, Klebsiella, and *Streptococcus* infect lung tissue, many times gaining access by hitching a ride on infected breathing tubes, oh-so-carefully inserted into patients by hospital staff. The bacteria cause pneumonia, often untreatable, in elderly patients in hospitals and nursing homes. Once known as the old person's friend (because it, relatively gently, eased the old into death), pneumonia was significantly reduced through antibiotic use but is now making a comeback as a leading cause of death in the elderly.

Pseudomonas and *Klebsiella,* traveling into urinary passageways on nurse-inserted catheters, initiate serious or intransigent urinary tract infections in many patients. They also gain entry into female nurses' urinary tracts through poor hygiene, where they rapidly mutate under the pressure of the free antibiotics dispensed to such hospital personnel. (Most nurses' and physicians' hands are covered in resistant bacteria whether they wash or not — hand disinfection and hand washing are not the same thing.)

> Complete and total antibiotic resistance of the [staph] organism is inevitable at this point.
> — *Eric Skaar*
> *Vanderbilt University*

Haemophilus and *Streptococcus* initiate serious ear infections (sometimes leading to meningitis) in pediatric wards, which multiple rounds of antibiotics often fail to cure. These organisms can also cause debilitating infections of the GI tract accompanied by severe, unremitting diarrhea. And they are not alone in this. One of the newer, more dangerous infectious organisms of the GI tract is *Clostridium difficile*. As the Infectious Diseases Society of America reports, "The rate of infections caused by *Clostridium difficile* in U.S. hospitals doubled between 2000 and 2003. Outbreaks of severe *C. difficile* disease among hospital patients and clusters of unusually severe *C. difficile* disease among previously low-risk patients have been reported from multiple states. Many of the changes in the behavior of this infection appear due to the spread of an epidemic strain of *C. difficile* with increased virulence and increased resistance to commonly used fluoroquinolone antimicrobials."[24]

According to the CDC, there were four times as many deaths from this disease in 2004 as there were in 1999. The organism has become so difficult to treat with antibiotics that Western doctors are turning to a new treatment: fecal transplants. Yes, you heard that right, they put someone else's poop into your bowel in hopes that a healthy bowel population might just reestablish itself. The new poop is fed into the body through a tube in the patient's nose. (This is *modern* medicine.)

The Return of Diseases Once Thought Cured

Tuberculosis (TB) is increasingly resistant and is spreading in inner cities, homeless shelters, and prisons. About two billion people worldwide are thought to have latent TB, about one in three people. Two hundred million of those will become infectious (15 million in the United States) while three million a year will die. About 80 percent of those infected show some signs of antibiotic resistance. Two percent, or 40 million people worldwide, currently have an untreatable, resistant strain. TB is, in fact, becoming so difficult to treat that older approaches, such as surgical removal of the diseased lung, are sometimes being utilized.

Gonorrhea has reemerged with a potent resistance it learned in brothels in Vietnam among prostitutes who were regularly given daily courses of antibiotics. It now causes 700,000 infections in the United States each year. Malaria, spread by mosquitos and once considered only a disease of the tropics, kills one million people a year worldwide and is resistant to pharmaceuticals over 85 percent of the time.

Cholera has also learned resistance to a number of antibiotics through improper dosing by physicians. Even more telling, it has learned resistance to the primary drug used to kill it in the wild — chlorine. Chlorine, though naturally present in the ecosystem, rarely exists in pure form. Generally, it is chemically bonded to something else, as in such things as table salt (sodium chloride). Industrial production is around 50 million pounds a year of chemically pure chlorine. It is used in products such as organochlorines (e.g., the PVCs used in medicine) and, commonly, in water supplies as an antimicrobial disinfectant. Both cholera and *E. coli* have developed resistance to chlorine as a result. Dangerous in and of itself but more so because *E. coli*, exposed to such large numbers of antibiotics in the human GI tract, is one of the principal bacteria that learns resistance and passes it on. This information exchange is especially easy with other types of GI tract bacteria, especially if they are Gram-negative, which cholera is. In 2000, when the first documented outbreak of simultaneous infection by enterotoxigenic *E. coli* and cholera occurred in India, both were resistant organisms.

Cholera lives in water, usually near human settlements, in a quiescent state between epidemics. During these lulls cholera encounters not only chlorine but the scores of other antibiotics that flow in sublethal doses into nearly all water supplies on Earth. Resistance determinants are widely shared between multiple serotypes of cholera. Like all pathogenic bacteria, the resistance curve of cholera organisms is exponential. In 1992, only 35 percent of cholera O1 serotypes were resistant to ampicillin. By 1997, 100 percent were.

Cholera epidemics tend to emerge in human populations when the fecal content of waste streams from population centers is high. The organisms follow the effluent upstream, seeking its source. They usually find it.

Antimicrobial pressure has caused *E. coli*, not normally pathogenic, to also develop unexpected virulence capacities in such forms as the potentially deadly *E. coli* O157:H7. Epidemiologists now know, through genetic markers, that it was taught its virulence by *Shigella* bacteria. Researcher and physician Marguerite Neill, a specialist in infectious medicine, observes that judicious reflection on the meaning of this finding suggests a larger significance — that *E. coli* O157:H7 is a messenger, bringing an unwelcome message that "in mankind's battle to conquer infectious diseases, the opposing army is being replenished with fresh replacements."[25]

How Hospitals Create the Problem

Hospitals, where large numbers of pathogenic bacteria and antibiotics come into frequent contact, give bacteria the most opportunity to develop resistance *and* virulence. Researchers examining the effluent streams from hospitals have found them to contain exceptionally large numbers of resistant bacteria as well as large amounts of excreted antibiotics. These antibiotics and resistant bacteria flow into the environment and spread everywhere. As Julie Gerberding of the Centers for Disease Control comments, "Once restricted to hospitals, where seriously ill patients are exposed to constant infusions of drugs, these [resistant bacteria] are now being found in the community."[26]

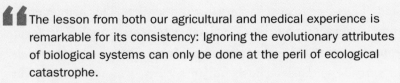

The lesson from both our agricultural and medical experience is remarkable for its consistency: Ignoring the evolutionary attributes of biological systems can only be done at the peril of ecological catastrophe.
— Marc Lappé, *When Antibiotics Fail*

The prodigious production of antibacterial soaps that end up going into the water are stimulating resistance among many classes of bacteria as well. Even though resistance dynamics were well understood long before antibacterial soaps were allowed on the market, under pressure from corporations they were still allowed in the United States. And like all other antibacterial substances, they have begun to confer unique forms of resistance on the planet's bacteria. The fear of microbes, so thoroughly leveraged by television advertising, has only hastened the resistance problem. The Centers for Disease Control in Atlanta, Georgia, found that the average amount of the antibacterial component of such soaps, triclosan, increased in Americans' urine by 42 percent between 2003 and 2006. Studies have shown that the chemical encourages bacterial resistance and that it disrupts hormone levels in regular users. Triclosan is common in many toothpastes, in nearly all antibacterial soaps, and even on knives and cutting boards.

These circumstances have increased the rate of resistance in bacteria exponentially. In 1999, 95 percent of *E. coli* was susceptible to ciprofloxacin but that had dropped to 60 percent by 2006; *Acinetobacter* susceptibility decreased by 70 percent in just 4 years; 36 percent of *Staphylococcus* organisms were resistant in 1992 but by 2003 64 percent were — the usual exponential learning curves. But these are only part of the story.

Factory Farms: The Story Gets Worse

The use of antibiotics by factory farms and wide antibiotic use by veterinarians for our pets has created a similar bacterial evolution in fast-forward. At least half, if not more, of all antibiotics used in the United States goes to huge factory farm operations. This has generated tremendously potent and quick resistance in a large range of bacteria. As reporter Brandon Keim comments, "Much of it is used to treat diseases spread by industrial husbandry practices, or simply to accelerate growth. As a result, farms have become giant petri dishes for superbugs, especially multidrug-resistant *Staphylococcus aureus* or MRSA, which kills 20,000 Americans every year — more than AIDS."[27]

Nicols Fox comments in her exposé of the problem in her book *Spoiled: The Dangerous Truth About a Food Chain Gone Haywire*:

> The conditions under which [farm animals were] raised presented all the conditions for infection and disease: the animals were closely confined; subjected to stress; often fed contaminated food and water; exposed to vectors (flies, mice, rats) that could carry contaminants from one flock to another; bedded on filth-collecting litter; and given antibiotics (which, ironically, made them more vulnerable to disease) to encourage growth as well as ward off other infections.... Every condition that predisposed the spread of disease from animal to human actually worsened. Farming became more intensive, slaughtering became more mechanical and faster, products were processed in even more massive lots, and distribution became wider.[28]

As with human diseases, pathogenic animal bacteria have specialized: *E. coli* O157:H7 in beef, *Salmonella* in chicken eggs, *Campylobacter* in chickens, *Listeria* in deli meat. (And there are others such as *Cyclospora*, *Cryptosporidium*, and *Yersinia*). Like the resistant bacteria emerging from our hospitals, bacteria from factory farms spread quickly into the wider world. And while factory farm owners deny their practices have *anything* to do with the problem, the only place where antibiotic-resistant organisms genetically identical to those from factory farming operations don't yet seem to exist is in indigenous animals in the northern arctic regions.

One of the early pioneers in antibiotic resistance is Stuart Levy, a professor who runs the Levy Lab at the Center for Adaptation Genetics and Drug Resistance at Tufts University School of Medicine. To trace the flow into the environment of resistant bacteria from farming operations, he took six groups of chickens and placed them 50 to a cage. Four cages were in a barn, two just outside. Half the chickens received food containing subtherapeutic doses of oxytetracycline. The feces of all the chickens as well as the farm family living nearby and farm families in the neighborhood were examined weekly. Within 24 to 36 hours of eating the first batch of antibiotic-containing food, the feces of the dosed chickens showed *E. coli*–resistant bacteria.

Soon the undosed chickens also showed *E. coli* that were resistant to
tetracycline. But even more remarkable, by the end of 3 months, the
E. coli of *all* chickens were also resistant to ampicillin, streptomycin,
and sulfonamides *even though they had never been fed these drugs*. Still more startling: At the end of 5 months, the feces of the nearby farm family (who had had no contact with the chickens) contained *E. coli* resistant to tetracycline. By the sixth month their *E. coli* were also resistant to five other antibiotics. A similar but longer study in Germany
found that this resistance eventually moved into the surrounding
community — taking a little over 2 years.

> At least half, if not more, of all antibiotics used in the United States goes to huge factory farms.

Salmonella, which is now genetically lodged *in the ovaries* (and
hence the eggs that come from them) of many agribusiness chickens,
can survive refrigeration, boiling, basting, and frying. To kill salmonella bacteria the egg must be fried hard or boiled for 9 minutes or
longer. *Listeria* in deli meat can survive refrigeration. *E. coli* can now
live in both orange juice and apple juice — two acidic mediums that
previously killed it. And a recent study (2011) found that nearly 50 percent of all store-bought meat and poultry tested were contaminated
with staph, and over half the bacteria tested were resistant strains.
Lance Price, the lead author of the study, remarked, "The fact that
drug-resistant *S. aureus* was so prevalent, and likely came from the
food animals themselves, is troubling."[29]

These food-borne bacteria are moving with greater frequency into
the human food chain and human populations. There were 23 recalls
by the U.S. FDA in 2010 for contamination from *Salmonella, Listeria,
Clostridium, E. coli*, and *Bacillus* organisms.

Recent research has found that one of the main vectors for the
spread of resistant organisms into the general community is flies.
At minimum, over 30,000 flies will visit a poultry farming operation
within any 6-week period. Researchers who studied groups of flies
from such operations found them to be infected with exactly the same

genetic variants of resistant bacteria as those found in the poultry wastes the flies were feeding on. This same phenomenon occurs at all large-animal factory farms, with both cattle and pigs.

The growth rate of resistance and virulence is so fast that 15 years ago Stuart Levy observed, "Some analysts warn of present-day scenarios in which infectious antibiotic-resistant bacteria devastate whole human populations.... This situation raises the staggering possibility that a time will come when antibiotics as a mode of therapy will only be a fact of historic interest."[30] To people such as David Livermore, MD, at the Antibiotic Resistance Monitoring and Reference Laboratory in London, it has now gone much further. "It is," he says, "naive to think we can win."[31]

In the first edition of this book I noted that bacteria are, in fact, learning resistance to new antibiotics in only a few years instead of the decades that it took previously. At the time of this second edition, that span has lessened to 6 months to a year. As infectious disease specialist Brad Spellberg has commented, "Resistance is inevitable."

Resistance in the Ecosystem

Though resistance in the bacteria affecting people and farm animals has been the most publicized and studied, these bacteria are not confined to people or their food animals. They move freely in the ecosystem and among species. Newer research has found that seagulls, and other birds, not only humans, are spreading resistant bacteria throughout the world. As Dr. Jeffrey Fisher, in his book *The Plague Makers*, notes:

> The resistant bacteria that result from this reckless practice do not stay confined to the animals from which they develop. There are no "cow bacteria" or "pig bacteria" or "chicken bacteria." In terms of the microbial world, we humans along with the rest of the animal kingdom are part of one giant ecosystem. The same resistant bacteria that grow in the intestinal tract of a cow or pig can, and do, eventually end up in our bodies.[32]

This is especially true if antibiotics flow into water. This promotes the transmission of resistant traits throughout the environment because bacterial growth is high wherever water-related biofilms occur: on the surface of water, on stones in water, and in the sediment of ponds, rivers, and oceans. Antibiotics given to fish contact all these regions, as does the antibiotic-rich effluent from factory farms and human waste treatment facilities. Resistance transfers in these biofilm regions from domestic to wild bacteria and it tends to persist in these natural ecosystems.

Researchers Christian Daughton and Thomas Ternes report that "a number of stream surveys documented the significant prevalence of native bacteria that display resistance to a wide array of antibiotics including vancomycin. Isolates from wild geese near Chicago, Illinois, are reported to be resistant to ampicillin, tetracycline, penicillin, and erythromycin."[33] Researchers have found 16 antibiotics commonly present in groundwater/surface waters that are detectable in the microgram-per-liter range. Some researchers report that these antibiotic compounds are showing genotoxicity; that is, they are affecting the integrity of genetic structures in other life-forms. Daughton and Ternes comment that this is indeed cause for concern, as the bacteria never seem to forget what has been done to them:

> Indeed, the rampant, widespread (and sometimes indiscriminate) use of antibiotics, coupled with their subsequent release into the environment, is the leading proposed cause of accelerated spreading resistance among bacterial pathogens, which is exacerbated by the fact that resistance is maintained even in the absence of continued selective pressure (an irreversible occurrence). Sufficiently high concentrations could also have acute effects on bacteria. Such exposures could easily lead to altered microbial community structures in nature and thereby affect the higher food chain.[34]

Salmon, catfish, and trout — all raised commercially — are heavily dosed with antibiotics and other drugs, which are often blended into their food. As the food gets wet, the antibiotics begin to leach into the water. Commercial salmon, unlike catfish and trout, are raised in the open sea in pens, speeding the flow of antibacterials throughout the oceans. Because of crowded conditions, the 55 million pounds of commercial U.S. salmon are frequently dosed with antibiotics for long periods of time — about 150 pounds of antibiotic per acre of salmon. Stuart Levy comments:

> Since they are deposited in the water, [antibiotics] can be picked up easily by other marine animals. Tetracycline is not rapidly degraded in fish. Thus, it is excreted in its active state in feces and deposited on the sea floor. Here, too, it remains relatively stable, out of direct sunlight, which can degrade it. Consequently, the ecological effect of this antibacterial agent in the sea is the same as it is in land animals: the long-term selection of resistant and multi-resistant bacteria in salmon and other marine life.[35]

Plant communities and soil are also exposed to direct antibiotic use, not just through effluent flows. To treat infections in mono-cropped fields, especially while attacking fire blight in apple and pear orchards, antibiotics such as streptomycin are sometimes sprayed in heavy doses directly on crops. In the United States, between 40,000 and 50,000 pounds of tetracycline and streptomycin are sprayed on fruit trees every year (1 pound of tetracycline will treat 450 people). This kills not only bacteria on the plants but all susceptible bacteria in the soil itself with cascading effects on soil integrity and health. While spraying allows potent doses of streptomycin to directly enter the eco-system, other antibiotics, like oxytetracycline, are sometimes injected, much as they are with people, directly into larger plants' trunks and roots. Not surprisingly, resistant pathogenic plant bacteria have been found in soil and plant communities wherever such practices occur. The bacterial transposon developed by leaf blight during resistance acquisition has been found in seven wild bacterial species in the soil. All these bacteria now have resistance to the streptomycin normally produced by the soil fungi in the region. This same dynamic has also been found occurring in the soil under wheat plants. The application or spread of antibiotic effluents in the environment is promoting resistance impacts in natural soil communities among wild bacteria, thus interfering with the normal balance of the soil biota. Agricultural practices such as liming fields and industrial heavy-metal pollution

31

have been found, as well, to increase the density of resistant pathogens in the soil. Researchers have also started to insert bacterial resistance factors directly into the genetic structure of some plants (e.g., sugar beets), and these resistance factors have also been found to move into ecosystem bacteria.

The immense production of antibacterial substances once found only in minute quantities in the environment — substances produced by soil fungi, bacteria, or plants to protect their territorial integrity — has begun to affect the life cycle of bacteria and thousands of other organisms in the ecosystem and subsequently is affecting the health of the soil and the planet itself.

We have, as Mark Lappé remarked in *The End of Antibiotics*, "let our profligate use of antibiotics reshape the evolution of the microbial world and wrest any hope of safe management from us."

Bacterial Partners

Bacteria are not our enemies, as some scientists have postulated, nor a dangerous life-form bent on sickening mankind, as so many television commercials would have us believe. They are our ancestors and we are very much alike; we both metabolize fats, vitamins, sugars, and proteins. Lynn Margulis comments succinctly, "The more balanced view of microbe as colleague and ancestor remains almost unexpressed. Our culture ignores the hard-won fact that these disease 'agents,' these 'germs,' also germinated all life. Our ancestors, the germs, were bacteria."[36] Bacteria are not germs but the germinators — and fabric — of all life on Earth. In declaring war on them, we declared war on the underlying living structure of the planet, on all life-forms we can see, on ourselves.

One of the few naturally sterile places on Earth is a woman's womb, and the gestation period prior to birth is the only time any human body is bacteria free. At birth, assuming it is a healthy one, the baby is immediately placed on the mother's chest near the nipple. As the first movements toward bonding are taking place, the bacteria that live on the mother's skin began to colonize her baby's body. When the infant begins to nurse, the interior of the baby's intestinal tract is colonized — from the skin around the nipple and the milk itself — and these bacteria are crucially important. Nursing introduces lactobacilli and other bacteria such as *Bifidobacterium bifidus* into the intestinal tract of newborns. This has significant effects on their health. *Lactobacillus acidophilus* bacteria create important vitamins and nutrients such as B_1, B_2, B_3, B_{12}, and folic acid in the intestinal tract. They help digest food and they also secrete natural antibiotic substances such as acidophilin, various organic acids, and peroxides that help prevent bacterial infections.

> In declaring war on bacteria we declared war on the underlying living structure of the planet, on all life-forms we can see, on ourselves.

One to two pounds of our adult body weight comes from our coevolutionary bacteria. The bacteria that colonize us as infants have an ancient, coevolutionary relationship with human beings; they are an integral part of our species' development and our body ecology. They are in fact our first line of defense against disease.

The skin of our bodies and the mucosal systems of our sinus passages and intestinal tracts are to bacteria much like fresh fertile black soil is to plants. Plow up the soil, disturbing the plants that grow there, and even if you don't plant anything, the soil will soon be covered with a profusion of new plant growth. The same thing occurs in our bodies if our bacterial ecology is disturbed, as it often is, by antibiotics.

Why We Need Bacteria

The bacteria that colonize our bodies are friendly, mutualistic bacteria. They take up all the space on and in our bodies on which bacteria can grow. By so doing, they leave no room for other, less benign bacteria to live. But the relationship goes beyond this. *All* of our coevolutionary bacteria generate antibiotic substances that kill off other, less friendly bacteria. The *Streptococcus* bacteria that normally live in our throats produce large quantities of antibacterial substances that are specifically active against the *Streptococcus pyogenes* bacteria that cause strep throat.

Regular exposure to pathogenic bacteria as we are growing teaches our bodies and our symbiotic bacteria how to respond most effectively to disease organisms. This produces much higher levels of health in later life. Research continually finds that children who are "protected" from bacteria by keeping them in exceptionally clean environments where they are constantly exposed to antibacterial soaps and wipes are not in fact healthier but much sicker overall than children not so protected. The constant exposure to a world filled with bacteria, the world out of which we emerged as a species, in fact stimulates the immune health of all of us as we grow. We actually *need* to come into contact with the microorganisms of the world to be healthy.

The truth is, we live in an ancient, healthy symbiosis with bacterial, viral, and microfaunal colonizers. Our bodies are much like the soil of the earth, covered inside and out with a broad diversity of microfauna providing an interdependent complex of support services. When we become ill, our symbiotic relationship with the healthy bacteria and other microfauna — our body ecology — is disturbed. The underlying factor that disrupts the body ecology is the illness, not the pathogenic bacteria that take advantage of it to occupy body sites. Antibiotics do not cure disease, they simply kill off opportunistic bacteria. Without the body's ability to restore a healthy ecology, people die anyway. More than any other disease, AIDS has taught us the limitations of antibiotics and the bacterial model of disease. Irrespective of the quantities of antibiotics used, when AIDS patients' bodies can no longer reestablish their internal ecology they die. As Marc Lappé says, "It is the *body* which ultimately controls infections, not chemicals. Without underlying immunity, drugs are meaningless."[37] Ironically, as many public health historians now know, the major decreases in human mortality and disease proclaimed to be brought about by antibiotics were due more, in fact, to better public hygiene.

Because they kill off so much of the internal symbiotic microfauna along with pathogenic bacteria, antibiotics create significant changes in human microfaunal ecology and makeup. The appearance of many diseases new to humankind such as certain nutrient deficiencies, candida overgrowth, certain chronic infections, allergies, and chronic immune suppression are now being directly linked to the distorted internal landscape antibiotics cause. Marc Lappé comments:

> Lincomycin eliminates virtually all of the bacteria that require oxygen, while neomycin and kanamycin decrease the number of oxygen-requiring germs and gram-positive anaerobic ones, leading to overgrowth of *Candida albicans* and *Staphylococcus aureus.* Polymyxin can reduce native *E. coli* to the point of extinction, leaving the terrain open for staph and strep organisms. Erythromycin has a similar favorable effect on streptococci, while bacitracin and damycin, by contrast, appear to favor the growth of *Clostridium difficile.*[38]

And it is not just humans that have coevolutionary bacterial partners but all plant, insect, and animal life. When these other life-forms encounter antibiotics, their interior and exterior ecologies are disturbed as well.

If bacteria had not learned how to develop resistance, all life on Earth, including humans, would already have died. When we try to kill all disease organisms on this planet, ultimately, we are acting to kill ourselves.

The situation is dire and there are solutions, but they are not easy ones. As David Livermore has said, "A lot of modern medicine would become impossible if we lost our ability to treat infections."[39] Routine surgeries would no longer be routine but nearly impossible to perform safely. Infectious diseases would regularly become epidemic, sweeping through whole communities. The use of quarantine, rare now, would become common. Mortality among the old and the very young would rise tremendously. An entire world view, commonly accepted by most people in Western countries, would begin to crumble. It would be (medically speaking), for all practical purposes, 1928 again.

In the first edition of this book, I, as many others have done, urged people to give up using antibiotics unless there were a serious threat of death or disability if they did not. (I also thought real estate in Nevada might be a good investment.) More than a decade later, it is clear that antibiotics are not going to be used any less and in fact are being used at far greater rates than they were 15 years ago. The human species, as a group, has never really been known for doing the sensible thing before it is too late. We will stop using antibiotics only when they truly fail to work. And even then most of the people in the Western world will still try to hold on to them and our fatally flawed approach to bacterial disease.

But for those who clearly understand what the word "exponential" means, who want to truly empower themselves and their families and prepare for the time that is so quickly approaching us, there are options.

You can take control over your own health and health care. You can prepare. You can learn to use herbal medicines to heal yourself from disease. And you can learn what to do if you find that one day you need to know how to treat a resistant infection.

The rest of this book is designed to help you do just that.

2

THE RESISTANT ORGANISMS, THE DISEASES THEY CAUSE, AND HOW TO TREAT THEM

The significant problems we face cannot be solved at the same level of thinking we were at when we created them.

— **Albert Einstein**

Included among the Gram-positive pathogens are methicillin-resistant Staphylococcus aureus *and* S. epidermidis, *vancomycin-resistant* Enterococcus faecium *and* E. faecalis, *and the rapidly growing mycobacteria. In the past five years, however, no fewer than four novel agents have been approved that have clinical activity versus these bacteria. It is really among the multidrug-resistant Gram-negative bacteria that we find growing unmet medical need, and only a single new agent has been approved in well over a decade.*

— **Steven Projan**, *Bacterial Resistance to Antimicrobials*

Many people believe that there will always be antibiotics and that if the ones we have now aren't working, others will be discovered that will work just as well, so no need to worry. The truth, unfortunately, is very different. There are virtually no new antibiotics in development, and there are unlikely to be. Pharmaceutical companies have almost completely given up the search for them. There are a number of reasons for this, the main one being, of course, financial.

In spite of cultural beliefs to the contrary, physicians can cure relatively few of the conditions that plague us. For high cholesterol they prescribe anticholesterol drugs, for arthritis anti-inflammatories, and so on. These drugs artificially alter the condition of the body, but they do not cure the underlying condition. In consequence, the drugs are often taken for decades; they are a never-ending source of money for the companies that make them. (And the profit of the top 12 pharmaceutical companies in the world in 2009? 100 *billion* dollars.)

Antibiotics, on the other hand, are too successful. They are used for a short period of time, the disease is eradicated, the patient cured. They are a victim of their own success. Brad Spellberg, author of *Rising Plague*, notes: "For many years now, leading members of the Infectious Diseases Society of America (IDSA) have been aware that antibiotics were no longer being developed by many pharmaceutical companies. Indeed, many pharmaceutical companies have actually completely eliminated their research and development programs for antibiotic drug discovery."[1] Stuart Levy, perhaps the foremost researcher on resistant organisms in the United States, comments that "the problem is the pharmaceutical industry has left the discovery field and so new antibiotics are not coming along."[2] He says, rather matter-of-factly, that it is just more profitable for the drug companies to develop medications for long-term conditions such as heart disease and arthritis than it is to find new antibiotics.

> "The money's not in the cure. The money's in the medicine."
> — *Comedian Chris Rock*

Research by Spellberg's group found that between 1983 and 2008, investment in antibiotic research and development in the United States fell by 75 percent. His team found only five to seven new antibiotics in the pipeline, most expected to reach the market by 2012, and all of them just slightly altered versions of existing antibiotics.

And no, biotechnology companies are not doing any better. In 2004 all biotech companies combined had only one antibiotic in any kind of development stage. Worse, *every* one of the antibiotics expected to reach market by 2012 are for Gram-positive bacteria. There are *none* in any stage of development that can treat Gram-negative organisms, the fastest growing category of resistant pathogens. After 2012? That's it. There are none in any stage of development and no plans for any, a fact that shocks most people. They just don't believe that the drug companies would be so complacent — or that they would care so little. I mean, they are in the business of helping people . . . aren't they?

Resistance: An Exponential Growth Curve

There is a very old story — it's about greed actually, and just a little bit about mathematics — of a king and the man who saved his life. The king was very grateful and told the man he would reward him with anything he wished. The man told the king that the only thing he wanted was some rice. He then asked the king if he played chess. The king replied that yes, he did. So the man said he would like to use the chess board to determine the amount of rice with which he would be rewarded. He wanted the king to put one grain of rice on the first square, then two on the second, four on the next, and so on. The king said sure, that sounds like a good idea, and he told his councilors to arrange it. They came back a bit later and very hesitantly told the king that they couldn't do it. The king was pretty upset and asked why and was told that by the last square the man would receive more rice than existed in the entire kingdom. (I'm not sure, but I think the king beheaded the man who made the request — nobody likes a smart-ass.)

Bacterial resistance grows exponentially, just like those grains of rice. In practical terms that means we will be fine for a while (say from 1945 to 2010) because, as you can see, it takes a while to get into the big numbers. Welcome to big-number territory.

MRSA, once limited to the very young, the old, and the immuno-compromised, has not only emerged in the general community; it is now exceptionally virulent and infecting the healthiest population of all — young adults. As Spellberg comments, "The highly publicized

39

outbreaks of MRSA infections are dwarfed by the enormous number of cases that occur every day across the United States and throughout the world. Overall, healthy children, adolescents, and teenagers have been particularly heavily hit by MRSA infections, and these cases had gone unheralded until very recently."[3]

Young people, completely healthy, begin to fall ill, enter emergency rooms, and are found to have out-of-control MRSA infections. After just a simple skin break, their arms swell with cellulitis, or the infection becomes systemic and infects the blood (bacteremia), the heart (endocarditis), spinal cord (myelitis), or bones (osteomyelitis). In 2007 the state of Virginia closed 21 high schools to try to stop an MRSA infection that had killed one student and sickened others.

The situation will only get worse. We are within 5 years of MRSA being completely untreatable by any antibiotics at all.

Thirty percent of all *E. coli* urinary tract infections are resistant to treatment, up from 5 percent 10 years ago. The resistance rate has increased 50-fold in the last decade. One of the more troubling resistance mechanisms in *E. coli* is what is called "extended-spectrum beta-lactamase" resistance, or ESBL. ESBL bacteria are highly virulent and strongly resistant to a class of antibiotics called beta-lactams, some of the most potent antibiotics still useful for Gram-negative bacteria. Beta-lactamase is an enzyme that the bacteria create and use to deactivate the antibiotics. *All* the bacteria in the Gram-negative family have begun acquiring that genetic resistance information. *E. coli* and *Klebsiella* are two of the forerunners.

ESBL resistance in *E. coli* in 1990 was only 3.6 percent, by 1993 it was 14.4 percent, by 1995 it was 25 percent in Europe and as high as 40 percent in France. The only antibiotic that until recently could still treat the ESBL-resistant strains of *Klebsiella* was carbapenem and a much older antibiotic, polymyxin, that is only partially effective and often causes severe kidney damage.

Fully resistant strains of *Klebsiella* have now (as of 2011) become common and are often, like MRSA, referred to by an acronym, CRKP. It stands for carbapenem-resistant *Klebsiella pneumoniae*. It is virtually untreatable; 40 percent of those infected with it die. "These are very serious infections, hugely complicated by the fact that the treatment options are severely limited," is how Dr. Ajun Srinivasan of the Centers for Disease Control in Atlanta, Georgia, puts it. The first isolated reports of CRKP occurred in 1999 in New Jersey. As of 2010, Srinivasan says, "we are seeing reports of this organism from all over the country."[4]

In March of 2010 a severe outbreak of CRKP occurred in Southern California (another occurred in March of 2011 in Los Angeles just as I was completing this manuscript). Brad Spellberg, speaking from the Los Angeles Biomedical Research Institute near Torrance, California, commented, "In the next decade there isn't going to be anything that becomes available that's going to be able to treat these bacteria. . . . [There] is no current treatment for CRKP bacteria, and there might not be any in the future either."[5]

Neil Fishman, president of the Society for Healthcare Epidemiology of America, is more blunt: "We have lost our drug of last resort."[6]

Pan-resistant *Pseudomonas* and *Acinetobacter* are similarly dangerous. *Pseudomonas* has also begun to develop resistance to carbapenem antibiotics; the bacteria are now reliably treatable only by polymyxin. *Acinetobacter*, *E. coli*, and *Klebsiella* have also been promiscuously sharing a new plasmid, NDM-1, that confers resistance along a wide range of antibiotics, including carbapenem. "In many ways, this is it," says Timothy Walsh, a microbiologist and resistant bacteria specialist at Cardiff University in the UK. "There are no antibiotics in the pipeline that have activity against NDM-1-producing Enterobacteriaceae. We have a bleak window of maybe ten years."[7]

Enterococcal organisms, once readily treatable, are so no longer. George Eliopoulos in the Division of Infectious Diseases at Beth Israel Deaconess Medical Center in Boston, Massachusetts, observes:

> Ominously, in recent years, enterococci resistant to multiple antimicrobial agents have become increasingly prevalent in the hospital environment. . . . More than half of these enterococcal isolates were resistant to tetracycline, levofloxacin, and quinupristin-dalfopristin; 28 percent were resistant

to ampicillin; and approximately 20 percent were nonsusceptible to vancomycin. From ICUs in the United States, even higher rates of vancomycin resistance have been reported. . . . Vancomycin resistance genes originating in enterococci have now been found in several clinical isolates of *S. aureus*. This validates concerns expressed more than a decade ago that VRE may serve as a reservoir of genes that could confer upon staphylococci resistance to glycopeptides, the principal antibiotics [remaining] for treatment of infections caused by methicillin-resistant strains [MRSA].[8]

There are *no* new antibiotics being developed to treat these resistant strains. The most recent, tigecycline, entered the market in 2005. It is active against resistant forms of *Acinetobacter* but not resistant *Pseudomonas*. Only tigecycline and that rather dangerous older antibiotic, polymyxin, can now treat *Acinetobacter*, and polymyxin itself has begun to encounter resistant forms of the bacteria. But then, so has tigecycline.

As Spellberg comments, "If we did not have tigecycline, these infections would be essentially untreatable." But as he continues, "tigecycline resistance spread within two years of the drug's availability. Indeed, on a recent trip to visit a hospital on the East Coast, I was told that nearly all the hospital's *Acinetobacter* is already fully resistant to tigecycline."[9]

People who now enter hospitals, even for very minor treatments, are at serious risk of contracting untreatable infections. Over 70 percent of all pathogenic bacteria in hospitals are at least minimally resistant; the ones discussed herein are considerably more so, being resistant to most major groups of antimicrobials. As oncology nurse Sue Fischer says, "These kids come in for a short treatment and the next day they complain about a pain in their side and the next day they're gone. We open them up and find their whole body shot through with resistant bacteria that have attacked nearly every organ. Nothing works to stop it and it happens as quick as that."[10]

Resistant Microorganisms: The Specifics

The first edition of this book covered 12 resistant pathogens that researchers were concerned about. There are 21 on this new list and that doesn't count the various subspecies in each genus that are now resistant (at least 40, not including variants) or several others that are lurking out there on the horizon. The problem, as many epidemiologists have warned, is increasing exponentially and there is no end in sight.

Some of these organisms, such as methicillin-resistant *Staphylococcus aureus* (MRSA), are already causing significant problems in hospitals and communities throughout the world. Others, such as *Clostridium difficile*, are becoming increasingly widespread and dangerous. And still others, such as *Stenotrophomonas maltophilia*, are just beginning their run as resistant organisms.

Most of the resistant pathogens are either Gram-positive or Gram-negative bacteria — a list is included under the respective headings that follow; there are, in addition, one parasitic protist (the malarial parasite), one mold (aspergillus), and one yeast (candida) that have now become dangerously resistant. The parasitic protist is *Plasmodium falciparum*, which causes malaria; the mold is *Aspergillus* spp. (*A. fumigatus, A. flavus, A. terres*); the yeast is *Candida* spp. (*Candida albicans* is dominant, but most species are now resistant).

Gram-positive and Gram-negative organisms are denoted as such because of their ability to take a Gram stain, one way of identifying

What's a Gram Stain?

Hans Gram (1853–1938) found he could see bacteria more clearly under a microscope if he applied a stain made from crystal violet to them. Different types of bacteria absorb the stain differently, enabling researchers to more easily identify them.

them. Of much more importance are the differences in their cellular structure.

Just as we have skin, bacteria have an external membrane surrounding their bodies, a.k.a. the cell wall. Their interior is called the *cytoplasm*; then there is the *cytoplasmic membrane*, which covers the cytoplasm, then the *cell wall*. The cell wall consists primarily of a polymer called peptidoglycan. If the bacteria happen to be Gram-negative, they will have a second wall called the *outer membrane*. Between the two membranes in Gram-negative bacteria is a compartment, the *periplasmic space*. Gram-positive bacteria, because they lack that other membrane, have much thicker cell walls to protect them from outside events.

Because Gram-positive bacteria have only a single cell wall, even though it's thicker, they are, in general, much easier to treat. With Gram-negative bacteria, two cell walls have to be penetrated, not just one. In essence, the bacteria have two chances to identify and deactivate an antibacterial that is hostile to them. Even if an antibiotic gets into the periplasmic space, it usually will not kill the bacteria. It still has to penetrate the second wall.

> Over 70 percent of all pathogenic bacteria in hospitals are at least minimally resistant.

Gram-negative bacteria have a series of highly synergistic reactions to antibiotics, in essence using three primary mechanisms, all highly coordinated, to resist antibiotics. The first is the double cell wall. The second is a special group of enzymes, beta-lactamases, that are especially effective in deactivating beta-lactam antibiotics (the antibiotics most often used against them). The third is a variety of multidrug efflux pumps. These efflux pumps essentially act like sump pumps; they pump out the antibiotic substances just as fast as they come in so that the bacteria are unaffected by them.

Gram-positive bacteria rely on their thicker cell wall and very, very fast efflux pumps since they don't have a periplasmic space in which to hold the antibiotics while they deal with them. Some Gram-positive bacteria, such as the staphylococci, have incorporated the use of beta-lactamases, which they learned about from Gram-negative organisms.

Resistant Diseases and How to Treat Them

Here are some general thoughts to keep in mind when you are approaching treatment of a resistant pathogen. Always remember that you are dealing with virulent, highly pathogenic microbial infections — your treatment must be focused and continual and unremitting until the outcome is decided, one way or the other.

As a general rule of thumb, follow these recommendations when dealing with a resistant infection.

Disease	Herbal Remedy
Systemic infection	Cryptolepis, alchornea, or sida will *almost* always work. (Bidens is very good, but you will need higher doses.)
Severe diarrhea, dysentery	A berberine plant will *almost* always work.
Urinary tract infection	Juniper berry combined with bidens will *almost* always work.
Infected surface or surgical wound	Honey has *always* worked.
Meningitis	Add piperine, isatis, and either Japanese knotweed or stephania to the herbal mix — they are exceptionally good for this.
Sepsis or bacteremia	Use *Echinacea angustifolia* in large doses.

Note: Gram-positive bacteria are often highly susceptible to hyaluronidase inhibitors. Echinacea is a potent one — if your treatment is going poorly, consider adding it.

RECOGNIZING ENDOTOXINS

Endotoxins generally come from the outer wall of Gram-negative bacteria and are released into the body when the bacteria die. In a number of diseases, bubonic plague for example, it is not the bacteria that kill you but the endotoxins that are released when they die. If you are treating a systemic infection by a Gram-negative bacteria, the use of an endotoxin scavenger and protectant is often important. Isatis (though not discussed in this book) is perhaps the best herb for this (ginger is also good). It should be included if endotoxin release may be a problem.

USING SYNERGISTS

If you are treating a difficult infection, especially if it is Gram-negative, use a synergist to enhance the treatment. There are two forms of synergists: the first is active against the efflux pumps in the bacteria, the second helps move the herbs across the intestinal membrane and strongly into the blood. Licorice is the best synergist for Gram-negative bacteria. Piperine will potently move herbal compounds across the intestinal membrane, significantly increasing their presence in the blood. See chapter 6 for more specifics.

INCREASING NATURAL IMMUNITY

Always work to increase the body's natural immune function through the use of immune herbs or an immune formulation. These should be taken daily. The formulations suggested in this section were generated by looking at immune herbs that were also active against the specific organisms — kind of a two-for-one thing. Nevertheless, don't get obsessed by these, as other immune herbs that don't have any specific antibacterial activity will work, often better than these, in increasing immune function. These are only guidelines.

A note about the suggested formulations: The formulations that I have included to treat the various bacteria and the types of infections they cause *are only suggestions*. They can be varied considerably. Don't get stuck in thinking that any of these formulations are the only way to go. *Read the book* and the monographs on the herbs themselves. Tremendous sophistication is possible. These are just guidelines.

Piperine Warning

Under no circumstances should you use piperine for severe intestinal infections such as *E. coli* O157:H7 or cholera. Piperine increases intestinal permeability, which can allow the resistant organisms access to the interior of your body in significantly greater numbers. It can make you much sicker.

Finally, don't forget that human love and caring are an essential part of the healing process — they are medicines that you must also dispense to those you are working to heal. There is perhaps nothing that the ill need more than to know that they are supported in their suffering. It is very difficult to live without love, and nearly impossible to truly heal without it.

Using This Book

The rest of this chapter is concerned with the individual resistant bacteria, what herbs are effective in treating them, and then some actual specific suggestions for treatment. These are the main ones you need to know about to be able to take care of yourself and your family.

Subsequent chapters explore the individual herbs in depth; examine what other organisms they are active against; explore what else they can do medicinally; and then show how to grow, harvest, and prepare them as medicines so that you can take complete charge of your own health care if you wish to do so.

Chapter 7 contains in-depth explorations on the immune-enhancing herbs that you can use to keep your immune system strong — a number of which are also potently effective against resistant pathogens. And chapters 8 and 9 will tell you more than you ever wanted to know about making just about any kind of herbal medicine you might ever need.

Dealing with Gram-Positive Bacteria

The major resistant Gram-positive organisms are:

- *Clostridium difficile*
- *Enterococcus* spp. (*E. faecalis, E. faecium*)
- *Mycobacterium tuberculosis*
- *Staphylococcus aureus*
- *Streptococcus* spp. (*S. pyogenes, S. pneumoniae*)

Note: *All* the formulations given for treating each type of bacteria are meant to be taken simultaneously. Some offer immune support, some are directly antibacterial, some are for a specific symptom picture.

Clostridium difficile

The *Clostridium* genus comprises about 100 different species of bacteria; four of them are human pathogens. They often form spores that, once they enter a cut or the GI tract, lead to a number of potentially dangerous diseases.

C. botulinum is the source of botulism poisoning in food (and of the drug Botox) and sometimes also causes infections in wounds; *C. perfringens* can cause anything from food poisoning to gas gangrene; and *C. tetani* is the cause of tetanus. *C. difficile* is the main resistant pathogen. The organism flourishes in people who have been on long antibiotic therapies, especially in hospitals, and because it is exposed to so many antibiotics, it is highly resistant to treatment. At the present most *C. difficile* infections are confined to hospitals, but their numbers are increasing exponentially. The disease causes severe diarrhea and inflammation of the colon and sometimes death.

The primary herbs to use to treat the condition, listed in order of strength against the organism, are the berberine plants, cryptolepis, isatis, usnea, lomatium, licorice, and echinacea. Because juniper berry is active against *C. perfringens*, I would suggest its use for *C. difficile* as well.

TREATING CLOSTRIDIUM DIFFICILE

Formulation 1 (antibacterial) Cryptolepis or any berberine plant tincture: 1 tsp–1 tbl, 3–6x daily, depending on severity of symptoms

Formulation 2 (immune support) Echinacea, ginger, and licorice (equal parts) tincture: 1 tsp, 6x daily

Formulation 3 (antidiarrheal/colon soothing) Blackberry root and marsh mallow root (equal parts) standard infusion: up to 6 cups daily (Note: Elm bark porridge will also help ease colon inflammation tremendously.)

Enterococcus spp.

This genus was considered to be part of the streptococcus genus until it was reclassified in the 1980s. Although both *E. casseliflavus* and *E. raffinosus* may sometimes cause human infections, the major problematical species are *E. faecalis* and *E. faecium*. These enterococcal organisms are often highly resistant to antibiotics, especially in hospitals. They don't respond very well to beta-lactam antibiotics (penicillins and cephalosporins), aminoglycosides, and, increasingly, vancomycin.

Enterococcal organisms cause urinary tract infections, bacteremia, bacterial endocarditis, diverticulitis, and meningitis. The primary herbs to treat them are sida, alchornea, cryptolepis, bidens, ginger, echinacea, juniper berry, usnea, *Artemisia annua*, honey (I know, it's not *exactly* an herb), licorice, oregano oil, and *Acacia aroma*. If you are treating a really tough vancomycin-resistant enterococcal infection, add ginger juice to your formulation; it strongly inhibits resistance mechanisms in these bacteria.

TREATING ENTEROCOCCUS INFECTIONS

Formulation 1 (antibacterial) Sida, alchornea, or cryptolepis tincture: 1 tsp–1 tbl, 3–6x daily, depending on severity of symptoms (Note: Bidens tincture will work but requires higher doses and must be prepared properly; see monograph, page 127.)

Formulation 2 (immune support) Licorice, astragalus, and rhodiola (equal parts) tincture: 1 tsp, 3x daily (Note: Echinacea tincture will also be of benefit for immune support.)

For systemic enterococcal infections, diverticulitis, and endocarditis: Formulations 1 and 2

For enterococcal UTI: Formulation 1 plus juniper berry–bidens tincture (1 part juniper, 2 parts bidens), 30 drops, 3–6x daily, depending on severity

For enterococcal bacteremia: Formulation 1 plus *Echinacea angustifolia* tincture, ½ tsp–1 tbl in minimal water, every half hour to hour

For enterococcal meningitis: Formulations 1 and 2, plus formulations 3 and 4 below

Formulation 3 Piperine: 20 mg, 2x daily, with the first dose in the morning 30 minutes before taking the other formulations, and the second dose at 4 P.M.

Formulation 4 Isatis leaf (or root) and either Japanese knotweed or stephania (equal parts) tincture: 1 tsp, 3–6x daily

Mycobacterium tuberculosis

This is the primary cause of tuberculosis (TB), which has become increasingly resistant and difficult to treat. There are, however, some 130 species of mycobacteria, a number of which can cause human disease. The members of this genus are a bit different than other Gram-positive bacteria. They don't stain well, but they also don't possess the double membrane structure of the Gram-negative bacteria. Their membrane is waxy and thicker than that of other Gram-positive bacteria, making them tougher overall. Of the 130 or so species, there are eight that can cause TB. *M. leprae* causes leprosy and the *M. avium* complex often causes pulmonary infections in AIDS patients and has been implicated in Crohn's disease.

Mycobacterium tuberculosis has been developing increasing resistance for decades. MDR-TB (multidrug-resistant TB) is resistant to the two main first-line drugs used to treat it, isoniazid and rifampicin. Some 450,000 people contract this disease each year. XDR-TB (extensively drug-resistant TB) is resistant to all of the most effective anti-TB drugs. About 45,000 people a year contract this form of the disease; the death rate is about 90 percent.

The herbs effective for treating resistant and nonresistant TB are cryptolepis, sida, bidens, piperine, *Artemisia annua*, berberine plants, juniper, usnea, lomatium, licorice, echinacea, and rhodiola.

TREATING TUBERCULOSIS

Formulation 1 (systemic antibiotic) Cryptolepis and sida (equal
parts) tincture: 1 tsp–1 tbl, 3–6x daily, depending on symptoms

Formulation 2 Piperine: 20 mg, 2x daily, with the first dose in the
morning 30 minutes before taking the other formulations, and the
second dose at 4 P.M.

Formulation 3 (immune support) Lomatium, licorice, and rhodiola
(equal parts) tincture: 1 tsp, 3x daily

Staphylococcus aureus

Methicillin-resistant *Staphylococcus aureus* (MRSA) has become
an increasingly common infectious disease. It is now present in both
hospitals and the general community and is passing between people,
wherever they congregate, with great abandon. Individuals with compromised immune function, even if they appear healthy, are at greater
risk of serious infections. There are numerous strains of the bacteria,
some more resistant than others. In many respects MRSA should
mean "multidrug-resistant," not merely "methicillin resistant."

Most MRSA infections in the general community initially present
as small red bumps that are similar to pimples or perhaps spider
bites or small boils. There may be fever or even a rash. As the disease
progresses, the bumps become larger and very painful, eventually
breaking open into deep, pus-filled boils. In those in whom antibiotic
treatment fails, the boils continue to spread and the infection goes
deeper, sometimes necessitating amputation of affected limbs.

In hospitals MRSA can infect open wounds, intravenous catheters,
the urinary tract, and the lungs; the infection can be quite dangerous,
spreading throughout the whole system. Unchecked, it can infect the
valves of the heart, the bones and joints, the organs, and the blood
(bacteremia or sepsis) and cause toxic shock syndrome and necrotizing (flesh-eating) pneumonia. Many people worldwide die from it
each year.

The main herbs to treat MRSA are cryptolepis, sida, alchornea,
bidens, black pepper, the berberines, usnea, juniper berry, isatis,

licorice, ginger, ashwagandha, echinacea, red root, reishi, honey, and *Artemisia annua*.

TREATING MRSA INFECTIONS

Formulation 1 (internal systemic antibacterial) Cryptolepis tincture: 1 tsp–1 tbl, 3–6x daily, depending on severity

Formulation 2 (immune support) Ginger, reishi, and licorice (2 parts ginger, 2 parts reishi, 1 part licorice) tincture: 1 tsp, 3x daily

For MRSA UTIs: Formulations 1 and 2 plus juniper berry–bidens tincture (1 part juniper, 2 parts bidens), 30 drops, 3–6x daily

Streptococcus spp.

The main species of streptococcal bacteria that cause disease in human beings are *S. pyogenes*, which causes strep throat, acute bacterial glomerulonephritis, and necrotizing (flesh-eating) fasciitis; *S. pneumoniae*, which causes bacterial pneumonia, otitis media, sinusitis, meningitis, and peritonitis; and *S. agalactiae*, which causes pneumonia, meningitis, bacteremia, intestinal infections, and infections of the female reproductive tract. Of these, the first two are the most common causes of infections in people.

The primary herbs used to treat streptococcal bacteria are cryptolepis, sida, alchornea, bidens (though you'll need to use larger doses, for longer), the berberine plants, juniper, usnea, lomatium, honey, echinacea, licorice, ginger, and red root.

TREATING STREP INFECTIONS

Formulation 1 (antibacterial) *Echinacea angustifolia* tincture: 1 tbl in minimal water, every hour

Formulation 2 Cryptolepis, sida, or alchornea tincture: 1 tbl, every hour

Formulation 3 Lomatium, rhodiola, and eleuthero (equal parts) tincture: 1 tsp, 4x daily

For streptococcal glomerulonephritis: Formulations 1, 2, and 3, plus juniper berry tincture, 10 drops, up to 6x daily

For streptococcal bacteremia, necrotizing fasciitis, pneumonia, peritonitis, and infections of the female reproductive tract: Formulations 1, 2, and 3

For strep throat: 1/2 tsp *Echinacea angustifolia* tincture, undiluted, held in the mouth until saliva is well stimulated, then allowed to dribble slowly down throat, over the affected areas; repeat *every* hour

For streptococcal necrotizing fasciitis (topical): Honey is best (see monograph, page 188). If it's not available, combine equal parts *Echinacea angustifolia* root powder, berberine plant powder, juniper berry powder, and lomatium root powder; mix well, apply as poultice, replace every 2 hours.

For streptococcal intestinal infection: Tincture of equal parts berberine plant, cryptolepis, and lomatium, 1 tsp–1 tbl, 3–6x daily, depending on severity of infection

For streptococcal meningitis: Treat as you would enterococcal meningitis (see page 50).

Dealing with Gram-Negative Bacteria

One of the most important things to remember in treating Gram-negative infections is that the use of a synergist will significantly increase the impact of the herbs on the bacteria. For instance, when treating diseases caused by *Shigella* spp., *Serratia marcescens*, *Salmonella* spp., *Klebsiella* spp., *Enterobacter* spp., or *E. coli*, add licorice to the mix. It strongly inhibits several of the main efflux pumps in this family of bacteria (AcrAB-TolC). You can use piperine when dealing with a *non–gastrointestinal tract infection,* but this is important: Don't use it with a GI tract infection such as *E. coli* or cholera. Piperine allows more of the herbs to pass through the GI tract, increasing the presence of their antibacterial compounds in the body.

The Gram-negative organisms are:

- *Acinetobacter baumannii*
- *Campylobacter jejuni*
- *Enterohemorrhagic E. coli* (*E. coli* O157, *E. coli* O157:HM, *E. coli* O157:H7)
- *Haemophilus influenzae*
- *Klebsiella pneumoniae*
- *Neisseria gonorrhoeae*
- *Proteus* spp. (*P. vulgaris, P. mirabilis*)
- *Pseudomonas aeruginosa*
- *Salmonella* spp. (*S. typhi, S. enteritidis, S. typhimurium*)
- *Serratia marcescens*
- *Shigella* spp. (*S. dysentariae, S. flexneri, S. sonnei*)
- *Stenotrophomonas maltophilia*
- *Vibrio cholerae*

Acinetobacter baumannii

Of the many species in this genus that can infect humans, *Acineto-bacter baumanii*, the most common, is multidrug resistant; its name is often abbreviated as MDRAB. As of this writing it has become resistant to nearly all the antibiotics that can affect it. The only drugs still useful for fully resistant MDRAB are the older polymyxins that have not been in use for decades due to their toxicity — tigecycline has been the most recent drug of choice but *Acinetobacter*'s resistance to it is increasing rapidly. In some hospitals it won't work at all. It is inevitable that as they are used more regularly to treat the bacteria, the polymyxins will also become ineffective.

Acinetobacter spp. are highly responsive to the exchange of DNA strands with other bacteria that contain both resistance and viru-lence factors. Many of the soldiers wounded in combat overseas tend to return with active MDRAB infections that then spread across hospitals. The bacteria enter the body through wounds, breathing tubes, catheters, injection sites, anything that breaks the surface and allows foreign pathogens in. They are generally spread by health-care workers and are especially troublesome because they can live on hospital surfaces (and the hospital staff's hands) for up to 5 months.

Most hospital infections from these bacteria, aside from those due to combat, come from the insertion of contaminated breathing tubes during hospital procedures; 82 percent of these patients develop severe pneumonia and die as a result. Catheter insertion can cause severe infections of the urinary tract. Injections, blood draws, intravenous lines, surgical drains, and open wounds invite infection of the bloodstream, a.k.a. bacteremia.

These bacteria like to live in aquatic conditions and are often found in the irrigating and intravenous solutions used by the physicians; they love the lungs. They may enter the peritoneal fluid during peritoneal dialysis and can also find their way into the cerebral spinal fluid under some circumstances.

The herbs active against *Acinetobacter* are alchornea, cryptolepis, sida, juniper, isatis, ginger, lomatium, honey, oregano essential oil, epigallocatechin, *Acacia aroma*, *Zuccagnia punctata*, and *Sechium edule* fluid extract.

Note: Ginger juice taken internally is especially effective in reducing the resistance of *Acinetobacter* organisms. It is crucial to use if the infection is serious and has not responded to antibiotics.

TREATING ACINETOBACTER INFECTIONS

Formulation 1 (antibacterial) Cryptolepis, alchornea, or sida tincture: 1 tsp–1 tbl, 3–6x daily, depending on severity of symptoms

Formulation 2 Lomatium, astragalus, and rhodiola (equal parts) tincture: 1 tsp, 6x daily

Formulation 3 (important) Fresh ginger juice, stabilized with 20 percent alcohol (see page 227): 1 tbl in hot water, 6x daily

Formulation 4 Oregano or juniper essential oil inhalation as aromatherapy: 3x daily

For *Acinetobacter* pneumonia: Formulations 1, 2, 3, and 4

For *Acinetobacter* surgical wound infections: Formulations 1 and 2, plus daily topical honey dressings (see monograph, page 188)

For *Acinetobacter* UTIs: Formulations 2 and 3, plus juniper berry–bidens tincture (1 part juniper, 2 parts bidens), 30 drops, 6x daily (or oregano essential oil, 3 drops in water, 3x daily)

For *Acinetobacter* septicemia: Formulations 1, 2, and 3, plus *Echinacea angustifolia* tincture, ½ tsp–1 tbl, every half hour to hour

Campylobacter jejuni

Campylobacter infections generally cause enteritis accompanied by abdominal pain, diarrhea, fever, and malaise. They are not usually fatal but can be debilitating. The organism is increasingly resistant to antibiotics.

The herbs for campylobacter are cryptolepis (strongly), sida, ginger, and the berberines.

TREATING CAMPYLOBACTER INFECTIONS

Formulation 1 (antibacterial) Cryptolepis or sida tincture: 1 tsp, 3x daily

Formulation 2 Any strong tannin-containing plant (oak, geranium, krameria, pine needles) as a decoction: 6 ounces, up to 6x daily

E. coli

There are, roughly, three kinds of *E. coli* to be aware of. The first is the enterohemorrhagic *E. coli* strains (*E. coli* O157, *E. coli* O157:HM, and so on). The second is the kind that cause urinary tract infections, especially ST131. And finally, there are the *E. coli* B2 strains that cause what are called extraintestinal infections.

Of the current strains of enterohemorrhagic *E. coli*, O157 is the best known. All of them create similar conditions after infection; that is, hemorrhagic diarrhea and occasionally kidney failure. The infection is generally foodborne, most frequently arising from contaminated ground beef. It can also be contracted by drinking contaminated water or juices, eating contaminated vegetables, or swimming in contaminated pools.

The early signs are abdominal cramps, then acute diarrhea, often hemorrhagic. In some cases the red blood cells in the body are destroyed and the kidneys fail. Death is most common in the very young and the elderly.

A number of *E. coli* strains, both O157 and non-O157 strains, produce a shiga toxin (very similar to those made by *Shigella* species — all named after Kiyoshi Shiga, who discovered the shigella bacteria in the late nineteenth century). The toxins cause hemolytic-uremic syndrome; hemolytic anemia, acute renal failure, and low platelet counts all occur. Sida is essential to use if there is anemia/red blood cell damage.

The *E. coli* strains that cause UTIs have been fairly easy to treat, but a new strain of *E. coli*, ST131, emerged in 2008 and has begun to spread widely. It is strongly resistant and extremely virulent. The strain is, at this writing, only one resistance gene short of being untreatable. Unlike O157, ST131 causes urinary tract infections, generally in hospital settings, that sometimes lead to death.

The B2 group causes extraintestinal infections in the body, things like sepsis, meningitis, bacteremic pneumonia, peritonitis, and ascending cholangitis.

The first two strains are relatively easy to treat, but severe extraintestinal infections call for much more focus and care.

The herbs that are effective for *E. coli* are the berberines, cryptolepis, sida, alchornea, bidens, nearly all artemisias, juniper, honey, usnea, lomatium, isatis, licorice, ginger, ashwagandha, and reishi. All oak species (*Quercus*) and pomegranate (*Punica granatum*) fruit rind or tree bark are also highly effective against the *E. coli* O157:H7 strains. They are highly bacteriostatic and bactericidal and are very effective in killing the organisms *and* correcting the diarrhea. If you can't find any of the other plants I've listed, use oak bark; oak species grow nearly everywhere.

TREATING ENTEROHEMORRHAGIC E. COLI INFECTIONS

Formulation 1 (antibacterial) Berberine plant tincture: 1 tsp–1 tbl, 3–6x daily, depending on severity

Formulation 2 Blackberry root or oak bark decoction: 3 tbl–½ cup, 2–4x daily (Note: If the intestines are highly inflamed and sore, add powdered elm bark gruel.)

For enterohemorrhagic *E. coli* with red blood cell damage:
Formulations 1 and 2 plus sida tincture, 1 tsp, 6x daily, along with ginger, licorice, and reishi (equal parts) tincture, 1 tsp, 3x daily

TREATING E. COLI ST131 INFECTIONS

Formulation 1 (antibacterial) Juniper berry–bidens tincture (1 part juniper, 2 parts bidens): 30 drops, 3–6x daily

Formulation 2 Cryptolepis and either sida or (if you can't get sida) berberine plant (equal parts) tincture: 1 tsp, 6x daily

Formulation 3 Ginger, licorice, and reishi (equal parts) tincture: 1 tsp, 3x daily

TREATING E. COLI B2 INFECTIONS

Formulation 1 (antibacterial) Cryptolepis and sida (equal parts; sida is important here) tincture: 1 tbl, 2–4x daily

Formulation 2 *Echinacea angustifolia* tincture: ½ tsp–1 tbl, every half hour to hour

Formulation 3 Ginger, licorice, and reishi (equal parts) tincture: 1 tsp, 3x daily

For *E. coli* B2 with sepsis: Formulations 1, 2, and 3

For *E. coli* B2 with meningitis: Treat as you would enterococcal meningitis (see page 50).

For *E. coli* B2 with bacteremic pneumonia: Formulations 1, 2, and 3, plus eucalyptus or juniper berry essential oil inhalation as aromatherapy, 4–6x daily

For *E. coli* B2 with peritonitis: Formulations 1, 2, and 3

For *E. coli* B2 with ascending cholangitis: Formulations 1, 2, and 3

Haemophilus influenzae

Four species in this genus are the main sources of *Haemophilus* infection in people, the primary one being *Haemophilus influenzae*, in specific *H. influenzae* type B. Widespread vaccination in the United States and Europe began in 1988 and rates of infection from this particular organism have since fallen, though it is still common in the rest of the world.

The four species that cause infections in people are *H. influenzae*, *H. parainfluenzae*, *H. aphrophilus*, and *H. ducreyi*. *H. influenzae* has a number of types that cause disease: the encapsulated types, identified as A through F (B being the most problematical), and the unencapsulated, non-typeable strains.

The encapsulated strains, especially type B, cause invasive infections: pneumonia, meningitis, epiglottitis, septic arthritis, osteomyelitis, facial cellulitis, and bacteremia, generally in children, generally under 5 years of age. Pneumonia and meningitis are the most common. These forms of infection are generally spread by inhalation of infectious respiratory droplets — in other words, someone coughs, someone else breathes in.

The unencapsulated strains generally cause otitis media (ear infections) in children and lower respiratory tract infections in both children and immunocompromised adults — often those with existing lung diseases such as cystic fibrosis. They can also cause acute sinusitis and acute exacerbations of chronic bronchitis. A unique form, *H. influenzae* biogroup *aegyptius*, causes purulent conjunctivitis and sepsis in children, usually 1 to 4 years of age, following conjunctivitis infection.

H. parainfluenzae typically has low virulence but does occasionally cause endocarditis and bacteremia. However, it carries resistance genes that help increase resistance in other members of this genus. *H. aphrophilus*, uncommonly, causes endocarditis and brain abscesses. *H. ducreyi* causes chancroid, a sexually transmitted disease accompanied by shallow and painful genital ulcers and inguinal lymphadenitis (buboes).

Haemophilus organisms are common in most people. They usually become a problem only when a person becomes immunocompromised. However, the genus is growing increasingly resistant to antibiotics; it appears that while type B is becoming less of a problem due to vaccination programs, the other types are growing more problematical. Resistant respiratory infections are more common every year and the organisms, once more invasive of children, have now shifted to infecting adults in nearly equal numbers.

An additional concern is that influenza viruses are highly synergistic with *Haemophilus*. Dual infection is considerably more dangerous than with either alone. There is some evidence that the 1918 influenza epidemic involved a highly activated synergy with *Haemophilus*; even immunocompetent individuals become highly susceptible to the bacteria when the two activate together. This synergistic capacity seems inherent in *Haemophilus;* other studies have found the same kind of synergy between it and other respiratory pathogens such as *Moraxella catarrhalis*, respiratory syncytial virus, human parainfluenza virus 3, and rhinovirus.

Importantly, *Haemophilus* are what are called fastidious bacteria, meaning they need an iron source to grow, and unlike most other bacteria, they usually get it from the hemoglobin in our blood to which iron is bonded (giving blood its red color). Protecting the blood cells through the use of something like sida is crucial in treating this kind of infection.

The herbs that have been found active against *Haemophilus* are ginger, licorice, isatis, lomatium, honey, eucalyptus essential oil, eucalyptus leaf, and basil essential oil. Unfortunately, cryptolepis, sida, and alchornea have not been tested against this organism. However, I believe that, due to their activity against similar Gram-negative bacteria, they are usable for *Haemophilus* infections, especially sida, given its strong protective effects on red blood cells. I would use them myself without hesitation.

TREATING HAEMOPHILUS INFECTIONS

Formulation 1 (antibacterial) Sida tincture: 1 tsp, 3–6x daily

Formulation 2 Isatis, ginger, licorice, and red root (equal parts) tincture: 1 tsp, 6x daily

Formulation 3 Fresh ginger juice tea (see page 228): 4–6x daily

For *Haemophilus* pneumonia: Formulations 1, 2, and 3

For *Haemophilus* epiglottitis and facial cellulitis: Formulations 1, 2, and 3

For *Haemophilus* chancroid: Formulations 1, 2, and 3. Add a topical wash of an infusion of eucalyptus and lomatium and honey 4x daily. If ulcers are severe, apply honey dressings after using the topical wash.

For *Haemophilus* meningitis: Formulations 1 and 2, along with piperine, 20 mg, 2x daily, with the first dose in the morning 30 minutes before taking the other formulations, and the second dose at 4 P.M. Also add isatis leaf (or root) and either Japanese knotweed or stephania (equal parts) tincture, 1 tsp, 3–6x daily. Echinacea will also be of benefit, as for bacteremia.

For *Haemophilus* bacteremia and osteomyelitis: Formulations 1, 2, and 3, along with *Echinacea angustifolia* tincture, 1/2 tsp–1 tbl, every half hour to hour

For *Haemophilus* septic arthritis: Formulations 1, 2, and 3, along with *E. angustifolia* and teasel root (equal parts) tincture, 1/2 tsp, 3x daily

For *Haemophilus* otitis media: Use Formulations 2 and 3 plus oil ear drops as follows: Make an oil infusion with lomatium. When done as per recipe, add 10 drops eucalyptus essential oil and 10 drops basil essential oil. Place 2–3 drops in ear 2x daily.

For *Haemophilus* purulent conjunctivitis: Use isatis or isatis-honey eyedrops.

Klebsiella

The main species that causes human infection is *K. pneumoniae*, but *K. oxytoca* and *K. rhinoscleromatis* occasionally do, too. Most infections occur in the lungs, but they also can occur in the urinary tract, the biliary tract, the lower respiratory tract, and surgical wounds. The organism can cause pneumonia, bacteremia, urinary tract infections, diarrhea, cholecystitis, osteomyelitis, meningitis, thrombophlebitis, and respiratory infections. Generally, infections are caused by hospital staff from bacteria on their hands or bacterial colonization of invasive apparatus, and sometimes patients' GI tracts are contaminated.

When *Klebsiella* infect the lung tissue, necrosis, inflammation, and hemorrhage often occur, giving rise to a thick, bloody mucus; it looks something like currant jelly (so they say).

Klebsiella organisms are often multidrug resistant, producing extended-spectrum beta-lactamases (ESBL). These strains are highly virulent and spread promiscuously. The mortality rate is around 50 percent, irrespective of antibiotic use. They are one of the fastest-growing resistant infections in U.S. hospitals and are common throughout the world. The newest resistant form is referred to as CRKP (carbapenem-resistant *Klebsiella pneumoniae*). Very dangerous.

The herbs useful for *Klebsiella* are cryptolepis, alchornea, bidens, black pepper, juniper, the berberine plants, *Acacia, Artemisia annua*, reishi, licorice, and honey.

TREATING KLEBSIELLA INFECTIONS

Formulation 1 (antibacterial) Cryptolepis and alchornea (equal parts) tincture: 1 tsp–1 tbl, 6x daily

Formulation 2 (to thin mucus) Ginger juice tea (page 228): 4–6x daily

Formulation 3 (immune support) Reishi, red root, licorice, and *Echinacea angustifolia* (equal parts) tincture: 1 tsp, 6x daily

Formulation 4 Juniper essential oil inhalation as aromatherapy: 4–6x daily

For *Klebsiella* **pneumonia and respiratory infections:** Formulations 1, 2, 3, and 4

For *Klebsiella* **osteomyelitis:** Formulations 1, 2, and 4, plus *Echinacea angustifolia* tincture, ½ tsp–1 tbl, every half hour to hour

For *Klebsiella* **meningitis:** Treat as you would enterococcal meningitis (see page 50).

For *Klebsiella* **surgical wound infections:** Formulations 1, 2, and 4, plus daily topical honey dressings (see monograph, page 188)

For *Klebsiella* **bacteremia:** Instead of the formulations above, use *Echinacea angustifolia tincture*, ½ tsp–1 tbl, every half hour to hour; cryptolepis tincture, 1 tbl, 6x daily; and piperine, 20 mg, 2x daily (the first dose in the morning 30 minutes before taking the other formulations and the second dose at 4 P.M.).

For *Klebsiella* **UTIs:** Instead of the formulations above, use juniper berry–bidens tincture (1 part juniper, 2 parts bidens), 30 drops, 3–6x daily; and cryptolepis–berberine plant tincture (equal parts), 1 tsp, 3x daily.

For *Klebsiella* **diarrhea:** Instead of the formulations above, use a berberine plant tincture, 1 tsp, 3–6x daily.

Neisseria gonorrhoeae

This organism causes gonorrhea, which is sexually transmitted. The main herbs effective for it are cryptolepis and sida.

TREATING NEISSERIA GONORRHOEAE

Formulation Cryptolepis and sida (equal parts) tincture: 1 tsp, 3x daily for 14 days

Proteus spp.

The two most troublesome *Proteus* species are *P. vulgaris* and *P. mirabilis*. Both are resistant. *P. mirabilis* generates 90 percent of *Proteus* infections in people. *Proteus* infections can cause alkaline kidney stones, but more seriously, when contracted in hospitals they can cause wound infections, urinary tract infections, septicemia, and pneumonia.

The herbs that are effective for proteus are cryptolepis, sida, alchornea, *Artemisia annua*, juniper, usnea, *Acacia aroma*, lomatium, ginger, and honey.

TREATING PROTEUS UTIs

Formulation 1 (antibacterial) Juniper berry and bidens tincture (1 part juniper, 2 parts bidens): 30 drops, 3–6x daily

Formulation 2 Cryptolepis, sida, or alchornea tincture: 1 tsp, 3–6x daily

Formulation 3 Ginger, rhodiola, and red root (equal parts) tincture: 1 tsp, 3x daily

Formulation 4 Piperine: 20 mg, 2x daily (the first dose in the morning 30 minutes before taking the other formulations and the second dose at 4 P.M.)

TREATING PROTEUS SEPTICEMIA

Formulation 1 (antibacterial) Cryptolepis, sida, or alchornea tincture: 1 tsp, 6x daily

Formulation 2 (to prevent septic shock) Isatis tincture: 1 tbl, 3–6x daily

Formulation 3 *Echinacea angustifolia* tincture: ½ tsp–1 tbl, every half hour to hour

Formulation 4 Lomatium, rhodiola, and red root (equal parts) tincture: 1 tsp, 3x daily

TREATING PROTEUS WOUND INFECTIONS

Formulation 1 (antibacterial) Cryptolepis, alchornea, and sida (equal parts) tincture: 1 tsp, 6x daily

Formulation 2 Lomatium, rhodiola, and red root (equal parts) tincture: 1 tsp, 3–6x daily

Formulation 3 Daily topical honey dressings (see monograph, page 188)

TREATING PROTEUS PNEUMONIA

Formulation 1 (antibacterial) Cryptolepis, alchornea, and sida
(equal parts) tincture: 1 tsp, 6x daily

Formulation 2 Ginger juice tea (page 228)

Formulation 3 (immune support) Lomatium, licorice, red root, and
Echinacea angustifolia (equal parts) tincture: 1 tsp, 6x daily

Formulation 4 Juniper essential oil inhalation as aromatherapy:
3x daily

Pseudomonas aeruginosa

This species is another opportunistic pathogen that takes advantage
of hospital settings. It can live, even thrive, on most surfaces and is
common on most medical equipment, including catheters, on which
it often enters the human body. It can grow in diesel and jet fuel and
survive temperatures up to 108°F, so fevers don't affect it much. It can
live in oxygen, partial oxygen, or no oxygen. It can even live in distilled
water in which virtually no nutrients exist. It's tough and very, very
resistant to antibiotics.

Pseudomonas can infect nearly any part of the body; all it needs is
an opening (which hospitals often give it). It causes pneumonia, septic
shock, urinary tract infections, otitis media, gastrointestinal infections, and skin and soft tissue infections. The most common infections
are from burns, surgical wounds, urinary tract infections, and otitis
media. Low phosphate levels in the human body are highly stimulatory
of its growth.

The primary herbs useful for treating *Pseudomonas aeruginosa*
are isatis, alchornea, bidens, cryptolepis, sida, black pepper, *Artemisia
annua*, the berberines, juniper, ginger, *Acacia aroma*, honey, lomatium,
ashwagandha, echinacea, and reishi.

TREATING PSEUDOMONAS PNEUMONIA

Formulation 1 (antibacterial) Cryptolepis and alchornea (equal
parts) tincture: 1 tsp–1 tbl, up to 6x daily

Formulation 2 Ginger juice tea (page 228)

Formulation 3 (immune support) Ginger, isatis, red root, and *Echinacea angustifolia* (equal parts) tincture: 1 tsp, 6x daily

Formulation 4 Juniper essential oil inhalation as aromatherapy: 3x daily

TREATING PSEUDOMONAS SEPSIS

Formulation 1 (antibacterial) Cryptolepis and alchornea (equal parts) tincture: 1 tbl, 6x daily

Formulation 2 (immune support) Ginger, isatis, and red root (equal parts) tincture: 1 tsp, 6x daily

Formulation 3 *Echinacea angustifolia* tincture: ½ tsp–1 tbl, every half hour to hour

Note: To reduce septic shock from endotoxin release, isatis tincture can be used in much larger doses: 1 tbl, up to 6x daily.

TREATING PSEUDOMONAS GI TRACT INFECTIONS

Formulation 1 (antibacterial) Cryptolepis and a berberine plant (equal parts) tincture: 1 tsp–1 tbl, 3–6x daily depending on severity

Formulation 2 Ginger, red root, and *Echinacea angustifolia* (equal parts) tincture: 1 tsp, 6x daily

TREATING PSEUDOMONAS UTIs

Formulation 1 (antibacterial) Juniper berry and bidens (1 part juniper, 2 parts bidens) tincture: 30 drops, 3x daily

Formulation 2 Berberine plant tincture: 1 tsp, 3x daily

Formulation 3 Ginger, licorice, and red root (equal parts) tincture: 1 tsp, 3x daily

TREATING PSEUDOMONAS INFECTIONS OF SURGICAL WOUNDS AND BURNS

Formulation 1 (antibacterial) Piperine: 20 mg, 2x daily, with the first dose in the morning 30 minutes before taking the other formulations, and the second dose at 4 P.M.

Formulation 2 Cryptolepis and alchornea (equal parts) tincture: 1 tsp, 6x daily

Formulation 3 (immune support) Ginger, licorice, and red root (equal parts) tincture: 1 tsp, 6x daily

Formulation 4 Daily topical honey dressings (see monograph, page 188)

TREATING PSEUDOMONAS OTITIS MEDIA

Formulation Ear formulation with lomatium, honey, berberine plant, or cryptolepis or use ear infection glycerite (page 345) with the addition of lomatium: 1–3 drops topically, up to 6x daily

Salmonella spp.

Closely related to both shigella and *E. coli*, salmonella organisms cause typhoid fever (*S. typhi*), paratyphoid fever (*S. paratyphi*), and salmonellosis, a.k.a. food poisoning. Most infections come from contaminated foods.

Salmonella can survive outside a host for years — active organisms have been identified in dried two-and-a-half-year-old feces. They are not destroyed by freezing and have to be heated to at least 130°F for 1 hour to kill them (or 10 minutes at 170°F). Poultry, pork, cattle, and many fruits and vegetables are now commonly infected with the bacteria. About 150,000 people in the United States sicken from eating infected chicken eggs each year.

The bacteria inhibit the innate immune system as they penetrate the body to better enable their survival. General symptoms are diarrhea, vomiting, fever, severe abdominal cramps. Sepsis and infection of other organs can occur in severe cases.

The organisms, due to heavy antibiotic use in both plant and animal agriculture, have developed multidrug resistance and are becoming much more difficult to treat.

The primary herbs effective for salmonella are cryptolepis, sida, alchornea, bidens, the berberines, juniper, honey, licorice, lomatium, and ginger.

TREATING SALMONELLA INFECTIONS

Formulation 1 (antibacterial) Cryptolepis, sida, or alchornea tincture: 1 tsp–1 tbl, 3–6x daily depending on the severity of the infection

Formulation 2 Berberine plant tincture: 1 tsp–1 tbl, 3–6x daily, depending on symptom picture

Formulation 3 (immune support) Licorice tincture, rhodiola tincture, and ginger juice (equal parts) combined: 1 tsp, 3x daily

Note: Juniper-evergreen and sida teas are especially useful for treating salmonella.

For salmonella with sepsis: Formulations 1, 2, and 3, and add *Echinacea angustifolia* tincture, ½ tsp–1 tbl, each half hour to hour.

Serratia marcescens

This is primarily a hospital-acquired infection. The bacteria can colonize the urinary tract (causing UTIs, from catheters), surgical wounds, the blood (bacteremia), the eye (conjunctivitis), the respiratory tract (pneumonia), the CNS (meningitis), the bones (osteomyelitis), and the heart (endocarditis). It is becoming highly resistant.

The primary herbs active against the organism are juniper, bidens, licorice, lomatium, *Coptis chinensis*, honey, oregano oil, *Tribulus terrestris*, and *Emblica officinalis*. The following plants are also active: *Trichosanthes cucumerina, Cassia didymobotrya, Blumea lacera, Moringa oleifera, Isodon* spp., *Dendrophthoe falcata, Zuccagnia punctata,* and *Phrygilanthus acutifolius.*

Note: For all *Serratia* infections, use piperine, 20 mg, 2x daily, with the first dose in the morning 30 minutes before taking the other formulations, and the second dose at 4 P.M.

TREATING SERRATIA UTIs

Formulation 1 (antibacterial) Juniper berry and bidens (1 part juniper, 2 parts bidens) tincture: 30 drops, 6x daily for 10 days

Formulation 2 Bidens fresh plant juice or tincture; or *Coptis chinensis* tincture; or *Tribulus terrestris* tincture; or a combination of the three (equal parts): 1/2 tsp, 3x daily

Formulation 3 (immune support) Ginger, licorice, and rhodiola (equal parts) tincture: 1/2 tsp, 3x daily

TREATING SERRATIA SURGICAL WOUND INFECTIONS

Formulations 2 and 3 for *Serratia* UTI infections (above), plus topical honey dressings daily (see monograph, page 188)

TREATING SERRATIA EYE INFECTIONS

Formulation 1 (antibacterial) Bidens fresh juice: 1–3 drops applied to the eye, up to 6x daily

Formulation 2 (immune support) Lomatium, licorice, and ginger (equal parts) tincture: 1/2 tsp, 3x daily

TREATING SERRATIA BACTEREMIA AND OSTEOMYELITIS

Formulation 1 (antibacterial) *Echinacea angustifolia* tincture: 1/2 tsp–1 tbl, every half hour

Formulation 2 (immune support) Lomatium, licorice, and ginger (equal parts) tincture: 1 tsp, 3x daily

Formulation 3 Bidens fresh juice or plant tincture: 1 tbl, 6x daily

TREATING SERRATIA PNEUMONIA

Formulation 1 (antibacterial) Bidens fresh plant juice or tincture: 1 tsp, 6x daily

Formulation 2 (immune support) Lomatium, ginger, licorice, and red root (equal parts) tincture: 1 tsp, 6x daily

Formulation 3 Juniper or oregano essential oil inhalation as aromatherapy: 3x daily

TREATING SERRATIA WOUND INFECTIONS

Formulations 1 and 2 for *Serratia* pneumonia (above), plus topical honey dressings daily (see monograph, page 188)

TREATING SERRATIA MENINGITIS
Formulations 1 and 2 for *Serratia* pneumonia (above), plus formulation 3 below:

Formulation 3 Isatis leaf (or root) and either Japanese knotweed or
stephania (equal parts) tincture: 1 tsp, 3–6x daily

Note: Echinacea will also be of benefit, as for *Serratia* bacteremia.

Shigella spp.

The main *Shigella* species are *Shigella dysentariae, S. flexneri, S. boydii,*
and *S. sonnei.* Shigella, *E. coli,* and salmonella are all closely related; all
usually cause some form of severe diarrhea. *S. flexneri* causes about 60
percent of the shigella infections in the nonindustrialized nations, and
S. sonnei about 80 percent of those in the industrialized. *S. dysentariae*
is the cause of most epidemics of dysentery.

Shigella organisms destroy the cellular lining of the intestinal
mucosa and invade the body; the disease is generally accompanied by
mild to severe diarrhea and/or dysentery. There are some 165 million
shigella infections a year and about a million deaths. The main route
of transmission is fecal/oral. There is frequent loose-stool diarrhea
consisting mostly of blood and mucus accompanied by fever, pain, and
bowel cramping. Sepsis, intestinal perforation, toxic megacolon, dehydration, hyponatremia, encephalopathy, hemolytic-uremic syndrome,
and pneumonia are common acute complications from the infection.
If untreated, persistent dysentery, severe protein loss, and malnutrition commonly occur, even in uncomplicated cases. Fever, malaise,
and body aches are common no matter the severity of the infection.
Some strains produce shiga toxins, which exacerbate the symptoms
considerably.

S. dysentariae is very prone to antimicrobial resistance and soon
passes the information on to the other species in the genus (as well as
to *E. coli* and *Salmonella* spp.). Most strains are now resistant to nearly
all low-cost antibacterials. The bacteria developed resistance in much
of the world to the last low-cost antibacterial, quinolone NA, within
6 months after it was used to treat an epidemic outbreak.

The herbs that are effective for shigella are cryptolepis, sida, alchornea, bidens, the berberines, juniper, honey, licorice, lomatium, and ginger.

TREATING SHIGELLA INFECTIONS

Formulation 1 (antibacterial) Cryptolepis, sida, or alchornea tincture: 1 tsp–1 tbl, 3–6x daily depending on the severity of the infection

Formulation 2 Berberine plant tincture: 1 tsp–1 tbl, 3–6x daily, depending on symptom picture

Formulation 3 (immune support) Lomatium tincture, licorice tincture, and ginger juice (mixed in equal parts): 1 tsp, 3x daily

Note: Juniper/evergreen needle and sida teas are especially useful for GI tract shigella infections.

For shigella with sepsis: To the above formulations, add *Echinacea angustifolia* tincture, 1/2 tsp–1 tbl, each half hour to hour.

Stenotrophomonas maltophilia

Once considered to be *Pseudomonas maltophilia*, then identified as *Xanthomonas maltophilia*, now this newly emerging resistant bacteria is called *Stenotrophomonas maltophilia*. It usually occurs in hospitals, where it can cause infections in surgical wounds, pneumonia, bacteremia, endocarditis, and meningitis. Few herbs have been tested for activity against it as of 2011. Here is what is known to be active so far: *Berberis* spp., alchornea, boneset, honey, epigallocatechin (green tea constituent), *Scorzonera sandrasica* (aerial parts), eucalyptus essential oil, eucalyptus leaf tincture, thyme essential oil, oregano essential oil, *Acacia aroma*, *Zuccagnia punctata*, *Sechium edule* fluid extract, *Salvia* spp., *Menyanthes trifoliata*, *Artemisia dracunculus*, *Mammea americana*, *Oedogonium capillare*, *Centaurea cariensis*, *Artemisia arborescens*, *Artemisia afra*, rosemary, garlic, and devil's claw (*Harpagophytum procumbens*).

TREATING STENOTROPHOMONAS MALTOPHILIA INFECTIONS

Formulation 1 (antibacterial) Alchornea tincture: 1 tsp, 3–6x daily,
  depending on severity of symptoms

Formulation 2 Fresh garlic juice: $1/4$–1 tsp, up to 4x daily

Formulation 3 Thyme, rosemary, eucalyptus, and oregano essential
  oils (blended in equal parts), inhalation as aromatherapy: 3–6x
  daily

Formulation 4 Eucalyptus leaf infusion: 8 ounces, up to 6x daily

Formulation 5 (immune support) Boneset, licorice, and red root
  (equal parts) tincture: 1 tsp, 6x daily

Formulation 6 Piperine: 20 mg, 2x daily, with the first dose in the
  morning 30 minutes before taking the other formulations, and the
  second dose at 4 P.M.

For *S. maltophilia* pneumonia: Formulations 1 through 6

For *S. maltophilia* bacteremia: Formulations 1, 2, 4, 5, and 6 (omitting formulation 3). Add *Echinacea angustifolia* tincture, $1/2$ tsp–
  1 tbl, every half hour to hour.

For *S. maltophilia* wound infections: Formulations 1, 2, 4, 5, and
  6 (omitting formulation 3). Add daily honey dressings (see monograph, page 188).

For *S. maltophilia* meningitis: Formulations 1, 2, and 6. Add tincture
  of isatis leaf (or root) and either Japanese knotweed or stephania
  (equal parts), 1 tsp, 3–6x daily. Echinacea will also be of benefit, as
  for bacteremia.

Vibrio cholerae

Cholera organisms infect the small intestine and cause extensive
watery diarrhea (10 to 20 quarts a day — usually without cramping),
generalized muscle cramps, and sometimes vomiting (clear fluid),
which in turn lead to dehydration and electrolyte imbalances. (One of
the most important interventions in cholera treatment is fluid replacement.) About five million people a year suffer from cholera, but before

antibiotics cholera epidemics were much worse. Generally, contaminated water or food is the culprit.

Prior to 1977, there were no reports of resistance in cholera organisms, but now they are common. Most cholera strains, including O1 Inaba, O139, O138, and El Tor, are now resistant to many antibiotics, including tetracycline, ampicillin, kanamycin, streptomycin, sulphonamides, trimethoprim, and gentamicin.

The herbs useful against cholera are the berberines, cryptolepis, licorice, ginger, *Geranium mexicanum* (or any of the geranium species' roots), *Psidium guajava* (guava) leaf and bark tea or ethanol extract, and *Punica granatum* (pomegranate) fruit peel or bark as tea or ethanol extract. Basil (*Ocimum basilicum*), nopal cactus (*Opuntia ficus-indica*), *Acacia famesiana*, and *Artemisia ludoviciana* are also very active against cholera organisms. Extracts of those four plants (and the geraniums as well) disrupt the cell membranes of the cholera organisms, increase membrane permeability, decrease cytoplasm pH and cell membrane hyperpolarization, and decrease cellular ATP concentration in all strains tested. In fact, nearly any of the acacias will do for this use.

TREATING CHOLERA

Formulation 1 (antibacterial) Cryptolepis and berberine plant
   (equal parts) tincture: 1 tsp, 6x daily

Formulation 2 Geranium root strong decoction: 3 tbl, every hour

Formulation 3 Guava leaf or bark and pomegranate peel or bark
   (equal parts) tea: as much as possible

Alternative Effective Decoction Acacia bark decoction: 3 tbl, every
   hour; basil and artemisia infusion: 8 ounces, every hour

Nonbacterial Variants

The three resistant nonbacterial variants are the candidas, malaria, and the aspergillus mold.

Candida spp.

Candida species are a type of yeast that form a normal part of the human intestinal and urinary tracts and skin flora. The main species is usually *Candida albicans*. Antibiotic overuse has stimulated tremendous problems with this organism. Overgrowth in the intestinal and urinary tracts is common. Candida has traditionally been treated with antifungals and azoles, but the last 20 years have seen significant resistance emerge across the entire genus.

Resistant candida infections cause urinary tract infections, vaginal infections, mouth infections (thrush) — they love mucous membrane systems. Itching, burning, soreness, irritation, and whitish patches or discharge are common symptoms. In some instances candida can become systemic and affect multiple organs. Infections are much more serious in people whose immune systems are compromised.

The herbs to treat candida are sida, alchornea, bidens, cryptolepis (minimally), *Artemisia annua*, the berberines, juniper, honey, usnea, black pepper, lomatium, isatis, licorice, red root flowers, reishi, echinacea, chaparro amargosa (*Castela emoryi*), and desert willow (*Chilopsis linearis*).

TREATING CANDIDA UTIs

Formulation Berberine plant, alchornea, or sida tincture: 1 tsp, 3x daily; or juniper berry–bidens tincture (1 part juniper, 2 parts bidens): 30 drops, 3x daily; or lomatium, isatis, and echinacea (equal parts) tincture: 1 tsp, 3x daily

TREATING CANDIDA VAGINAL INFECTIONS

Formulation 1 (antibacterial) Alchornea or sida tincture: 1 tsp, 3x daily

Formulation 2 Lomatium, isatis, and echinacea (equal parts) tincture: 1 tsp, 3x daily

Formulation 3 Berberine tincture diluted in water, used as a douche (see page 162): 2x daily, in the morning and again in the evening

TREATING CANDIDA MOUTH INFECTIONS
Formulation 1 (antibacterial) Lomatium, isatis, and echinacea
(equal parts) tincture: 1 tsp, 3x daily
Formulation 2 One ounce berberine tincture diluted in 6 ounces water,
take 1 tablespoon to wash mouth and gums thoroughly: 3x daily

TREATING SYSTEMIC CANDIDA INFECTIONS
Formulation 1 (antibacterial) Alchornea or sida tincture: 1 tsp,
3x daily
Formulation 2 Licorice, reishi, and echinacea (equal parts) tincture:
1 tsp, 3x daily
Formulation 3 Desert willow and chaparro amargosa (equal parts)
tincture: 1 tsp, 3x daily

Plasmodium spp.

There are some 200 or more species of plasmodia, parasitic protists
that infect red blood cells. Eleven of the species infect people. The disease is transmitted by mosquito bites. The organisms grow in the liver,
then infect the red blood cells. Fever, shivering, shaking, muscle pain,
headache, anemia, enlarged spleen and liver, and malaise are typical
symptoms. Vomiting is sometimes present. In severe infections brain
damage, convulsions, and death can occur. Given their life cycle, latent
parasites can emerge later. This is why treatment for *Plasmodium* is
often repeated after 14 days.

Worldwide, there are some 250 million cases of malaria each year,
resulting in nearly a million deaths, and 80 percent of them come from
Plasmodium falciparum. The malarial organisms are often resistant
to antibiotics, hence the development of artemisinin from *Artemisia
annua*. However, the use of that isolated constituent is now provoking
resistance worldwide, so the constituent is often combined with antibiotics to retard resistance development. In the treatment of malaria,
the whole herb or mixtures of herbs are preferable for just that reason.

The herbs effective for malaria are cryptolepis, sida, alchornea,
bidens, *Artemisia annua*, juniper, isatis, and licorice.

TREATING MALARIA

Formulation Cryptolepis, sida, or alchornea tincture: 1 tbl, 3x daily
for 7 days, repeat in 14 days; or artemisinin: 1,000 mg the first day,
500 mg daily for 4 more days, repeat in 14 days

Aspergillus spp.

Aspergillus, especially *A. fumigatus*, is an increasing source of resistant infections. This rather common mold can cause bronchopulmonary infections and chronic sinusitis. In hospital settings or among the immunocompromised it usually causes pulmonary disease and to a lesser extent surgical wound infections. It is resistant to most available drugs — polyenes, azoles, and echinocandins. Mortality rates in hospitals run 50 percent to 60 percent on average and as high as 90 percent in some populations (such as leukemia patients).

The herbs effective for aspergillus are sida, alchornea, cryptolepis, juniper, lomatium, isatis, ginger, honey, *Artemisia giraldii*, and *Sechium edule* fluid extract.

TREATING ASPERGILLUS INFECTIONS

Formulation 1 (antibacterial) Cryptolepis, sida, or alchornea tincture, or a combination of the three: 1 tsp, 3x daily

Formulation 2 (immune support) Ginger, licorice, and rhodiola (equal parts) tincture: 1 tsp, 3x daily

Formulation 3 Nasal spray formula for sinus infections (see page 181) prepared with *just* juniper essential oil; or juniper essential oil inhalation as aromatherapy: 3–6x daily

For sinusitis and bronchopulmonary conditions: Formulations 1, 2, and 3

For systemic treatment in the immunocompromised, pulmonary infection, or pneumonia: Formulations 1, 2, and 3; increase the dosage for formulations 1 and 2 to 1 tsp–1 tbl, up to 6x daily

For surgical wound infections: Formulations 1 and 2, plus topical honey dressing daily (see monograph, page 188)

3

ABOUT HERBAL ANTIBIOTICS

Facts are subversive of lies, half-truths, myths;
of all those easy speeches that comfort cruel men.
— **Timothy Garton Ash**

In 1998, when I wrote the first edition of this book, the Internet was very new; the world was a different place. A lot has changed.

For one thing, the Internet has become the greatest reference library human beings have ever known. A tiny part of that library, though enormously huge compared to what was available in the past, has to do with medicinal plants and the vast amount of research now being conducted on them. This facilitated the revision of this book enormously. During my research for the first edition, despite the size of my personal library (huge) and my access to a great university library at the University of Colorado in Boulder, I had access to only a tiny portion of the research and other material on medicinal plants that existed in the world. Now I have access to a great deal more; it's as close as my office computer.

But that is only a small part of the changes that have taken place over the past 15 years; something a great deal more interesting has been happening. As I spent weeks on the Web, following the scent of medicinal plants through the Internet forest, what struck home the most was a deep and visceral impact of just how much the human world itself has changed.

It is a new world out there. And it is a world with which the United States has an increasingly tenuous connection. The rest of the

Western nations are nearly as lost. During the past 15 years nations on the African continent, in Asia and South America, within the Russian sphere, and in most of the old Eastern bloc have realized that the medical model used by the West is unworkable, and to a great extent, they have begun abandoning it as the dominant approach to their people's health care.

Nations in those regions, especially in Africa, Asia, and South America, have realized they can't afford a pharmaceutical/techno-logical medical model as their primary approach to health care. They know that the problems of antibiotic resistance, petroleum depletion (most pharmaceuticals and all medical technology are made from or highly dependent on petroleum products), population expansion, top-down care models, and most especially cost and cost inflation cannot be solved and are only going to worsen over time. With that realization, they have begun abandoning industrialized medicine as a legitimate model for providing health care to their populations. (Industrialized medicine will still play a part but a much smaller, more affordable, and considerably less dangerous one.)

Unlike in the United States, researchers in those nations aren't exploring *whether* plant medicines work (nor are they spending their time and money trying to discredit what they feel is "primitive" medicine or unscientific quackery); they are exploring which herbal medicines work best and in what form and at what dosage. Their research and their journal papers are looking for the herbs that can treat malaria most successfully (for example) and how those plants, once identified, can be grown by the people who need them so they can be used when, and where, and by whom they are needed.

Many non-Western researchers are actively addressing the health problems of their populations with little if any profit motive. They have simply realized that corporate profit making and human health are not compatible. Shorthand: they are tired of seeing their cultures get screwed by international corporations that make billions out of the misery of others. They want to solve the problems facing them, simply, repeatedly, cheaply, ecologically, and with a great deal of personal empowerment for the people who are most directly affected. Reading the journal articles of U.S. researchers and comparing them with those of other nations and cultures is an illuminating and sobering experience.

The African and Asian journal articles tend to have titles like this: "Antibacterial activity of guava (*Psidium guajava* L.) and neem (*Azadirachta indica* A. Juss.) extracts against foodborne pathogens and spoilage bacteria" or "Evaluation of antimicrobial activities of extracts of five plants used in traditional medicine in Nigeria" or "Antimicrobial activity of ethanolic and aqueous extracts of *Sida acuta* on microorganisms from skin infections."

The U.S. journal articles are more along these lines: "Severe hypernatremia and hyperosmolality exacerbated by an herbal preparation in a patient with diabetic ketoacidosis" or "Metal content of ephedra-containing dietary supplements and select botanicals" or "Hypereosinophilia associated with echinacea use."

The abstract for that last study contains the kind of commentary common to many Western researchers, especially in the United States:

> Echinacea, believed by herbal practitioners to enhance the immune system, is one of the most widely used herbal supplements in the United States. Like most herbal products, it lacks strict FDA regulation and more information is needed about its potential adverse reactions. Here, we report the case of a patient with eosinophilia of unclear etiology whose condition resolved after cessation of this supplement. We feel this likely represents an IgE-mediated allergic process to echinacea.[1]

The article ignores the in-depth research on echinacea done in Germany over decades and the fact that it is a part of primary care medicine in that country. It uses words and phrases such as "believed by" and "we feel" and "likely." Its writers *assume* that the echinacea is the cause of the eosinophilia even though they have conducted no research to make sure of it. It's not science, not research, but rather guesswork and opinion that reflect the orientation, and bias, of the technologically focused, pharmaceutically dominated medical world, especially in the United States.

Now compare that with this abstract from an article by Nigerian researchers, "Antimicrobial activity of ethanolic and aqueous extracts of *Sida acuta* of microorganisms from skin infections."

The antimicrobial effect of the ethanolic and aqueous extracts of *Sida acuta* was investigated. Phytochemical analysis revealed the presence of saponins, tannins, cardiac glycosides, alkaloids and anthraquinones. The test isolates from human skin infections were *Staphylococcus aureus, Bacillus subtilis, Pseudomonas aeruginosa, Escherichia coli, Scopulariopsis candida, Aspergillus niger* and *Aspergillus fumigatus*. The zone of inhibition for the ethanolic extract varied from 10 mm for *P. aeruginosa* to 43 mm for *S. aureus* and from 4 mm for *P. aeruginosa* to 29 mm for *S. aureus* in the aqueous extract. Though the zone of inhibition increased with increase in the concentration of the extract, the highest concentration of the ethanolic extract revealed a higher significant (P. 0.05) inhibition against *S. aureus* and *B. subtilis* compared to the inhibition effect on these organisms by gentamicin used as control. The aqueous extract had no significant effect on the test organisms. The extracts had no inhibitory effect on the fungi isolates. This study has shown that the extract of *S. acuta* if properly harnessed medically will enhance our health care delivery system.[2]

This herb "will enhance our health care delivery system." I have never seen that sentiment in a research article in the United States and I've read thousands of them. (Gentamicin, by the way, is what is called an aminoglycoside antibiotic, often used to treat Gram-negative bacteria. *Sida acuta* at higher doses was more active against the test organisms than the antibiotic was.)

The authors of this study tested both aqueous (water) and ethanolic (alcohol) extracts of the plant — essentially infusions and tinctures — to see which were most effective. Most plants are used by indigenous cultures as water infusions (strong teas) or in whole form of one sort or another, either eaten or placed directly on the affected area of the body. Some cultures do use simple alcohol extractions. Of the active ingredients in plants, some are soluble in water, some in alcohol, and the researchers clearly wanted to find out which form of preparation was the most effective for this plant. It's *usable* information they were after. And they found it. They came to *Sida acuta* by looking at what traditional healers and herbalists in Nigeria were using in their practice and they decided to test it for activity. If it was effective they wanted to find out how it was *most* effective. And they planned then on supporting the use of that plant widely throughout Nigeria to enhance their country's health care system. Nothing could be more alien to the medical establishment in the United States.

To be fair, there are some good studies occurring in the United States, but to be clear, virtually *none* of them support the use of herbal medicines by the general populace or even by educated herbal practitioners. Their focus, rather, is on the identification of an "active" constituent that can then be modified chemically, patented, and subsequently produced by a pharmaceutical company for profit. U.S. researchers, in spite of often being affiliated with universities, generally work for or in concert with pharmaceutical companies. They are not looking for something the general populace can use without a prescription; they are not working to empower self-care. In most instances they don't trust the general populace to be intelligent enough to provide their own health care, nor do they want to interrupt their own financial income stream.

We in the Western world, especially in the United States, are being left behind in an outmoded model that has no effective place in the real world. By the time we realize it, the rest of the world will be generations ahead. The rest of the world has abandoned our approach; they understand the problems they face and what lies ahead. In the meantime, we spend our time making better and better buggy whips, not realizing the automobile really is here to stay.

Some Comments on the Herbs Discussed in This Book

To find the top herbs that can be effectively used for treating antibiotic-resistant organisms, I have relied on decades of my own experience, the cumulative experience of a great many other practitioners, many thousands of journal papers of very good research by committed researchers from many countries around the world, and the history of use of these plants by local peoples over centuries.

I have put the herbs in this book into three categories: systemic antibacterials, localized antibacterials, and facilitative or synergistic herbs.

Systemic antibacterials are herbal medicines that are broadly systemic, that are spread by the bloodstream throughout the body, thus affecting every cell and organ within the body, and that are active against a range of bacteria. These herbs are good for treating infections such as MRSA that have spread throughout the body and are not responding to multiple antibiotic protocols.

Localized antibacterials are those that do not spread easily throughout the body but are limited in their movement. Because they don't easily cross membranes, they are effective in the GI and urinary tracts and for external infections. These kinds of herbs are useful for infections such as *E. coli* O157:H7 or cholera or for infected skin wounds that refuse to heal.

Facilitative or synergistic herbs are just that: plants that facilitate the action of other plants or pharmaceuticals. They either enhance the action of the antibacterial being used or affect the bacteria so that the antibacterial is more effective. Most plants contain both antibiotic substances *and* a potent synergist, quite often one or more efflux inhibitors. Goldenseal, which contains berberine, is an example.

Berberine, a strong antibacterial, is very active against a number of resistant organisms. It is considerably more active, however, in the presence of another constituent in goldenseal, 5'-methoxyhydnocarpin (5'-MHC), which is a multidrug efflux pump inhibitor. It reduces or eliminates MRSA's ability to eject antibiotic substances that might harm it from inside its cellular membrane. 5'-MHC has no known function other than to do exactly this, and it is one of the reasons goldenseal is so effective in the treatment of resistant infections of the GI tract.

Compounds such as 5'-MHC are why plants are often more effective than single constituents in treating disease conditions. Other compounds in plants do still other things; some have no known function in the plant other than to reduce the side effects of the more pharmacologically active constituents. This is one of the reasons plants tend to be strange medicines in the minds of medical reductionists — they can't understand that kind of complexity or see the reason for its existence. Nevertheless, newer generations of researchers have grasped that the old paradigm is unworkable and they are looking toward plants with new eyes. They are understanding that plant medicines are much more sophisticated than pharmaceuticals (something those in older cultures innately understand).

As some specific examples: The anticonvulsant actions of yangonin and desmethoxyyangonin, kavalactones found in *Piper methysticum*, are much greater when the lactones are used in combination with other kava constituents. Concentrations of yangonin and another lactone, kavain, are much higher in the brain when the whole plant extract is used rather than the purified lactones themselves. In other words, some of the other constituents in kava help move the bioactive lactones across the blood-brain barrier into the brain. Blood plasma concentration of kavain is 50 percent less if the purified compound is used rather than an extract of the plant itself. Plant compounds in *Isatis tinctoria*, a potent antiviral and anti-inflammatory herb, are highly synergistic. Tryptanthrin, a strong anti-inflammatory in the plant, possesses very poor skin penetration capacity. However, when the whole plant extract is applied to the skin, penetration of tryptanthrin is very good. In other words, applying a salve of pure tryptanthrin to the skin, despite how anti-inflammatory that compound is, won't do you much good. But if you make the plant itself into a salve, the tryptanthrin moves rapidly into the skin and helps reduce skin inflammation.

Artemisinin is much more active against malarial parasites if administered with artemetin and casticin, flavonoids normally contained in the artemisia plant. Additional flavones in the plant, chrysophlenetin and chrysospenol-D, also act as potent synergists in this way. They are also permeability glycoprotein (P-gp) inhibitors (see monograph on piperine, page 236), thus facilitating the movement of artemisinin and the plant's other constituents through the intestinal membrane and into the blood.

As a final example, side effects such as tinnitus and stomach ulcers that can occur from the use of acetylsalicylic acid don't occur if whole extracts of willow bark are given rather than that purified constituent; other compounds in the plant specifically ameliorate its side effects.

Combining Plants for Greater Effect

When it comes to plant combinations, things get even more complex. For example, constituents from licorice (glycyrrhizin and its related compounds) significantly enhance the solubility of other plant compounds, such as the saikosaponins from Asian ginseng, in water. Thus, combining plants *during the medicine-making process* — a field almost completely unexamined in Western herbal approaches — can produce much stronger tinctures than when they are produced singly.

Quercetin (an anti-inflammatory and moderate anticancer flavonol found in many plants and vegetables) is poorly soluble in water, but that solubility is strongly enhanced by complex mixtures of saponins if plants containing them are added to the mix when the medicine is being made.

So . . . while some plants such as goldenseal are synergistic within themselves from the presence of efflux inhibitors and potent antibacterial constituents, other plants, such as *Dalea spinosa*, are relatively mild as antibacterials but contain compounds that are multidrug resistance (MDR) inhibitors, making them synergists for other plants. Adding synergists to a systemic antibacterial when creating an herbal compound increases the potency of the primary herb being used, sometimes considerably. (This has long been recognized in the actions of such plants as licorice and western red cedar, though the reasons *why* were not known.)

Synergists, while known throughout herbal history, have been only mildly recognized for their actions, usually in the Chinese and Ayurvedic systems, but they have not been accepted as a legitimate and unique category of herbal medicines that should be studied in their own right. Given the seriousness of emerging resistant pathogens, it is time to begin developing this category of herbal medicines in more depth, to begin to understand how to use them in practice, and to find the most potent ones that can be used for healing. The material in this book is, I hope, the beginning of that development.

The Importance of Preparation Methods

I remember, growing up, how often the physicians in my family made fun of the old plant doctors and herbalists insisting that some plants must be harvested only at such and such a time or they would be too weak to work or their insistence that certain plants must be used together to work. Turns out there is a great deal to those old assertions. So . . . considerable attention is paid within this book to *how* and *when* the plants should be harvested, prepared, and made into medicine.

There are other complexities that come into play when it comes time to actually make your plants into medicine. There is a synergy between the plant and the medium in which it is extracted. Regrettably, there has been an unfortunate lack of attention paid to this in much of the world, especially among us American herbalists. For example: The word *alkaloid* means *alkaline-like*, a clue that has been overlooked in every herbal preparation manual I have read over the past 30 years. In practical terms: Plant alkaloids won't extract easily in alkaline waters; they need more acidic waters to do so. Extracts of plants with highly bioactive alkaloids increase in strength if the plants are extracted in liquid mixtures that are at least minimally acidic. The water being used to make extracts (tinctures and infusions) needs to be "soft," or else an acid such as vinegar needs to be added in minimal amounts to make it so (see box, page 92).

Understanding these kinds of complexities in plants and the medicines they become comes from long exposure to them, from the same kind of intuitive sensing (holistic nonlinear perception) that all artisans use (in things from writing to house building to making music), and, most importantly, from a lack of intellectual hubris. If you understand up front that plants are highly complex living beings that are a great deal older than the human species, it is much more difficult to place an intellectually reductionistic paradigm on them. *You can't see what you assume is not there.*

Herbalism is an art; it is, and always will remain, much too complex to be approached from a reductionist and linear orientation with any expectation of success. "Phytorationalism" is an oxymoron. A practitioner with such an orientation will never grasp the essential nonlinearity of the world, of healing, of plant medicines.

The synergy within and among plant medicines, a prime example of the nonlinear complexity in this field, *means* that the combined effect of different substances will be greater than that which can be expected from the individual components alone. Combination produces outcomes beyond rational expectation. To face the challenges before us, we ourselves have no choice but to synergize within ourselves: to develop our abilities to feel and think *simultaneously*, neither in competition with the other, and blend those capacities together into a unique perceptual tool of tremendous elegance. I am talking about developing forebrain elegance here, not just tentative understandings of the hindbrain. As Erich Fromm once commented: "Reason flows from the blending of rational thought and feeling. If the two functions are torn apart, thinking deteriorates into schizoid intellectual activity and feeling deteriorates into neurotic life-damaging passions."[3]

4

HERBAL ANTIBIOTICS: THE SYSTEMICS

Our epitaph [as a species] may well read: "They died of a peculiar strain of reductionism, complicated by a sudden attack of elitism, even though there were ready natural cures close at hand."

— Gary Paul Nabhan, *Cultures of Habitat*

Most herbalists, irrespective of culture or country, do know of the antibacterial activity of plants and they do use them to heal bacterial disease on a regular basis, but, in general, our understanding of herbal antibiotics has been thin. By *thin* I mean we've been stuck in a paradigm of "take this for that" or "what's that plant good for" or even (among the reductionist herbal schools that have adopted the medical model; that is, the phytorationalists) "the active constituent of *Hypericum perfoliatum* should be standardized in order for the plant to be effective in the treatment of mild depression." Given the seriousness of the emerging bacterial diseases, we need to have a more comprehensive paradigm in place, one that takes into account the potential sophistication of herbal medicine as a very ancient art form of healing, one that uses both perceptual and intellectual awareness, as well as a focus on outcomes, in its expression.

The importance of systemic herbal antibacterials cannot be overstated.

Many resistant diseases, such as staph, are widely spread throughout the body. They can affect internal organs, invade difficult-to-reach parts of the body, or, very commonly, infect the skin (from the inside rather than outside), appearing as skin ulcerations in various locations. To treat a systemic infection like staph, an herbal antibiotic that is systemically spread throughout the body is necessary.

I remember the first time someone told me she had a community-acquired systemic staph infection; it was a woman who'd come to hear me teach. She said that she had undergone numerous courses of antibiotics, and that after the last one failed the physicians had told her, "Well, let's just observe it and see what happens." Her furious response was, "I know what's going to happen, I'm going to lose my foot."

I began to understand then just how important systemic antibacterials are in herbal practice. With resistant bacterial infections spreading at the rate they are, we *need* systemics — we need to know them as a category and we need to *really* know how to use them. We need to move from herbalism as a kind of "let's-eat-organic-today" choice (unless we're really sick; then we'll go to the emergency room) to a "we-can-depend-on-this-for-our-life" form of healing.

When herbs are taken into the body, some just stay pretty much in the GI tract, whereas others cross the intestinal membranes and circulate in the body, often concentrating in particular locations; the liver or kidneys, for instance. But one class of herbs is always broadly systemic. Once ingested they concentrate in the bloodstream (and sometimes the liver) and are widely circulated, reaching every cell that needs a constant blood supply, which is pretty much every cell in the body. These are the herbs that have traditionally been used to treat malaria. Many, if not most of them, also tend to possess rather strong antibacterial actions, sometimes broadly so. It is important, however, to make a distinction between the two common types of malarial herbs, for not all malarial herbs are true antimalarials.

Some malarial herbs are widely systemic and actually do kill the parasites responsible for malaria, but others only treat some of the symptoms of the disease such as fever or chills. Many researchers have not understood the distinction and so they may list an herb as being used for malaria when in fact it is *only* being used as an adjunct herb to treat one of the symptoms of malaria; for instance, when yarrow is used to treat malarial fevers.

Yarrow isn't a systemic antimalarial (even though it does have some mild actions against the parasite) but, rather, is a diaphoretic adjunct. It helps reduce fevers because it induces sweating, which cools the body. When researching the ethnobotanical literature, it is crucial to understand this distinction between the different kinds of malarial herbs. Once you do, their study begins to open up the wider world of systemic antibacterials. Systemic antibacterial herbs have often been used for centuries in the treatment of malaria simply because one of their antimicrobial actions is against malarial organisms. But they are often widely active against other organisms and can be very powerful. (Systemic antibacterials may also be found in a particular category of Chinese medicine — plants for toxic blood.)

The first systemic herbal antibiotic I began to understand was *Cryptolepis sanguinolenta,* a traditional herbal medicine from Ghana. I was introduced to it by a healer from Ghana, Nana Nkatiah, and it was this herb that I recommended to the woman who approached me at the workshop. Her family had become infected through exposure to her and at this point they were all ill. They used cryptolepis and it worked very well. Since then I have used cryptolepis on numerous occasions to treat systemic staph infections that have not responded to multiple antibiotic regimens. It has, so far, never failed. I consider this plant, along with alchornea, sida, and bidens, to be *the* primary systemic herbal antibiotics for use in treating resistant organisms at this time.

While cryptolepis is sometimes hard to find, many of the other herbs in this section are not — at least in the wild. They are often widely distributed throughout the world; a number of them are considered invasive plants, which is a plus.

Invasive plants — Earth's way of insisting we notice her medicines.

Cryptolepis

Family: In flux, given the propensity of botanical PhD students to write dissertations on minutiae; probably Apocynaceae (subfamily Periplocoideae) or perhaps Asclepiadaceae

Common Names: *Cryptolepis (in the West)* • *delboi* • *gangamau (among the Hausa)* • *Ghanian quinine* • *kadze (among the Ewe)* • *koli mekari (among the Mpiemo peoples in the Central African Republic and the eastern part of Cameroon)* • *nibima (among the Twi-speaking people of Ghana)* • *ouidoukoi* • *yellow dye root*

Species Used: There are about 20 or maybe 30 (taxonomists are so irritating) species of cryptolepis, 10 or more in Africa, two in Madagascar, four in Asia, three in Papua New Guinea, and one in Australia, and probably others elsewhere if that larger number is accurate. The primary systemic antibacterial among the genus is *Cryptolepis sanguinolenta.*

The potency of *C. sanguinolenta* has generated a lot of interest in this genus of plants. *C. triangularis*, native to Angola, Lagos, Belgian Congo, and Gambia, has, like *C. sanguinolenta*, been found to contain cryptolepine, one of the more potent antimalarial alkaloids known. (Some sources consider these two to be the same plant; others list them as distinct species.) Some sources say that *all* the members of this genus contain the antibacterial alkaloids cryptolepine, quindoline, and neocryptolepine. I have been unable to verify this by finding any in-depth chemical analysis of the other species. A number of sources do list cryptolepine and similar alkaloids as present in *C. buchanani*, a traditional Ayurvedic plant, commonly used as a medicinal in Thailand, Nepal, and India. It may be true; the traditional uses of *C. buchanani* show the same range of action as that of *C. sanguinolenta*,

The Top 5 Systemic Herbal Antibiotics
Cryptolepis
Sida
Alchornea
Bidens
Artemisia

so I tend to give the reports credence. *C. hypoglauca* is reported in one study to contain cryptolepine, but I can't find anything definitive on that either.

Of all the plants in the genus, *C. buchanani* and *C. obtusa* have stimulated the most interest outside *C. sanguinolenta*. Given the importance of *C. sanguinolenta*, in-depth chemical research needs to be done on the entire genus to determine whether the other species within it can be used as effectively.

Parts Used

The root is usually the part used medicinally (or in dyeing). The leaves *can* be used medicinally (see the description of the plant's chemistry below) but rarely are. The root of the plant is generally about the thickness of a pencil, appears to be fairly consistent in thickness over long lengths, and has a light tannish color on the thin exterior bark and a brilliant yellow on the interior. It's pretty. The root is exceptionally bitter due to the many alkaloids present.

Preparation and Dosage

Cryptolepis can be prepared as powder, capsules, tea, or tincture.

POWDER

For bacterial infections of the skin and wound sepsis, liberally sprinkle cryptolepis powder on the site of infection as frequently as needed.

TINCTURE

1:5, 60 percent alcohol, 20–40 drops, up to 4x daily

For resistant staph: In the treatment of severe systemic staph infection, the usual dose is $1/2$ tsp–1 tsp, 3x daily. In very severe cases increase the dose to 1 tbl, 3x daily. (I prefer to not use dosages this high for longer than 60 days. That is usually sufficient.)

For malaria: 1 tsp–1 tbl, 3x daily for 5 days, repeat in 14 days

TEA

Use 1 teaspoon cryptolepis in 6 ounces water to make a strong infusion.

As a preventive: Drink 1 or 2 cups daily.

In acute conditions: Drink up to 6 cups daily.

Note: While the herb will work if infused in cold water, studies have found that the hot-water extraction is more effective. It is nearly as strong as the alcohol tincture.

CAPSULES

As a preventive: Take 3 "00" capsules 2x daily.

In acute conditions: Take up to 20 capsules daily.

Side Effects and Contraindications

None noted. Considerable research has taken place to determine the potential adverse reactions from using the plant, and none have been found, either in human clinical use or with in vivo testing on mice, rats, and rabbits. The herb is taken as a regular tonic for years at a time in some parts of Africa and India. One or two cups of the tea or two or three droppers of the tincture (60 to 90 drops) a day are fine for extended, long-term use.

Check the pH of Your Water

The alkaloids in cryptolepis are water soluble, but if the pH of the water is alkaline, the alkaloids will not dissolve well. The pH scale ranges from 1 to 14, where 1 is the most acidic, 14 the most alkaline, and 7 is neutral. The word alkaloid means "alkaline-like." The more alkaline water is, the less well alkaloids will dissolve in it. You have to have a pH of at least 6 for the alkaloids to dissolve in water. "Hard" water is alkaline. (A water softener makes hard water soft; that is, acidic rather than alkaline.) If you have hard water (you can call your city's water department to find out the average pH) or if you don't know, add a teaspoon of vinegar or lemon juice to the boiling water you are using to make your cryptolepis tea.

Researchers in some instances have noted that people taking cryptolepis have elevated levels of ALP (alkaline phosphatase) and uric acid, which return to normal after the herb is discontinued. There have been no reported side effects from this. And though there is one report in the literature of adverse effects of cryptolepis in mouse pregnancy, I can find nothing in traditional use that substantiates an extrapolation to humans nor any studies in the literature that show negative effects in pregnancy in people.

Cryptolepine has been found to be cytotoxic, which raises concerns in some people. A few points:

- Cryptolepine is an isolated constituent, and like most isolated constituents that are made into pharmaceuticals, it produces side effects that don't appear when the whole herb is used. *Cryptolepis itself has not been found to be cytotoxic to people.*
- The word *cytotoxic*, when used in reports, generally means it kills cancer cells, and indeed, cryptolepine does.
- Cryptolepine is cytotoxic because it intercalates DNA. DNA is a double helix, two joined twisted ladders. Cryptolepine inserts itself between the two ladders — that is, intercalates — and as a result interferes with cellular division, which is why it is useful in cancer treatment. Cryptolepine is a potent inhibitor of topoisomerase II, which it inhibits once it intercalates. The function of topoisomerase II is to allow DNA replication by unwinding the DNA helix, using it as a template, then winding it again after replication. If topoisomerase is inhibited, DNA replication, and cellular division, can't occur.

Herb/Drug Interactions

None noted. However . . . cryptolepis has been used in traditional medicine to help rectify insomnia. One mouse study has supported that effect of the plant. There is some potential for the plant to synergize with hypnosedatives or central nervous system depressants. Caution should be exercised, although there have been no reported adverse effects in these situations to date.

Properties of Cryptolepis

Actions

Antibacterial	Antimuscarinic	Antiviral (mild)
Anticomplementary activity	Antiparasitic	Hypoglycemic
Anti-inflammatory	Antiprotozoal	Hypothermic
Antimalarial	Antipyretic	Noradrenergic
Antimicrobial	Antithrombotic	Renal vasodilator

Active Against

Aspergillus spp.	*Escherichia coli*	*Proteus vulgaris*
Babesia spp.	*Herpes simplex*	*Salmonella* spp.
Bacillus subtilis	*Klebsiella* spp.	*Shigella dysentariae*
Campylobacter spp.	*Mycobacterium* spp.	*Staphylococcus aureus*
Candida spp.	*Neisseria gonorrhoeae*	*Streptococcus pyogenes*
Entamoeba histolytica	*Plasmodium* spp.	
Enterobacter cloacae	*Proteus mirabilis*	

Tests have found the plant to be a stronger antibacterial than the pharmaceutical antibiotic chloramphenicol. Generally, it is more broadly active against Gram-positive bacteria (which are usually easier to treat due to their cellular structure), but it does have potent activity against a number of Gram-negative bacteria.

A number of studies have found cryptolepis active against *Pseudomonas aeruginosa*; other studies have found it ineffective. A balanced review of the journal papers, in my opinion, indicates that it is active against *Pseudomonas*. Examination of the studies does not give an easy clue as to the discrepancy in findings, but preparation differences seem to be involved.

Cryptolepis possesses little antifungal activity, though again, some studies have found it effective against candida while others have not. Again, a review of the studies, in my opinion, indicates that it is effective against candida and that preparation problems are the source of the discrepancy.

Use to Treat

Systemic infections, especially malaria, MRSA, streptococcus, babesia, campylobacter, urinary tract infections, tuberculosis, wound sepsis. It is very good for several Gram-negative bacterial infections: klebsiella, salmonella, shigella, *E. coli*, enterobacter, gonorrhea, and most likely pseudomonas

Other Uses

The root has long been used as a brilliant yellow dye in the regions in which it grows; hence its common name, yellow dye root. The dye is usually used for dying leather, generally goat skins. The roots are gathered, dried, then ground in a wooden mortar. The powdered root is blended with hot water in a large vessel. The goat skin is coated with groundnut oil and then dipped in the dye bath. The extract is hand-rubbed into the leather during soaking. Then a tamarind fruit paste is added and rubbed in. The skin is exposed to air for a few minutes, then reimmersed in the bath and rubbed once more. The fruit paste purifies the color.

Though the roots are the primary part of the plant used (both for dye and medicine), the leaves are used as a vegetable in Burkina Faso.

Finding Cryptolepis

The herb is somewhat difficult to obtain in the United States. The only tincture I currently know of is available from Woodland Essence. *Cryptolepis buchanani* may (I repeat, *may*) be a decent substitute for *C. sanguinolenta*, and it is somewhat easier to find. Raksa Thai Herbs is a good source.

Habitat and Appearance

Cryptolepis sanguinolenta is a slender, thin-stemmed climbing shrub whose stem produces a blood-red to deep orange juice when cut (*sanguinolenta* means "tinged or mixed with blood; bloody"). Essentially it's a tropical plant that likes it hottish and a bit humid. It is common from sea level to 2,500 feet (800 m) in altitude in savanna, dry forest, and gallery forest — that is, the riparian forests that develop along rivers and wetlands.

Cultivation and Collection

From reports, though it is usually wildcrafted, cryptolepis seems fairly easy to cultivate from seed and root cuttings. The seeds can be broadcast if desired. Due to its climbing nature, the plant needs a trellis to do well. Because of the growing international interest in the plant, commercial planting in Africa is on the increase.

The seeds are collected when semi-ripe and red/black in color. Normally they are then planted in raised mounds to facilitate harvesting of the roots. The seeds lose viability fairly quickly; they have a 90 percent to 100 percent germination rate for 4 weeks after harvesting and then begin to decline.

Roots can be collected after the plant is 1 year old, at any time of year. The side of the mounds are dug into and the root harvested. Up to one-third of the root from an individual plant can be taken without damaging the plant or its growth.

Cryptolepis would probably grow well in the American South, the northwest Olympic Peninsula, and parts of the West, or in any climate similar to its natural home. Given its importance, it should be cultivated wherever and whenever it can grow.

Plant Chemistry

There is some confusion in the naming of some of the more potent alkaloids in *C. sanguinolenta*, as researchers in different parts of the world named them with different names at about the same time. It still isn't sorted out. However, the primary ones are cryptolepine, neocryptolepine (a.k.a. cryptotackieniene, quinindoline), several other forms of neocryptolepine, hydroxycryptolepine, cryptolepine hydrochloride, isocryptoline (a.k.a. cryptosanguinolentine), quindoline, crypto-heptine, biscryptolepine, cryptoquindoline, cryptospirolepine, and cryptomisrine.

Most cryptolepis species contain phenolic compounds but *C. sanguinolenta* does not. Screening has found alkaloids (numerous), polyuronoides, and reducing sugars but little else. Polyphenols, saponins, flavonoids, and cyanogenic glycosides have been reported in at least one study. Cryptolepine is considered to be the strongest constituent (see the sida monograph, page 102, especially the "Scientific Research" section), though many of the others are nearly as potent.

An analysis of the leaves has found many of the same alkaloids that are present in the root, including cryptolepine. Aqueous and ethanolic extracts of the leaves are highly active against malaria (and presumably other microorganisms), giving a 90 percent inhibition of multidrug-resistant malarial strains in vitro. The leaves contain at least two novel alkaloids not present in the roots: cryptolepinoic acid and methyl cryptolepinoate, as well as the usual cryptolepine, hydroxycryptolepine, and quindoline.

C. buchanani, C. hypoglauca, and *C. triangularis* have all been listed as containing similar alkaloids as *C. sanguinolenta*. The research is thinner than I would like and *triangularis* may be a synonym of *sanguinolenta*. *Buchanani* has been studied in the most depth. It's a traditional herb in Ayurvedic practice (see that description, page 98). Several sources list it as containing cryptolepine and quindoline as well as sarmentogenin, sarmentocymarin, nicotinoyl glucoside, glucopyranose, buchananine, buchanin, n-triacontanol, n-triacontanoic acid, alpha-amyrin, beta-sitosterol glucoside, cryptosin, cryptanoside A-D, germinocol, cryptolepain, sarverogenin, and isosaverogenin. These latter two compounds appear to have potent antibacterial and antiparasitic properties. Given its traditional uses in India, it appears that *C. buchanani* may in fact be a good substitute for *sanguinolenta*.

C. obtusa contains some novel steroidal alkaloids, but not much work has been done on this plant — and on the rest of the family even less.

Traditional Uses of Cryptolepis

Cryptolepis has been successfully used for centuries by traditional African healers in the treatment of malaria, fevers, and diarrhea, as shown in the chart below.

Country/Region	Use Cryptolepis For
Congo	Amoebic infection, including dysentery
DR Congo	Colic, stomach complaints
Ghana	Malaria, fever
Guinea-Bissau	Fever, hepatitis, jaundice
Nigeria	Urinary tract infections, upper respiratory tract infections, colic, stomach complaints, venereal disease, rheumatism, as a general tonic
Senegal	Colic and stomach complaints, venereal disease, rheumatism, as a general tonic
Uganda	Colic and stomach complaints, wounds, snakebite, hernia
Zaire	Stomach and intestinal diseases

AYURVEDA

Cryptolepis buchanani has been used in traditional Ayurvedic practice for millennia. It is widely distributed throughout Pakistan, India, Nepal, Bhutan, Myanmar, China, Thailand, and Sri Lanka. It is considered an invasive weed in many areas (a useful sign of medicinal importance). There are a multitude of local names for the plant in those regions, 60 that I have identified so far. *Maranta* is a common one. It's been used as an antidiarrheal, antibacterial, anti-inflammatory, antiulcerative, blood purifier, demulcent, diaphoretic, and diuretic, and for treating paralysis and rickets and as a general tonic for overall health. It is commonly used for urinary tract infections, for coughs as an expectorant, as a febrifuge (antipyretic), and for abdominal disorders such as dysentery.

In Thailand alcohol extracts of the plant have been used as a primary anti-inflammatory in the treatment of arthritis, muscle and joint pain, and rheumatism.

Scientific studies of *C. buchanani* conducted in India and based on traditional use have found it is strongly antibacterial, effective against *Staphylococcus aureus, E. coli, Salmonella typhimurium, Klebsiella pneumoniae, Proteus vulgaris*, and *Bacillus subtilis*. Research has found it to possess immunopotentiating properties (useful in immunodeficiency), to act as a cardiotonic and cardio-protector, to be hepatoprotective, and to be strongly anti-inflammatory. It has shown some hypotensive actions and is considered to be, in one study, antiamphetaminic (a truly strange category — I gave him the amphetamines but they didn't work because . . .).

A Clinical Trial

Parameters: 44 outpatients with uncomplicated malaria were given a strong tea (steeped for 5 to 10 minutes) three times daily for 5 days, with posttreatment follow-up for 28 days.
Results: More than half cleared the malarial parasite from their blood within 72 hours (mean clearance time was 82.3 hours). Fever clearance time was 25.2 hours compared with chloroquine's clearance time of 48 hours. Chills, vomiting, and nausea were cleared in all patients in 72 hours. There were two instances of late recrudescence (return of the disease), but the researchers are unsure whether this resulted from reinfection or relapse; no genetic testing was done on the initial infection. Overall the cure rate was 93.5 percent. Nii-Ayi Ankrah, of the Department of Clinical Pathology at the University of Ghana, remarked (in a separate article), "The present result is indeed welcome news since it advances the vision to incorporate plant medicine into the health care delivery system in Ghana."[1] How different than in the United States.

Other studies, in mice, have found that the intake of a cryptolepis tea prior to inoculation with the malarial parasite does confer some degree of protection against infection. Taking it daily as a preventive as so many in Africa do seems to work well.

TRADITIONAL CHINESE MEDICINE

Given the plant's presence in China and nearby countries, it is certain that it is used in TCM, but none of my sources, though rather extensive in places, give a listing for the plant.

WESTERN BOTANIC PRACTICE

Until recently, this plant was not known to Western practice.

....

Scientific Research

Cryptolepis was discovered by the West because of the resurgence of pharmaceutically resistant plasmodial parasites. In an attempt to find new treatments for malaria, researchers began looking at traditional treatments. Initial studies revealed both *Cryptolepis sanguinolenta* and *Artemisia annua* (see monograph, page 140) to be powerfully active against resistant strains. Artemisia was the first to be developed into a drug (with the same predictable problems ensuing). Cryptolepis lagged behind, but in the past 15 years a tremendous amount of research has been conducted on the plant. Initially, most of it was concerned with malaria.

Cryptolepis is potently active against the malarial parasite, *Plasmodium falciparum*. (It is also active against other members of the genus: *P. berghei berghei, P. berghei yoelii,* and *P. vinckei petteri.*) Scores of studies have found it to be effective against the malarial parasite *no matter the degree of its resistance to pharmaceuticals.* Five of the plant's constituents — cryptolepine, cryptolepine hydrochloride, hydroxycryptolepine, cryptoheptine, and neocryptolepine — have been found to be exceptionally active against the parasite, and one

other, quindoline, is also active, though not as strong. Studies looking solely at inhibition of beta-haematin formation, which is one of the primary ways that antimalarials deal with malarial infection of blood cells, have found that seven compounds in cryptolepis are active in that respect.

The herb has been remarkably potent against malaria in human clinical trials. One such trial compared the effectiveness of cryptolepis (a hot water infusion of the powdered root) with chloroquine, the usual synthetic drug for malaria treatment, in comparative patient populations at the outpatient clinic of the Centre for Scientific Research into Plant Medicine at Mampong-Akuapem in Ghana, West Africa. Clinical symptoms were relieved in 36 hours with cryptolepis, and 48 hours with chloroquine. Parasitic clearance time was 3.3 days in the cryptolepis group, and 2.3 days in the chloroquine group — a remarkably comparable time period. Forty percent of the patients using chloroquine reported unpleasant side effects necessitating other medications, whereas those using cryptolepis reported *no* side effects.

Because many of the antimalarial compounds in cryptolepis are water soluble, and water-soluble extracts have worked well in clinical trials, a local company in Ghana hopes that a premade tea of cryptolepis will work well against malaria. Using 2.5 grams of powdered root per tea bag, the preparation is called Phyto-Laria and can be purchased over the counter in Ghana. (Similar products, Malaherb and Herbaquine, are also available in Ghana, and one called Malarial is sold in Mali.)

Pharmaceutical companies have created a number of cryptolepine analogues in an attempt to generate a patented drug they can control. Side effects from these analogues are unknown (isolated cryptolepine, unlike the plant it comes from, has shown a number of serious side effects during in vitro and in vivo studies), and like artemisinin and artesenuate (constituents isolated from *Artemisia annua*; see monograph, page 140), these analogues are likely to prove futile in the long run since the malarial parasite does develop immunity to single chemical compounds with regularity. Even though the analogues are molecularly close to cryptolepine, studies have found their mode of action to be different from cryptolepine's — the researchers really don't know what they do in the body or the likely long-term impacts. Because the herb itself is so tremendously safe and effective, I would not recommend the use of analogues if they do in fact ever come on the market.

ANTIBACTERIAL AND OTHER PROPERTIES

Cryptolepis is also broadly antibacterial. It has been tested against over 100 strains of campylobacter bacteria and found strongly effective against all of them. The tincture is more effective than co-trimoxazole and sulfamethoxazole, and equal to ampicillin. Cryptolepis is active against cholera but is not as strong in its effects as tetracycline. It has been found to be broadly active against a number of enteropathogenic microorganisms including *Shigella dysentariae, Entamoeba histolytica*, and *E. coli*. It is especially potent in the treatment of resistant staph, *Streptococcus pyogenes*, numerous strains of tuberculosis (*Mycobacterium* spp.), and urinary tract infections caused by enterobacter and klebsiella bacteria. The activity against such a wide range of organisms bears out its traditional use for many of the diseases that these organisms cause.

Cryptolepis also possesses antihyperglycemic properties, making it a potential antidiabetic herb. The isolated constituent cryptolepine lowered glucose levels in mouse models of type 2 diabetes, caused a decline in insulin levels, and enhanced glucose uptake. Several patents have been granted in this area.

The herb is strongly hypothermic, which means it lowers body temperature, a main reason why it has been found so effective in the treatment of fevers. It is also hypotensive due to its vasodilating effects, and it has been found to be active against a number of cancer lines and is stimulating interest as a potential anticancer agent.

Sida

Family: Malvaceae

Common Names: *Most of the species in this genus are commonly called something to do with "fanpetals," and in fact the sidas are sometimes referred to as the fanpetals.* S. cordata, *for example, is heartleaf fanpetals,* S. neomexicana *is New Mexico fanpetals,* S. spinosa *is prickly fanpetals, and so on. If it has fanpetals as part of its common name, it is probably a sida.*

Oddly, the most medicinally inclined tend to be called something else: S. cordifolia *is country mallow,* S. rhombifolia *is Cuban jute,* S. acuta *is common wireweed or teaweed or ironweed — all of which give an indication as to its nature, as does the Australian common name: spinyhead sida. Sometimes it is called hornbeam-leaved sida, morning mallow, or broomweed (the immensely durable branches are used everywhere the plant grows to make brooms), but most prefer a nastier name.*

The sidas are so widely distributed around the world and used in so many medicinal traditions that their non-English common names are legion. (See the Traditional Uses section on page 113 for some examples.)

Species Used: There are 125 or 150 or 200 species of the genus *Sida* (taxonomy is an *exact* science). They are distributed throughout the world, mostly in the tropics and subtropics, but some species extend into temperate regions.

The main medicinal species that has been studied is *Sida acuta.* However, as research has deepened on this species, other sidas are coming to light as similarly potent, particularly *S. rhombifolia* and *S. cordifolia.* Two other species, *S. tiagii* and *S. spinosa,* have not been studied as extensively, but their traditional uses, and some research, indicate they may possess the same medicinal actions.

Given the potency of some of this genus, it makes sense for more research to occur. As far as I can determine, little has been done along this line, but it may well be that many sidas contain similar constituents. If so, given their wide range, they would be one of the world's most accessible systemic herbal antibacterials.

This section will primarily concentrate on where the most research has been done: *Sida acuta*, with some depth on *S. rhombifolia*, *S. cordifolia*, *S. spinosa*, and *S. tiagii*.

Note: *Sida carpinifolia* is considered to be a synonym of *S. acuta*.

Parts Used

The whole plant — roots, leaves, stems, seeds. Most people tend to just use the aerial parts for the simplicity of harvest and ecological soundness. More practically, harvesting the root of a mature plant in this genus is as difficult as conveying to a politician the meaning of the word *integrity*. It is a tough, tough root to dig up. Nevertheless, *S. acuta* is considered an invasive botanical in many countries and most people are happy if you just take the whole damn thing.

Preparation and Dosage

The tincture and the hot-water extract are the strongest medicinal forms of sida for internal use. The plant can be prepared as powder, capsules, hot tea, or alcohol tincture. Most people use the leaves.

POWDER

For bacterial infections of the skin, wound sepsis, and eczema, liberally sprinkle the powder on the site of infection as frequently as needed.

CAPSULES

As a preventive: Take 3 "00" capsules 3x daily.
In acute conditions: Take up to 30 capsules daily. Or you can just use
1–3 tablespoons powder in water or juice.

TINCTURE

1:5, 60 percent alcohol, 20–40 drops, up to 4x daily

For resistant staph: In the treatment of severe systemic staph infection the usual dose is ½ tsp–1 tbl, 3–6x daily. (I prefer to not use dosages this high for longer than 60 days. That is usually sufficient.)

TEA

Use 1–2 teaspoons of the powdered leaves in 6 ounces water; let steep 15 minutes.

As a preventive: Drink 1 or 2 cups daily.

In acute conditions: Drink up to 10 cups daily.

For eye infections: Use the cool tea as eyedrops, 1–3 drops as needed, 3–6x a day.

Note: While the herb will work if infused in cold water, studies have found that the hot-water extraction is more effective. It is nearly as strong as the alcohol tincture. Also, because the plant's primary active constituents are alkaloids, the water used for the infusion must be acidic; see the box on page 92.

Side Effects and Contraindications

None noted, known, or reported; however . . .

- The herb is traditionally used to prevent pregnancy. It does interfere with egg implantation in mice. The herb should not be used in patients who are trying to get pregnant or are newly pregnant.

Not Good for Goats

The plant is a good forage plant for all animals except goats. Goats react negatively to swainsonine and will develop ataxia, hypermetria, hyperesthesia, and muscle tremors of the neck and head. Essentially the plant induces alpha-mannosidosis in goats, something other animals get if they eat too much "locoweed" — usually that is swainsonine-containing plants of the *Oxytropis* or *Astragalus* genera. This constituent does not affect people. Oddly enough, many foraging animals tolerate sida very well; the only report of adverse effects has been in goats.

- Even though the herb is traditionally used in later pregnancy, caution should be exercised with pregnant patients. I would be uncomfortable using it if I were pregnant, but then I would be uncomfortable anyway if I were pregnant.
- Since the herb contains cryptolepine, it is a DNA intercalator and interferes with DNA replication. (See page 93 in the cryptolepis monograph, for more.)
- The herb contains ephedrine, although not in large quantities (see Plant Chemistry, page 111, for an explanation of just how minute those amounts are). There has been a lot of inaccurate, hysterical reporting on ephedra, even among researchers who should know better. Weight loss and "natural energy" companies marketed supplements containing the herb (usually along with caffeine and other stimulants). People wanting to lose weight or increase their energy took the supplements — often in huge doses, far beyond sanity. Herbalists did not support this use of the herb. Ephedra is very safe when used properly; it really didn't need to be banned. The companies using it improperly just needed to be prohibited from doing so. Nevertheless, be aware that sida contains minute amounts of ephedra and that a mild raciness or wakefulness may occur from using the herb — but it probably won't. (See more in Finding Sida, page 108.)

Herb/Drug Interactions

None known or reported; however . . .

- Since the herb is hypoglycemic, it *may* affect medications for diabetes. Just watch blood sugar levels of diabetic patients.
- Since the herb contains ephedrine, it probably should not be used with pharmaceuticals that possess similar effects.

Properties of Sida

Actions

Adaptogenic
Analgesic
Anthelmintic
 (fresh leaf juice)
Antiamoebic
Antibacterial
Anticancer
 (antineoplastic,
 antiproliferative)

Antifertility activity
 (inhibits egg
 implantation in mice)
Anti-inflammatory
Antimalarial
Antimicrobial
Antioxidant (mild)
Antiprotozoal
Antipyretic

Antiulcerative
Antivenin activity
Hematoprotectant
Hematoregenerator
Hematotonic
Hepatoprotective
Hypoglycemic
Insecticidal

Active Against

Sida acuta is active against:

Babesia spp.
Bacillus spp.
Escherichia coli
Herpes simplex
Listeria innocua

Mycobacterium phlei
Pasteurella multicocida
Plasmodium spp.
Salmonella typhimurium
Shigella boydii

Shigella dysentariae
Shigella flexneri
Staphylococcus aureus
Streptococcus pyogenes

The plant is apparently less active against *Pseudomonas aeruginosa*, *Candida* spp., *Aspergillus niger*, and *A. fumigatus* (however, see the Scientific Research section on page 116).

Sida rhombifolia is active against:

Aspergillus niger
Bacillus spp. (various)
Candida albicans
Entamoeba histolytica
Escherichia coli
Klebsiella pneumoniae
Micrococcus luteus
Morganella morganii
Proteus vulgaris

*Pseudomonas
 aeruginosa*
Salmonella enteritidis
 (mildly)
Salmonella paratyphi
Salmonella sonnei
Salmonella typhi
Shigella boydii
Shigella dysentariae

Staphylococcus aureus
Vibrio mimicus
Vibrio parahaemolyticus

Use to Treat

Anemia	Eye infections	Skin rashes such
Cancer of the blood	(as eyedrops)	as eczema and
Diarrhea	Fevers	impetigo
Dysentery	Infected wounds	Systemic staph
	Malaria	infections
		Tuberculosis

Early indications are that sida is moderately virucidal against herpes viruses and can help prevent outbreaks. It is also useful as an adaptogenic in long-term debilitating infections such as Lyme, malaria, and dysentery.

Other Uses

Sida is very high in protein, being 16 percent to 25 percent protein depending on how it is grown. Some cultures use it as a pot herb; it is possible to use it as a primary protein source, especially if you are an "invasivore." Yes, they do exist. Invasivores eat only invasive species — though none have yet (publicly) admitted to consuming *Homo sapiens*.

I have not eaten sida, but the tincture is delicious, one of the few that delights the tongue. If you do try the herb as a vegetable, let me know what you think.

Many cultures use the plant's twigs in making brooms. From all reports they are exceptionally long lasting and useful given the hardiness of the wood. The bark from the stems of most species has been used for making cords, ropes, and twine; the bark from *S. acuta* can be used for making canvas and fishnets as well, hence the "jute" designation for some of the species.

Finding Sida

From what I can tell, based on traditional use and what research there is, *Sida acuta*, *S. cordifolia*, and *S. rhombifolia* can all be used similarly, and most likely *S. spinosa* and probably a number of others can as well. My preference is for *S. acuta* if you can get it, as the most research has been done on that species, then *S. rhombifolia*, then *S. cordifolia*.

Sources for the seeds in-the-year-of-our-plant-2012 are rare, but hopefully the material in this book will stimulate enough interest to make them more easily available. They are certainly available in quantity wherever the plant grows. Seeds of *Sida acuta* can be ordered from e*species Tropical Seeds. Horizon Herbs has *Sida cordifolia* seeds.

Because a number of weight loss companies are adding it to some of their "lose-weight-while-eating-all-you-want" formulations and bodybuilder supplement companies are also going gangbusters with it, some of the sidas may be banned. At this writing the only one that I have heard *may* be illegal in the United States is *rhombifolia,* but I have been unable to confirm that. If you search for *S. cordifolia,* you will find a number of capsule forms of it for sale. Use only the pure herb — many of those weight loss formulas have adulterants or other herbs mixed in. Again, I think the tincture and hot-water extracts are the most potent forms to use for healing, especially with resistant bacteria.

Unfortunately, due to the ephedra content in some of the sida species, at least one, *Sida rhombifolia*, has been reported to be illegal to harvest. Entheogenic adherents have also, sigh, been using the plant to get high by smoking it. (It is reputed to be an aphrodisiac stimulant in a number of cultures.)

Habitat and Appearance

Many of the sidas are typical-looking mallow-like plants with the usual five-lobed pale yellow to orange flowers. They get their name from the spreading or fanning of their flower petals. Some of the species are ground covers, while others grow into sturdy bushes as much as 6 feet (2 m) tall. They can be perennials, annuals, or biennials — and I am talking about the same plant here; they alter their behavior depending on where they are growing and the climate. They are often considered wasteland weeds irrespective of the species.

Sida acuta grows from 3 to 6 feet tall and may appear as either an annual or a perennial. It is a *potently* invasive medicinal wherever it gets established. In general, when the sidas get loose, they just keep on going, and they don't like to be controlled once they're established.

S. acuta has a very deep and strong taproot that endures droughts, mowing, and tillage with impunity. The plant easily survives extensive foraging by animals. With age the stem gets tough and woody, which helps the plant resist the phytopolice who wish to send it back to Mexico. Once established, the plant is highly competitive, loves and spreads easily into disturbed ecosystems, and doesn't share or play well with others. It can be found as high as 5,000 feet (1,500 m) and is often found in pastures, wastelands, cultivated farmland, roadsides, lawns, forests, and any human-planted or disturbed environment. It grows well in clay soils and desert as well as your typical black humus and survives heavy rainfall as well as drought. The seeds (spinyhead) adhere well to clothing and animals, are picked up in mud on tires and shoes, hide in hay and grass bales, and germinate easily wherever they end up. They are very sharp and puncture the skin, and feet, with abandon.

Truly one of the great invasives.

NORTH AMERICAN RANGE

Sida acuta can be grown in much of the United States and should be cultivated wherever it can be. It has been reported in Alabama, Florida, Georgia, Hawaii, Louisiana, Mississippi, New Jersey, Pennsylvania, South Carolina, Texas, Puerto Rico, and the U.S. Virgin Islands. Although it is said to grow most easily in zones 8 to 11, given that it grows in New Jersey and Pennsylvania, there is no reason it cannot grow throughout that region as well as in Northern California, Oregon, and the Olympic Peninsula and most likely other regions as well.

Sida cordifolia grows in Alabama, Hawaii, Florida, Texas, Puerto Rico, and the U.S. Virgin Islands.

Sida rhombifolia is widely distributed: Alabama, Arizona, Arkansas, California, Florida, Georgia, Hawaii, Kansas, Kentucky, Louisiana, Maryland, Mississippi, New Jersey, North Carolina, Oklahoma, Pennsylvania, South Carolina, Tennessee, Texas, Virginia, Puerto Rico, and the U.S. Virgin Islands.

Sida spinosa grows throughout those states and also in Connecticut, D.C., Delaware, Illinois, Indiana, Iowa, Maine, Massachusetts, Missouri, Nebraska, New York, Ohio, West Virginia, and Ontario, Canada.

WORLDWIDE RANGE

Sida acuta is considered to be native to Mexico and Central America, but it has spread around the world with great abandon (the seeds are great hitchhikers — the Spanish colonizers in South America and Mexico took some with them everywhere they traveled). In Australia's northern territories biological control has been instituted to try to stop its spread, with only mixed success.

This species is common in China, Japan, Taiwan, the Philippines, Malaysia, Singapore, Indonesia, Papua New Guinea, Fiji, Tonga, Tahiti — it's common throughout the entire Pacific Rim and Pacific Islands, in fact — India, Sri Lanka, Thailand, Cambodia, Vietnam, Burkina Faso, Togo, Nigeria, Kenya, Peru, western Colombia, Panama, Honduras, El Salvador, Guatemala, Mexico, and other similar places and regions around the world. In most places where it has been introduced it is considered invasive and noxious and is often deeply disliked (the seeds, rather nasty, contribute to its poor reputation). It is considered a plant threat to Pacific ecosystems. However, in some regions (Florida) people grow it as an ornamental. Go figure.

Sida rhombifolia is even more widespread than *S. acuta*. It is invasive throughout the Pacific Rim and Islands, Australia, and New Zealand. It is widely found in China, Japan, Taiwan, Thailand, Cambodia, Vietnam, Malaysia, Indonesia, the Indian Ocean chain, Peru, Ecuador, Colombia, Costa Rica, Nicaragua, Honduras, El Salvador, Guatemala, and Mexico.

Sida cordifolia also grows widely throughout the Pacific Rim and Islands (invasive status) as well as in Japan, Taiwan, Australia, El Salvador, and Honduras.

Sida spinosa is invasive throughout the Pacific Rim and Islands and grows widely in Japan, Australia, Chile, Peru, and Mexico.

Cultivation and Collection

Sida acuta grows well from seed. In fact, its seeds are very hardy, with at least a 30 percent survival rate over several seasons of drought. Each plant produces several hundred seeds every year. They attach to any passing animal and drop off later to spread the plant even further. The seeds need a period of high temperature to break their seed coat and do best if there is a period of alternating high and low temperatures.

The seeds are collected in the fall and can be top-seeded where you want them to grow, with average watering.

Note: *Sida acuta* is as good at healing damaged land as it is ill people; it is exceptionally good at detoxifying polluted soils. It removes cadmium, lead, nickel, iron, zinc, cobalt, mercury, molybdenum, copper, manganese, arsenic, and chromium from industrially polluted or dump sites. It is particularly good at scavenging lead, zinc, iron, nickel, cadmium, chromium, molybdenum, and arsenic. The plant should *not* be harvested for medicine from such sites as it will contain high levels of heavy metals.

Plant Chemistry

Sida acuta (and several others in the genus) is one of the few medicinals known besides *Cryptolepis sanguinolenta* to contain cryptolepine. This is one of the more potent constituents in the plant. The plant, like *C. sanguinolenta*, also generates a number of cryptolepine derivatives: quindoline, quindolinone, cryptolepinone, and 11-methoxy-quindoline.

Other constituents include ecdysterone, beta-sitosterol, stigmasterol, ampesterol, evofolin A and B, scopoletin, loliolide,

4-ketopinoresinol, ephedrine, beta-phenethylamine, quinazoline, carboxylated tryptamine alkaloids, alpha-amyrin, hentriacontane, hypolaetin-8-glucoside, campesterol, heraclenol, acanthoside B, daucoglycoside, choline, betaine, trans-feruloyltyramine, vomifoliol, ferulic acid, sinapic acid, syringic acid, syringaresinol, vanillic acid, swainsonine, vasicine, vasicinol, vasicinone, and peganine.

The seeds of both *Sida acuta* and *Sida rhombifolia* contain numerous ecdysteroids including ecdysone and 20-hydroxyecdysone. *Sida filicaulis* seeds contain lesser amounts. There is some indication that the plants, as opposed to the seeds, contain these compounds as well. This is the presumed source of the adaptogenic actions of the sidas when used as medicine. *Sida acuta* plants also contain alkaloids, flavonoids, steroids, tannins, cardenolides, polyphenols, terpenoids, and cardiac glycosides.

Sida acuta and *Sida rhombifolia* contain a number of cycloprope-noid fatty acids.

The same alkaloids present in *Sida acuta* have been found in *Sida humilis, S. rhombifolia*, and *S. spinosa*.

Not a Good Source of Ephedrine

The ephedrine content of *Sida acuta* and the other sidas is tiny compared to that of the true ephedra species. *S. acuta* has 0.006 percent in the roots and 0.041 percent in the leaves and stems. *S. cordata* has 0.005 percent and 0.036 percent; *S. cordifolia* has 0.007 percent and 0.112 percent; *S. rhombifolia* has 0.031 percent and 0.017 percent. In contrast *Ephedra distachya* contains about 3 percent in the plant; *E. sinica* has about 2.2 percent. *Sida cordifolia* root at 0.112 percent is the closest in strength to the ephedras' percent. Essentially, *S. cordifolia* has about 1/20th the ephedrine content of *E. sinica*. Nevertheless, companies are once again selling the sidas for weight loss and energy, and for weight lifters — a practice I consider to be unscrupulous.

Traditional Uses of Sida

Sida acuta is widely used in traditional medicinal practice around the world to treat malaria, fevers, headache, skin diseases, infected wounds, diarrhea, dysentery, snake bites, asthma, GI tract problems, systemic infections. James Duke's database lists 12 species of sida that have been used in traditional medicine, all for a similar range of complaints. The heaviest hits occurred with *acuta, cordifolia, rhombifolia,* and *veronicaefolia. S. acuta* and *rhombifolia* are sometimes smoked in Mexico for their euphoric effects.

Country/Region	Use *Sida* For
Australia	Aborigines use to treat diarrhea and indigestion
Burkina Faso	Fever, diarrhea, pulmonary infection, snake and insect bites
Colombia	Snakebite
Guatemala, Nicaragua	Asthma, renal inflammation, colds, fever, headache, ulcers, intestinal worms
Hawaii	Used by native islanders for vaginal infections, the flowers chewed as a laxative, the whole plant pounded and the juice taken for asthma or for general debility
Kenya	Tonic and common plant food
Malacca	Influenza, wounds, toothaches, ulcers, chest pains, scabies, abscesses, impotence, gonorrhea, and rheumatism
Nigeria	Malaria, typhoid fever, toothache, sore gums, teeth cleaning, ulcer, fever, gonorrhea, abortion (but also to stop diarrhea during pregnancy), hysteria, bruises, eye infections (as eyedrops), nosebleeds (fresh leaf juice), breast cancer, poisoning, inflammation, and sores and wounds, to stop bleeding, and as an antipyretic and emollient
Sri Lanka	Hemorrhoids, fevers, impotency, gonorrhea, and rheumatism; *S. acuta* is used in the treatment of neuralgia, *S. cordifolia* for hysteria, *S. rhombifolia* for fever
Togo	Eczema, kidney stones, headache
Trinidad and Tobago	Eczema

AYURVEDA

Various sida species have been used in India for over five thousand years; some species are native, others were introduced from the Americas. The primary species used is *Sida cordifolia,* but all are common medicinals. *Sida acuta* is considered an invasive menace by some and listed as such in some government writings. Practitioners in India commonly use the various species interchangeably, which has led to calls for stricter identification of which sidas are being used and for what. Species commonly used are *S. acuta, S. carpinifolia, S. cordifolia, S. humilis, S. indica, S. rhombifolia,* and *S. spinosa.*

Bala is the primary term in Sanskrit for the main medicinal species — *acuta* and *cordifolia* — while lesser species are distinguished by a linguistic modification of that term: *S. carpinifolia* is *bala phani-jivika, S. rhombifolia* is *atibala* (or *mahabala*), *S. spinosa* is *nagabala, S. humilis* is *bhumibala.* However, every local ethnic group that uses the genus for medicine has its own local name for the plants. There are scores of them. The plants, again, are considered to be interchangeable for the most part in practice; the roots, leaves, seeds, and stems are all used.

Sida cordifolia is considered to be cooling, astringent, stomachic, tonic, aromatic, bitter, febrifuge, demulcent, diuretic. The seeds are used as an aphrodisiac and to treat gonorrhea, cystitis, hemorrhoids, colic, and tenesmus. The leaves are used for strangury, hematuria, gonorrhea, cystitis, leukorrhea, chronic dysentery, nervous diseases, facial paralysis, and asthma, and as a cardiac tonic. They are cooked with rice and used for bloody diarrhea and bleeding hemorrhoids. An infusion of the roots is effective for nervous and urinary diseases and disorders of the blood and liver, while a decoction of the root (with ginger) is used for fever accompanied by cold shivering fits (essentially malarial fevers). The root juice is good for wounds, and an infusion of the dried root for bloody diarrhea, dandruff, and scalp problems. The juice of the plant is used for spermatorrhoea, rheumatism, and gonor-rhea. All parts of the plant are used as a stomachic and cardiac tonic.

Sida acuta is used as a diaphoretic and antipyretic and to treat fevers, dyspepsia, and lingering debility from previous illnesses. The juice of the root is used for intestinal worms, an infusion of the root for intermittent fever and chronic bowel complaints and for asthma, and the powdered root is made into a paste and applied to boils and abscesses. The leaves are used as a demulcent and diuretic and to treat chronic diarrhea and dysentery, rheumatic conditions, and gonorrhea. It is a common food plant in some districts.

Sida rhombifolia is used as a diuretic and aphrodisiac and to treat hemorrhoids, gonorrhea, rheumatism, kidney stones, fever, and scorpion sting. An infusion of the root is used for asthma.

Sida spinosa is used for cooling fevers (as a decoction, 2x daily) and to treat gonorrhea, gleet, scalding urine, debility. It was used as a primary trauma medicine in Chhattisgarh, India, during the wars of the twentieth century. The leaf juice was used to stop bleeding, decrease pain, prevent infection, and hasten healing time.

Other Ayurvedic uses of sida include the treatment of eye problems (infections), sinusitis, cramps, joint pain, fracture, swelling, Parkinson's disease, colic, whooping cough, uterine problems, vaginal infection, bronchitis, TB, emaciation, and cystitis. All the sidas are used as veterinary medicine for treating diarrhea in farm animals throughout India.

TRADITIONAL CHINESE MEDICINE

Sida acuta — huanghuaren or *huang hu aren* — is used in Chinese medicine, as is *Sida rhombifolia — huan hua mu* — and presumably other sidas as well. I can find little on the plants even though they seem to have a longish history of use there. The plants are usually used as decoctions, with a dosage range of up to 30 grams, or about 1 ounce. The Chinese consider sida to clear heat and benefit dampness. They have found it to be antibiotic, anti-inflammatory, analgesic, diuretic, and tonic.

Sidas are commonly used for depression, bronchitis with cough and wheezing, and urinary tract inflammations. Less common uses are for dermatosis, itching, eczema of the scrotum, sores and boils, stomach pain, dysentery, gastritis, enteritis, tonsillitis, liver problems, jaundice, cervical tuberculous lymphadenitis, malaria, colds and flu, and kidney stones.

WESTERN BOTANIC PRACTICE

Sida (*S. rhombifolia* primarily) was apparently introduced into the United States in the nineteenth century as a fiber plant, but it wasn't much used as a medicinal. The Eclectics listed it in a tiny reference under *Althea*, a.k.a. marsh mallow, as being highly mucilaginous, useful as a poultice, and effective for respiratory complaints.

Scientific Research

The recent focus on cryptolepine-containing plants as well as traditional malarial plants has stimulated a lot of interest in *Sida acuta* and some of the more commonly used Asian sidas. Most of the scientific studies have focused on phytochemical analysis and in vitro studies of the plants' antimicrobial actions, with a smattering of in vivo studies. The scientific exploration of these plants is still in its infancy and no clinical trials have been conducted that I am aware of.

There have been a number of studies of the antimicrobial activity of *Sida acuta*, and while they do give a good indication of its potency, nearly all the studies are flawed. Inexplicably, very few of the researchers appeared aware of the importance of proper preparation of the plant extracts. Looking only at the ethanol and water extract preparations in the studies, the problems are twofold. First, they tended to use 90 percent to 95 percent pure alcohol to make the ethanol extracts. This means that *only* the alcohol-soluble constituents would be present in the extract. (There would be a tiny amount of water-soluble constituents from the 5 percent to 10 percent water that was present in the alcohol.) Many of the most potent constituents in the plant, such as

cryptolepine, are only water soluble, so the preparation method will affect the impact of the extract on microorganisms.

Second, when making the water-based extracts many of the researchers used a neutral-pH distilled water. Additionally, some made it as a cold maceration. This is problematical for several reasons. Firstly, the alkaloids in the plant, most importantly cryptolepine and its derivatives, are primarily soluble in water that is somewhat acidic. Secondly, the plant constituents are less soluble in cold water than in hot. For the studies to be truly relevant, the water extracts should have used water with a pH of from 1 to 6 to make sure they were acidic enough to extract the alkaloids and the water should have been hot. With the ethanol extracts, preparation should have been made using half water and half pure grain alcohol; the water should have been hot, the herb inserted, the mixture allowed to cool, and then the alcohol added. The differences in preparation techniques are the most likely reason that the antimicrobial actions of the plant vary as much as they do from study to study.

Nevertheless, in all studies *Sida acuta* has been shown to be potently active against malarial parasites, staph bacteria, and TB, though beyond that there is a lot of variance. The best study took these factors into account but was exploring *only* alkaloid activity.[2] That study found more activity from the alkaloids against Gram-negative bacteria than previous research, which makes sense, as cryptolepis has been found to be active against Gram-negative bacteria simply due to the presence of crypto-lepine and its derivatives. In fact the alkaloidal extract of *Sida acuta* was nearly as effective against Gram-negative as Gram-positive bacteria.

A close examination does indicate, however, that both cryptolepis and sida more easily kill Gram-positive organisms than Gram-negative. This does not mean they are not active, it simply means that the dose needs to be higher if you are dealing with Gram-negative organisms, an observation confirmed by studies on both plants. The plant should also be taken for a longer duration — the Gram-negative bacteria did need a longer exposure to the herb than the Gram-positive. The use of a synergist that enhances antibacterial activity against Gram-negative bacteria would be helpful. (See piperine monograph, page 236.)

In spite of the problems in the in vitro studies, tests for antimicrobial activity have borne out the traditional uses of the plants against microbial diseases. They have found sida strongly active against *Plasmodium* spp., *Staphylococcus aureus*,

Neutralizing Hemotoxins

Importantly, sida has been found in vivo to neutralize venom from the snake *Bothrops atrox*, a common and very poisonous pit viper in South America. The snake's venom is a hemotoxin that destroys red blood cells (rather than the neurotoxin more common to cobras and rattlesnakes). The constituents in sida are particularly protective of red blood cells, which is one reason they are effective for treating malaria and babesia. With the snake venom, compounds in the plant neutralize a hemotoxic compound, rather than the plant's antimicrobial actions killing an infective organism. In this sense sida represents a unique category of herbal medicines: hematotonic, hematoregenerator, and hematoprotectant. It is especially useful for treating anemia and I believe there are strong indications that the herb will be significantly useful for the treatment of certain forms of myeloma — cancer of the red blood cells. It is the only herb I know of that is specific in this way for red blood cells.

Given that the actions of cryptolepis are similar to sida's and that it contains some similar constituents, it makes sense to explore cryptolepis for similar protectant actions; e.g., from hemotoxins.

and *Mycobacterium phlei*, resistant and nonresistant strains. It is highly active against *Streptococcus pyogenes*, *E. coli*, *Bacillus subtilis*, *Pasteurella multicocida*, and *Salmonella typhimurium*. It is also active against herpes simplex, *Shigella boydii*, *S. flexneri*, *S. dysentariae*, and *Listeria innocua* and less active against *Pseudomonas aeruginosa*, *Candida* spp., *Aspergillus niger*, and *A. fumigatus*, but still effective, especially if the dosage is increased. In many instances the plant was more effective against the bacterial strains than pharmaceutical antibiotics.

Sida increases glutathione levels in the blood, increases red blood cell numbers (making it good for treating anemia), and increases total white blood cell count, indicating an immune potentiation effect that may tie in with its reported adaptogenic actions in traditional practice.

In vivo studies have found *Sida acuta* to have a strong and reliable antiulcerative effect; that is, it protects the stomach lining from the formation of induced ulcers. In vivo research has also found a strong analgesic action.

Another in vivo study found sida hepatoprotective against induced liver damage (the plant is used in India for liver disease among other things). Several compounds from the plant have been found to inhibit induced preneoplastic lesions in mouse mammary tissue. In vivo studies have also found sida to be hypoglycemic, lowering blood sugar concentrations in diabetic mice, and to be antihyperlipidemic, lowering blood cholesterol and triglyceride levels, again in diabetic mice.

An analysis of four sidas — *S. acuta, humilis, rhombifolia*, and *spinosa* — found them to have similar alkaloidal constituents, including cryptolepine.

An analysis of five sidas — *S. acuta, alba* (a synonym of *spinosa*), *cordifolia, rhombifolia*, and *urens* — found varying levels of polyphenols in the plants (see chart at bottom of page).

The antioxidant activity of the plants followed that order as well, with *Sida alba* having the highest, *S. urens* the lowest. The plants were tested for anti-inflammatory activity, exploring their lipoxygenase (LOX) and xanthine oxidase (XOX) inhibition. For LOX, *alba* inhibited 80 percent, *acuta* 79 percent, *cordifolia* 21 percent, *rhombifolia* 52 percent, *urens* 47 percent; for XOX *alba* inhibited

Species	Compound			
	Phenolic (mg GAE/100mg extract)*	Flavonoid (mg QE/100mg extract)**	Flavonol (mg QE/100mg extract)**	Tannin (mg TAE/100 mg extract)***
S. alba	32.53	5.17	2.33	25.83
S. acuta	15.35	4.36	1.95	9.30
S. cordifolia	10.25	1.92	0.57	7.83
S. rhombifolia	5.75	1.02	0.68	4.35
S. urens	4.21	0.43	0.31	2.28

*Gallic acid equivalents   **Quercetin equivalents   ***Tannic acid equivalents

47 percent, *acuta* 43 percent, *cordifolia* 13 percent, *rhombifolia* 46 percent, *urens* 35 percent.

All these species of sida are successfully used to treat liver diseases including hepatitis B in Burkina Faso; the authors of the study were exploring some of the mechanisms that might explain their effectiveness.

Sida alba (i.e., *S. spinosa*) is fairly high in ecdysteroids, which are adaptogenic and explain, in part, the plant's use for debility in traditional practice.

Numerous studies have found *Sida cordifolia* to possess very potent anti-inflammatory and analgesic activities. An alkaloid with a tremendously long name, one of the quinazoles — a group of which cryptolepine is a member — was found to be the most potent

source of the activity. In vivo studies: An aqueous extract of *cordifolia* stimulated liver regeneration in 67 percent partial hepatectomy in rats; birds treated with cyclophosphamide, which causes immunosuppression, experienced a reversal of that condition when given *cordifolia*. In vitro studies: The plant is strongly antimicrobial and acts as an antistressor/adaptogenic in stressed mice; use of the plant after myocardial injury showed significantly increased endogenous antioxidants in heart tissue; other studies found evidence of a protection from neurotoxicity caused by quinolinic acid.

Sida tiagii during in vivo research has been found to have antidepressant and antiseizure effects in mice.

Alchornea

Family: Euphorbiaceae

Common Name: *Christmas bush*

Species Used: The genus *Alchornea* is a pan-tropical group of plants comprising some 60 species, six of which are indigenous to Africa. *Alchornea cordifolia* is the main medicinal species, though *A. laxiflora* is a reliable substitute. Regrettably, there has been little study on the members of this genus other than *A. cordifolia*.

Parts Used

Mostly the leaves, but the stem bark, pith, root bark, roots, and fruits are all used.

Preparation and Dosage

TEA

Add 7 grams (¼ ounce) of herb per cup of liquid, one ounce per quart. Boil for 20 minutes. Strain, then drink 6–8 ounces of the tea every 4 hours. Studies have shown that the tea takes about 3 hours to begin getting into the blood, and it tends to hit peak presence 1 to 2 hours after that depending on the dose; dosage presence lasts about 4 hours. This means that if you are using the tea you need to have another cup every 4 hours or so. Recommended dosage times: 8 A.M., 12 P.M., 4 P.M., 8 P.M., or beginning whenever you rise and then going to a 4-hour period. **For eye disease:** Use the cool tea as eyedrops, 1–3 drops every 3–4 hours.

TINCTURE

1:5, 50 percent alcohol, 50 percent water; take ¼ teaspoon of the tincture every 4 hours

POWDER

For wounds and infected skin, liberally sprinkle the powder on the site as frequently as needed.

Side Effects and Contraindications

None noted, and no toxicity has been found. There are no reports in the literature or by traditional practitioners of side effects, although large doses may have a sedative or depressant effect on the central nervous system.

Herb/Drug Interactions

None noted; however, large doses should not be taken along with CNS depressants or sedatives.

Note: Some people indicate that *Alchornea castaneifolia* can be used interchangeably but I can't see this as accurate — I would never recommend using it interchangeably. See Beware of *A. castaneifolia,* opposite page.

Habitat and Appearance

Alchornea cordifolia is a common plant throughout much of the largish middle of Africa, from Senegal to Kenya and Tanzania and from just north of South Africa to Angola. It's a straggly shrub or small tree up to 25 feet in height. It is widespread in secondary forest and likes riparian habitat and marshy areas but does spread into drier ecosystems, especially in disturbed soils. It will grow in terrain up to 5,000 feet (1,524 m) in altitude. It likes acid soils and is an active soil modulator, restoring calcium levels to depleted soils. *Alchornea laxiflora* grows in the same regions and has virtually the same appearance.

Cultivation and Collection

Propagates well from cuttings; they root solidly in a few months. The seeds are considered to be difficult germinators, needing to be scarified and tended diligently. Germination takes up to 3 months.

The plant can be harvested at any time. The leaves are taken when healthy and vital in appearance. The plant is normally wildcrafted as

Beware of *A. castaneifolia*

A few normally reliable companies list scientific studies on the activities of *Alchornea cordifolia* under an entirely different plant — *Alchornea castaneifolia*. *A. castaneifolia* has become popular because it is sometimes used in indigenous ayahuasca ceremonies. The Internet now has scores of sites selling it under the identifier *iporuru* or some version of that name.

Unfortunately most of the sites selling *A. castaneifolia* indicate that it has the same actions as *A. cordifolia* and point to studies on *A. cordifolia* to prove it. This just isn't accurate. The plants are definitely *not* interchangeable. There is very, very little research on the pharmacology of *A. castaneifolia*, and while there may be some overlap in actions — for instance, it *may* be useful for staph infections — there probably is not. Under no circumstances should you believe that *A. castaneifolia* will act as a reliable systemic antibacterial for resistant infections.

Properties of Alchornea

Actions

Amoebicidal
Anthelmintic
Antiamoebic
Antianemic
Antibacterial
Antidiarrheal
Antidrepanocytary

Antifungal
Anti-inflammatory
Antimalarial
Antimicrobial
Antioxidant
Antiprotozoal
Antiseptic

Antitumor
Antiviral
Bronchial relaxant
Smooth muscle tissue
  relaxant
Trypanocidal

Active Against

Aspergillus spp.
Babesia spp.
Bacillus subtilis
Candida albicans
Entamoeba histolytica
Escherichia coli

Helicobacter pylori
Klebsiella pneumoniae
Plasmodium spp.
Proteus mirabilis
Proteus vulgaris

*Pseudomonas
  aeruginosa*
Salmonella enteritidis
Salmonella typhi
Shigella flexneri
Staphylococcus aureus
Streptococcus pyogenes

Use to Treat

Malaria, systemic staph infections, pseudomonas, anemia, fevers, infections from *Streptococcus pyogenes*, and diarrhea and dysentery from such things as severe *E. coli*, *Salmonella*, *Entamoeba*, *Shigella*, or amoebic organisms. Generally, resistant Gram-positive and Gram-negative infections, systemic or of the GI tract. Infected wounds. Sickle cell anemia, sleeping sickness, resistant respiratory infections, conjunctivitis (as an eyewash), UTIs.

Other Uses

Alchornea is a potent alley-cropping plant and soil restorer: Rows of the trees are planted as windbreaks to protect other crops while returning calcium to depleted soils. The fruits produce a black dye traditionally used for fishing nets, cloth, pottery, and leather. The wood is used for construction and crafts.

it is widespread and vigorous once established. It is not yet an agricultural crop.

It coppices well and is very hard to get rid of once established.

Plant Chemistry

A. cordifolia contains the usual terpenes, sterols, flavonoids, tannins, carbohydrates, glycosides, saponins, and alkaloids. It also has alchorneine, alchornine, and alchornidine (all are imidazopyrimidine alkaloids), several guanidine alkaloids, gallic acid, gentisic acid, anthranilic acid, protocatechuic acid, ellagic acid, hyperoside, various quercitrins, daucosterol, acetyl aleuritolic acid, beta-sitosterol, epoxy fatty acids (in the seeds, lots), and a lot of other stuff no one has discovered yet.

Traditional Uses of Alchornea

A. cordifolia is widely used throughout every region of Africa in which it grows. It is used as a wash for eye infections and powdered for ringworm and other skin infections. It is an anti-inflammatory, a carminative, an anodyne, a diuretic, an emmenagogue, a blood purifier, and a tonic and has antitumor actions. See chart on next page for a comprehensive list of traditional uses.

Finding Alchornea

The herb is not readily available in the West. I have found only one supplier (Woodland Essence) that carries the herb in tincture form. Part of the point of listing this wonderful plant here is to stimulate suppliers to import it or for gardeners to begin planting it in the United States. It would do well here. If you can plant alchornea in your region, do so; it will be worth the effort.

Seed stock is available from the National Forestry Seeds Centre of Burkina Faso (Centre National de Semences Forestières de Burkina Faso) at $14 per kg (about 2.2 pounds). The website is www.cnsf.bf. The primary government language is French, but an English version of the website was under construction as this was being written.

Traditional Uses of Alchornea		
Amoebic dysentery	Epilepsy	Snakebite
Anemia	Fever	Sore throat
Asthma	Gastro-intestinal disorders	Tachycardia
Bronchitis	Gonorrhea	Thrush
Buccal ulceration	Headache	Toothache
Chancre	Hemorrhoids	Trypanosomiasis
Chills	Jaundice	Tuberculosis
Conjunctivitis	Leprosy	Ulcers
Constipation	Malaria	Urinary disorders
Cough	Mouth ulcers	Urogenital infections
Dental caries	Myalgia	Worms
Diarrhea	Postpartum hemorrhage (topical)	Wounds
Edema	Respiratory	Yaws
Enlarged spleen	Rheumatism	

AYURVEDA

Not known as far as I can tell.

TRADITIONAL CHINESE MEDICINE

Not known as far as I can tell.

WESTERN BOTANIC PRACTICE

Not known as far as I can tell, though some species have been used for a long time in South American indigenous practice. They don't seem to be similar in action to the two African species discussed here.

Scientific Research

In vitro studies have found *Alchornea cordifolia* active against 15 MRSA isolates and to be strongly active against *Pseudomonas aeruginosa*. Low concentrations of the herb are active against *E. coli, P. aeruginosa, Staphylococcus aureus*; it is as or more active than pharmaceutical antibiotics such as gentamicin and ampicillin. In vivo studies have confirmed the MRSA action in mice. A 50 percent ethanol extract (normal tincture) of alchornea was tested against 74 microbial strains: aerobic, facultative, anaerobic, and fungi. It was active at low concentrations against all except three strains, all filamentous fungi. Like most systemic antibacterial herbs, it was a bit stronger against Gram-positive strains than Gram-negative. It has been found to be active against *Helicobacter pylori, Salmonella typhi, Shigella flexneri, Salmonella enteritidis,* and enterohemorrhagic *E. coli* (EHEC), bearing out its traditional uses for treating dysentery and diarrheagenic bacterial pathogens. Ethanolic and water extracts have been found to be equally active except that only the ethanolic extract was active against EHEC. Other studies have found the ethanolic extract reliably effective in vitro for *E. coli, Pseudomonas aeruginosa, Staphylococcus*

aureus, Klebsiella pneumoniae, Proteus mirabilis — at the proper dosage, it is as effective as ciprofloxacin.

In vitro screening of 45 Congolese medicinal plants found alchornea to be highly antiamoebic, with strong activity against *Entamoeba histolytica.* Other studies have confirmed this, including finding a strong spasmolytic action. The plant exhibited a more than 70 percent reduction of spasms in guinea pig ilea.

A. cordifolia has been found to produce its activity in the treatment of dysentery and diarrheal diseases through three mechanisms: antibacterial, antiamoebic, and antispasmodic actions that are apparently

Treating Sickle Cell Anemia

Sickle cell anemia is a genetic disease resulting from a mutation in the hemoglobin structure. The cells undergo alterations, ending up as a sickle shape rather than round. This reduces the ability of the cells to carry oxygen and starves the body of enough oxygen to function. About 25 percent of people in sub-Saharan Africa have the disease, which is passed from parent to child genetically; half of those in whom the disease becomes active die before the age of five, about 60,000 in Nigeria each year. Traditional healers have used *Alchornea cordifolia* for centuries in the treatment of the disease, and recent scientific study has found it highly effective. Essentially the plant prevents sickling of the cells (antidrepanocytary activity) and reverses cells that have already transformed. Of all the plants tested for sickle cell treatment, *A. cordifolia* was the most potent. In Lagos a relative, *A. laxiflora*, has been found to have the same activity. The use of *A. cordifolia* reduced sickling by 85 percent and reversed 69 percent of sickled cells. The pharmaceutical approaches normally used for sickle cell anemia are highly toxic, but researchers commented that with this herbal preparation "toxicity . . . is not a problem." The herb is sold as a standardized product, as a tea or capsules, in Lagos and called Cellod-S. Good outcomes have been reported in clinical practice.

synergistic. In vivo study has found the plant to be highly antidiarrheal against castor-oil-induced diarrhea in mice.

Given the traditional use of alchornea for treating malaria across Africa, it is odd that only two in vitro studies have been conducted on its activity against *Plasmodium falciparum*. One study found it potently active, the second mildly so. *A. cordifolia* is fairly high in ellagic acid, which has been found to be strongly active, in vivo and in vitro, against the malarial parasites. The former study also found it strongly active against *Trypanosoma brucei*. (*A. cordifolia* is used in ethnoveterinary practice to treat that disease, and studies have found it active against both resistant and nonresistant forms.)

Like a number of plants in this chapter, *Alchornea* appears to be hemotonic, a hemoregenerator, and hemoprotectant, but the research has not focused that broadly. It does have a long history of use against anemia, malaria, and sickle cell anemia, as well as for trypanosomiasis (a.k.a. African sleeping sickness), which is also a parasitic disease of the bloodstream, similar in some respects to malaria and babesia.

The research on *Alchornea laxiflora* is limited, but both its traditional use and the studies that exist seem to confirm that its actions are very similar to those of *A. cordifolia*. It grows in the same eco-ranges and is considered interchangeable by the traditional practitioners. In vitro studies have found that the plant has anticonvulsant and sedative actions (in vivo studies have found this action in *A. cordifolia* as well) and is strongly anti-

oxidant, anti-inflammatory, antimicrobial, and antibacterial against both Gram-positive and Gram-negative bacteria. The chemistry of the two plants is very similar.

One study found *A. laxiflora* strongly active against HIV-1 and HIV-2 in vitro, more so than AZT. Another found the plant to possess immune modulatory and stimulant actions. It generates a lymphoproliferative effect on naive murine splenocytes and thymocytes and modulates the effects of the phagocytic and lysomal enzyme activities of murine macrophages. It increases phagocytosis and intracellular killing capacity. Lysosomal phosphatase activity of peritoneal macrophages increased significantly.

Of 42 plants tested in one study, *Alchornea cordifolia* was found to have the most potent antioxidant effects. In vitro study found that the plant was highly protective of rat liver against hepatotoxins. In vivo study in mice found the same.

A number of in vivo studies have found the plant to be strongly anti-inflammatory and very effective in the treatment of induced edema in rats. In vitro studies have found *Alchornea cordifolia* strongly anti-inflammatory by inhibiting human neutrophil elastase and superoxide anion.

Histological changes occur in rat pancreas after use of an ethanolic extract of the plant — 28 days of use resulted in regenerative alterations. Islet cells in the pancreas of rats with induced type 1 diabetes regenerated. Quiescent cells proliferated and replaced lost cells. The plant also decreased blood glucose levels and increased B-cell levels in other studies.

The plant is used as an antiasthmatic in Ghana, and an in vivo study found it to act similarly to isoprenaline, which is sometimes used in bronchial inhalers for asthma. Another study found the plant to have a marked effect on the aorta of Wistar rats, essentially inducing elastogenesis.

Bidens

Family: Asteraceae (Compositae)

Common Names: *Spanish needles, beggarticks, demon spike grass, needle grass, *$%#*%!, and a lot of other names in hundreds of languages. It appears to grow everywhere and people either hate it or loathe it or both. They certainly do name it.*

Species Used: There are 200 species in the *Bidens* genus. Maybe. Anal-retentive phytospecific maniacs are continually messing about with which species belong in the genus and, as usual, making problems for everyone. In consequence, the taxonomy of *Bidens* is considered "unsatisfactory," which is a massive understatement.

Bidens pilosa is the main species used medicinally (or at least on which most of the studies have been done), but there do seem to be a number of others in the genus that historical use and early research indicate can almost certainly be used similarly: *B. frondosa, B. tripartitus, B. ferulaefolia, B. alba* are all fairly potent, *frondosa* and *tripartitus* more so than *pilosa* in their antimalarial effects. *B. maximovicziana, B. pinnata,* and *B. campylotheca* are all fairly strong as well but, in terms of impact on the malarial organism, a bit less strong than *pilosa*.

Note: *Bidens leucantha* is a synonym for *B. pilosa.*

Parts Used

Usually the aerial parts, but the entire plant is active, and in some instances the roots seem to be a bit stronger as a medicinal. Normally, however, the leaves tend to be the most potent part of the plant, followed by the roots. The fresh leaves are often used and a number of studies show the fresh leaves and juice of the plant to be the most antimicrobial. Drying the plant reduces its antimicrobial action considerably.

Preparation and Dosage

There are some important things to know about using and preparing bidens:

- The most potent forms of this herb are alcohol tinctures and the fresh juice.
- The most potent constituents are considerably more soluble in alcohol than in water. Water infusions have a decent range of potency (as can be seen from the plant's traditional uses as a tea in Africa) but are not nearly as effective as a cold alcohol/water maceration.
- Some of the plant's most potent constituents oxidize easily and begin to degrade as soon as the plant is dried. Heat also destroys them.
- Expect about a two-thirds reduction in antimicrobial activity if the plant is not prepared fresh.
- The older the dried plant is, the less potent it will be in either water or alcohol. The fresher the dried plant material, the better.
- Water infusions lose potency fairly rapidly; they should be made and used daily. The rapidity of degradation of the plant chemicals is, in part, why so many cultures that don't normally make alcohol tinctures resort to using the juice of the leaves of this plant, internally and externally, for disease.
- Water extractions of the plant (teas, infusions, decoctions), especially if it is dried, possess about half the antibacterial activity of an alcohol tincture (depending on how old the extractions are), but they do possess most or all of the other actions described in this material (anti-inflammatory, antiallergenic, immune-modulating, and so on), especially the anti-inflammatory and antipyretic actions.
- A tincture is the strongest form of the herb as medicine. The use of piperine as a synergist will increase the potency of the plant considerably.

TINCTURE

Fresh plant, 1:2, 95 percent alcohol, 45–90 drops in water, up to
4x daily. Tincture made from the dried plant, if you must, would be
1:5, 50 percent alcohol, triple the dose.

For acute conditions (malaria, systemic staph): $1/4$–1 tsp and up to
1 tbl in water, up to 6x daily for up to 28 days, depending on severity.
The tincture can also be used topically on infected wounds.

WATER EXTRACTION

Possible, but not really recommended.

Tea: 1 teaspoon herb in 8 ounces hot water; let steep 15 minutes. Drink
2–4 cups daily.

Decoction: Not recommended; heat degrades the herb. But if you
must: For external use, boil 1 ounce herb in 1 quart water for
20 minutes, then strain. Cool and use on skin inflammations. For
internal use, boil 2–4 ounces herb in 1 quart water for 20 minutes,
then strain. Drink by the cup 2–4x daily.

Cold infusion: Steep 2–4 ounces herb in 1 quart cold water overnight.
Drink by the cup 2–4x daily.

FRESH JUICE

You can run the leaves through a juicer to obtain a decent quantity of
the fresh juice — the plants are pretty prolific. Be aware that they have
strong fibers that will bind the juicer and you'll have to clean it often.
Use the juice on infected wounds, for eye infections, or internally for
systemic infections. If you want, you can stabilize the juice with the
addition of 20 percent alcohol so that it will keep (see page 227). It
can then be taken internally much like the tincture, though it will be
more potent in its actions. Dosages are similar to those listed for the
tincture.

Properties of Bidens

Actions

Antibacterial	Blood tonic	Mucous membrane tonic
Antidiabetic	Carminative	Neuroprotectant
Antidysenteric	Diuretic	Prostaglandin synthesis inhibitor
Anti-inflammatory	Galactagogue	Styptic
Antimalarial	Hepatoprotective	Vulnerary
Antimicrobial	Hypoglycemic	
Antiseptic	Hypotensive	
Astringent	Immunomodulant	

Active Against

Bacillus cereus	*Escherichia coli*	*Plasmodium* spp.
Bacillus subtilis	Herpes simplex 1 and 2	*Pseudomonas aeruginosa*
Candida albicans	*Klebsiella pneumoniae*	*Salmonella* spp.
Human cytomegalovirus	*Leishmania amazonensis*	*Serratia marcescens*
Entamoeba histolytica	*Mycobacterium tuberculosis*	*Shigella flexneri*
Enterococcus faecalis (Streptococcus faecalis)	*Neisseria gonorrhoeae*	*Staphylococcus aureus*
		Staphylococcus epidermidis

Bidens is not very active against *Aspergillus*.

Like a lot of studies for antimicrobial activity, a number of those on *Bidens* are contradictory. For every study that finds it active against *E. coli,* another says it is not. Same for *Pseudomonas, Klebsiella, Streptococcus,* and *Candida*. Some studies show very strong activity, others mild, others none at all.

The differences come from the time of year the plant was gathered, the ecosystem in which it was found, whether wild or domesticated plants were used (wild plants have been found to be much stronger antibacterials), and differences in how the plants were prepared — the main problem being preparation. (See Preparation and Dosage, page 128.)

For this plant to act as a potent antimicrobial, it must be prepared as a tincture of the fresh plant or the fresh juice must be used.

Use to Treat

In order of potency:

1) *Any* systemic infections that are accompanied by problems in the mucous membranes anywhere in the body, especially chronic diarrhea, dysentery, UTI, vaginitis, and inflamed respiratory passages
2) Systemic staph
3) Malaria, babesia, leishmania
4) Any of the other resistant organisms bidens is active against

Other Uses

As a pot herb. The plant comes up early in the spring, is very hardy, and is used by many cultures as a food staple. However, see Side Effects and Contraindications (page 132) for a caveat on the plant as food.

Finding Bidens

Look outside in the yard. If for some reason the plant has overlooked you, ask around and you can probably find someone to send you some seeds. Soak them in some water for a day or two, then scatter them outside on the ground and cover with a bit of soil. Don't tell your neighbors.

Side Effects and Contraindications

None noted; however, be aware that *Bidens pilosa*'s leaves have numerous sharply pointed microhairs around the margins that are very high in silica. This kind of silica formation has been linked to esophageal cancer in certain domesticated animals (cows) and humans. Tribal cultures that eat large quantities of the plant as a primary food source show increased levels of that type of cancer. Cultures that use the plant only sporadically for food do not have an increased incidence of cancer. Exercise caution if using bidens as a food plant; it appears fine for occasional use but not as a steady diet.

Note: *Bidens pilosa* is a toxic-waste reclamation plant. Unless you want more heavy metals in your body, be careful where you get the plant. It should not be harvested from sites where there is heavy metal contamination. Numerous studies have found it to be a potent phytoremediation plant for cadmium and one study showed the same for arsenic; another indicates it may have an affinity for heavy metals in general.

Herb/Drug Interactions

None noted, although one study does show it potentiating tetracycline.

Caution should be exercised when using the plant with people on diabetic medications as it will alter blood glucose and insulin levels.

Habitat and Appearance

A native of South America, *Bidens pilosa* is a world-class invasive species. Spread by the Spanish during colonization, it is now widespread seemingly everywhere. If it does not currently grow someplace, it eventually will.

Bidens grows from sea level to 10,000 feet (3,600 m) in altitude. It tolerates moist soil, sand, clay, lime rock, infertile soil, drylands. It thrives best in high sunlight, dry soils, and disturbed areas but has been found in nearly every type of eco-range on the planet. It can withstand long periods of drought and survives temperatures as low as 5°F (–15°C). It isn't fire tolerant but rapidly invades burned areas and is quite happy about any opportunity to do so.

It loves the southern and southwestern United States and has spread up the West and East Coasts into eastern Canada.

It is found throughout the Caribbean, Central America, South America, Europe, Russia, China, most of Africa, Southeast Asia, southern India, Japan, the Pacific Islands, and Australia. It may not grow in Ulan Bator or Nebraska, but then again, it may.

At its initial appearance in spring, bidens is quite a beautiful ground-coverish sort of plant, but as the season develops and it grows taller, it develops a rather straggly, weedy appearance. The flowers are the usual white, five-petaled things with an orange interior. The seeds are longish, thin, black needles with a sharp, extended pronged tip. There are often three or four prongs in spite of the fact that *Bidens* means "two-toothed" (*bi* means two and *dens* — as in dental — being tooth). The seeds can attach themselves to about anything, hence the name beggarticks. If you walk through a patch of bidens during seeding season, your shoelaces and pants to the knees will be covered with hundreds of the hard-to-remove seeds — a thousand seeds weigh only about 1 gram. They take hours to pick out, hence the name *$%#*%!

The plant loves disturbed places, especially agriculturally disturbed fields, and actively tries to colonize cultivated land. It is allelopathic (toxic to other plants) and can reduce domesticated crops up to 50 percent once it invades a planted field. It is considered highly noxious in scores of countries just for that reason. The plant has very few natural predators.

I like it.

Cultivation and Collection

Bidens grows best from sea level to 10,000 feet (3,600 m) within a temperature range of 75°–90°F (25°–30°C) during the growing season. The edges of its growing temperature are from about 55° to 115°F (15° to 45°C).

Bidens grows easily from seed and is a tenacious grower. The seeds can still be viable after 3 years. The plant grows very fast, flowering as few as 6 weeks after its emergence from the ground. The first seeds mature just 4 weeks after flowering. Each plant produces a minimum of three thousand seeds a year and in some climates will reproduce four times before dying back.

The seed germinates best if buried about 4 cm in the soil; deeper than 6 cm and it won't germinate at all. Soaking the seed in water prior to planting increases germination rate and numbers. The seed can be broadcast or sown in rows.

The plant is an annual and can be harvested within 4 to 6 weeks of its emergence in the spring; it is generally considered to be harvestable until it sets seed (unless of course you are interested in making medicine from the seeds). The older the leaves, the more bitter and astringent they become. If you are using it for its astringency, gather late in the year. If you are gathering it for food, get it early in the year.

If you are growing it as a medicinal, remove the flowers to retard old age and stimulate leaf growth. The leaves can be harvested throughout the year as long as you don't allow the plants to go to seed early on. If the plants are topped, you can get up to six harvests a year depending on your climate.

If you must dry bidens, do so out of the sun. And collect a lot of it, as it dries to almost nothing; a big bag of the fresh plant will give you a handful of dried powder. The plant will oxidize, so keep it in paper bags or, if well dried, in plastic, inside a plastic bin out of the sun. Replace every year or two, depending on how you store it. But ideally it should be used fresh.

A great deal of research has found that the plant leaves if used fresh or tinctured fresh possess significantly stronger antimicrobial activity than if dried. The herb's ability to inhibit malarial parasites drops from 90 percent in the fresh leaf tincture to 38 percent in the dried (in vivo studies). If you are using the plant as an antimicrobial for resistant pathogens, harvest the leaves before flowering and tincture them fresh.

If you do grow bidens intentionally, you may irritate your neighbors. Nevertheless, its ease of growth, widespread habitat, and medicinal nature make it an essential herb to know, grow, and use for the treatment of resistant pathogens.

Plant Chemistry

There has been a lot of work on the constituents of *Bidens pilosa*, and around 100 different plant chemicals have been identified so far. There are numerous aurone flavonoids, butoxy lipids, coumaric acids, and erythronic acid phenylpropanoids, a number of heptaphenyl and phenylheptatriyne benzenoids, a lot of okanin flavonoids, numerous stigmasterol steroids, a lot of quercetin flavonols, daucosterol, and a whole lot more. A very comprehensive plant in terms of flavonoids, terpenes, phenylpropanoids, lipids, and benzenoids.

The most active constituents are thought to be the polyacetylene compounds and the flavonoids. The acetylenes have shown the broadest-spectrum antimicrobial activity.

Traditional Uses of Bidens

The plant is one of the great easily available systemic antibacterial herbs. It does not appear to have as wide a range of action as *Sida* or *Cryptolepis* and is definitely not as strong. But it is reliable for the treatment of a number of resistant bacterial infections and is very simple to use. Because it grows so easily and is so prevalent in so many countries, it is a crucial herb to know about as resistant organisms extend their reach.

Wherever the plant grows it is often used by the local peoples for similar problems: to treat mouth and stomach ulcers, headaches, ear infections, hangovers, diarrhea, kidney problems, malaria, jaundice, dysentery, burns, arthritis, ulcers, abdominal problems, swollen spleen, coughs, colds and flu, rheumatism, boils, diabetes, skin rashes, and infected wounds. It is also used as an anesthetic, a coagulant, a poison antidote (especially for snakebite), and to ease childbirth.

AYURVEDA

Bidens pilosa grows primarily in the south of India, where it is known as *ottrancedi*. It is frequently used for glandular sclerosis, wounds, colds, flu, acute or chronic hepatitis, and urinary tract infections. Another species, *Bidens trifada*, is used for chronic dysentery, eczema, skin problems, ulcers, headache, earache and ear problems, toothache, cough, inflammation, and leprosy.

TRADITIONAL CHINESE MEDICINE

Called *xian feng cao* (abundant weed), *gui zhen cao* (demon needle grass), or *nian shen cao* (I don't know but probably unflattering) by the locals, all parts of the plant are used to clear heat and toxins. Dosage runs from 15 to 60 grams ($\frac{1}{2}$ to 2 ounces) per day, or as high as 120 grams (4 ounces) in acute conditions such as appendicitis.

It is used for treating cardiac spasm, itching, gastroenteritis, appendicitis, colitis, irritable bowel syndrome, hemorrhoids, diarrhea, dysentery, difficulty swallowing, sore throat, tonsillitis, esophageal enlargement, jaundice, acute or chronic hepatitis, malaria, boils, abscesses, infections, fever, chills, joint pain, traumatic injury, sprains, swelling, contusions, rheumatoid arthritis, gastric and esophageal cancer, epilepsy in children, infantile fever with convulsions, malnutrition in infants, colds and flu, bronchitis, chest congestion, hemoptysis, allergies, lung irritation, pneumonia, insect bites, scorpion sting, and snakebites.

WESTERN BOTANIC PRACTICE

Herbalists in the United States have consistently failed to understand this species, generally listing it as of little importance and having only minimal medicinal uses. The Eclectics knew it but used it little, primarily as an emmenagogue and expectorant, for amenorrhea, dysmenorrhea, uterine problems, severe cough, asthma, and as an infusion. An infusion of the seeds sweetened with honey was used for whooping cough. The plant was thought useful for heart conditions including palpitation, for colds, and for acute bronchial and laryngeal attacks.

The Seminole tribe used bidens similarly, as did the native Hawaiians. Numerous tribes used it as a pot herb.

Michael Moore was the first contemporary herbalist to begin to understand its actions and he wrote about it extensively in the early 1990s. He didn't explore its antimicrobial activity but rather focused on its potency as a mucous membrane tonic. In his words, bidens "is probably the best herbal therapy we have for irritation, inflammation, pain, and bleeding of the urinary tract mucosa."[3]

The plant is a mucous membrane tonic and not only stops the inflammation and acts as a potent antibacterial in UTI infections but also heals the mucous membranes themselves. Moore felt it good for recurrent UTI infections and inflammations that didn't respond to antibiotics. The pain will usually go away in a day or two if you use bidens; he recommends using it an additional few days to completely clear up the problem.

Moore also considered bidens specific for reducing elevated levels of uric acid in the blood; i.e., for treating gout or urate-based kidney stones. It is a decent diuretic and does in fact stimulate uric acid elimination in the urine.

Because it is a mucous membrane tonic and is astringent, powerfully anti-inflammatory, and strongly antibacterial, it is specific for a number of troublesome diseases caused by resistant pathogens: UTIs, chronic diarrhea and dysentery, gastritis and ulcers (anywhere in GI tract, from mouth to anus), inflamed mucous membranes in colds and flu and respiratory infections of any sort, sore throats from coughs or infection or even overuse of the throat, and vaginal infections.

Moore notes that bidens has the "ability to tighten, shrink, and tonify the structural cells of the mucus membranes, thereby preventing congestion and edema, while simultaneously increasing the circulation, metabolism, and healing energy of the functional cells of those tissues."[4]

It's a good plant, too often overlooked.

Scientific Research

Bidens pilosa is highly active against the malaria parasite in in vivo and in vitro studies, bearing out its traditional use for that disease. The linear polyacetylenic diol extracted from bidens was found to be highly active against the malarial parasite in vivo and in vitro, especially in the fresh plant. The constituent is unstable in the dried state.

It is generally felt that the polyacetylenes in the plant are the most active constituents, the most potent antimicrobials. The research seems to bear this out. Alcohol tinctures of the fresh plant showed a 90 percent inhibition of the malarial parasite in vivo, while dried plant tinctures ran about 65 percent and water extracts about 38 percent. That activity is the same whether resistant or nonresistant strains are tested. In comparison, chloroquine-susceptible strains, when treated with chloroquine, will show a 99.2 percent inhibition of the malarial parasite. So the plant is nearly as strong as the pharmaceutical but not quite. It is definitely not as potent a plant as sida or cryptolepis, so larger doses need to be taken and for longer if you are using this plant for malaria.

An interesting in vivo study comparing the effectiveness of wild bidens versus domesticated found the wild species to be consistently stronger in its actions (the domesticated worked, just not as well).

As noted earlier, bidens possesses good antibacterial activity, as many antimalarials do. It has been found active against a wide range of microbial organisms, but some of the results are contradictory. (See Active Against, page 130, for more depth.)

Several of the plant's isolated polyacetylenes were found to be more active than ampicillin, tetracycline, norfloxacin, and amphotericin B during in vitro studies. Ciprofloxacin and ofloxacin were more potent than the plant extracts. In one study, water extracts of the plant were found to be more effective against *E. coli* and *Bacillus cereus* than gentamicin.

Bidens has been found to potentiate the activity of tetracycline if taken along with that pharmaceutical.

It is effective against herpes simplex 1 and 2 in in vitro studies, being nearly as strong as acyclovir but without the side effects.

Bidens pilosa during in vitro testing was found more active than metronidazole in the treatment of *Entamoeba histolytica*, a cause of amoebic dysentery around the world. The organisms weren't completely inhibited but were significantly reduced in number. *B. pilosa* was also found to be highly active in the treatment of the parasite *Leishmania amazonensis*. An ethanolic extract inhibited both the intracellular amastigotes and the promastigote form. The extract had very low toxicity.

Bidens pilosa is as effective as atropine, promethazine, neostigmine, and hydrocortisone in protecting mice from the venom of *Dendroaspis jamesoni*, a snake in Cameroon whose venom contains a potent neurotoxin. The plant extract also potentiated the antivenom normally used to treat those snakebites (as did atropine and promethazine). It is a very potent protector against neurotoxins. However, the plant is only weakly effective against viper venom, which causes hemorrhage and necrosis.

A number of in vivo studies reveal the herbal tincture to be highly anti-ulcerogenic, inhibiting gastric lesions induced by alcohol, and to be more effective than sucralfate. The herb significantly protected gastric mucosa and initiated mucosal healing through a number of mechanisms. (See Western Botanic Practice, page 136.)

A number of studies have found the plant to possess antitumor activity. It inhibits angiogenesis (the formation of abnormal blood vessels, common in cancer and certain forms of macular degeneration), is antiproliferative, and directly reduces viable tumor cells (stimulates apoptosis). It possesses a strong antileukemic activity and numerous cell regulatory actions that normalize cellular function and growth.

The plant also has a strong anti-pyretic effect, comparable to acet-aminophen. It is specific for lowering fever during acute infections.

Bidens has been found to be a strong antioxidant and anti-inflammatory. A double-blind, randomized crossover trial with 20 participants found the herb effec-tive in the treatment of allergic rhi-nitis. In vitro and in vivo studies have found it highly effective in protecting erythrocytes from oxidative damage. The water-soluble fractions are more antioxidative than the ethanol-soluble fractions. The plant inhibits COX-2 expression (similarly to ibuprofen) and prostaglandin production by inhibiting prostaglandin synthesis. It's a significant free-radical scavenger, comparable to alpha-tocopherol. It inhibits histamine release.

A number of in vivo studies note bidens to be an effective hepato-protector. It protects the liver from chronic obstructive cholestasis and decreases the rate of necrosis and liver fibrosis. It normalizes liver enzyme levels and restores superoxide dismutase and glutathione peroxi-dase levels in liver-injured mice. It is strongly protective against induced liver damage.

The plant possesses oxytocic-like actions on the uterus, tones the uterine muscle, and helps in labor contractions (in vivo studies).

It possesses relaxant activity on vascular tissue, is a vasodilator, and relaxes cardiac action. It reduces the aorta resting tone and inhibits KCL- and CaCl2-induced contractions by 95 percent. The effects are relatively long lasting. It attenuates high-fructose and salt-loaded hypertension in rats and reduces insulin levels in their blood. The effects are marginal in normotensive rats, but marked in hypertensive ones.

The plant possesses antidiabetic properties: It lowers glucose levels in the blood of mice, increases insulin sensitivity, and stimulates the release of insulin from the pancreas. A single daily dose for 28 days (in mice) also was found to protect islet structure in the pancreas and potentiate its activity. It was successfully used to reverse type 2 diabetes in mice. It reduces hypoglycemia. One of the herb's constituents, cytopiloyne, a polyacetylene, has been found to pre-vent type 1 diabetes in nonobese mice.

Bidens pilosa is a strong and reli-able immune modulator. It has been found to modulate the differentiation of helper T cells and prevent Th1-mediated autoimmune diabetes in nonobese diabetic mice. This has been attributed to a number of polyacetylenic compounds and a butanol fraction. The butanol fraction also reduces Th2-mediated airway inflammation in mice. Hot-water extracts of the plant stimulate interferon-gamma expression. The plant will increase immune action if such action is low, and decrease it if it is high.

Artemisia

Family: Asteraceae

Common Names: *Sweet Annie • sweet wormwood*

Species Used: There are around 400 artemisias in the genus, but *Artemisia annua* contains the most artemisinin — a potent antiparasitic — and this section will focus primarily on that species. Artemisinin is famous for its effectiveness in treating malaria. Many other artemisias contain artemisinin (contrary to earlier reports saying they did not) and I will discuss some of them in this section.

All the plants in the genus do have some antibacterial and antimicrobial actions; however, those constituents are not nearly as systemic as those in the other plants in this chapter. *Artemisia annua*, artemisinin, and its related constituents are best thought of as systemic antihematoparasiticals; that is, specific for killing blood parasites, rather than systemic antibacterials. Nevertheless, for treating diseases in their range of action, they are great.

Parts Used

The aerial parts, including the flowers, which have the highest artemisinin content.

ANTIBACTERIAL ACTIVITY

The whole herb has a much broader range of actions than the isolated constituent artemisinin.

Because the studies are few and plant preparation differs from study to study, the outcomes in the antibacterial studies of the artemisias are contradictory. They do find a range of antibacterial activity across the artemisias — bearing out traditional uses of the genus — but the studies tend to vary on which bacteria the species are active against, leading to confusion. There is a tendency to extrapolate the clinical use of the plant based on its in vitro antibacterial activity, but that is a mistake, as it is with numerous other plants.

This same problem exists with goldenseal. Goldenseal is highly active against a number of bacterial organisms, but berberine, the strongest constituent, does not make it across the GI tract membrane in any quantity so the plant (and the constituent) is not a systemic antibacterial; it is mostly limited to the GI tract. Artemisinin, and some of the other antiparasitics in artemisia, are strongly systemic, but they have limited antibacterial activity. They are primarily anti-parasitics for the blood and liver and antitumor agents.

The activities of the essential oils are more broadly antibacterial, but they are primarily confined to the GI tract when the plant is taken internally. This makes them useful for GI tract infections — or for use directly on the skin — but useless as systemic antibacterials. The traditional use of *Artemisia annua*, which gives a very good indication of its range of medicinal activity, has been primarily:

- For reducing fever — the plant stimulates sweating
- For topical use — it's useful for infected wounds and skin infections
- For GI tract problems and infections
- For female reproductive problems — primarily as an emmenagogue
- For liver problems
- As a steam inhalant for respiratory problems — which utilizes the essential oils
- For parasitic diseases of the blood and liver

Most of the antibacterial studies have been on the essential oils of various species but again, these oils do not disseminate widely in the bloodstream, which means they will be useful only for respiratory infections when used as steam, internally in the GI tract when prepared as a cold infusion (which keeps the oils in the liquid), or topically when used as a poultice or cold infusion wash. Nevertheless, when used in these ways the artemisias are very good medicines for resistant organisms other than blood parasites.

A study of *Artemisia nilagirica* leaf extracts found the plant active against a range of both Gram-positive and Gram-negative organisms: *Bacillus subtilis, Clavibacter michiganensis, Enterobacter aerogenes, Pseudomonas aeruginosa, Pseudomonas syringae, Salmonella typhi, Shigella flexneri*, and *Yersinia enterocolitica*. It was not active against *Enterococcus faecalis, E. coli, Klebsiella pneumoniae*, or *Staphylococcus aureus*. A number of studies have found most artemisias inactive against *E. coli, Klebsiella, Pseudomonas*, and staph, but others, such as one looking at the activity of *Artemisia anomala* against *Bacillus subtilis, E. coli, Proteus vulgaris, Salmonella typhi*, and *Staphylococcus aureus*, have found the plant to be active. In that example a methanol extract was used. Given the solubility dynamics of artemisia constituents (including artemisinin), it seems likely that the variability in the studies is coming from solubility differentials (hexane, for example, is a much better solvent for artemisia constituents than anything else and artemisinin is much more highly soluble in fat — whole milk — than water).

Preparation and Dosage

Artemisinin: The effective dosage for malaria is 500 to 1,000 mg on the first day and 500 mg daily thereafter for 2 to 4 more days. This will completely clear the malarial parasite from the blood. However, at 400 mg per day for 5 days, the recrudescence rate is 39 percent. Dosage at 800 mg drops the rate nearer to 3 percent. Chinese dosage runs from 500 mg to 1,600 mg for 3 days, repeated in 2 weeks (to treat newly hatching parasites). I do think there is some evidential support for 800 to 1,200 mg for 5 to 7 days, repeated for another 5 to 7 days in 2 weeks. The relapse rate is definitely smaller at the higher dose.

Note: Artemisinin becomes less present in the blood the longer it is taken, so that by day 7 the constituent is present at only 24 percent of its day-1 levels. *The isolated constituent is not very effective if taken for longer than 7 days at a time for parasitical infections.* If it doesn't work for babesia, for instance, within a few weeks, it is not going to. Pulsing will not help.

There are several things to keep in mind when preparing the whole herb for use:

- The fresh plant is the strongest.
- Whether fresh or dried, the plant should never be boiled.
- Fat helps extraction of the active constituents.
- The plant, while still potent for blood parasites, loses a lot of its antioxidant activities if dried.
- Dosage and length of use are crucial.

Traditional Chinese texts, thousands of years old, recommend preparation of the fresh herb, infused in room-temperature water, then pounded and wrung out to extract the plant juice as well. Examination has indeed shown that this produces the most potent infusions.

Many of the constituents in artemisia are not very water soluble, including the artemisinin. However, they are highly soluble in fats and alcohol.

FRESH HERB INFUSION FOR MALARIA

Place 100 grams (about 4 ounces) of fresh herb (leaves and flowers) cut into pieces in a container, pour ½ quart (2 cups) hot water over the herb, cover, and let stand 12 hours. Wring out; drink it all. Do this daily for 7 days. Repeat after 2 weeks.

FRESH HERB JUICE FOR MALARIA

Run the fresh plant through a juicer. Take 1 tablespoon of the fresh juice every day for 7 days — you can stabilize the juice with the addition of 20 percent alcohol (see page 227). Repeat after 2 weeks.

Note: The fresh juice is 6 to 17 times more potent than pure artemisinin; this and the tincture are the two most potent forms of the herb.

Properties of Artemisia

Actions

Antibacterial	Antiparasitical	Immunomodulant
Antifungal	Antitumor	Plasmodicide
Anti-inflammatory	Antiviral	Schizonticide
Antimalarial	Calcium antagonist	

Active Against

Babesia spp.	Epstein-Barr virus	*Opisthorchis viverrini*
Bovine diarrheal virus	*Fasciola hepatica*	*Plasmodium* spp.
Clonorchis sinensis	Hepatitis B and C	*Schistosoma* spp.
Eimeria acervulina	*Leishmania* spp.	*Toxoplasma gondii*
Eimeria tenella	*Neospora caninum*	*Trypanosoma* spp.

Also active against various cancer cell lines. Broadly active against dermatophytes — fungi that cause infections in hair, skin, and nails. *A. annua* is active against a number of bacteria in vitro, but the data in the various studies is contradictory, as usual. Specific for parasitic infections in the blood and liver and to some extent in the GI tract.

Decoctions of the herb are active against *Bacillus cereus, Bacillus subtilis, Bordetella bronchiseptica, E. coli, Klebsiella pneumoniae, Micrococcus flavus, Proteus vulgaris, Pseudomonas aeruginosa, Salmonella typhi, Salmonella typhimurium, Sarcina lutea, Staphylococcus aureus, Staphylococcus epidermidis,* and *Streptococcus mutans.*

A different extract (type not stated) was found to be active against *Mycobacterium avium.* Methanol extracts were found active against *Bacillus cereus, Bacillus pumilus, Bacillus subtilis, E. coli, Micrococcus luteus, Pseudomonas aeruginosa, Salmonella* spp., and *Staphylococcus aureus.*

The essential oil has been found active against *Candida albicans, Enterococcus hirae, E. coli,* and *Staphylococcus aureus* but not *Pseudomonas aeruginosa.*

Other Actions

The oil of *Artemisia tschernieviana* has been found active against *Bacillus cereus*, *Bacillus subtilis*, *Candida albicans*, *Enterobacter aerogenes*, *E. coli*, *Klebsiella pneumoniae*, and *Staphylococcus aureus*. This same antibacterial activity has been found in other artemisias: *A. absinthium*, *A. douglasiana* and *A. ludoviciana* (also *Helicobacter pylori*), *A. echegarayi* (also active against *Proteus mirabilis* and various *Listeria* species), *A. gilvescens* (also MRSA), *A. giraldii* (also *Aspergillus* spp., *Proteus* spp., *Sarcinia lutea*, *Trichoderma viride*), *A. herba-alba*, *A. iwayomogi*, *A. kulbadica*, *A. leucodes*, *A. monosperma* (also TB and staph), and *A. princeps* var. *orientalis* (also *Bacteroides fragilis*, *Bifidobacterium*, *Clostridium perfringens*, and staph), *A. vulgaris* (also *Streptococcus mutans*).

The artemisias in general are considered to be active against intestinal parasites, but again, little actual study has occurred. *A. absinthium* is often considered the most potent against intestinal parasites in historical practice. Leaf extracts are active against *Syphacia* parasites, nematodes that infect the intestinal tracts of mice; the plant is also active against multi-drug-resistant malarial parasites in vivo.

Artemisia maciverae is active in vivo against *Trypanosoma brucei*, showing complete clearance after 7 days of treatment (10 mg/kg body weight). The same plant is also strongly antiplasmodial at the same dosage, clearing the parasites from mice in 3 days.

Various artemisias have been found active against plant pathogens (which is why artemisias are used to protect crops in some locations) and various fungi.

Use to Treat

Any parasitic infection in the blood and liver or for systemic cancers (artemisinin does have good activity as an antitumor drug). These are the real strengths of the plant if it is being used as a systemic. There is nothing else comparable in potency for these uses. The plant, if properly prepared, is also active against microbial and parasitic infections, especially in the GI tract (see Preparation and Dosage, page 142) and on the skin.

DRIED HERB INFUSION FOR MALARIA

Pour 1 quart hot water over 100 grams of dried herb (leaves and flowers), and let stand 12 hours. Strain and drink. Do this daily for 7 days. Repeat after 2 weeks.

INFUSION IN MILK FOR MALARIA

Pour 1 quart hot, whole milk over 100 grams fresh or dried herb, cover, and let stand 4 hours.

Note: This will extract 80 percent of the artemisinin in the herb while water infusions extract much less (about 25 percent in dried herb formulations).

TINCTURE FOR MALARIA

Chop fresh herb finely, and measure its weight in ounces. Place the herb in twice that amount (now using liquid ounces) of pure grain alcohol. (For example, you'd mix 1 ounce of herb with 2 ounces of alcohol; see Fresh Plant Tinctures, page 339, for more depth on this). Let stand 2 weeks. Press out the liquid. Take 1 tablespoon twice daily for 7 days. Repeat after 2 weeks.

TINCTURE WITH SIDA AND CRYPTOLEPIS FOR MALARIA

Take 2 ounces each of the tinctures of sida, cryptolepis, and *Artemisia annua* and combine together. Take 2 tablespoons of the mix each day for 7 days. Repeat in 2 weeks.

Finding Artemisia

The herb grows pretty much everywhere it is planted; seeds are widely available (try Horizon Herbs for some of the best). It is a good herb to have growing in the garden — as are any of the other artemisias that contain artemisinin, such as *Artemisia absinthium*.

Artemisinin is, currently, easily found for sale everywhere, and an online search will turn up sources for both the herb and the supplement. However, there is a movement to prohibit over-the-counter sales of the supplement due to over- and improper use. The overuse of the supplement is already beginning to stimulate resistance in malarial organisms.

The herb is very effective if used properly. The dose can be increased fairly high, as it is a very safe herb. Remember: The reason that this herb was discovered was that in the region of China where it is used there were few or no incidences of malaria. The secret is in the dose, as with all medications.

Side Effects and Contraindications

About 25 percent of people using *Artemisia annua* as an antimalarial report a mild nausea, which does not progress to vomiting. It may also cause occasional dizziness, tinnitus, pruritus, and mild abdominal pain.

Artemisinin itself can cause gastrointestinal upset, loss of appetite, nausea, cramping, diarrhea, vomiting. About 4 percent of people who take it experience these symptoms, usually in a more severe form than that experienced from ingesting the herbal infusion. Very high doses (5,000 mg per day of artemisinin for 3 days) have caused liver inflammation, which corrects upon stopping the supplement. Artemisinin has a slightly chronotropic effect on the heart. It causes mild hypotension. This has not been, apparently, a problem in any users.

Both the herb and the constituent should be used with caution in pregnancy, especially in the first trimester. In vivo studies have found a number of adverse effects in rats and mice if the herb is used in the first trimester. However, one clinical trial with 16 patients in the first trimester of pregnancy taking the herb found the miscarriage rate to be the same as that for the general population.

Herb/Drug Interactions

Artemisia annua, like many antimicrobial plants, contains synergists that make its compounds more active against microbial organisms. In this instance, chrysospenol-D and chrysophlenetin, two flavonols in the plant, have been found to potentiate the activity of berberine and norfloxacin against resistant staph. Artemisinin does induce certain liver enzymes and may interact with drugs such as omeprazole.

Habitat and Appearance

A. annua is native to China, western Asia, northern India, Japan, Korea, Vietnam, Myanmar, southern Siberia, and southeastern Europe. An emerging invasive plant species, it is naturalized in the United States and many other countries. It loves waste places — roadsides, fallow fields, neglected gardens — especially in eastern North America. It can grow pretty much anyplace but is stronger and more aromatic when grown in poor, dry soil. Its artemisinin content is about 20 percent higher when it grows in mildly potassium-deficient soils.

The plant, once established, grows into a large straggly bush. The leaves look a bit like celery's leaves, though *A. annua*'s are much broader, bushier, and more extensive in their growth. The plant grows 4 to 6 feet (1.2 to 2 m) tall with a typical attractive, weedy, bushy look. It blooms in late summer.

Cultivation and Collection

Artemisia annua is an annual (hence its species name) and cultivates easily from seed. Sow the tiny seeds outdoors in the fall or seed them indoors before the last frost. They like it best on top of well-aerated soil; they need light to germinate. Once established, the plant self-sows and will never go away.

The aerial parts should be harvested just after flowering. The flowers and leaves both contain artemisinin. The artemisinin content is higher in the fall than in spring; it takes the plant time to create the chemical. The longer you wait, the better the yield, so take even the older, dying-back leaves. The stems and root contain only very low amounts of the compound and aren't generally worth the trouble.

Once the plant is picked, let it dry in the sun for a week. The light helps the artemisinin precursors keep producing after the plant is harvested. After a week, the sun does more harm than good, so finish drying in a dry, dark spot inside.

Several hybrid plants (*Artemisia annua* var. *artemis*, var. *campinas*, var. *anamed*) have been bred for higher artemisinin content. They are available from Anamed (*www.anamed.org*) as part of an artemisia antimalarial starter kit that includes a lot of useful information on growing and using the plant. One problem with the hybrids is that they don't reseed themselves well and the artemisinin content of those that do is poor (so it is not as sustainable an alternative as it should be). If you want a continual supply of the plant, non-hybrids are the way to go.

Plant Chemistry

Artemisia annua contains a great many chemical constituents, over 150 at last count, and that is most likely just a tiny fraction of the total. There are a minimum of 28 monoterpenes, 30 sesquiterpenes, 12 terpenoids and steroids, 36 flavonoids, 7 coumarins, 4 aromatics, and 9 aliphatic compounds.

Artemisinin is considered to be the active antiplasmodial compound but numerous other compounds with malarial activity have been found. Others, such as arteannuin B and artemisinic acid, are antibacterial and antifungal. Arteannuin B, while found to be ineffective against malarial parasites, strongly potentiates the activity of artemisinin. Many of the flavonoid compounds have been found to be antimalarial in vitro. Some of them (artemetin, casticin, chrysophlenetin, chrysosplenol-D, and cirsilineol) have been found to also potentiate artemisinin's ability to kill plasmodial parasites. Many of these

Lyme Disease Caution

I have heard from several people with Lyme disease that they have been taking artemisinin for 1 to 2 years at relatively high doses. This is highly contraindicated and should *not* be done under any circumstances. I repeat: This is a really bad idea. Artemisinin is extremely safe when used appropriately; That is, in doses around 1,200 mg daily for 7 days. If it is used long term in high doses, there is significant risk of neurotoxicity; that is, damage to the central nervous system and brain. Sida, alchornea, cryptolepis, and bidens are all much safer alternatives for long-term use, especially if you are treating babesia.

149

flavonoids are abundant in the plant; they induce a three- to five-fold reduction in the amount of artemisinin needed to kill malarial organisms. Some of the sesquiterpene lactones are also antiplasmodial, with ridentin, some of the guainolides, and germacranolides being the most important.

The artemisinin content of *A. annua*, if the leaves and flowers are harvested in the fall before the plant goes to seed, can run anywhere from 0.75 percent to 1.4 percent (several high-yield varieties are in development or are just on the market).

A relatively new development is the finding of another strongly active antiplasmodial constituent, tehranolide, in a number of artemisia species. In vivo studies show it to be strongly antiplasmodial. Treatment with the tehranolide extracts of *Artemisia diffusa* resulted in complete clearance of parasites from the blood in mice at similar dosages to artemisinin.

Traditional Uses of Artemisia

Artemisia annua (and many of the other artemisias) is somewhat unusual in its actions. The *systemic* constituents of the plant primarily act in two ways: 1) as highly potent antiparasitics for blood and liver parasites; and 2) as antitumor agents. These same constituents have two other actions that are useful: 1) they stimulate sweating and thus help reduce fever; and 2) they are emmenagogues; that is, they stimulate menstruation. The emmenagogue action is why the plant is generally not recommended in the first trimester of pregnancy. Caveat: *Artemisia annua* has much less emmenagogue activity than some of the other artemisias; the stimulatory activity has been found to be only minimal.

Although other artemisias have been used to effectively treat malaria and other blood parasites, the most potent species for this, at this time, is *Artemisia annua.*

The plant has been used in Chinese medicine for over two thousand years, but its current status as an antimalarial emerged from its use by the North Vietnamese during the Vietnam War. Malarial infections were exceptionally high among the North Vietnamese troops. Appeals to the Chinese leader Mao for help resulted in the discovery of *Artemisia annua* for use as an antimalarial.

Chinese researchers had discovered that in one region of China the people had little incidence of malaria infection. Looking closer they discovered that the local people took the herb at the first sign of symptoms. In 1972 Chinese researchers isolated artemisinin.

AYURVEDA

This plant is unknown in India, though a number of other artemisias are used. *Artemisia absinthium* is used for intermittent fevers, for stomach complaints (as a bitter and digestive), as a vermifuge for intestinal worms, and for nervous system complaints (from hysteria to depression). *Artemisia maritima* (wormseed) is specific for intestinal worms, especially ascarides and oxyuris. Most of the other artemisias are used similarly.

Artemisinin in Other Artemesias

A number of other artemisias do contain artemisinin (18 identified so far), none to the degree of *Artemisia annua*, though some are close. The flowers of *A. bushriences* have nearly as much artemisinin as *A. annua* (about 80 percent), then the leaves of *A. dracunculus* (about 60 percent), then flowers of a number of species (in descending order): *A. roxburghiana* (about half), *A. vestita* and *A. sieversiana* (40 percent), and *A. moorcroftiana* and *A. absinthium* (about 30 percent). Most species do have about 10 percent to 15 percent of the amount of artemisinin as is found in *A. annua*. Other species that contain artemisinin are *A. vulgaris*, *A. indica*, *A. roxburghiana* var. *gratae*, *A. japonica*, *A. tangutica*, and *A. lancea*. An exception is *A. desertorum*, which has virtually none. As usual, in the species that contain artemisinin, the flowers and leaves will have the most. Again, skip the roots and stems.

TRADITIONAL CHINESE MEDICINE

Called *qing-hao* in traditional Chinese medicine, *Artemisia annua* is used for clearing fevers from the blood, especially in conditions with headache, dizziness, low fever, and a stifling sensation in the chest. Also for febrile diseases, for malaria, and for scabies, pruritus, and malignant ulcers.

WESTERN BOTANIC PRACTICE

For many years *A. annua* was unknown, although many other artemisias have long been used. *Artemisia absinthium* was a primary herb among the Eclectics in the late ninteenth century in the United States. The herb was used for intermittent fevers, for malaria, as a vermifuge in the treatment of intestinal worms, for dyspepsia, nervous conditions, diarrhea and liver complaints, for amenorrhea and leukorrhea, for jaundice. Other artemisias were used similarly.

The indigenous peoples throughout the United States used the plants similarly.

Scientific Research

There have been hundreds of in vitro and in vivo studies and clinical trials on the antiparasitical actions of artemisinin (and its analogues), most on malaria and schistosomiasis. I will just touch on them here.

Every one of the several hundred clinical trials shows the effectiveness of artemisinin in the treatment of malaria. (There have been a number of clinical trials with the whole herb as well; see Whole Herb vs. Artemisinin, page 154.)

Artemisinin has become the choice for malarial treatment worldwide because it is effective against resistant strains of the organism. Ninety-eight percent of malarial parasites are generally killed within 24 hours with use of the herb or its isolated constituent. If low, short-term doses are used (less than 5 days), however, relapse rates can be as high as 39 percent. Higher dose ranges for a longer period of time (5 instead of 3 days) lower the relapse rate considerably. Clinical trials with as many as 2,000 people (with both low and high dosages) have found 100 percent clearance rates for all participants if artemisinin is taken for 5 to 7 days. There are very few side effects when used properly in short-term treatment.

The constituents of the herb that are antiparasitic are exceptionally systemic in that they spread quickly throughout the body and easily cross the blood-brain barrier. Artemisinin is considered specific for cerebral malaria. Because it infuses the blood, it is carried throughout the body to every cell, all of which need blood to live.

A slightly modified form of artemisinin — artesenuate — has been found effective for babesia organisms in vitro. Relatively low concentrations of the compound are effective; complete inhibition of *Babesia equi* and *B. caballi* occurred at 0.2 and 1.0 micrograms/ml respectively. (To make artesenuate, artemisinin is modified slightly in order to get patent protection.)

Use of artemisinin in clinical practice, however, has shown only moderate success for this organism; it seems to be effective in about half the people who use it for babesia. Sida and cryptolepis appear to be better alternatives.

A number of clinical trials have occurred with a synthetic form of artemisinin, artemether, in the treatment of schistosoma infections. Schistosoma are a type of blood fluke — and are a major infectious parasitic organism, second only to malaria in

numbers of those infected, totaling hundreds of millions worldwide.

Artemether is normally given in a single dose of 6 mg/kg every 2 weeks. It is primarily active against the juvenile form of the parasite rather than the adult. Repeated dosing results in parasite reductions of 90 percent to 98 percent. Artesenuate has been found just as effective.

Artemisinin is also effective against *Neospora caninum*, another type of protozoa that affects both endothelial cells and macrophages. CNS involvement and carditis are common. Artemisinin is effective against a number of other organisms such as *Eimeria tenella*, *Leishmania major* (which infects macrophages), *Toxoplasma gondii*, *Schistosoma mansoni* (liver flukes), and *Clonorchis sinensis* (liver flukes), all parasitical organisms. It is antispirochetal against leptospire organisms, killing them in vitro. Artemisinin does appear to possess broad antiparasitical actions.

ANTICANCER PROPERTIES

Artemisinin is also stimulating interest as an antitumor and anticancer compound. It has shown effectiveness as an anticancer agent both in vitro and in vivo. In vitro studies have found artemisinin effective against human leukemia cells, breast cancer, and colon cancer. Treatment of both bone cancer and cancer of the lymph nodes in dogs was effective with 10 to 15 days of treatment. The use of artemisinin in people with cancer has shown effectiveness as well; Vietnamese doctors have found it successful in curing 50 percent to

60 percent of several different types of cancer patients.

Clinical practice reports indicate the use of artesenuate in the successful treatment of non-Hodgkin's lymphoma (60 mg IM for 14 days), artemisinin for small-cell lung carcinoma (500 mg BID for 4 months), artesenuate (IV) and artemisinin (300 mg BID) for 4 months in the treatment of stage 4 breast cancer with metastases, topical artemisinin in the treatment of multiple skin cancers, oral artemisinin in the treatment of breast cancer with metastases to the spine, and artesenuate in the treatment of stage 4 uveal melanoma.

A number of studies have found the herb to possess anti-inflammatory and antioxidant activity.

Artemisinin is immunostimulatory in vivo. It stimulates phagocytosis, and macrophages become more potent; they are better at phagocytosing malarial-infected erythrocytes.

ARTEMISININ RESISTANCE

There is increasing evidence that using the single compound artemisinin or any of its derivatives is stimulating resistance in the organisms it is being used to treat. Resistant malarial organisms have been found in Cambodia and are beginning to spread worldwide.

A recent study found that malarial organisms go into a dormancy state upon encountering artemisinin and then recover after dosing has ceased.

In consequence, many groups are beginning to use combination therapies to treat susceptible parasites, essentially artemisinin plus a pharmaceutical. It's known as artemisinin combination therapy or ACT.

WHOLE HERB VS. ARTEMISININ

The increasing resistance to artemisinin and its synthetic derivatives is a problem that cannot be solved through multidrug therapy: single constituent pharmaceuticals will *always* end up promoting resistance in disease organisms. A different approach is essential.

As I have already mentioned, there is a conflict between two ideologies in health care and medicine: 1) sustainable, affordable health care that empowers the people who use it; and 2) health care controlled by corporations for their own profit, a model that is designed to keep the people who use it dependent on specialists and corporate manufacturers. There is no way to avoid encountering, or dealing with, this conflict in some form if you explore the use of herbal medicines for your own health.

While the cost of artemisinin is low when viewed from Western, industrialized perspectives, in Africa it is prohibitively high. In 2004 the cost of a course of artemisinin was $2.40, more than most people in Africa can afford. As a result artemisinin forgery has become a lucrative business in Africa. Products that contain no artemisinin are widely available; they do nothing to cure malaria.

A number of NGOs (nongovernmental organizations) such as ANAMED (Action for Nature and Medicine), of which I am an admirer, have begun to address the problem in a simple and direct manner — they are providing artemisia seeds to anyone in Africa who wants them, teaching them how to grow the plant and how to use it to treat malaria. This has resulted in rather predictable responses from Western researchers, physicians, and corporate scientists. They oppose it and sometimes work quite strongly to stop it.

The primary argument being made is that the plant is not very effective against malaria, which of course ignores the reason artemisinin was discovered in the first place — people who used it for medicine had little or no incidence of malaria in their communities. Some researchers go so far as to say the plant does not work at all, *only* the isolated constituent is effective. Jansen (2006) is a perfect example. He comments, "The herbal tea approach to artemisinin for malaria is totally misleading and should be forgotten as soon as possible."[5]

Thankfully, the reaction to such antiquated thinking has been strong.

RITAM (Research Initiative on Traditional Antimalarial Methods), a partnership between the Global Initiative for Traditional Systems of Health at Oxford University and hundreds of international researchers from over 30 countries who are exploring malaria treatment with traditional plants, responded to Jansen's comment this way: "We believe that this statement is totally misleading and should be forgotten as soon as possible."[6] Their article then explains in depth how most Western researchers, in looking at *Artemisia annua* tea formulations, consistently fail to understand the plant or how it should be used in practice to be effective. It points out, as well, how Hansen's comments are fatally flawed.

Extensive work by RITAM and ANAMED has resulted in comparable tea preparations that are as effective in use as artemisinin.

The artemisinin content in the plant is strongly stable if it is properly stored (out of the sun in foil or plastic bags inside plastic tubs). Even after 1 year in storage, the artemisinin content is nearly identical to that in the freshly harvested plant. (Ceiling-hung plants will begin to degrade after 3 months.) The artemisinin is held in the glandular trichomes of the plant's leaves and flowers, where the essential oils of the plant are also held. These oils protect the artemisinin from degradation, oxidation, fungi, and molds.

Numerous researchers are suggesting that artemisinin combination therapy (ACT) is the best approach to treating malaria as the recrudescence rates are smaller and the parasite has a harder time developing resistance. But the plant already is an ACT substance. Researchers, using identical tiny amounts of *Artemisia annua* and artemisinin, found that these tiny amounts of *A. annua* reduced parasitemia in vivo by 50 percent at day 4, while the artemisinin was no more effective than placebo.

Other researchers, removing the artemisinin from the plant, found it still effective for malaria treatment.

There are other constituents in the plant that have been found to be synergists with artemisinin. Several flavonols have been found to be potentiating synergists with both berberine and norfloxacin in the treatment of MRSA, for instance. They apparently act as a multidrug-resistance efflux pump inhibitor (see chapter 6). These same flavonols have also been shown to potentiate the action of artemisinin against the malarial parasite. And both *Artemisia annua* and *Artemisia dracunculus* contain an essential oil, piperitone, that acts as a potentiator of nitrofurantoin against *Enterobacter cloacae*.

The number of synergists and potentiators in the artemisias seems large. The complex combination of multiple antiplasmodium constituents and synergists makes the plant a potent choice for an, essentially, free treatment for those who need it, or want it as the treatment of choice.

There have been a number of clinical trials in the use of the tea (or whole herb or tincture) in treating malaria. Studies have shown that the pharmacokinetics of the herb's artemisinin when taken as a tea are identical to those of artemisinin taken as an isolated constituent:

Clinical trial with tincture: 72 grams of crude extract in divided doses over 3 days in the treatment of 485 cases of *Plasmodium vivax* and 105 cases of *P. falciparum*. Clearance rate was 100 percent, but the patients were not followed for recrudescence.

Clinical trial with whole-herb infusion: 93 percent clearance rate in 254 patients using a 7-day course of whole herb infusion (tea) in the treatment of *P. falciparum*. Recrudescence rate was 13 percent after 1 month.

Clinical trial with capsules: Clinical trial of 165 people infected with *Plasmodium vivax*. Fifty-three were given capsules of *A. annua* that also contained oil (COEA) for 3 days (the oil enhances absorption of the artemisinin). Another 50 received the herb capsules with oil (COEA) for 6 days. Forty-one received capsules without the oil (QHET). Twenty-one received chloroquine. Dosage was 36.8 grams on the first day, 18.4 on subsequent days. Parasite clearance and fever reduction were faster with

the capsules than with chloroquine. There was a 30-day follow-up with blood checks every 10 days. About one-third of those who took the COEA herb capsule for only 3 days or who took the non-oil capsules (QHET) experienced recrudescence. Those who took COEA for 6 days experienced about 8 percent recrudescence. There was no recrudescence in the chloroquine group.

Clinical trial with infusion: An aqueous infusion for 5 days in a small trial of five people found 100 percent clearance; no follow-up occurred to check for recrudescence.

Clinical trial with infusion and decoction: A trial using infusions (254 people) and decoctions (48 people) with 5 grams herb in 1 liter of hot water, infused for 15 minutes or boiled for 5 minutes, found both forms effective. Dose was 250 ml (about 8 ounces) four times daily for 7 days in the infusion group and 4 days in the decoction group. Clearance rate was 93 percent and 92 percent respectively. There was a 13 percent recrudescence rate in the infusion group. Recrudescence in the decoction group was not checked.

Early indications are that if the plant is properly prepared and used it can be as effective as artemisinin or its analogues in the treatment of malaria and other blood parasites. It will be especially effective if combined with other plants described in this chapter, especially sida and cryptolepis.

5

HERBAL ANTIBIOTICS: THE LOCALIZED NONSYSTEMICS

Each tree, each shrub, and herb, down even to the grasses and mosses, agreed to furnish a remedy for some one of the diseases [of humankind] and each said: "I shall appear to help man whenever he calls upon me in his need."
— **The oral teachings of the Cherokee Nation**

Localized nonsystemic antibacterial herbs do not easily cross the GI tract membrane and concentrate in the bloodstream. They are almost always limited to the GI tract itself, the skin, or certain organs of the body. In the latter instance, it is because those constituents that do make it through the intestinal membrane are eliminated from the body through a particular organ (e.g., garlic through the lungs, juniper berry through the kidneys).

> ## The Top 4 Localized Nonsystemic Herbal Antibiotics
> The Berberines
> Juniper
> Honey
> Usnea

The localized antibacterials need to be used with that in mind; they generally do not act as systemics, even if they are being sold as if they do. Nevertheless, they can be exceptionally potent in the treatment of resistant disease organisms if used properly. Here are four of the best of them.

The Berberines

For the purposes of this book, most berberine-containing plants can be used as analogues for each other in the treatment of resistant bacterial and fungal infections of the GI tract and skin. I prefer the use of invasive species, however, primarily because they tend to be easily found in the wild, are ubiquitous around the globe, and can be harvested with abandon. They are free to those who know them and harvesting them does not create the ecological problems that wildcrafting and large agricultural production of plants such as goldenseal and coptis do.

Berberine-containing plants grow nearly every place on Earth. *Phellodendron amurense, Hydrastis canadensis, Mahonia aquifolium, Berberis vulgaris,* and *Coptis chinensis* are only a few of the major species used medicinally.

However, given their prolific natures, I believe that if you are wild-crafting, the *only* genera that should be used as berberine antibacterials are (in the following order) *Phellodendron, Berberis,* and *Mahonia.*

If you are buying, look for *Hydrastis, Tinospora, Coptis,* and *Corydalis,* which are established agricultural crops. The latter two genera are major agricultural products in China and are thus sustainable in a nonwildcrafted sense. *Hydrastis* is being grown in the United States, and it is possible to buy organically grown roots. If you do decide to use any of these species, make sure you are getting commercially grown and not wildcrafted plants.

Personally, I prefer the wildcrafted species. In my opinion they are the strongest — domesticated plants have a tendency to get a bit wimpy over time — and I particularly like the idea of using invasive species for invasive diseases. I think it particularly interesting that *Phellodendron* and *Berberis* species are invasive in the same bio-region in which goldenseal was once prevalent. It points up the rather neglected understanding that plants and their constituents perform specific functions in the eco-ranges in which they grow. The loss of a particular medicinal species always leads to ecosystem degradation and weakness. But then, the planet has a long history of engaging in correctives to such damage, invasives being just one of them.

Phellodendron amurense is invasive, especially in the eastern United States, and I believe that it should be the main species used if it is at all available. The plant is a large tree that grows quickly, producing huge amounts of berberine and other alkaloids and synergistic constituents in its inner bark. Branches can be harvested to supply large quantities of medicinal herb with little or no damage to the tree. You can get several years' supply in a short afternoon.

Here is a more inclusive list of the berberine genera, and some of the species, that are known to date.

Hydrastis canadensis, the American goldenseal, is perhaps the best known and most commonly used berberine-containing plant in the United States, but it is rather limited in its range and is endangered in the wild from overharvesting. The root is generally used, which, obviously, kills the plant, contributing to its difficulties in surviving in the wild. It has become a decent agricultural crop in the United States and organically grown roots are easily found these days. Wildcrafted plants should never be bought. The leaves are weaker and can be used as well as the root, but hardly anyone does. It is the only member of its genus.

Mahonia, a genus comprising 70 or so species, is common throughout the world. Plant classification freaks really want the mahonias included in the genus *Berberis*, which is why you might see *Mahonia aquifolium*, a.k.a. Oregon grape, perhaps the best known of the mahonias, also identified as *Berberis aquifolium*. The lower branches of the mahonias tend to have berberine in them, but the roots are much higher in the alkaloid. Several mahonias are considered invasive in the United States, making them perfect for wild harvesting.

Berberis, a genus of about 500 species of plants, also has a number of species that contain berberine. Barberry, *Berberis vulgaris*, is perhaps the best known. While the branches (especially the lower) contain berberine (scratch the stem — if it's yellow underneath the outer bark, it's got berberine), the roots have a much higher berberine content, by at least a factor of 10. Several species of berberis are considered invasive in the United States, particularly *Berberis thunbergii*, Japanese barberry.

Coptis, a genus of 15 or so species, also has a number of plants whose roots (rhizomes actually) contain berberine. *Coptis chinensis*, a.k.a. goldthread, is probably the best known. The genus is used for a number of reasons, one of which is that it is relatively high in berberine content, up to 9 percent by weight. The root on this genus is tiny (hence "thread") and it takes a lot of harvesting to get much usable material. The wild species in the United States are at risk and should not be harvested commercially. *Coptis chinensis* is a major agricultural crop in China and is available in bulk, though it is rather expensive.

Phellodendron (*not* the houseplant, which is spelled differently) is a genus of 4 to 10 species (arguments are ongoing) of trees whose bark contains berberine. The best known is probably *Phellodendron amurense*. A great invasive.

Tinospora, a genus of 40 or so twining species of plants, contains berberine. The best known is probably *Tinospora cordifolia*. The bark and stems of this genus are used.

Corydalis, a genus of some 470 species (this genus is sometimes considered to be part of the poppy family), has several that contain berberine, as well as hydrastine. The medicinal varieties contain a number of opioid alkaloids (try saying that 10 times fast), though in lesser concentration than the opium poppies (about one-tenth as much), and are used in part for their analgesic activity. The best known are probably *Corydalis chaerophylla*, *C. yanhusuo*, and *C. longipes*. The herb is a major agricultural crop in China and bulk purchase is pretty easy.

Argemone is a genus of about 30 species of plants, generally called the prickly poppies. Many of the species contain berberine, the best known of which is the Mexican poppy, *Argemone mexicana*. The aerial parts are used; they contain the berberine (as does the resin), so it is a sustainable-use plant. But the berberine content is rather small and

I would not use the plant as a berberine antibacterial myself — even though it has been traditionally used along berberine lines of function; its medicinal functions are more subtle.

Nandina domestica, the only member of its genus, is a suckering shrub, also in the barberry family. It is a rather common ornamental and I think a good choice for a berberine medicinal if you have it in your yard. The lower branches and roots are highest in berberine. Treat it as a *Mahonia/Berberis* species if you are harvesting and making medicine from it; it is pretty much identical.

The genus *Eschscholtzia*, the California poppies, is also reputed to contain berberine, but I can't find much research on it. Berberine and similar alkaloids are also present in a number of other genera such as *Coelocline, Archangelisia, Chelidonium, Toddalia*, and *Thalictrum*.

In this section I will concentrate mostly on *Phellodendron amurense* — and to some extent on *Berberis* and *Mahonia* — however, if you take a look at the traditional uses of the berberines, you will see that they are all used similarly.

Parts Used

Bark, root bark, stems, roots, leaves, resin.

Preparation and Dosage

The alkaloids in the berberine plants, including berberine, are not very water soluble. (So if you see a study showing an aqueous extract of a berberine plant to be not as effective as an antimicrobial, you now know why.) Tinctures need to use a higher alcohol content (generally 1:5, 70 percent alcohol, 30 percent water), and the water needs to be acidic, with a pH of 1 to 6. The addition of 1 tablespoon of vinegar to the tincture mix is recommended if your water is alkaline (hard) or if you don't know. (See chapter 9 for an extensive listing of berberine plants and their alcohol-to-water ratios.)

The berberine plants may be used as a powder for topical application, as a douche, as a wash, as a tincture, in capsules, or as a snuff.

POWDER

Apply to cuts, scrapes, or infected wounds.

TINCTURE

Dried bark of phellodendron: 1:5, 70 percent alcohol, 20–50 drops, up to 4x daily (the taste is exceptionally strong)

In acute dysenteric/diarrheal conditions: Take 1 tsp–1 tbl morning and evening until symptoms subside. Improvement should be seen within 2 days; usually there will be some improvement within 8 hours.

Note: The berberine plants are only about 50 percent active against cholera in clinical trials, as compared with enterotoxogenic *E. coli*, which they completely inhibit. However, if you combine the berberine plants with the root of *any* geranium species, the bark of pomegranate or the peel of the fruit, or the leaf or bark of guava the cholera organism will be completely inhibited.

As a douche: Add ⅓ ounce tincture to 1 pint water and douche once or twice daily.

As a wash: Add 1 ounce tincture to 2 pints water and wash the affected area morning and evening — especially good for helping acne and infected wounds.

CAPSULES

For non-acute conditions: Take 1 or 2 "00" capsules, up to 4x daily.

In acute dysenteric/diarrheal conditions: Take up to 25 "00" capsules daily for up to 10 days.

SNUFF

Place two thin lines of root powder on a table and snort them vigorously — each line into a different nostril like those cocaine addicts on television, up to 3x daily for up to 7 days.

Side Effects and Contraindications

Caution is advised in pregnancy.

Properties of the Berberine Plants

Actions

Analgesic	Anti-inflammatory	Expectorant
Antiamoebic	Antisecretory	Febrifuge
Antibacterial	Antiseptic	Mucosal anti-inflammatory
Anticholeric	Antitumor	
Antidiarrheal	Astringent	Mucosal stimulant
Antidysenteric	Diaphoretic	Mucosal tonic
Antifungal		

Berberine interferes with adherence of bacteria such as *Streptococcus* spp. to mucous membranes by stimulating the release of lipoteichoic acid from bacteria or by stopping the formation of complexes between the microbial surface and host cells. It inhibits the intestinal hypersecretion (by about 70 percent) induced by cholera, *E. coli,* and other intestinal disease organisms. Berberine targets the assembly of the *E. coli* cell division protein FtsZ. Basically, it is an FtsZ inhibitor, stopping replication of the bacteria.

Some studies have found berberine to be cardioprotective, antimalarial, antioxidative, cerebroprotective, antimutagenic, vaso-relaxing, anxiolytic, and anti-HIV, but these studies are all in vitro; they don't translate well and the berberine would tend to work in most of those instances only if injected.

Active Against

Berberine-containing plants are active against a wide range of microorganisms. Berberine has been the most intensively tested of the plants' alkaloids, though a number of others such as hydrastine, jatrorrhizine, and palmatine have also undergone a fair amount of study. The various antimicrobial alkaloids in the berberines tend to be active against different organisms and are highly synergistic with each other and additionally benefit from other compounds in the plants whose only known functions are to disable antibiotic-resistance mechanisms in microbial organisms. Thus, whole plant extracts, rather than isolated constituents, tend to have a greater range of action and, in my opinion, are much more effective.

This is borne out by numerous studies. As an example, researchers in Italy commented in their research paper, "The crude extract [of *Berberis*

CONTINUED ON NEXT PAGE

PROPERTIES OF THE BERBERINE PLANTS, CONTINUED

aetnensis root extracts] was active against Candida species, this activity being higher than that of the alkaloidal fraction and berberine."[1] The berberine-containing plants are very good at what they do — if they are prepared and used properly (i.e., ethanolic extracts or powders used for direct-contact disease treatment rather than systemic disease conditions).

The following list is comprised of microorganisms that have been found susceptible to either individual constituents of the berberine-containing plants or crude extracts of the plants themselves (e.g., *Mahonia, Berberis, Hydrastis, Coptis, Phellodendron*). As an example, the ethanolic extract of *Mahonia aquifolium* (as well as two of its constituents) was tested on 20 strains of coagulase-negative staphylococci, 20 strains of *Propionbacterium acnes* isolated from skin lesions of patients with severe acne, and 20 strains of *Candida* spp. isolated from chronic vulvovaginal candidiasis and found active against all of them. The Slovakian researchers comment, "The results indicate a rational basis for the traditional use of *Mahonia aquifolium* for localized skin and mucosal infection therapy."[2] This kind of finding and commentary, at least in cultures other than the United States, is not uncommon.

Aspergillus spp.
Aureobasidium pullulans (black and white strains)
Bacillus cereus
Bacillus subtilis
Blastocystis hominis
Candida spp.
Chlamydia spp. (including *C. trachomatis*)
Corynebacterium diphtheriae
Cryptococcus neoformans
Dengue virus
Entamoeba histolytica
Enterobacter aerogenes
Epidermophyton floccosum
Erwinia carotavora

Escherichia coli
Fusarium nivale
Fusobacterium nucleatum
Giardia lamblia
Helicobacter pylori
Hepatitis B
Herpes simplex 1 and 2
Human cytomegalovirus
Klebsiella pneumoniae
Leishmania spp.
Malassezia spp.
Microsporum spp.
Mycobacterium tuberculosis
Propionbacterium acnes
Pseudomonas aeruginosa
Salmonella paratyphi

Salmonella typhimurium
Shigella spp.
Staphylococcus aureus
Staphylococcus epidermidis
Streptococcus mutans
Streptococcus pyogenes
Streptococcus sanguinis
Trichoderma viride (green strain and brown mutant)
Trichomonas vaginalis
Trichophyton spp.
Trypanosoma cruzi
Vibrio cholerae
West Nile virus
Xanthomonas citri
Yellow fever virus
Zoogloea ramigera

Use to Treat

Internally: Dysenteric diseases of all sorts, especially those caused by resistant bacteria, as well as cholera (better used in combination with geranium root, pomegranate bark or fruit peel, or guava leaf or bark), giardia, bloody stools

Externally: Topically for infected wounds from bacterial and fungal organisms; conjunctivitis and other eye infections, especially trachoma

Mouth, throat, vagina: As a tincture or spray, or as a douche, for bacterial, fungal, and yeast infections of the mucous membranes of the throat, mouth, vagina

Finding Berberine Plants

Phellodendron amurense bark, *Coptis chinensis* root, and *Corydalis yanhusuo* root are available in bulk from 1st Chinese Herbs. *Berberis vulgaris* and *Mahonia aquifolium* root bark and organically grown *Hydrastis canadensis* root are available from Pacific Botanicals. *Tinospora cordifolia* is available from Banyan Botanicals. *Argemone mexicana* seeds grow easily and are available many places if you Google them. The "resin" is often sold as a psychoactive (sigh), which makes it easily found at usually ridiculous prices. What this "resin" should in fact be is the dried latex, but it generally is not for, as most confess, it is very time intensive to gather. Usually the "resin" is a concentrated extract of the plant. It will work as a berberine, but there are much cheaper alternatives. The latex itself is actually fairly high in berberine and was once a staple of regular practice botanical medicine in the United States but is nearly impossible to find now. The dried plant is a bit hard to find as well.

There is a tendency, because of the berberine plants' poor absorption across the intestinal mucosa, to increase the dose of the plants substantially to try to get more alkaloids into the bloodstream. *This is a very bad idea.* Abdominal cramping, nervous tremors, and, most importantly, excessive drying of the mucous membranes will occur at high doses. Do not attempt to use these herbs as systemics.

Herb/Drug Interactions

The berberines are synergistic (or additive) with a number of pharmaceuticals such as fluconazole, ampicillin, and oxacillin. Repeated use of berberine *may* reduce the GI tract absorption of permeability glycoprotein (P-gp) substrates including chemotherapeutic agents such as daunomycin. Berberine intake will *increase* the absorption of cyclosporine A if it is taken after long-term berberine use: One study showed that 3 mg/kg of berberine in six human volunteers taken twice daily for 10 days increased the bioavailability of cyclosporine A by 19 percent. A randomized, clinical trial of 52 renal transplant patients for 3 months found that constant berberine intake significantly increased the amount of cyclosporine A in blood plasma.

Conversely, P-gp inhibitors, such as piperine, will substantially increase (by six times) the uptake of berberine across the intestinal mucosa. Sodium caprate, for example, will do so as well.

Glutin, a fraction isolated from gluten, *increases* the transport of berberine alkaloids across the mucosa. Eating gluten-rich foods *may* increase the amount of berberine-type alkaloids moving across the intestinal mucosa. Gum arabic inhibits the crossing of most alkaloids other than berberine. Coptis interferes with the movement of constituents from radix scutellariae (*Scutellaria baicalensis*) across the intestinal membrane.

Habitat and Appearance

I will primarily look at just three plants here: *Phellodendron, Berberis, Mahonia.*

PHELLODENDRON

Phellodendron amurense is a rather impressive deciduous tree (*deciduous* simply means "falling" because it loses its leaves in the fall); it is a native of Manchuria. It was introduced into the United States as an ornamental in the 1870s and escaped into urban fringe forests in New York State and Pennsylvania. It easily moves into multiple forest types and densities. It is now considered invasive in Illinois, New York, Pennsylvania, Massachusetts, Connecticut, and Virginia.

The tree grows to 60 feet tall (largest found was 90 feet, or 30 m) with a fairly short, wide trunk from which the tree begins branching almost immediately, giving it a widely spreading full canopy to 40 feet in diameter. The trunk has a deeply ridged and corky outer bark. The name *phellodendron* means "cork tree" (*phellos* meaning "cork," *dendron* meaning "tree"). So the plant is sometimes referred to as the corktree or the Amur corktree (from the region in Manchuria from which it comes). The female tree produces clusters of grape-like fruits (each containing two to five seeds) that possess a strong odor so that often only the male plants are cultivated, usually as a sterile cultivar, the so-called macho hybrid (rather oxymoronic).

The fruits have a high sugar content and are good food sources for birds and other animals, who routinely spread the seed far and wide. The leaves are edible and sometimes used in salads, soups, stews, and as a tea. The tree's primary use in the United States has been as a shade tree and ornamental. The bark has been used as a cork source (though a poor one); the tree is often used for lumber in China; the berries and inner bark are the source of several dyes; the fruits are used in insecticides, soaps, and lubricants. The inner bark is what is used medicinally. It is a good tree for bees and helps restore damaged soils when planted along with *Pinus sylvestris*.

BERBERIS

Both *Berberis thunbergii*, Japanese barberry, and *B. vulgaris*, common barberry, are introduced plants. Both are invasive here and there, Japanese barberry the most so. It is considered an invasive throughout the upper Midwest and Northeast — 20 states and the District of Columbia altogether. Both it and common barberry outcompete the only native barberry, *Berberis canadensis*, which is slowly disappearing. Nor do wildlife like to browse the introduced species. *Berberis* species are abundant in nearly every state, except Texas, Florida, Nevada, Arkansas, Louisiana, Mississippi, and Oklahoma.

Japanese barberry forms dense stands in woodlands, canopy forests, wetlands, pastures, and meadows. The leaves are prickly (hence "barb" berry) and look a bit like holly leaves, and whitetail deer studiously avoid the plant. The plant grows up to 15 feet in height. The fruits are edible and were often used for jams.

MAHONIA

Mahonias are very similar in appearance. *Mahonia aquifolium* is mostly found on the East Coast, from Georgia up into Canada, and on the West Coast from California up into Canada and eastward into Montana. *Mahonia repens* is widely spread from the Mississippi River west, from Texas into Canada and a bit around the Great Lakes. *Mahonia fremontii* is in the southwest, Colorado, New Mexico, Arizona, Utah, Nevada, California. *Mahonia bealii* is located throughout the Southeast. It is strongly present in most states except the extreme Northeast and the central plains into Louisiana and Mississippi.

Mahonias and the barberries, one or the other, grow in nearly every state in the United States. If you add in the phellodendrons, you can find a berberine plant just about anyplace. And, of course, all three genera are common in much of the world. The *Berberis* genus is very prolific, with a lot of diversity, in Africa, South America, and Asia. The mahonias are prolific in eastern Asia, North America, and Central America and have been widely planted throughout Europe. *Phellodendron* is widely dispersed in Asia, Russia, Europe, and North America.

Cultivation and Collection

Phellodendron tolerates a great many soil types and transplants easily. It does take a while to recover from transplanting, so it is usually planted in spring. Most people buy saplings for planting, but the seeds germinate easily (better with stratification) and sprout well; the plant is a strong grower. The seeds are highly allelopathic, killing off competing plants and protecting their growing zone. The tree spreads fairly easily once established — if you don't get the sterile cultivar. ("Macho" — how can it be macho? I don't get it.)

The root system is fairly shallow, so it needs room to spread. The tree loves disturbed areas and full sun, and it will tolerate most soils (sand, loam, clay, acidic, alkaline) and likes them well drained, occasionally wet. It is highly tolerant of drought and cold, resistant to nearly all pests, and likes it in Zones 3 through 7, which includes most of the United States except for the extreme South, Southwest, and Pacific coastline. The tree takes 7 to 13 years to set seed.

The inner bark may be harvested for medicinal use at any time, but when harvested in spring (April 4 through 20 in China), the inner and outer bark is more easily removed. Cut limbs are the best source of the bark unless for some reason you need to cut a whole tree. In regions where purists are trying to exterminate *Phellodendron* as an alien invader, you may be able to obtain whole trees from which to harvest considerable amounts. The outer bark is removed and abandoned and then the inner bark peeled off, cut into slices, and dried. Sometimes, no one knows why, the Chinese fry it with salt during the drying process (studies have found no difference in the strength of the resulting herb). In China they dry it in the sun, but I prefer it in a shady, dry location in the herb room myself.

Japanese barberry is shade tolerant, is drought and cold resistant, loves disturbed ecosystems, loves sunlight, and can seemingly grow just about anyplace. The plant spreads by seeds (which are themselves spread by birds and animals eating the fruit and excreting the seeds over a wide range), root and branch cuttings, live branches touching the ground, and root spread. Any root left in the ground will resprout. It is a prolific seed producer; the seeds have a 90 percent germination rate. It forms dense stands wherever it takes root in the wild and is very hard to eradicate. Ticks infected with *Borrelia* (Lyme disease) love the thick stands of the plants and are often densely present in them.

The plant's wood is very strong, so it has to be cut into small (1 inch or less) segments while still fresh. Don't do it later unless you have a dedicated wood chipper to use for your medicinals (or a meth addict friend with an axe — well, better stick with the chipper). Scrape your fingernail along the bark of the sections you intend to harvest. When the outer bark scrapes off, the inner bark should be yellow; if not, don't use it. The roots are tough to dig but have the highest alkaloid content. Use a tough, indestructible shovel (no wooden handles), long-handled clippers, a pickaxe, sweat, determination, and profanity. The outer bark of the roots is the most potent, but many people use the whole thing, chopped small and then cut and sifted, to make tinctures. It's easier.

Harvest the plant in autumn. With a good-sized plant, the roots and lower branches should last you a very long time. Dry well in the shade, and store in plastic bags inside plastic tubs, in a dark, dry location.

Mahonias are handled identically to barberries for medicine making, harvesting, and cultivation.

Plant Chemistry

The chemistry of the various berberine-containing plants differs a bit even though they are all used similarly. Over time, familiarity with the individual species allows a much more sophisticated use of the plants. This section will only highlight some of the major plant constituents in some of the species, beginning with the berberine content.

Coptis teeta has about the highest percentage of berberine of all plants — from 8 percent to 9 percent in the rhizome. *C. chinensis* runs 4 percent to 8 percent. *Berberis aristata*, as far as I can tell, has the most berberine in its genus, about 5 percent in the roots and 4 percent in the lower stems. *B. vulgaris*, the most commonly used species, has 1 percent to 1.5 percent berberine in its roots, about one-tenth of that in its stems, even less in the leaves. *B. croatica* is about the same. *Hydrastis canadensis* root contains about 3.4 percent berberine and

2.5 percent hydrastine. The leaves contain about 1.5 percent berberine and 0.5 percent hydrastine. The older the *Hydrastis* plants, the more they contain. Fall plants are stronger.

Phellodendron amurense bark runs about 3 percent to 4 percent berberine. *P. wilsonii* and *P. sachalinense* are reputed to contain the most berberine, followed by *P. chinense*.

Phellodendron species contain berberine, oxyberberine, epiberberine, caffeic acid ethyl ester, isovanillin, ferulic acid, dimethoxy-lariciresinol, methyl-beta-orsellinate, limonin (about 1 percent of the plant) and various other liminoids (obakunone, nomilin, etc.), 12-alpha-hydroxylimonin, gamma-fagarine, cathin-6-one, 4-methoxy-N-methyl-1-quinoline, palmatine, oxypalmatine, lyoniresinol, beta-sitosterol, stigmasterine, amurenlactone A, amurenamide A, phellodensins, various phellodenols, magnoflorine, jatorrhizine, various coumarins, phellodendrine, phellodendric acid, various quercetins, platydesmin, skimmianine, chilenine, and pteleine.

The five major alkaloids in the plant are considered to be berberine (about 80 percent of total alkaloids), palmatine, jatrorrhizine, phellodendrine, and magnoflorine.

The other berberine-containing plants have just as complex a chemistry though their alkaloids tend to be a bit different. They all do similar things.

Traditional Uses of the Berberines

The plants are used around the world in very similar ways, the main differences being that both *Corydalis* and *Argemone* species contain either opioid or opioid-like constituents, making them very useful for pain relief in addition to their other functions.

Although the different berberine-containing plants will have unique applications when you get more sophisticated in their use, for my purposes here — the treatment of resistant GI tract infections with presenting dysentery or severe diarrhea (bloody or not), resistant infections of the mouth and throat, and skin infections — all the plants work similarly. From a look at their traditional uses, you can see that healers for the past several thousand years in every geographical region have found similar uses for all the berberines.

Hydrastis canadensis: As a bitter tonic, mucous membrane tonic; for skin disorders including infection and inflammation, eye and ear infections, mouth ulcers, throat and mouth infections, fever, diarrhea, dysentery, catarrh, vaginal discharges, liver congestion and gallbladder problems, menstrual irregularities, ulcerative colitis, cancer.

***Mahonia* spp.:** As a bitter tonic, mucous membrane tonic; for liver and blood stagnation, skin problems including inflammation and infections, GI tract infections, ulceration, fever.

***Berberis* spp.:** As a bitter tonic, mucous membrane tonic; for skin inflammation and infection, GI tract problems, cholera, dysentery, diarrhea, fever, cancer, liver stagnation, poor blood, gout.

***Coptis* spp.:** For abdominal problems, GI tract problems, dysentery, cholera, enteritis, typhoid, respiratory tract infections, UTIs, gynecological inflammations, ear/nose/throat infections, jaundice, fever, blood problems, eye inflammation, insomnia, abscesses, skin problems.

***Corydalis* spp.:** As a bitter tonic, analgesic, mucous membrane tonic; for liver stagnation, spleen stagnation, stagnant blood, menstrual irregularities, ulcers.

***Phellodendron* spp.:** As a bitter tonic; for GI tract problems, dysentery, jaundice, vaginal inflammation and discharges, urinary tract infections, pain, swelling in knees and feet, boils, sores, abscesses, ulcers, eczema, canker sores, burns, fever, night sweats.

***Argemone* spp.:** As a sedative, laxative; for jaundice, skin diseases, cough, venereal disease, vaginal discharge, arthritis, kidney pain, postpartum difficulties, dropsy, swelling of the legs, malaria, fever.

Many of the other berberine-containing plants have been used similarly.

AYURVEDA

The phellodendrons are not that common in India, but the barberries are and have been used for millennia. Five species are commonly used, the main ones being *Berberis vulgaris* and *Berberis aristata*. They are used just as all berberine-containing plants are. See Traditional Uses of the Berberines, page 171.

TRADITIONAL CHINESE MEDICINE

Phellodendron, known as *huang bo* or *huang bai,* is considered to be one of the 50 fundamental herbs of traditional Chinese medicine (TCM). It has been used for millennia and appears in medical texts as early as 300 BCE. It is considered bitter and cold, affecting urinary bladder, kidney, and large intestine meridians. It is used to clear heat and dry dampness, to reduce fire and release toxins. See Traditional Uses of the Berberines, page 171, for specific TCM uses. Normal dosage in China is 3 to 10 grams of the dried herb ($1/10$ to $1/3$ ounce). The plant has also been a part of traditional Korean and Japanese medicine for a very long time, used for similar diseases and conditions.

Coptis, Corydalis, Mahonia, and *Berberis* species have all been a part of TCM for millennia and are used in similar ways.

WESTERN BOTANIC PRACTICE

Phellodendron has been unknown until now. *Hydrastis, Berberis* species, and *Mahonia* species were all used for a very long time, in just the same ways all berberine plants are.

Scientific Research

All the berberine plants, and berberine (in vitro studies), are highly active against a wide range of microorganisms, especially bacteria. There are literally scores if not hundreds of such studies on the compound.

Part of the problem with berberine as a systemic is that it does not move across the GI tract membranes very well; it tends to be limited to where it can touch for its activity. Researchers have been trying for years to find a way to make it broadly systemic but have not succeeded. Most of the pharmacokinetic studies have focused on injectable forms of berberine or other, similar, alkaloids. Oral administration of crude plant preparations has shown some movement of alkaloids, e.g., berberine and palmatine, into blood plasma in rats, but the amounts are tiny, 0.31 ng/ml as compared to 18.1 ng/ml if pure berberine is injected. Tiny amounts of berberine have been found in the pancreas, heart, kidney, spleen, lung, testes, and uterus. This does have some tonic and stimulatory effects on those systems, which is reflected by the plant's traditional uses. The tiny systemic amounts do provide *some* systemic antimicrobial help, just not very much and certainly not enough to treat a resistant systemic disease.

In human volunteers (China), normal dosing produced about 0.020 ng/ml in plasma, very large doses got it up to 3.0 ng/ml in the blood, still not enough for systemic treatment of serious diseases, and this was from ingesting pure berberine. Oral intake of goldenseal (product contained 77 mg hydrastine, 132 mg berberine) produced only 0.1 ng/ml of *both* constituents (combined total) in blood plasma of human volunteers. Berberine (and presumably many of the other alkaloids in these plants) just doesn't transfer well across the GI tract membranes; however, the amounts that do are very quickly expressed into the urine for excretion, into the mucous membranes for excretion by that route, or routed to the liver, where they are expressed into the bile. The amounts expressed in the urine (about 5 percent) are what account for the use of berberine plants in the treatment of urinary tract infections (for which they do work to some extent). The amounts concentrated in the liver and then expressed into the bile (0.5 percent) are what account for

the traditional uses of the herbs for sluggish liver and as a bile stimulant. Berberine is metabolized in the liver and the metabolites excreted into the bile, which then expresses them into the GI tract. The gut bacteria play a role then in the enterohepatic circulation of the metabolites. These metabolites remain more prominently in the body than berberine itself, however still at fairly low levels.

The particular substance, pervasive in the intestinal epithelium (and hepatocytes), that keeps berberine from circulating widely in the body is permeability glycoprotein, a.k.a. P-glycoprotein. P-glycoprotein distributes a great many substances across the mucous membranes of the intestinal tract, including herbal constituents. However, it is also responsible for transporting substances the body identifies as toxic out of the body, often through urine and bile — the berberine-plant alkaloids are some of them. Because P-glycoprotein (or its directors) identifies berberine-like alkaloids as toxic, they are not allowed to cross the intestinal barrier to circulate in any concentration in the bloodstream.

However, the tiny amount of alkaloids that do circulate in the bloodstream increases the level of the active immunoglobulin A antibodies (IgA) in the mucous membranes — though this action is much, much higher in the intestines because the herb is actually able to touch the membranes there. IgA is one of the most potent antibodies in the human body and it infuses the mucous membranes in order to fight infections that seek to gain entry there. In this instance the body is identifying the berberine alkaloids and their metabolites as an infectious agent and producing IgA antibodies in response. Stimulation of the mucous membranes and the IgA antibodies helps prevent infections. This is the main source of the immune-modulating and immune-potentiating actions of the berberines and is why the herbs, if used properly, help prevent and can effectively treat viral and bacterial infections of the mouth, throat, and sinuses. Synergistically, berberine also interferes with the adherence of bacteria, e.g., *Streptococcus pyogenes*, to epithelial cells, thus reducing disease incidence.

The berberine plants are, however, most specific for intestinal infections from pathogenic organisms. That is where their great strength lies. Berberine reduces the intestinal secretion of water and electrolytes caused by infectious intestinal bacteria such as cholera and *E. coli* organisms, inhibits cholera and other bacterial entertoxins, reduces smooth muscle contraction and intestinal motility (thus reducing cramping), delays intestinal transit time, reduces inflammation in intestinal tissues, and is directly bactericidal to cholera and other dysenteric/diarrheal organisms. Berberine specifically inhibits bacterial adherence to mucosal or epithelial surfaces, thus stopping the infection.

Because berberine is so widely antimicrobial, many people have used berberine plants (and many companies have touted them) as systemic antibacterials. They are not and are only partially effective for colds and flu, their other main use. (They are active against some viruses and do potentiate mucous membrane function, which helps the membranes fight off microorganisms.) Goldenseal is the primary berberine plant used medicinally in the United States and it is ridiculously overused, usually for the wrong things. There are much better plants for colds and flu.

Many of the berberine-containing plants have been found to contain multidrug-resistance (MDR) reversal activity, usually inhibiting efflux pumps in resistant bacteria. *Berberis* species and *Hydrastis canadensis* contain 5'-methoxyhydnocarpin-D (5'-MHC) and pheophorbide A, which inhibit the NorA efflux pump in *Staphylococcus aureus*. This is part of what makes the plants so effective in treating resistant organisms, especially MRSA. There are numerous other compounds in the berberine plants that show this kind of MDR inhibition.

The MDR inhibitors in the berberine plants have been found to be synergistic with the alkaloids in the plants. They have also been found to be synergistic with pharmaceuticals, increasing their activity and effectiveness in treating resistant organisms and lowering the necessary dose for antibacterial, antifungal, and anti-amoebic action.

In this section I am only going to look in any depth at research on the phellodendrons and berberine as an isolated constituent.

PHELLODENDRON

An in vivo trial in the treatment of both acute and chronic induced inflammation using an ethanol extract of *Phellodendron* and *Coptis* (in a

2:1 ratio) found the tincture to be as potent in its effects as celecoxib and dexamethasone in reducing inflammation. In vitro studies on human osteoarthritis cartilage found that the plant significantly inhibited collagen and chondrocyte destruction by inhibiting proteoglycan release and type II cartilage degradation; down-regulating aggrecanases, matrix metalloproteinase (MMP) activity, and phospho-ERK $\frac{1}{2}$, JNK, and p38 MAP kinase signaling; and up-regulating TIMP-1 activity. Another found potent antioxidant activity by the plant.

Eighty people (45 completing) were enrolled in an 8-week, placebo-controlled, randomized, double-blind study of the effects of a *Phellodendron amurense* bark and *Citrus sinensis* peel combination capsule (740 mg, twice daily) on primary osteoarthritis of the knee in both overweight and normal-weight persons. Overweight participants lost an average of 5 percent of body weight, and lipid levels, blood pressure, and fasting blood glucose levels normalized. There was significantly less inflammation and fewer symptoms of osteoarthritis in all those who used the herb combination.

A clinical trial with 28 participants (premenopausal women), double-blind, placebo-controlled, and randomized, testing a combination extract of magnolia and *Phellodendron* bark found no weight gain in the extract group but gains in the placebo group. The extract group had lower cortisol levels in the evening (the placebo group, higher) and lower levels of stress.

A combination blend of *Phellodendron* and magnolia, in a randomized, parallel, double-blind, placebo-

controlled, clinical trial with healthy, overweight women (40 participants, 26 completing) found the extract effective in reducing temporary, transitory anxiety.

Phellodendron has been found effective in treating periodontal disease.

Extracts of *Phellodendron* (Nexrutine) fed to TRAMP mice for 20 weeks significantly inhibited prostate cancer cell proliferation and progression. There have been a number of studies that found similar antitumor activity of the plant for the prostate. It's strongly active on the prostate gland in vitro, inhibiting contractility. Dietary berberine and dietary *Phellodendron* extract were found to inhibit cell cycle progression and lung tumorigenesis in mice.

In vivo studies with hyperuricemic mice found a decrease in uric acid levels in mice ingesting a high-dose *Phellodendron* extract. Other studies found that the plant constituent phellodendrine suppresses autoimmune responses in mice and guinea pigs. Unlike prednisone and cyclophosphamide, the extract did not affect antibody production.

Phellodendron extracts prevent ethanol-, aspirin-, stress-, and pylorus-ligated-induced ulcers in mice. Extracts of *P. wilsonii* were highly protective of mouse liver in CCl4-induced hepatotoxicity. Other species provided only moderate protection.

During in vitro studies *Phellodendron* was found to be antioxidant, antitumor, anti-inflammatory, antimicrobial (plaque), anti–herpes simplex 1, and antibacterial against a wide range of bacteria.

Clinical (and a few other) studies with other berberine-containing plants:

123 people with acute bacillic dysentery were treated with a decoction of Sankezhen (any of four *Berberis* species used in China: *soulieana, wilsoniae, poiretii,* or *vernae*). Of them, 113 were cured, 4 improved. In another trial with 94 people, 88 were cured.

A trial used tablets prepared from *Berberis poirettii* decoction in the treatment of 228 cases of chronic bronchitis. Of them, 12.3 percent experienced cure, 39 percent marked effects, 38 percent improved. (A tincture would have worked better.)

An in vivo trial with goldenseal found that the plant was helpful in treating liver cancer in rats. The plant's constituents do possess some antitumor actions and their concentration in the liver was found to be useful in the treatment of liver cancer, primarily as a supportive therapy.

Berberis vulgaris, when used instead of antibiotics in chicken feed, substantially increased the birds' weight, just as antibiotics do.

BERBERINE (AND OTHER BERBERINE-PLANT ALKALOIDS)

Quite a number of the in vivo studies of the effectiveness of berberine as an antimicrobial use injectable forms of the compound. I am omitting most of these here (even though some of them are included in the bibliography). They don't in any way indicate the actions of the compound when used as an herbal preparation. Injection is one of the ways researchers are trying to make the compound systemic. There has been some success at this but there is a rather high toxicity when the isolated constituent is used that way, a toxicity that does not occur when crude extracts of the plants are used.

I am also skipping most of the in vitro studies, which are voluminous. Berberine's antimicrobial actions have already been mentioned throughout this section. Quite a few references are in the bibliography. Here are just a few clinical results of berberine's use.

A clinical trial with children suffering from giardia (ages 5 months to 14 years) was conducted in India. Berberine, administered orally, 10 mg/ kg/day, was effective in eradicating the infection, comparable to quinacrine hydrochloride, furazolidone, and metronidazole.

Four hundred adults presenting with acute watery diarrhea were treated in a randomized, placebo-controlled, double-blind trial of berberine. Berberine combined with tetracycline was potently effective. Berberine alone reduced diarrheal stools and cyclic adenosine monophosphate concentrations in stools by 77 percent; another study found that berberine reduced diarrheal stools in cholera and/or enterotoxigenic *E. coli* (ETEC) up to 50 percent and that it was more potently effective in treating ETEC than cholera; another trial in a randomized, controlled trial of 165 adults with either ETEC or cholera found that in those with cholera berberine significantly reduced the mean 8-hour stool volume; however, with ETEC berberine completely inhibited diarrhea in half the participants within 24 hours.

Clinical (human) trials — placebo-controlled, randomized, double-blind — with 63 men with enterotoxigenic *E. coli* diarrhea found 400 mg of berberine sulfate to have dependable effectiveness, surpassing pharmaceuticals. In the 8 hours following treatment those in the berberine group experienced significant decrease in stool volume. Within 24 hours 42 percent of the participants in the berberine group stopped having diarrhea, versus 20 percent in the placebo group.

Another trial in the treatment of giardia in India found that berberine improved gastrointestinal symptoms and reduced giardia-positive stools. Berberine was found as effective as metronidazole at only half the dose.

In a clinical study with 51 people of an aqueous berberine preparation versus sulfacetamide in the treatment of *Chlamydia trachomatis* eye infections, berberine was found to be slightly less effective than the drug. However, the drug did not completely eradicate the organism and relapses occurred. In the berberine group there were no relapses of those cured, even after 1 year. Other clinical studies have found similar outcomes. The crude extracts of berberine plants have consistently been found more effective than berberine.

Palmatine was used to treat 1,042 cases of gynecological infection, upper respiratory infection, surgical infection, tonsillitis, enteritis, and bacillary dysentery with good effect. In the treatment of 200 cases of vulvovaginal candidiasis, 171 were cured, 24 improved.

Numerous in vivo studies have found berberine to be tonically antitumor for a number of different kinds of cancers, from breast to bladder to gastric to liver. It down-regulates metalloproteinases 1, 2, and 9 and is a potent COX-2 inhibitor.

Berberine, in vivo, oral administration, has been found to reduce insulin resistance in rats and to lower blood glucose levels and correct blood lipid metabolism disorders. In essence it suppresses intestinal disaccharidases, benefitting diabetic states while also improving glucose metabolism through the induction of glycolysis and increasing insulin sensitivity.

It has also been found to be immunomodulatory (rather than stimulatory). It does increase IgA antibodies in mucosal tissue but it also reduces the overactivity of various aspects of the immune system. In other words if the immune system is ramped up by an autoimmune dynamic or hyperactivated by something like phytohemagglutinin or phorbol dibutyrate plus ionomycin, berberine modulates the response, suppressing the overactivity.

Juniper

Family: Cupressaceae

Species Used: There are 50 or 59 or even 67 species (taxonomists have to use their fingers and toes to count) in the *Juniperus* genus; all of them can be used similarly.

Parts Used

Usually the berries and needles, but the bark, wood, and root are all active.

Preparation and Dosage

The constituents in the junipers are readily soluble in alcohol but vary in water depending on what part of the plant you are using. The berries must be tinctured in alcohol or eaten whole to be effective. The needles will work to some extent in water (but are better in alcohol — the monoterpenes just aren't that water soluble as numerous studies have found), the bark not so well.

   Use: The berries for urinary tract infections. The berries or needles for upper respiratory or GI tract infections. The heartwood, roots, bark, berries, or needles for skin infections and infectious dysentery. The essential oil for airborne and upper respiratory infections.

TINCTURE

Berries: 1:5, 75 percent alcohol, 5–20 drops, up to 3x daily.

INFUSION

Chopped or powdered needles prepared as a standard infusion, covered, 4–6 ounces, 3–6x daily.

DECOCTION

A strong decoction of the herb has been traditionally used in many cultures to sterilize brewing equipment, cooking utensils, surgical

Properties of Juniper

Actions

Antibacterial	Antinociceptive	Digestive
Anticatarrhal	Antioxidant	Diuretic
Antifungal	Antirheumatic	Hypoglycemic
Anti-inflammatory	Antiseptic	Hypolipidaemic
Antimicrobial	Antiviral	Radical scavenger
Antineoplastic	Carminative	Stomachic

Active Against

Alcohol extracts of juniper show activity against 57 strains of 24 bacterial species in the following genera:

Acinetobacter	*Enterobacter*	*Staphylococcus*
Bacillus	*Escherichia*	*Xanthomonas*
Brevundimonas	*Micrococcus*	
Brucella	*Pseudomonas*	

They have been shown to inhibit, as well, 11 *Candida* species. They are also active against biofilm formation. Some antimicrobial specifics:

Acinetobacter baumannii	*Helicobacter pylori*	*Rhodotorula* spp.
Actinomyces bovis	*Klebsiella oxytoca*	*Salmonella typhi*
Aspergillus fumigatus	*Klebsiella pneumoniae*	*Serratia marcescens*
Aspergillus niger	*Leishmania donovani*	*Shigella dysentariae*
Bacillus brevis	*Listeria monocytogenes*	*Shigella sonnei*
Bacillus cereus	*Micrococcus flavus*	*Staphylococcus aureus* (including resistant strains)
Bacillus megaterium	*Micrococcus luteus*	
Bacillus subtilis	*Microsporum gypseum*	*Staphylococcus epidermidis*
Caenorhabditis elegans	*Mycobacterium* spp. (including *M. tuberculosis*, even resistant strains such as H37Rv, and seven non-tuberculosis types)	
Candida spp.		*Staphylococcus intermedius*
Clostridium perfringens		*Streptococcus durans*
Cryptococcus neoformans		*Streptococcus faecalis*
Enterococcus faecalis	*Plasmodium falciparum*	*Streptococcus mutans*
Escherichia coli	*Proteus mirabilis*	*Streptococcus sanguinis*
Fusobacterium necrophorum	*Proteus vulgaris*	*Trichophyton mentagrophytes*
Geotrichum candidum	*Pseudomonas aeruginosa*	*Trichophyton rubrum*
Hansenula anomala		*Yersinia enterocolitica*

Juniper is also active against various cancer cell lines, SARS coronavirus, and herpes simplex 1.

instruments, hands, counters, etc. The decoction is also effective as a wound wash to either prevent or cure infection. Use 1 ounce herb per quart of water, boil 30 minutes, then turn off the heat and let steep overnight.

BERRIES

In whole form, for gastric problems: eat 1–5 berries per day for 2 weeks.

POWDER

Add any part of the plant to wound powders or use alone to prevent or cure infection in wounds.

STEAM

Any part of the plant, but usually the needles or berries. Use in sweat lodge or sauna directly on the stones or boil 4 ounces of needles in 1 gallon water, pour the resultant tea on stones, and inhale steam. Or just inhale the steam as it boils.

ESSENTIAL OIL

For sinus and upper respiratory infections, 8–10 drops in water in a 1-ounce nasal spray bottle, 4–6x day; shake well before use. Or use the essential oil in a diffuser for helping prevent and cure upper respiratory infections. Moderate amounts can be mixed in water for use as steam inhalant or in a sweat lodge for upper respiratory infections.

Side Effects and Contraindications

There has been a long-standing assertion in scores of herbals that the use of this plant may cause kidney irritation and that it is highly contraindicated in kidney disease. (Guilty of this myself.) I have used the plant for over two decades and have never seen any problems. The phytomedicalist Kerry Bone and others have tracked back the emergence of this belief; it began in the latter part of the nineteenth century, apparently from the administration of large doses of the essential oil to animals. Recent studies with rats have found, contrary to popular belief, a kidney-protecting effect from the use of the plant. This bears out the long use by the Eclectics of the berries in the treatment of active kidney disease and inflammation. I no longer consider the herb contraindicated in kidney disease, nor do I feel that kidney irritation can occur from normal use.

The only side effect I have ever seen from use was a mild diarrhea when the essential oil (15 drops in 1 ounce of olive oil) was used in the treatment of an ear infection. The mix was applied three times daily with a cotton swab. The diarrhea stopped upon discontinuance of the herb.

The essential oil is not really for internal use other than as a steam inhalant or for aromatherapy. Neither the plant itself nor the berry appears to produce any side effects, nor have I ever heard of any.

Caution should probably be exercised by diabetics in any long-term use of the plant as it affects blood glucose levels and may alter insulin requirements. It should probably not be used long term with pharmaceutical diuretics. *However*, almost no one uses the plant long term for healing; usually it is a short-course herb for UTI.

Herb/Drug Interactions

None noted.

Habitat and Appearance

Generally, there are two main types of junipers. The first is a typical sort of evergreen tree (sometimes shrubby looking) growing up to

Finding Juniper

It probably grows someplace near you. Go and pick the blue/purplish berries and use them, or buy them . . . they are available from herb suppliers everywhere.

Alternatives: Any evergreen species, especially thuja, cedar, pine, fir, and spruce in that order. Thuja, cedar, and pine have shown significant antibacterial activity in laboratory study against antibiotic-resistant bacteria, as has fir and, to a lesser extent, spruce. This tends to bear out their long traditional use for healing infectious disease. Dosages for all the evergreens are comparable.

50 feet tall. The second is a low, spreading shrub, usually with nasty, prickly needles that will easily penetrate clothing and skin. It is often intentionally planted along walkways and near the front doors of houses. And of course, to make things difficult, many of the tree species start out with needles very much like the low-spreading shrubs and only develop their scale-like needle structure as they age.

The trunk and branches of both types tend to have a reddish look to them, the outer bark peeling off in strips all on its own, giving the plant a rather shaggy, disreputable look. The needles on the shrubby species, primarily *Juniperus communis*, are exceedingly sharp, a bit blue-green in color, and somewhat similar to the needles on pines, firs, and spruce species. The needles on the tree species are more similar to those on some types of true cypress and cedar species, having an overlapping, scale type of growth, really not much like those of the pines, spruce, and firs.

Both species are readily identifiable due to the presence of their "berries," which are actually small cones that form after fertilization of the flowers. Like everyone else, I just call them berries. (Yes, I know tomato is a fruit, but no one cares.) The berries are green when first formed, then turn purplish during the winter, after a good frost.

Juniperus communis is a circumpolar species of the northern hemisphere. It and its high-altitude relations (*J. sibirica, J. montana*) are generally found from 8,000 feet (2,400 m) up to timberline. The tree species grow lower, up to about 8,000 feet, and are widely spread throughout the world; various species can be found in Africa as far south as Zimbabwe, and also in Australia and South America. The genus has been widely planted as ornamentals throughout the world. All of the species can be used for medicine.

Cultivation and Collection

Given that the berries of the junipers do contain seeds, there is no doubt that the trees propagate that way. Information on starting them from seed, however, is very hard to find. Everyone apparently plants seedlings — I just can't find out where the seedlings come from (storks maybe or perhaps Hogwarts). In any event, the seedlings need a well-drained soil in which to grow.

You can gather the needles, bark, roots, or heartwood at any time. First-year berries (they are green) should be gathered after the first frost, second-year berries (they are bluish-purple) at any time. Basically, the berries should be purplish before you use them for medicine — the frost is what does it.

Plant Chemistry

There are some 80 to 100 different compounds that have been identified in the junipers so far. Generally, alpha-pinene, junipene, eicosane, hexadecane, stenol, heptacosane, aromadendrene, germacrene, alpha-copaene-8-ol, ledol, elemol, trans-caryophyllene, epoxy caryophyllene, amorphene, and limonene are the major constituents. There is also totarol, ferruginol, longifolene, trans-communic acid, cedrol, alpha-cedrene, beta-cedrene, alpha-cedrol, 3-carene, terpinen-4-ol, beta-pinene, sabinene, myrcene, mycene, thujone, caryophyllene, cadinene, elemene, linalool, piperitone, gamma-terpinene, trans-pinocarveole, rho-cymene, alpha-terpineole, gamma-cardinene, beta-carophyllene, bornyl acetate, germacrene B, germacrene D, verbenol, camphene, tricyclene, beta-eudesmol, humulene, borneol, nerol, geraniol, carvacrol, and so on.

The constituents differ not only in species, but in species' location and in their age. Century-old trees have markedly different chemical profiles than those a decade old. The primary constituents in all species are monoterpene hydrocarbons, which are highly bioactive, strongly antimicrobial compounds.

Traditional Uses of Juniper

Juniper, and all the evergreens, have been used in every culture on Earth for purifying and cleansing — physically, emotionally, and spiritually. They have been used in sweat baths and saunas throughout time to help prevent or cure illness.

One of the often overlooked attributes of the evergreens is their vitamin C content. All animals except the higher primates synthesize their own vitamin C. The new spring growth of the evergreens is lighter in color, less astringent, and decidedly more citrus-tasting than older growth (it has a definite lemon-lime flavor). This new growth has traditionally been used in the human diet in scores of cultures to treat scurvy.

AYURVEDA

There are five species of juniper used in India, *Juniper communis* being the most common. Called by a variety of names, depending on which local language is being used, it is *hapusha* in Sanskrit. The berries are the main part of the plant used for medicine, though the leaves and wood are sometimes used as well.

Juniper is considered aromatic, carminative, stimulant, emmenagogue, digestive, stomachic, strongly antibacterial, and diuretic. It is used for scanty urine, chronic Bright's disease, hepatic dropsy, coughs and pulmonary disease, fever, gonorrhea, leukorrhea, catarrh, arthritis, amenorrhea, tuberculosis, diabetes, and improving digestion and appetite.

TRADITIONAL CHINESE MEDICINE

There are 23 primary species of juniper in China with numerous subspecies. Most of them are designated by a phrase ending in *bai* (or beginning with *bai*, depending on whether you read left to right or right to left); e.g., *chui zhi bai* for *Juniperus recurva*, or *bei mei yuan bai* for *Juniperus virginiana*. The junipers *are* used in Chinese medicine; it's just that none of my sources have much about it. "Used similarly to thuja," says one fairly rare book, "see that listing." The book then stops at the letter "N." And, of course, I haven't been able to find volume two anyplace. Irritating. And wouldn't you just know it, none of my other Chinese herbals list thuja either. Increasingly irritating.

However, the tiny amount I can find lists juniper as traditionally used for treating bleeding from coughs, for colds, for hemorrhage, as a general tonic, and for convulsions, detoxification of the blood, hepatitis, and sweating. It is used in the treatment of chronic obstructive pulmonary disease in situations where there is phlegm overproduction and congestion, blood stasis, and spleen deficiency.

WESTERN BOTANIC PRACTICE

Junipers were extensively used by indigenous cultures in the Americas for the exact same conditions as those in China and India. Additionally, they used them for diarrheal conditions, colds and flu, ulcers, throat infections; as an aromatic for lung conditions; for vaginal infections and scanty menses, especially after childbirth; as a primary tuberculosis medicine, a wash for skin infections, an anthelmintic, and a general disinfectant to prevent disease or to clean rooms after disease.

The Eclectic physicians in the United States used the berries as a potent diuretic, for dropsy, for ascites, as a specific for infected mucous discharges from the urethra, and for cystitis, pyelitis, pyelonephritis, and renal hyperemia. They were also used for leukorrhea, gleet, gonorrhea, scorbutic diseases, skin infections, eczema, psoriasis, and skin parasites. They were used similarly in Europe. Juniper is still official in German medical practice.

Scientific Research

There has been little scientific study on juniper, other than some rather extensive explorations of its constituents and their antimicrobial activity. A few in vivo studies do exist.

In vitro studies have found that extracts of the heartwood of various juniper species are comparable in their antimicrobial effects to streptomycin. Leaf extracts are comparable in potency to amphotericin B. Other in vitro studies found that leaf extracts were very active against resistant staph and bacillus bacteria, as potent as ampicillin and erythromycin in their zones of inhibition. Juniper inhibits the NorA efflux pump in staph organisms, making them more susceptible to the antibacterial compounds in the plant.

In vivo studies: Tacrolimus, a drug used for immunosuppression after organ transplants, can cause, among other things, severe kidney damage. Tacrolimus-induced kidney damage in rats was completely reversed by the use of juniper oil. The renal cell membranes incorporated vasodilatory prostanoids, the herb elevated PGF2-alpha urinary excretion, and the precipitous fall in inulin clearance usually caused by the drug was completely prevented. (This bears out the Eclectic use of the herb in treating kidney disease.) Additionally, the kidneys and livers of mice injected with CCl4 who had previously been given an oral extract of juniper were strongly protected from injury. The researchers commented that *J. phoenicea* leaf extracts "show a remarkable effect in enhancing liver and kidney functions and may thus be of therapeutic potential in treatment of hepatotoxicity and nephrotoxicity."[3]

Juniper berry oil is high in 5,11,14-eicosatrienoic acid, a polyunsaturated acid similar to that found in fish oil; it is highly resistant to peroxidation. Hepatic reperfusion injury in rats fed the oil as a regular part of their diet was significantly minimized. (This bears out the traditional tonic use of the herb for treating digestive/liver problems.)

Juniper extracts showed potent anthelmintic activity against pinworm infections in mice; they are strongly anti-inflammatory to induced edema in mice and antinociceptive to induced pain; they significantly lower blood glucose levels in induced-diabetic mice while also increasing zinc levels in the liver.

Juniper extracts, and various compounds in juniper species, are potently active against a wide range of *Mycobacterium* organisms, bearing out the plant's traditional use for treating TB.

Juniper also contains, as do nearly all evergreens, a rather amazing constituent called totarol. Like many of the constituents in juniper (longifolene, alpha-pinene), totarol is strongly antibacterial. Totarol is antimicrobial against a wide range of microorganisms, including the mycobacteria, enterococci, staphylococci, streptococci, *Pseudomonas*, plus a variety of other Gram-negative organisms, and a number of parasitic organisms. It is potently synergistic with the other antibacterials in juniper; studies have found that it potentiates a wide range of pharmaceutical antibiotics as well. It is highly active at tiny doses and is a main part of the synergistic potency of the plant as an antimicrobial, antioxidant, antitumor, hepatic protector, and cholesterol-lowering herb. The constituent is also highly effective in the treatment of skin diseases such as severe acne. It is a fairly strong NorA efflux pump inhibitor.

A number of compounds in the plant, especially the berries, most especially terpinen-4-ol, substantially increase the output of urine without reducing either potassium or electrolyte levels in the body. Kidney filtration rate is also enhanced. The reasons why the highly antibacterial monoterpenes in the plant work so well is that the body immediately works to excrete them through the urinary passages. This has the effect of disinfecting the whole system. If you have a resistant UTI, this is the one plant you want to be sure to use for it.

Honey

Any organic wildflower honey can be used effectively in the treatment of antibiotic-resistant skin and wound infections. There is some evidence that large-scale agricultural honeys and single-plant honeys are less potent than wildflower honeys. There are a few exceptions. Manuka honey from New Zealand, produced mainly from the flowers of *Leptospermum scoparium*, is very potent (which is why you will see it for sale all over the Internet at indecent prices — about four times the cost of locally produced wildflower honeys).

The belated recognition of the potency of honey in treating resistant bacterial infections of the skin, especially those acquired in hospitals, has led to significant study, clinical use, and trial of honeys in medical practice since the first edition of this book in 1999, primarily in the UK. Predictably, a pharmaceutical honey has been produced (which is, of course, tremendously expensive compared to local honeys). Called Medihoney, it is the only honey allowable for use in the medical system in the UK. (A brand called Revamil is used in the Netherlands.) The USFDA has also accepted the use of a pharmaceutical honey by clinicians in this country, again very expensive — though, of course, almost no U.S. hospitals are using it. Nevertheless, *any* wildflower honey will do. The more plants the bees collect nectar from, the more potent it will be. If it is organic, it will tend to be relatively free of agrochemical pollutants. Also important.

Other bee products such as propolis and royal jelly are also highly effective against resistant organisms. Studies have found them stronger in some instances than honey, but they are more difficult to apply. Royal jelly, when added to honey, increases its effectiveness.

Preparation and Dosage

Honey can be applied directly to wounds or used internally for immune stimulation, overall health improvement, and treatment of colds, flus, and respiratory infections.

Properties of Honey

Actions

Potent antibiotic against all known forms of resistant bacteria that infect the skin and wounds. In addition:

Antiallergenic	Anti-inflammatory	Laxative
Antianemic	Antiviral	Tonic
Anticarcinogenic	Expectorant	
Antifungal	Immune stimulant	

Promotes healing for wounds, moist wounds, peptic ulcers, and bacterial gastroenteritis; reduces plaque; good for gingivitis; facilitates debridement; soothes inflamed tissues; acts as a wound barrier; and stimulates skin and muscle regeneration.

Active Against

Acinetobacter spp.
Alcaligenes faecalis
Aspergillus niger
Bacillus stearothermophilus
Bacillus subtilis
Burkholderia cepacia
Candida spp.
E. coli O157:H7 (25 strains)
Enterobacter cloacae
Enterococcus faecalis (essentially any vancomycin-resistant enterococci)
Extended-spectrum beta-lactamase (ESBL) bacteria

Haemophilus influenzae
Helicobacter pylori
Herpes simplex
Klebsiella oxytoca
Klebsiella pneumoniae
Listeria monocytogenes
Malassezia spp.
Micrococcus luteus
Morganella morganii
Mycobacterium spp.
Proteus spp.
Pseudomonas aeruginosa (152 isolates)
Rubella virus
Salmonella enteritidis
Salmonella typhimurium (49 strains)

Serratia marcescens
Shigella dysentariae
Staphylococcus aureus (58 isolates and all MRSA strains tested)
Staphylococcus spp. (coagulase-negative species)
Stenotrophomonas maltophilia
Streptococcus spp.
Trichosporon spp.

Honey is also highly effective against bacterial biofilms.

CONTINUED ON NEXT PAGE

PROPERTIES OF HONEY, CONTINUED

Use to Treat

Use for prevention and treatment of all infected skin wounds: cuts, abrasions, leg and skin ulcers, gangrene, diabetic ulceration of the foot, all fungating wounds (skin ulceration with necrosis and bad smell), necrotizing soft-tissue infections, postsurgical wound infections, burns (first through third degree), cellulitis, furunculosis, abscesses, necrotizing fasciitis, conjunctivitis, radiation burns and wounds, gingivitis, dental plaque, and helicobacter infections of the stomach and duodenum. Use it prophylactically at the exit sites of medical devices to prevent infection. To prevent infection from catheter insertion, the catheter should be coated with honey before insertion. May be used similarly with all medical equipment that is being inserted into the human body.

Finding Honey

There is almost always someone in every local area that produces local wildflower honey. Many grocery stores carry it. However, recent research on store-bought honeys in the United States has found that up to 75 percent of them cannot genuinely be considered "honey." Many manufacturers remove all pollen from the honey. Sometimes it is then adulterated with corn syrup. Researchers found, however, *all* honey from farmers' markets, food co-ops, and natural food stores to be the real thing. Good honey should *always* contain a bit of pollen, which will make it appear slightly cloudy to the eye.[4]

DIRECT APPLICATION

For burns (first, second, and third degree): Direct application full
    strength, covered by sterile bandage, changed once or twice daily.

For ulcerations, bedsores (even to the bone): Same as for burns.

For infected wounds: Same as for burns.

For wounds: Same as for burns.

For impetigo: Dilute honey enough to use as a wash, then apply
    2x daily.

For seborrheic dermatitis: Same as for impetigo.

INTERNAL USE

As a preventive: Take 1 tablespoon, undiluted or in tea, 3x daily.

For acute conditions: Take 1 tablespoon honey each hour, or 1 table-
    spoon in tea 6–10x daily.

Best colds and flu tea: 2 tablespoons ginger juice, juice of ¼ lime,
    pinch cayenne pepper, 1 tablespoon honey, hot water.

Side Effects and Contraindications

External use: None.

Internal use: Mild to severe anaphylaxis in rare instances for those
    with allergic reactions to bee stings.

Traditional Uses of Honey

I have used honey in healing for over 20 years now; there is nothing
comparable for treating wounds of any sort, no matter how infected or
bad they are. It is *the* premier wound healer on this planet.

    Honey is the nectar of the flowers of plants, gathered by the bee,
and stored in its stomach for transport to the hive. Natural honeys are
from a profusion of wildflowers, whatever grows locally. With natural
honeys it is exceedingly uncommon to have a honey gathered from
a single species of plant such as the alfalfa or clover honeys of today
unless that plant species exists in great abundance (as heather does in
Scotland). As such, natural bee honeys generally possess the essence
of a multitude of wild plants — all of them medicinal. Honeybees have

a strong attraction to many strongly medicinal plants: vitex, jojoba, elder, toadflax, balsam root, echinacea, valerian, dandelion, wild geranium; in fact almost any flowering medicinal herb, as well as the more commonly known alfalfas and clovers. The nectar from a multitude of medicinal plants is present in any wildflower honey mix and so are whatever chemical constituents were present in the nectars. In addition to the plants' medicinal qualities, the plant nectars are subtly altered, in ways that modern science has been unable to explain, by their brief transport in the bees' digestive system. Before regurgitation the nectars combine in unique ways with the bees' digestive enzymes to produce new compounds. Honey, often insisted to be just another simple carbohydrate (like white sugar), actually contains, among other things, a complex assortment of enzymes, organic acids, esters, antibiotic agents, trace minerals, proteins, carbohydrates, hormones, and antimicrobial compounds. One pound of the average honey contains 1,333 calories (compared to white sugar at 1,748 calories), 1.4 grams of protein, 23 mg of calcium, 73 mg of phosphorus, 4.1 mg of iron, 1 mg of niacin, and 16 mg of vitamin C, along with vitamin A, beta-carotene, the complete complex of B vitamins, vitamin D, vitamin E, vitamin K, magnesium, sulphur, chlorine, potassium, iodine, sodium, copper, manganese, and high concentrations of hydrogen peroxide and formic acid. Honey, in fact, contains over 75 different compounds. Many of the remaining substances in honey (comprising 4 percent to 7 percent of the honey) are so complex that they have yet to be identified.

Scientific Research

In the years since the first edition of this book was published, honey has become a significant medical treatment for surgical wounds, wound healing, and burns in hospitals, especially in the UK. It has become, in fact, a major part of standard-practice medicine there — in part because of the spread of resistant organisms, against which honey is reliably effective. Many clinical trials (over 30) have been conducted on its use. Here are a few of them, from the UK and elsewhere.

Thirty-two children with pyomyositis abscesses were split into two randomized treatment groups. The abscess cavities were packed twice daily with either honey- or Eusol-soaked gauze. Honey-treated wounds healed faster, and length of time in the hospital was shorter, than those treated with Eusol.

Eighty-eight people were enrolled in a nonrandomized, open-label, side-by-side comparison of various forms of second-intention healing of donor site for split-thickness skin grafts. Honey-impregnated gauzes showed faster epithelization time and a lower level of pain than the other methods used.

A trial with 60 patients with chronic complicated surgical or acute traumatic wounds found that honey was easy to apply, kept the wounds clean, stopped infection, and was exceptionally safe.

One hundred and five people participated in a single-center, open-label, randomized, controlled trial in the treatment of honey for wounds. The honey-treated group's wounds healed significantly faster, in 100 days compared to 140 for the control group.

One hundred and eight people with venous leg ulcers engaged in a multicenter, open-label, randomized, controlled trial of honey treatment compared with IntraSite Gel. There was increased incidence of healing, effective desloughing, and lower infection rates in the honey-treated group. Other trials have found similar outcomes.

Fifteen people with pressure ulcers were treated with honey and 11 with ethoxy-diaminoacridine plus nitrofurazone dressings. Honey group healing was approximately four times that of the pharmaceutical group.

Only one of 20 patients in a honey group developed intolerable oral mucositis when receiving radiation, a better outcome than with lignocaine.

Other studies have replicated this.

Thirty infected diabetic foot wounds were treated with honey for 3 months. Complete healing was achieved in 43 percent of wounds treated, and decrease in size of ulceration and healthy granulation were observed in another 43 percent. The bacterial load in all ulcers was significantly reduced after the first week of honey dressing. Failure of treatment occurred in 6.7 percent. A number of other studies have been conducted on the treatment of diabetic foot ulcers and all have found comparable outcomes. For example: 60 people with limb-threatening diabetic infections were split into three groups: 1) full-thickness skin ulcer; 2) deep-tissue infection and osteomyelitis; 3) gangrenous lesions. All ulcers in group 1 healed and 92 percent of those in group 2 healed. All people in group 3 healed after surgical excision, debridement of necrotic tissue, and treatment with honey ointment (which also included royal jelly).

Seventy-eight people (ages 10 to 50) with burns on less than 50 percent of the body were split into two groups, one receiving honey dressings, the other silver sulfadiazine (SSD). Average healing duration in honey-treated patients was 18 days, with SSD it was 33 days. Wounds in all who received treatment within 1 hour of the burn and were treated with honey became sterile in less than 7 days. None in the SSD group did. All honey-treated wounds became sterile within 21 days but only 36 percent of those in the SSD group did within that time span. Outcomes were significantly better for the honey group. There was faster healing, no infection, less scarring and postburn contractures, and significantly decreased need for debridement irrespective of when the patients was admitted for treatment.

A randomized, double-blind, clinical trial among goldmine workers in South Africa was carried out using honey to treat shallow wounds and abrasions. Honey was found to be just as effective as IntraSite Gel in healing. The cost of the honey was approximately 49 cents (South African rand) versus 12.03 for the pharmaceutical.

In a clinical trial using honey to treat labial herpes, the duration of attacks, degree of pain, occurrence of crusting, and mean healing time with honey were found to be 35 percent, 39 percent, 28 percent, and 43 percent better respectively than with acyclovir treatment. With genital herpes the results were 53 percent, 50 percent, 49 percent, and 59 percent better respectively.

Thirty people (20 male, 10 female) with seborrheic dermatitis and dandruff were treated with a topical application of raw honey. The patients had presented with scaling, itching, and hair loss. Diluted raw honey (90 percent honey diluted with warm water into a manageable wash) was used every other day for 4 weeks and left on for 3 hours before rinsing with warm water. Half the patients acted as controls. In all the people using honey, itching was relieved and scaling disappeared, all within 1 week, and hair loss was reduced. Within 2 weeks skin lesions healed and disappeared. The honey-treated patients were treated prophylactically for 6 months afterward with one application of honey per week. None of the 15 patients treated with honey relapsed.

In a clinical trial of 139 children, honey was found to be more effective than dextromethorphan and diphenhydramine in alleviating nighttime cough due to upper respiratory infections. (Other studies have found the drugs and honey to be relatively equal in their effects. Parents, though, have generally reported honey to be better than the pharmaceuticals.)

Honey as a consistent additive to food has shown remarkable results in medical trials. Of one group of 58 boys, 29 were given 2 tablespoons of honey each day (one in the morning and one in the evening), and the other 29 boys were given none. All received the same diet, exercise, and rest. All were the same age and general health. The group receiving honey (after 1 year) showed an 8.5 percent increase in hemoglobin and an overall increase in vitality, energy, and general appearance.

Honey has been effectively used clinically for the treatment of ulceration to the bone the size of a human fist and third-degree burns. Complete healing has consistently been reported without the need for skin grafts and with no infection or muscle loss. Additionally honey has outperformed antibiotics in the treatment of stomach ulceration, gangrene, surgical wound infections, surgical incisions, and the protection of skin grafts, corneas, blood vessels, and bones during storage and shipment.

Honey is also exceptionally effective in respiratory ailments. A Bulgarian study of 17,862 patients found that honey was effective in improving chronic bronchitis, asthmatic bronchitis, bronchial asthma, chronic and allergic rhinitis, and sinusitis. It is effective in the treatment of colds, flu and respiratory infections, and general depressed immune problems.

Results have been good in clinical practice as well. The department of pediatric oncology at Children's Hospital at the University of Bonn regularly uses honey in the healing of wounds impaired by chemotherapy and has found it highly successful.

There have been a number of clinical reports of the use of honey by physicians in the treatment of various wounds:

Treatment of eight patients with leg ulceration used honey. Ulcer size decreased by 60 percent, odor was eliminated, pain reduced.

A chronic wound in a patient with dystrophis epidermolysis bullosa was treated. The wound, despite many treatments, had never closed in 20 years. A honey-impregnated dressing closed and healed the wound in 15 weeks.

Treatment of a patient with long-standing venous leg ulcer resulted in total healing. The honey was effectively antibiotic, anti-inflammatory, and deodorizing.

Six patients with chronic venous leg ulcers who underwent split-skin grafts experienced healing in 22 days without complications.

Two nursing-home patients with pressure ulcers were treated with honey. There was a rapid healing of the ulcers, and pain and odor were significantly reduced.

Twenty-eight cases of Fournier's gangrene were treated. Honey was found to accelerate wound healing in the six patients in whom it was used.

A woman with extensive phlegmonous and necrotic lesions in the abdominal integuments after a traumatic rupture of the colon was successfully treated with honey. Complete wound healing was achieved.

A man with pyoderma gangrenosum and ulcerative colitis (in the tropics) had his skin lesions successfully treated with honey.

Seven people with MRSA-infected wounds were treated with honey after antibiotics failed to eradicate the infection. All were successfully treated.

There have been scores of in vivo studies on the wound-healing actions of honey, with some 600 animals. In the treatment of auricular burn, induced wounds (incision, excision, burn, dead-space wounds), surgical wounds, bacterial infection of burns, burn contraction, and bite wounds, honey was found to be exceptionally effective. Intraurethral honey application healed urethral injury in Wistar male rats. It promotes angiogenic activity in rat aorta. The immune systems of rats fed fennel honey, propolis, and bee venom were more protected against induced staph infection than those of controls. Intraperitoneal honey administration prevents post-operative peritoneal adhesions. Honey promotes intestinal anastomotic wound healing in rats with obstructive jaundice. Following bowel resection, oral honey was effective in stimulating healing and reducing infection.

Honey has been found in vitro to be immune stimulating, skin regenerating, anti-inflammatory, antibacterial, antiviral, antifungal, antioxidant, free-radical scavenging, immunomodulatory, and antimutagenic. Antibacterial activity has been found effective with as little as a 4 percent honey solution. Full strength is better.

Salves made with honey, beeswax, and olive oil have been found effective against staph and *Candida* organisms.

Note: Raw wildflower honey should be used, *not* the clover or alfalfa honey readily available in grocery stores. Alfalfa and clover crops are heavily sprayed with pesticides *and* they do not have the broad activity available in multiple-plant honeys. Further, large commercial honey growers may often supplement their bees' food with sugar water, which dilutes the honey's power. Pure wildflower honey should lightly burn or sting the back of the throat when taken undiluted.

Usnea

Family: Parmeliaceae, but some people insist the usneas are in their own family, the Usneaceae. Most sources consider that to be unacceptable as well as completely wrong. (Fisticuffs at 10:00 P.M.)

Common Names: *Old man's beard or a number of similar phrases to do with hair or beard*

Species Used: There are 600 or so species of usnea. *Usnea barbata* and *U. longissima* are the most common, but any *Usnea* species will do. I prefer the smaller, tufted species (generally *Usnea hirta*) rather than *longissima*; I feel they are stronger in their actions; however, due to the larger size of *longissima*, it is the most commonly harvested species. (The others take hours.) *Usnea barbata* is also fairly good-sized, but there is currently some potential for that species to be banned for use in the United States even though it is a very safe plant (see Side Effects and Contraindications, page 200).

Part Used

Whole lichen.

Preparation and Dosage

It has taken some time to learn how to properly prepare *Usnea* for use. Ryan Drum, an herbalist in Washington State, was most responsible for providing understanding of how to generate the best immune-stimulating activity of the plant.

Properties of *Usnea*

Actions

Analgesic
Antibacterial
Antifungal
Anti-inflammatory
Antimitotic
Antineoplastic (cancer)
Antioxidant

Antiparasitic
Antiproliferative
  (cancer)
Antiprotozoal
Antiseptic
Antiviral

Drug synergist
  (potentiates
  clarithromycin
  against *H. Pylori*)
Immunostimulant
Inhibitor of biofilm
  formation

Active Against

Primarily Gram-positive bacteria, and very strongly so, both resistant and nonresistant strains:

Bacillus megaterium
Bacillus subtilis
Bacteroides spp.
Clostridium spp.
*Corynebacterium
  diphtheriae*
Enterococcus faecalis

Enterococcus faecium
Listeria monocytogenes
Micrococcus viridans
*Mycobacterium
  tuberculosis*
Propionbacterium acnes
Staphylococcus aureus

*Staphylococcus
  simulans*
Streptococcus faecalis
Streptococcus mutans
Streptococcus pyogenes

A number of these bacteria cause diseases of the GI tract, others of the skin.

Usnea species have been found active, in a number of in vitro studies, against a few Gram-negative bacteria: *Helicobacter pylori*, *E. coli*, *Yersinia enterocolitica*, and *Proteus mirabilis*. Interestingly, the first three of these cause infections in the GI tract, for which *Usnea* will be useful as it is not a highly systemic herb. The latter bacteria generally cause urinary infections.

Usnea is active against a number of viruses: herpes simplex, polyoma-virus (a tumor virus), Junin virus, Tacaribe virus, and Epstein-Barr.

It is active against a number of parasitical disease organisms: *Trypanosoma cruzi*, *Echinococcus granulosus* (and its cysts), and *Toxoplasma gondii*. And some yeasts: *Malassezia* yeasts, *Microsporum gypseum*, *Trichophyton mentagrophytes*, *T. rubrum*, and several *Candida* species.

Usnea and usnic acid are active against a number of cancer cell lines: lung and breast, malignant mesothelioma cells, and vulvar carcinoma cells.

CONTINUED ON NEXT PAGE

PROPERTIES OF USNEA, CONTINUED

Use to Treat

Resistant Gram-positive bacterial skin infections, vaginal infections (as a douche), resistant Gram-positive bacterial or TB infections of the GI tract and throat, fungal skin infections, resistant bronchial and pulmonary infections caused by Gram-positive bacteria or TB, conjunctivitis (as eyedrops).

Finding *Usnea*

It grows in nearly every forest or orchard if you just look for it. It is widely available on the Internet through herbal suppliers.

In essence, the polysaccharides in the inner cortex of the lichen contain the immune-potentiating compounds. These are much more efficiently extracted by heat. Given that the plant possesses a unique synergism — both immune-potentiating and antibacterial, antiviral, and antimicrobial actions — it makes sense, if you are using the plant to treat disease (rather than infected wounds or vaginal infections), to make sure the immune fractions of the plant are extracted along with the antibacterial fractions.

Additionally, while the polysaccharides are water soluble, many other compounds, including usnic acid, are not. The plant needs to be tinctured for optimum outcomes if you are treating disease conditions.

The plant appears rather delicate, but it is not. The plant must be ground well in a grinder or pestle before tincturing. Once it is ground you will find that you now possess a greenish powder and a bundle of white threads. The white threads are the inner cortex, the green powder the outer sheath.

WOUND POWDER

If you are treating wounds with *Usnea,* run the ground herb through a fine mesh or strainer. You can place the resulting powder directly on the wound or mix with other powdered herbs for a stronger blend. (You will have a bunch of white threads left over.)

TINCTURE

Again, the immune-stimulating polysaccharides are most efficiently extracted with heat. To do this, when you are making your tincture, heat the herb first in the water you are going to use for tincturing. The best way is in a slow cooker (or, failing that, on low heat, covered, overnight in the oven).

Use a tincture ratio of 1:5 (1 part herb to 5 parts liquid). (See chapter 8 for more on this.) The liquid should be composed of half water and half pure grain alcohol. So if you have 5 ounces of herb, you will use 25 ounces of liquid — 12.5 of water, 12.5 of alcohol.

Put the powdered herb in the slow cooker, add the 12.5 ounces of water, and stir well. It will turn into a kind of mush. Cover and then cook on low heat for 48 hours. Let cool enough to work with it without burning yourself, then pour into a heat-tolerant jar (Mason or equivalent), add the alcohol when the mix is still warm but not hot, and then put on the lid and shake well. Let macerate for 2 weeks, then decant and strain out the herb. Bottle and store out of the light.

Tincture dosage: 30–60 drops, up to 4x daily; or in acute conditions, ½–1 tsp, 3–6x daily.

As a douche: Add ½ ounce tincture to 1 pint water, and mix well. Use as douche or skin wash. Douche twice daily, upon rising and before retiring, for 3 days.

As a wash: For impetigo (staph or strep infections of the skin), put the tincture, or a 1:1 dilution of the tincture with water, directly on the site of infection (using a cotton ball or cloth). Wash the site upon rising and before bed.

As a nasal spray: Combine 10 drops of tincture with water in a 1-ounce nasal spray bottle. Use as needed for bacterial infections of the nose and sinuses.

TEA

Combine 1 teaspoon herb with 6 ounces hot water; let steep 20 minutes.

For disease prevention or immune stimulation: Drink 2–6 ounces, up to 3x daily.

In acute conditions: Drink up to 1 quart a day.

Note: Usnea is only partially water soluble. To make the strongest tea or decoction: Grind the herb first, then add enough alcohol to wet the herb and let it sit, covered, for 30 minutes to an hour. Then add hot water and let steep for 15–30 minutes.

Side Effects and Contraindications

Should not be used internally during pregnancy. May cause contact dermatitis.

Usnea has been found to readily absorb heavy metals in potentially toxic amounts. This has been noted as particularly problematic in extreme northern latitudes. Generally, the amount of usnea taken internally will not contain sufficient amounts of heavy metals to present a problem. In order to avoid problems, harvest usnea at least 300 feet (90 m) from roads, factories, polluted areas.

Note: There has been concern expressed in a number of forums about the toxicity of usnic acid. The problem, once more, has arisen through the improper use of an isolated constituent for weight loss. This has led to calls for the banning of usnea as an herb in the United States.

As usual, the promoters of the isolated constituent for weight loss were engaging in practices that are highly questionable ethically. They sold , and heavily hyped, the isolated constituent of usnea, usnic acid, as a weight-loss product. Unfortunately usnic acid in isolation and in large doses is very toxic to the liver. Several people died, others needed liver transplants. As a result the National Toxicity Program recommended a review of the toxicity of not only usnic acid but also *Usnea barbata*. Unfortunately, given the bias of the FDA, the odds are high that *Usnea barbata* will also be found to be unsafe for general use — when it in fact is not.

Usnic acid should never be used in isolation. The usnea lichens, however, are extremely safe for herbal use. More on the controversy can be found in "Safety Issues Affecting Herbs," by S. Dharmananda (see the bibliography).

Herb/Drug Interactions

Usnea is synergistic with clarithromycin, increasing its effectiveness.

Habitat and Appearance

Usnea grows on trees throughout the world, on every continent. Generally prefers conifers (pine, spruce, juniper, firs), deciduous hardwoods (oak, hickory, walnut, apple, pear, and so on), and the odd variant such as coconut palms.

Collection

Usnea is an extremely prolific though slow-growing, long-lived, gray to yellow-green lichen growing on trees throughout the world. The whole lichen may be harvested at any time. Again, I prefer the small, tiny tufted species that grow in the forests around where I live. They take longer to harvest, but they are not endangered and, I feel, are more potent than *U. longissima* and *U. barbata*.

Endangered status: While *Usnea longissima* is prolific in some areas, in others (California, northeast United States, Europe, Scandinavian countries) it is endangered. Logging and development have destroyed its main habitat, old-growth forests. It is also very sensitive to pollution and climate change. *U. longissima* is the *Usnea* species most often sold by herbal companies and most commonly wildcrafted because of its size, which ranges up to 3 feet (1 meter) in length. This species should *not* be sold by commercial companies nor bought from them by anyone. It should be harvested only for personal use from regions where it is in abundance. Again, *any* species of *Usnea* will do.

Lichen Chemistry

Usnic acid is the main constituent that everyone talks about; it is a potent chemical, highly antibacterial. *Usnea* species contain anywhere from 0.22 to 6.49 percent usnic acid. *U. longissima* is reported to have the most usnic acid content. However, many of the other constituents of the usneas are strongly antibacterial; hirtusneanoside and vulpinic acid are a couple of them.

In addition to usnic acid, usnea contains vulpinic acid, protolichesterinic acid, a number of orcinol derivatives, longissiminone A and B, glutinol, ethyl hematommate, friedelin, beta-amyrin, beta-sitosterol, methyl-2,4-dihydroxy-3,6-dimethylbenzoate, barbatinic acid, zeorin, ethyl orsellinate, 3-beta-hydroxy-glutin-5-ene, oleanolic acid, methylorsellinate, benzaldehyde, dibenzofuran, anthraquinone, hirtusneanoside, menegazziaic acid, stictic acid, glyceryl trilinolate, numerous polysaccharides including isolichenin, raffinose, numerous phenolic compounds, usnaric acid, thamnolic acid, lobaric acid, stictinic acid, and a lot of other stuff. About 50 percent of the plant is water-soluble polysaccharides.

One of the more interesting developments in the medicinal chemistry of lichens is the recognition that lichens often harbor diverse fungi that themselves are highly bioactive. Some of the fungi are harbored on the outside surfaces, others are lichenicolous — they fruit from the lichen thalli. But some of the most interesting are endolichenic fungi — they live within the lichen thalli. One lichen, *Letharietum vulpinae*, has over a thousand fungal strains living on and within it. Usneas also contain numerous fungal strains and these strains also possess bioactivity when used medicinally. An associated fungus from *Usnea cavernosa*, for example, has been found to contain some unusual compounds: corynesporol, dehydroherbarin, and herbarin. Dehydroherbarin potently inhibits the migration of cancer cell lines in vitro and, along with herbarin, possesses weak antiamoebic and antimicrobial activity.

Again, plants (or lichens as in this case) are exceptionally complex; their full chemical range is unlikely to ever be completely understood. Nevertheless, they are potently synergistic in their chemical actions. Some of the actions attributable to usnea are likely from associated fungal strains.

Traditional Uses of Usnea

Commonly called old man's beard, a name derived from its appearance, usnea is a lichen that grows on living and dead trees throughout the world. It is quite common in North America, Europe, Asia, and Africa (less so in South America and Australia) and this wide availability and its strong antibacterial properties make it a significant herb in treating resistant bacteria.

Usnea ranges in size from a small tuft to large hanging strands resembling hair. It may be a gray-green in the smaller species and a mild yellow-green in the larger hanging strands. As a lichen, the herb is in actuality a symbiote composed of two plants intertwined. The inner part of the plant (the cortex) is a thin white thread (a filamentous fungi) that, when wet, stretches like a rubber band. The outer part — the sheath or thallus — (an algae) gives the herb its color and grows round the inner rubber-band-like cortex. The algae (cyanobacteria in some types of lichen) is a photobiont, providing photosynthesis for the symbiotic organism. The filamentous fungi (a mycobiont) provides water and minerals.

The distinctive method of identifying usnea is wetting it and stretching it to see if it is springy and, when it snaps apart, looking for the distinctive white thread of the inner plant. This inner band is strongly immune stimulating; the outer sheath is where most of the plant's (yeah, I know, it's a lichen) other actions (e.g., antibacterial) come from.

Usnea has been traditionally used throughout the world for skin infections, abscesses, upper respiratory and lung infections, vaginal infections, and fungal infections. The lichen (*U. longissima* in this case), sometimes soaked in garlic juice or a strong garlic decoction (sometimes not), is an older medical method of treating large gaping wounds in the body (Spanish moss was also used this way). The moss absorbs blood and provides, along with the garlic, antibacterial, anti-inflammatory, antiseptic, astringent, analgesic, and wound-healing actions directly inside the wound.

Usnea is used for abscesses in veterinary practice in Canada.

AYURVEDA

There are some 30 species of usnea that grow in India, among them *Usnea complanata, U. ghattensis*, and *U. emidotteries*. They have been used in traditional practice, but I can find little on the particulars.

TRADITIONAL CHINESE MEDICINE

Generally called *songluo* (sometimes *haifengteng*), usnea species, primarily *diffracta* (sometimes *longissima*), are used to clear heat in the body and to clear the liver of sthenic heat. Usnea is used for the treatment of cough due to hot phlegm, conjunctivitis, headache, carbuncle, lymph node TB. It is considered to be antipyretic, mucolytic, detoxicant, anti-inflammatory, and analgesic.

WESTERN BOTANIC PRACTICE
Of ancient use in Europe but unknown in the United States until relatively recently. Indigenous cultures in the Americas used the usnea lichens primarily for wound dressings.

Scientific Research

Most of the scientific studies have focused on usnic acid — essentially trying to develop pharmaceutical drugs given the constituent's strong antibacterial activity. Nearly all the work has been in vitro. There have been no clinical trials using the herb and very few in vivo studies. There have been a few clinical trials in China using either usnic acid or its sodium salt, sodium usnate.

In clinical trials with sodium usnate in the treatment of pulmonary and intestinal TB, clinicians found that there was rapid improvement of cough, anorexia, fever, and diarrhea. Microscopic examinations after 14 days were negative for the tubercule bacillus. In one trial with 30 cases of pulmonary TB using sodium usnate, 24 were cured, 1 had marked improvement, 5 improved. Average treatment length was 71 days, dosage was 30 mg three times daily.

In another trial, 203 cases of chronic bronchitis were effectively treated with either usnic acid or sodium usnate. The compounds showed strong antitussive, expectorant, and antiasthmatic effects.

In the treatment of surgical suppurative wounds, sodium usnate stimulated the separation of necrotic tissue and the growth of new tissue. It was strongly disinfectant and anti-erosive, stimulating the healing of second- and third-degree burns, cervical erosion, and cracked nipples. It was found effective in the treatment of trichomonas vaginitis.

In veterinary practice a 1 percent alcohol solution of usnic acid was used effectively for treating suppurative conjunctivitis, endometritis, mastitis, and suppurative wounds in cows and horses.

Usnic acid, at a dose of 20 mg once or twice daily for 6 days, then 10 mg daily for an additional 25 days, stopped the development of experimental TB in guinea pigs. It stopped the development of pathological tissues in spleen, liver, and lungs of guinea pigs who had usnic acid added to their diet.

Two studies focused on the gastric-mucosa-protective actions of two of the plant's constituents: usnic acid and diffractaic acid. Diffractaic acid inhibited gastric mucosal lesions, oxidative stress, and neutrophil infiltration. Usnic acid prevented indomethacin-induced gastric ulcers in mice and was found to be highly antioxidant. A water extract of *U. longissima* also prevented that form of induced gastric ulcer in rats and was found to be a strong antioxidant. A methanol extract of *U. longissima* prevented pulmonary thrombosis in rats, and prevented platelet aggregation in vitro. In other studies, the anti-inflammatory activity of various usnea species has been found to be as strong as, and sometimes superior to, that of phenylbutazone and hydrocortisone hemisuccinate, the analgesic action as strong as that of noraminophenazone, and the antipyretic activity as strong as (or stronger than) that of aminophenazone. Usnea is active in both acute and chronic inflammation in rats and significantly accelerates skin wound healing, again in rats. The methanolic extract of *U. ghattensis* was found to be hepatoprotective in rats against ethanol-induced toxicity.

Usnea possesses antioxidant actions, is a strong superoxide and free radical, and is active in preventing lipid peroxidation. *Usnea barbata* extracts inhibit prostaglandin E2 synthesis and COX-2 expression in vitro and appear to be protective of keratinocytes when exposed to ultraviolet B. Usnea possesses strong wound-closure activity in vitro. Both usnic and diffractaic acid have shown antipyretic and analgesic actions in vivo.

Usnea and usnic acid, in vitro and in vivo, inhibit cancer cell formation and proliferation in breast and pancreatic cell lines and in induced colorectal cancer in rats. Crude extracts of *Usnea fasciata* showed up to 90 percent inhibition of sarcoma 180 and Ehrlich tumor cells in vitro.

In general, there has been little clinical research on the effectiveness of traditional uses of usnea. In clinical practice, however, I have found the herb very effective for topical use in the treatment of resistant bacteria, as a douche, and for urinary tract infections.

6

HERBAL ANTIBIOTICS:
THE SYNERGISTS

Sometimes it seems as if doses of supposed active constituents are too low to have an effect, and in the absence of clinical proof this has led sceptics to dismiss these medicines as mere placebos. . . . It is still routine to investigate and extract medicinal plants with a view to finding the single chemical entity responsible for the effect, and this may lead to inconclusive findings. If a combination of substances is needed for the effect, then the bioassay-led method of investigation, narrowing activity down firstly to a fraction and eventually a compound, is doomed to failure, and this has led to the suggestion that the plants are in fact devoid of activity. . . . When activity is thought to be lost through purification, synergy should be suspected.
— **Dr. Elizabeth Williamson, "Synergy and Other Interactions in Phytomedicines" (*Phytomedicine* 8, no. 5 [2001])**

All investigations have shown that most of the extracts and individual constituents thereof exert multivalent or pleiotropic pharmacological effects (this multivalance of pharmacological activities can generate additive or overadditive, potentiated synergistic effects). . . . The synergistic effects that have been measured exceed the effects of single compounds, or mixtures of them at equivalent concentrations, by a factor of two to four, or more.
— **Dr. Hildebert Wagner, "Natural Products Chemistry and Phytomedicine in the 21st Century" (*Pure and Applied Chemistry* 77, no. 1 [2005])**

Synergy, in its simplest definition, means that the combination of two (or more) things produces outcomes greater than the sum of the individual parts and, additionally, that those outcomes *cannot* be predicted from a study of the individual parts themselves. Individual plants, because of their complex chemistry, are highly synergistic organisms by themselves. If plants are used in combination, the complexity, and resultant synergy, increases substantially.

Within older healing traditions such as traditional Chinese medicine (TCM) and Ayurveda, the inherent synergistic nature of plant medicinals and plant combinations is an integrated aspect of healing. Those systems, over millennia, developed their own language and understanding of plants as synergists. A similar understanding, using our own Western terminology and perspectives, has been lacking in our medical approaches — herbal or otherwise.

Medical technologists (usually from the younger generations) have slowly begun to move away from the dogma of monotherapy — that is, the use of a single compound to treat disease. It's not that they inherently wanted to or that they innately understood that the system in which they were trained was flawed. Their change, as it is with most of us, was driven by events occurring in the outside world that they could no longer ignore; mainly, the emergence of multidrug-resistant microorganisms and AIDS.

AIDS (along with cancer), because of its spread, its disease dynamics, and its amazing adaptability, has forced a shift from a monotherapy frame to that of a multi-target paradigm of therapeutics. Multi-target therapies not only focus on killing the disease organism — which with AIDS and cancers are often futile — but also focus deeply on activating the natural defense, protective, and repair mechanisms in the body. In other words they also stimulate immune responses to disease and, as well, the body's own highly elegant repair mechanisms.

The emergence of multidrug-resistant bacteria has also been a factor in challenging the monotherapy paradigm. As fast as new pharmaceuticals were developed for resistant organisms, new resistance emerged. Physicians learned, eventually, that if they combined therapies, for example if they used antimalarial drug combinations, the development of malarial resistance could be delayed. (Not stopped, mind you, just delayed.) But that recognition opened up the understanding that complex drug therapies were much more effective against the disease and, as well, could slow down and, presumably if they were elegant enough, stop resistance development altogether. The use of artemisinin combination therapy (ACT) is a product of that understanding. At a very crude, simplistic level these approaches by medical technologists are beginning to mimic the actions of plant medicines, as well as older systems of healing such as TCM.

Changes in Western Monotherapy

Western herbalists have never been completely captured by the monotherapy paradigm, though they have often been strongly influenced, and sometimes fully seduced, by it. Medical (and naturopathic) herbalists, for example, since they often tend to mimic a medical reductionist model, generally lean much more strongly toward monotherapeutic thinking. They often lose sight of plant complexities in the search for "active" constituents and standardized herbs.

Community herbalists, like their counterparts in all third- (and some second-) world countries, tend to be more cognizant of plant complexities and subtleties, in part simply because they haven't been trained to believe they know some ultimate truth about the nature of plant medicines or reality as a whole. Most of them consider plants to be an expression of the general intelligence and livingness of Nature. They never have felt plants to be insentient substances that can be analyzed and completely understood by science and then used however human beings wish.

All Western herbalists, no matter their orientation, do know that plants are much safer than pharmaceuticals, that they tend to produce more complex effects in the body than pharmaceuticals, and that they need to be part of a more complex treatment regimen, one that also includes immune regeneration and support for the body's natural repair mechanisms. Herbalists just naturally tend to be more multi-target-therapy oriented than the majority of physicians. And most Western herbalists, not all, understand that whole-plant extracts are often more effective than isolated constituents and that plant combinations are often more effective than single-plant extracts.

In spite of this, Western herbalists as a group have nearly no understanding of synergy in plant medicines. Those few that do have some sense of it tend to speak of it in such vague terms that the concept is virtually useless. Part of the problem is simply that the concept hasn't had any developed presence in the herbal literature. It is hard to think about something you have never heard about. Another very common problem is the fear of sounding too "New-Agey" or "airy-fairy" — translation: not "scientific" enough. Herbalists, like all other people on the planet, do want to be accepted by their culture; the pervasiveness of such a widespread reductionist paradigm has had the (often intended) effect of causing people to censor their own thoughts. Thus the long-term herbal mimicry of the monotherapy paradigm in both the United States and Europe that has had such a tenacious and negative influence on the field.

> Medical herbalists often lose sight of plant complexities in the search for "active" constituents.

More deeply problematical, the majority of Western herbalists simply have not spent much time developing *their own* particular in-depth understanding of plant medicines, nor have they trusted themselves enough to support the modern development of *their own* unique system — a system that has very old roots in numerous indigenous cultures in the Americas, the older European cultures (Greek and Roman, for instance), and that of community herbalists nearly everywhere. Instead, most have mimicked older systems (TCM, for instance) or taken on the trappings of the newer system of technological medicine. They have spent decades trying to force their unique Western system, a system of which they have some sense every day of their lives, into those forms. (The American herbalist Michael Moore was a major exception to that trend.) Square peg into round hole living. It is time to *own* our own unique system, without embarrassment, without pretending or trying to be what we are not.

There are many aspects to our emerging Western herbal paradigm that need to be developed in depth; one of those is the understanding of plant synergy. This chapter is an early beginning, however brief or incomplete, in attempting to address it.

Understanding Plant Synergies

In the sense I am using the concept here, plant synergists act to increase the activity of other plants used for healing while affecting the body itself through a number of other, supportive actions. They do this through a wide range of mechanisms:

- They act to reduce toxic side effects of primary constituents.
- They increase depth and broadness of constituent penetration by among other things increasing intracellular transport.
- They enhance constituent activity by acting at different points of the same signaling cascade.
- They decrease the effective dose needed for cure.

Certain plant compounds alter the pharmacological actions of others, change their physicochemical properties, influencing biochemical parameters such as solubility, bioavailabilty, and activity. Some compounds enhance immune responses while others attack microbial organisms, weakening them and making them more susceptible to the heightened immune system. And still others specifically work to reduce viral and bacterial defenses to antimicrobial plant constituents so that the plant's antibacterial and antiviral compounds are more effective.

Plants suffer bacterial and viral infection, just like we do. One of the things they do to deal with bacterial infections is produce antibacterial substances such as berberine in order to deal with them. Correspondingly, all bacteria, to differing degrees, have learned to deal with antimicrobial substances, most simply, to protect themselves from antimicrobial attack. One way they do this is to utilize multidrug-resistance pumps. MDRs act to pump antibacterial substances that get into a bacterial cell out again. In response, plants, over time, innovated chemical constituents that would deactivate MDRs.

Berberis fremontii (also known as *Mahonia fremontii*), one of the berberine-containing plants, for example, contains a compound, 5'-methoxyhydnocarpin (5'MHC), that is a potent MDR inhibitor of the efflux pump found in some Gram-positive bacteria, especially staphylococci. The plant then, when used medicinally, acts synergistically. One compound, 5'MHC, inactivates the MDR in the staph organisms, and another, berberine, kills the bacteria. (And yet another compound in the plant, porphyrin pheophorbide A, acts synergistically with both of them to kill MRSA organisms.) Sublethal doses of berberine, in numerous experiments, when combined with 5'MHC, become decidedly lethal. The compound 5'MHC itself has no antibacterial activity at all. Not surprisingly 5'MHC is common among the berberine-containing plants.

Because of the nature of this book, I am going to primarily explore plants that contain potent efflux inhibitors that deactivate those particular bacterial resistance mechanisms and, as well, plants that allow more effective penetration of plant compounds into the body. The field is still new; there isn't a lot to work with yet, but I hope that this chapter will give you a good idea of the complexity that is possible when looking at synergists. I hope it will stimulate you to deepen the work yourself, for all of us are going to need to know these things.

Something to keep in mind: herbalism is and always will remain an art. Analytical knowledge, while important, has to be combined with a *feeling* for the craft, for the plants, for the people who come to us for help, and . . . for the bacterial organisms themselves. From this comes art . . . and the ability to truly reason while at the same time developing a genuine capacity to heal.

As I've said before, we need both feeling *and* thinking for this craft to flourish inside us, and behind it all, a deep and abiding love for the plants and the earth from which they, and we, come.

To begin I'll just look briefly at a few of the synergists that have promise for the future, then I will get into several in more depth and explore how to use them for the treatment of resistant bacterial infections.

A Quick Look at Some Synergistic Plants

Most of the current synergy research taking place is looking at plants and plant compounds that can reverse drug resistance. Unfortunately, for my purposes anyway, most of the resistance-modifying studies that have taken place are looking at reducing the resistance of various forms of cancer to pharmaceuticals. I am not covering those here but am focusing solely on those that have been found to modify resistance in bacteria. MRSA is the bacteria upon which most study of medicinal plants' ability to modify resistance has occurred.

In the list that follows, most of the plants were tested by using an antibiotic on a resistant organism, then adding the plant to the mix and seeing what happened. Once the herb, or its constituent(s), were combined with the antibiotic, the antibiotic either became effective or was so at much reduced levels, usually by a factor of four to eight, though in the case of thyme, the effectiveness threshold of tetracycline against MRSA went from 4 to 0.12 mg/L. Further tests were then conducted to find out just which bacterial efflux pumps were inactivated by the plant.

> Plant synergists increase the activity of other healing plants while supporting the body itself.

Dalea versicolor and ***Dalea spinosa*** both contain substances that are mildly antibacterial but others that specifically inhibit a particular efflux pump (NorA) in multidrug-resistant *Staphylococcus aureus*. They also inhibit the Bmr efflux pump found in *Bacillus subtilis*.

Ipomoea murucoides, Mexican morning glory, contains a number of compounds that are also potent inhibitors of the NorA efflux pump in resistant staph. These are, to date, the most potent inhibitors of NorA found, increasing the effectiveness of antibiotics 16-fold.

Geranium caespitosum also has a potent efflux inhibitor active against MRSA. It potentiates the activity of the plant antimicrobials berberine and rhein as well as the antibiotics ciprofloxacin and nor-floxacin. Other geraniums act similarly; these plants are exceptionally good to combine with berberine in the treatment of GI tract infections such as *E. coli* and cholera.

Cymbopogon citratus, lemongrass, while having only mild anti-bacterial activity itself, is an exceptionally potent synergistic activator of antibiotics against MRSA.

Rauwolfia serpentina and *R. vomitoria* are active against the Bmr efflux pump in *Bacillus subtilis*, the NorA and Tet(K) pumps in MRSA, the PmrA pump in *Streptococcus pneumoniae*, and an ABC transporter that is associated with ciprofloxacin resistance.

Epicatechin gallate and **epigallocatechin gallate**, both in green tea (*Camellia sinensis*), have been found to be highly potent efflux inhibitors for both MRSA and *Staphylococcus epidermidis*. They inhibit both NorA and Tet(K) efflux pumps.

Rosmarinus officinalis (rosemary), *Thymus vulgaris* (thyme), and *Lycopus europaeus* (gypsywort, bugleweed) have been found effective against the Tet(K) efflux pump in *E. coli* and MRSA and the Msr(A) pump in MRSA.

Prosopis juliflora (and other *Prosopis* species — the mesquites), a very good medicinal tree and intense invasive, contains a number of potent piperidine alkaloids, one of which has been found to be a very potent inhibitor of the NorA pump in MRSA.

Extracts of myrrh gum (*Commiphora*), gotu kola (*Centella asiatica*), wild carrot (*Daucus*), licorice, and bitter orange (*Citrus aurantium*) are all effective in inhibiting the AcrAB-TolC efflux transporter that is present in a number of Gram-negative bacteria. (They are especially effective against multidrug-resistant *Salmonella enterica* var. *typhimurium*.) This efflux mechanism is a homologue of the MexAB-OprM efflux transporter that is widely present in resistant

Gram-negative organisms. Both pumps affect a wide range of antibacterials. When used with pharmaceuticals, these plants reduced the MIC (minimum inhibiting concentration) by factors of 4 to 32.

Thymus vulgaris, thyme, inhibits the MexAB-OprM efflux pump and its gene expression. MexAB-OprM is heavily involved in the removal of tetracycline, beta-lactams, fluoroquinolones, chloramphenicol, novobiocin, macrolides, ethidium bromide, aromatic hydrocarbons, and homoserine lactones. Thyme essential oil, in tiny doses, one or two drops, when taken directly by mouth will enter the bloodstream immediately. If combined with herbs such as cryptolepis, it will potentiate their action against Gram-negative bacteria. Remember: *Tiny* doses.

The problem with most of these plants (gotu kola and licorice are exceptions) is that they are not highly systemic; that is, they are only moderately, if at all, present in any quantity in the blood. This makes their use as systemic synergists difficult — though of course they can be used topically and directly in the GI tract.

The next two are *most likely* systemic, though I don't know them well enough to say, and the final one *is* systemic and could be used to a limited extent as a systemic synergist for some resistant bacteria.

Caesalpinia benthamiana (syn. *Mezoneuron benthamianum*) and ***Securinega virosa*** are two fairly important but relatively unknown (to Western herbalists) medicinal plants. The first has a wide activity against both Gram-negative and Gram-positive bacteria and is used to treat dysenteric diseases, and early indications are it may be systemic in nature. The second plant has some similar actions, especially in its wide use for dysenteric diseases. Both are efflux inhibitors. They definitely warrant further study.

Punica granatum (pomegranate), the final plant in this list, is synergistic with ampicillin, chloramphenicol, gentamicin, tetracycline, and oxacillin against 30 different MRSA and MSSA (methicillin-sensitive *Staphylococcous aureus*) strains. The plant extracts inhibit ethidium bromide efflux mechanisms in a number of different types of bacteria. There is also some evidence, not conclusive, that it is effective against the MexAB-OprM efflux pump in Gram-negative bacteria.

Pomegranate is systemic in that many of its constituents are circulated widely in the blood (peak in 1 hour, lasting about 4 hours), but how effective it would be to use it in practice, I don't know. The plant has not been considered to be a synergist in any culture that uses it and really not much as an antibacterial in any of the healing systems I have looked at. It has been used for millennia in Ayurveda but primarily as an astringent (juice) somewhat like cranberry juice, or for intestinal worms (bark/root).

However, recent research is showing some interesting activity in the plant in the treatment of high blood pressure, the prevention of normal cellular degeneration that accompanies aging, reducing DNA damage, and reducing stress levels in the body.

An In-Depth Look at Three Plant Synergists

I will now explore three synergistic plants in detail: licorice, ginger, and black pepper and its primary constituent, piperine.

Licorice

Family: Leguminosae

Species Used: There are 18 or 20 or 30 species in the genus *Glycyrrhiza* (this gets tiresome — make up your minds). They are native to Europe, North Africa, Asia, Australia, and North and South America. All species have been used medicinally, but the two most common are *Glycyrrhiza glabra* (the European licorice) and *Glycyrrhiza uralensis* (the Chinese). Russian licorice, *G. echinata*, is often used in that region; the American licorice *G. lepidota* is rarely used these days in spite of its wide native range but was frequently used as a medicinal by the indigenous peoples in the Americas. (And, yeah, they used it just the same way.)

In this section I will refer to both the European and Chinese species herein as "the plant" or as "licorice," sometimes as "it." They are used pretty much interchangeably. If I talk about another species' actions, I will list it by name.

Licorice is an unusual medicinal. It is potently antiviral, moderately antibacterial (but fairly strong against a few bacterial species such as *Staphylococcus* and *Bacillus* spp.), and moderately immune potentiating. But one of its real, and generally overlooked, strengths is that it is a very potent synergist. In fact, it should be considered one of the primary synergists in any herbal repertory.

Parts Used

The root, though the leaves do have similar but much milder actions.

Preparation and Dosage

Used as tea, in capsules, as tincture. Again: This herb is best used with other herbs in a combination formula.

TINCTURE

Dried root, 1:5, 50 percent alcohol, 30–60 drops, up to 3x daily.

TEA

Add ½ to 1 tsp powdered root to 8 ounces water, simmer 15 minutes, strain. Drink up to 3 cups a day.

CAPSULES

Take 2–8 "00" capsules per day.

Side Effects and Contraindications

Because of licorice's many strengths, a lot of people overuse it, with sometimes serious side effects. *This herb should rarely be used in isolation or in large doses or long term. Long-term use is especially discouraged.* The side effects are many, specifically: edema, weak limbs (or loss of limb control entirely), spastic numbness, dizziness, headache,

hypertension, and hypokalemia (severe potassium depletion) —
especially in the elderly. Additional problems are decreases in plasma
renin and aldosterone levels, and at very large doses decreased body
and thymus weight and blood cell counts.

Because of licorice's strong estrogenic activity, it will also cause
breast growth in men, especially when combined with other estrogenic herbs. Luckily all these conditions tend to abate within 2 to
4 weeks after licorice intake ceases. Caution should be used, however,
in length and strength of dosages.

A number of studies have found that large doses of licorice taken
long term during pregnancy have detrimental effects on the unborn
children. Low doses are apparently safe. Again, this plant should not
be used in large doses or for lengthy periods of time *especially if you
are pregnant.*

The herb is contraindicated in hypertension, hypokalemia, pregnancy, hypernatremia, and low testosterone levels. However, for short-
term use (10 days or less), in low doses combined with other herbs, it is
very safe.

Herb/Drug Interactions

The plant is highly synergistic. It is also additive. It should not be used
along with estrogenic pharmaceuticals, hypertensive drugs, cardiac
glycosides, corticosteroids, hydrocortisone, or diuretics such as thia-
zides, spironolactone, or amiloride.

Habitat and Appearance

The *Glycyrrhiza* genus is a member of the pea family with the usual
pea-type leaves — a bunch of oval leaflets running along a central stem.
The plants are perennials, can grow to 6 feet (2 m) in height, and bush
out to 3 feet (1 m). The plants produce spikes of the usual pea-family
flowers during the summer. They range in color from yellowish to
blue to purple in the various species. The plant sends out both roots
and rhizomes, the roots thick and fleshy, up to 4 inches in diameter,
going as deep as 3 feet (1 m). The creeping rhizomes spread out from

the primary root up to 26 feet (8 m) in length, often sending up shoots of new plants far from the original. The roots and rhizomes of the cultivated species are light in color, the wild species darker. The inside of most of the species is yellowish, and, in the European and Chinese species at least, quite sweet. The American species is not very sweet, though a lot of sources say it is (I have eaten it; still waiting for that sweet taste to emerge on my tongue). The American species, though low in sweetness, possesses many of the same medicinal actions as the more prominent medicinal species. I've not encountered any of the other less common species in practice.

The licorice flowers mature into clusters of spiky brown seed capsules each about the size of a grape (at least in the American species — the only one I have seen).

The genus ranges from semi-arid desert to lush, wet climes such as Yorkshire, England, and from sea level to 8,500 or so feet (2,500 m) in altitude. When wild, the plants often like growing along waterways in sandyish soil. The American species is endemic throughout Canada and most of the United States excluding the Southeast. The European species is cultivated many places in the Americas but has escaped and can be found here and there in California, Nevada, and Utah. I can't find a record of any wild species in mid- to southern Africa (even though it is most likely grown there), but the genus seems to have spread pretty much everywhere else. If you look around you will probably find a licorice native in your eco-range someplace.

Cultivation and Collection

The plants grow fairly easily from root cuttings; the seeds are more demanding. The seeds need to be stratified for several weeks, then scarified and soaked for 2 hours in warm water before sowing if you want an easy germination. Treated seeds will germinate at about an 80 percent rate, and untreated at around 20 percent. Once started, the plants are pretty intent on remaining and spreading wherever they want to. Make sure you want it where you plant it — you won't be able to get rid of it if you change your mind. A few places here and there consider it an invasive, because, well, it is.

Both the European and Chinese varieties warrant planting in the wild and letting them go; they are well able to look after themselves if released from captivity. As they are a major medicinal, the more they spread, the better off we will be.

The plants like a free-draining friable soil with a pH between 6 and 7, but they can take on a greater range than that and do quite well. They are drought tolerant and like the sun but do need a bit of water; they often grow wild along streambeds, where they are very tenacious.

It takes a few years for the plants to establish themselves (2 to 3 years is a good minimum period of time), but once they do, you will be able to harvest from them pretty much forever. You will rarely, if ever, be able to dig up the entire root system of an established plant, and it will continue to grow and spread from what is left. Commercial growers generally achieve somewhere between 15 and 50 tons per hectare of roots once the plants have matured. The older the plants and the deeper the dig, the bigger the yield. The plants produce a lot of root mass. You can get enough medicine for an entire family from just one established plant, pretty much forever.

The plant roots and rhizomes should be harvested in the fall or early spring and dried out of the sun. The larger roots should be cut into smaller sections before being dried.

Plant Chemistry

There are hundreds of compounds in licorice, many of which have been intensively studied. The main one is glycyrrhizin, which makes up to 24 percent of the root by weight. Also: glabrin A and B, glycyr-rhetol, glabrolide, isoglabrolide, scores of isoflavones, coumarins, triterpene sterols, saponins, and so on and on and on.

Properties of Licorice

Actions

Adrenal cortex stimulant	Antitussive	Laxative (gentle)
Adrenal tonic	Antiulcerative	Mucoprotective
Analgesic	Antiviral	Prevents biofilm formation
Antibacterial	Cardioprotective	Protects from effects of radiation exposure
Anticancer/tumor inhibitor	Demulcent	Smooth muscle relaxant
Antihyperglycemic	Estrogenic	Stimulates pancreatic secretions
Anti-inflammatory	Expectorant	Synergist (potent)
Antioxidative	Gastric secretion inhibitor	Thymus stimulant
Antispasmodic	Hepatoprotective	
Antistressor	Immunomodulant	
	Immunostimulant	

Licorice is a fairly potent synergist (see page 217). It is specifically called for in treating resistant Gram-negative infections as it is most potent against that family of efflux mechanisms. In general, it increases the action of other herbs and pharmaceuticals, and if added to a mixture prior to tincturing it will enhance the extraction. It also acts as a detoxicant, and, most importantly, licorice is an inhibitor of one of the main efflux mechanisms in Gram-negative bacteria. As an antiviral, it prevents viral replication across a wide range of viruses, inhibits viral growth, inhibits neuraminidases in numerous influenza strains, inactivates virus particles, and inhibits RANTES secretion. As an immunostimulant, it stimulates interferon production, enhances antibody formation, and stimulates phagocytosis.

It takes about 4 hours for licorice's glycyrrhizin to reach maximum serum concentration after oral ingestion; then it is slowly excreted, and eventually eliminated at 72 hours after ingestion. It stays in the body a long time.

Active Against

Arboviruses	Bacillus stearothermophilus	Chaetomium funicola
Arthrinium sacchari	Bacillus subtilis	Clostridium sporogenes
Bacillus coagulans	Candida albicans	Cytomegalovirus
Bacillus megaterium		Enterococcus faecalis

CONTINUED ON NEXT PAGE

PROPERTIES OF LICORICE, CONTINUED

Enterococcus faecium

Enterotoxigenic
Escherichia coli

Enterovirus 71

Epstein-Barr virus

Haemophilus influenzae

Helicobacter pylori

Hepatitis B and C

Herpes simplex

HIV-1

Influenza A (various
strains, H1N1,
H2N2, H9N2,
novel H1N1 [WT],
oseltamivir-resistant
novel H1N1, and
so on)

Japanese encephalitis
virus

Klebsiella pneumoniae

*Mycobacterium
tuberculosis*

Newcastle disease
virus

Plasmodium spp.

Pseudorabies virus

Respiratory syncytial
virus

Salmonella paratyphi

Salmonella typhi

Salmonella typhimurium

Sarcina lutea

SARS-related
coronavirus (FFM1,
FFM2)

Shigella boydii

Shigella dysentariae

Staphylococcus aureus

Streptococcus lactis

Streptococcus mutans

Streptococcus sobrinus

Toxocara canis

*Trichophyton
mentagrophytes*

Trichophyton rubrum

Vaccinia virus

Varicella zoster virus

Vesicular stomatitis
virus

Vibrio cholerae

Vibrio mimicus

Vibrio parahaemolyticus

Use to Treat

Use in cases of respiratory viral infections and oral bacterial problems
(for gums and mucous membranes). Use as an adjunct for bacterial infections, especially of the GI tract and respiratory tract, especially if there
is cramping or ulceration. But primarily, in the context of this book, use
licorice as a synergist in systemic bacterial infections.

Note: Licorice should be used in combination rather than alone. See
Side Effects and Contraindications (page 217). I would not recommend
that this plant be used as a single medicinal.

Other Uses

As a sweetener. *Glycyrrhiza glabra* is also a potent plant remediator for
reclaiming saline-heavy soils.

Finding Licorice

You can buy very good quality European licorice from Pacific Botanicals, my preferred source. 1st Chinese Herbs has the Chinese variety. Seeds can be had from Horizon Herbs or Richters, an international seed merchant.

Note: Some of the licorice in commerce comes from eastern Europe, which possesses some of the highest levels of soil and air pollution in the world. It makes no sense to buy potentially contaminated herbs to use for their broad-spectrum immune and liver actions. Organically grown licorice is much better. If you buy both and compare them, you will find a significant difference in quality.

Traditional Uses of Licorice

Licorice has been used as a food plant and medicinal for between four and five millennia. The genus name, *Glycyrrhiza*, is Greek in origin, *glykys* meaning "sweet" and *rhiza* "root." The root's main constituent, glycyrrhizin, is 50 times sweeter than sugar. All the species have been used in medicine in any geographical region they grew and by any culture that had access to them.

AYURVEDA

Variously known as *mulethi, yasti-madhu, jasti-madhu, madhuka, mithiladki,* and so on. The plant is considered cooling, tonic, demulcent, expectorant, diuretic, and a gentle laxative. It's used for treating poisoning, ulcers, diseases of the liver, bladder, and lungs. Any inflammation in the mucous membranes anywhere in the body. For cough, sore throat, hoarseness, fever, and as a general tonic in debility from long-term disease conditions, especially those that are pulmonary or of the GI tract.

Licorice is considered a synergist, a specific additive to other herbal formulations.

TRADITIONAL CHINESE MEDICINE

Known as *gancao* in Chinese medicine, licorice has been used in China for three thousand years or so. The herb is considered sweet and mild, to regulate the function of the stomach, and to be qi tonifying, lung demulcent, expectorant, latent-heat cleansing, antipyretic, detoxicant, anti-inflammatory and spleen invigorative and is a synergist in many herbal formulations. The herb is used in pharyngolaryngitis, cough, palpitations, stomachache due to asthenia, peptic ulcer, pyogenic infection, and ulceration of the skin.

WESTERN BOTANIC PRACTICE

The ancient Egyptians used the plant as a major medicinal; the plant has often been found in their tombs. The Greek Theophrastus, in the third century BCE, noted the plant's use for asthma, dry coughs, and respiratory problems. The Romans called the plant *liquiritia*, which eventually was corrupted to the word *licorice*. It was a primary medicine in ancient Rome for coughs. It was used throughout Europe as a primary medicinal and although harvested in the wild originally, it has been a main agricultural crop for over a thousand years.

The American Eclectics used it intensively, as did most medicinal practitioners in the Americas. The Eclectics used it for coughs, catarrhs, irritation of the urinary passages, diarrhea, and bronchial diseases. It was an early agricultural medicinal, grown by most people in their medicinal gardens. The indigenous tribes of the Americas used the indigenous species similarly; that is, for sore throat, chest pains, swellings, coughs; as an antidiarrheal; for stomachache, fevers, toothache, skin sores, spitting blood; and as a general tonic.

Scientific Research

The medicinal species have been intensely studied for years. This look will be brief, as a full monograph would run to hundreds of pages.

As an immune stimulant: A double-blind, repeated (within subject), randomized trial with *Echi-nacea purpurea, Astragalus membranaceus*, and *Glycyrrhiza glabra* found that licorice significantly increased CD25 expression on T cells. It also increased CD69, CD4, and CD8 expression on T cells.

Postoperative sore throat:
Forty adults about to undergo elective lumbar laminectomy were split into two groups. One received water, the other water with licorice. The use of licorice gargle performed 5 minutes before anesthesia was effective in reducing or eliminating the incidence and severity of postoperative sore throat in patients.

Tuberculosis: A randomized, double-blind, placebo-controlled study with 60 people with sputum-positive pulmonary tuberculosis was conducted. They were split into two groups, one taking placebo, the other licorice — in addition to their regular therapy. Sputum conversion was seen in 80 percent of the licorice group, and 70 percent in the placebo group. Fever was relieved in all in the licorice group, and 80 percent in the placebo group. Cough was relieved in 96 percent of the licorice group, and 81 percent of the placebo group. GI side effects were seen in 20 percent of the placebo group, and none of the licorice group. ALT and AST levels were raised in 6 percent of the licorice group, and 30 percent of the placebo group. Elevated uric acid in serum was observed in 3 percent of the licorice group, and 16 percent of the placebo group.

Hepatitis: A single compound, an interferon stimulator, from licorice was used to treat patients with sub-acute hepatic failure. The survival rate was 72 percent compared to 31 percent in those who received traditional therapies.

Atopic dermatitis: A licorice gel was used to successfully treat atopic dermatitis in a double-blind clinical trial, 30 people in each group. The gel significantly reduced erythema, edema, and itching over the 2-week trial.

Aphthous stomatitis: Bioadhesive patches containing licorice were used to control the pain and reduce healing time in recurrent aphthous ulcer. Licorice patches caused a significant reduction in the diameter of the inflammatory halo and necrotic center compared with placebo. (There have been three of these trials, all successful.)

Pharmaceutical side effects:
In a comparative trial, licorice, when used along with spironolactone in the treatment of polycystic ovary syndrome, significantly reduced the side effects from spironolactone when used alone.

Peptic ulcer: Licorice was found in a trial with 100 people with peptic ulcer (86 of whom were unresponsive to conventional treatment) to be effective: 90 percent experienced good effects, 22 were cured, 28 were significantly improved.

Hepatitis A: In 13 cases of infectious hepatitis treated with licorice, the icterus index normalized in 13 days, urinary bile pigments were negative in 10 days, marked reduction of hepatomegaly took 9 days, pain over the liver disappeared in 8 days.

Hepatitis C: Glycyrrhizin has been used in Japan for more than 60 years in the treatment of hepatitis C. In several clinical trials it has been found to significantly lower AST, ALT, and GGT concentrations while reversing histologic evidence of necrosis and inflammatory lesions in the liver.

Lichen planus: In a clinical trial, 66 percent of people with lichen planus who took glycyrrhizin were cured.

Oral herpes: Glycyrrhizic acid cream, applied six times daily in people with acute oral herpetic infections (HSV1), resolved pain and dysphagia within 24 to 48 hours.

There have been a number of trials using licorice in combination with other herbs. It reduced risperidone-induced hyperprolactinemia in patients with schizophrenia. Reduced hyperuricemia in vegetarians. Was effective in the treatment of advanced pancreatic and other gastrointestinal malignancies. Was successful in the treatment of 138 cases of intestinal metaplasia and 104 of atypical hyperplasia of the gastric mucosa.

In vivo studies have found licorice to be potently antioxidant, to stimulant immune activity, to be anticonvulsant, to be potently anti-inflammatory on skin eruptions, to be hepatoprotective, to be cerebroprotective, to heal aspirin-induced ulcers, to be antispasmodic to the lower intestine, to be strongly antitussive, and to protect the mitochondria from damage.

SPECIFIC ACTIONS AS A SYNERGIST

Licorice is a fairly potent synergist through a number of avenues. Importantly, it is directly active against the efflux mechanism AcrAB-TolC in the Enterobacteriaceae family of bacteria, which are Gram-negative organisms. This efflux mechanism can extrude many diverse antibacterials including tetracyclines, fluoroquinolones, and chloramphenicol. Licorice, then, can effectively be added to formulations treating infections from that Gram-negative family, including, among others, *Yersinia, Shigella, Serratia, Salmonella, Morganella, Klebsiella, Enterobacter,* and *Escherichia.*

Licorice increases the potency of both herbs and pharmaceuticals when used with them. It has been found, for example, to enhance the action of anti-tuberculosis drugs, increasing positive outcomes in treatment; to increase the action of hydrocortisone; and to potentiate oseltamivir against resistant influenza strains. Chinese trials have shown that it increases the potency of other herbs in the treatment of rheumatoid arthritis and increases the antioxidant actions of other herbs such as astragalus and the isolated compound lycopene. Licorice enhances the anticancer activity of various herbs against prostate cancer cell lines; increases the effect of the neuromuscular blocking agent paeoniflorin; and significantly increases the immune-stimulating action of herbs such as *Echinacea purpurea* and *Astragalus.*

Licorice increases the strength of tincture formulations if added to the herbs prior to tincturing. For example, it enhances the solubility of compounds from other plants (e.g., the sapogenin isoliquiritigenin, the saikosaponins from ginseng) by a factor of up to 570.

Licorice also reduces toxicity in other plants; it prevents toxicity from aconite alkaloids and reduces the toxicity from a number of herbs used to treat rheumatoid arthritis in Chinese clinical trials.

Ginger

Family: Zingiberaceae. There are about 1,400 members of the family, of which the genus *Zingiber* is usually referred to as the *true* gingers. The species in the *Alpinia* genus are probably the other most commonly used medicinals in the family.

Species Used: There are 85 or maybe 100 species of plants in the genus *Zingiber*. (Why have taxonomy anyway?) *Z. officinale*, the common food ginger, is the most famous and the one generally used for medicine. Many of the species in this family contain similar constituents and can be used medicinally, but their actions do differ. This short monograph looks only at the culinary ginger, *Z. officinale*.

Part Used

The root. The root of ginger is really a rhizome, but nobody cares about the distinction but phytogrammarians, so I will just call it a root, as nearly all people who use language do.

Preparation and Dosage

The best form of the herb is the fresh juice of the root taken as a hot tea; it is most potent like this. Large quantities of the juice can be stabilized with alcohol (in an 80:20 juice-to-alcohol ratio) and then added to herbal combinations to blend the juice's synergistic actions into the formula. *If you are using the plant to treat resistant infections, this is the way to do it in tincture combinations.* Fresh tincture of the root is nearly as good. Dried root is relatively useless.

The hot tea from the fresh juice is exceptionally potent in serious infection. It takes about 30 minutes after drinking the fresh juice hot tea for ginger's compounds to enter the bloodstream; they reach peak concentration in about 60 minutes and then begin to decline. The fresh juice tea should be consumed every 2 to 3 hours in acute conditions to keep the constituents at high levels in the blood.

FRESH GINGER JUICE TEA

Juice one or more pieces of ginger, in total about the size of a medium to large carrot, or four pieces the size of your thumb. *Save the plant matter that is left over* (for making an infusion; see below).

Combine ¼ cup fresh ginger juice with 12 ounces hot water, 1 tablespoon wildflower honey, the juice from ¼ lime (squeeze the juice into the cup, then drop in the rind), and ⅛ teaspoon cayenne.

Drink 4–6 cups per day. (If you don't own a juicer, use infusion method two, below.)

In acute conditions: Drink 6 cups per day minimum.

INFUSION

Method One: The leftover plant matter from juicing ginger can be put into 1–2 cups hot water, depending on how much you have left, and allowed to steep for 4–8 hours, covered. Strain, and use the infused liquid as you would fresh ginger juice in making fresh ginger juice tea (above). It will be almost as useful as the fresh juice but not quite.

Method Two: Grate or chop gingerroot (a piece about the size of your thumb) as finely as you can. Steep in 8–12 ounces hot water for 2–3 hours, *covered* in order to preserve the essential oils in the tea. Drink 4–6 cups daily.

TOPICALLY

Ginger juice is exceptionally good (sometimes) in relieving the pain of burns and speeding up healing. Apply the fresh juice topically to the affected area with a cotton ball. It is also a good antibacterial and antifungal when applied to skin infections.

TINCTURE

Fresh root, 1:2, 95 percent alcohol, 10–20 drops, up to 4x daily. (I do not prefer this approach, as the fresh juice is much, much better — nevertheless it is a million . . . well, okay, a billion . . . times better than using the dried root.)

AS FOOD

In everything and anything, often.

Side Effects and Contraindications

Large doses should be avoided in pregnancy due to the plant's emmen-agogue effect, though the dried root can be used to help morning sickness in moderate doses. May aggravate gallstones, so caution is advised. Rarely: bloating, gas, heartburn, nausea — usually when using the dried, powdered root.

Herb/Drug Interactions

The root is synergistic with a number of antibiotics, especially the aminoglycosides, increasing their potency, especially against resistant organisms.

Habitat and Appearance

The exact geographical location of the original ginger plant is unknown — most likely someplace in Asia. It has been cultivated for four thousand or more years in China and India and reached the West around two thousand years ago. The genus name *Zingiber* is of ancient Hindu extraction; it means "horn-shaped." ("They" say it's from the shape of the root, but I don't believe it; I've seen gingerroot roots.) The roots form dense clumps as they grow and that is what everyone harvests.

The plant is a perennial and likes warm, humid climates from sea level up to about 5,000 feet (1500 m) in altitude. It is rarely found wild; it's a cultivated medicinal.

The plant grows 2 to 3 feet (up to 1 m) in height and looks like sort of a shortish bamboo with a thin central stalk. *Zingiber* plants look much alike and are often confused with the alpinias, another genus in the family.

Cultivation and Collection

Ginger is almost always cultivated from pieces of the living root, like potatoes. Simply allowing some gingerroot to begin budding, then cutting it into pieces, each with a bud, and planting them is usually how it is done. Most ginger plants on Earth are rootstock clones. And it is one of the most heavily cultivated plants on Earth. *Everybody* loves it. The plant is considered a perennial, but it generally depletes the soil in which it is grown so it's usually rotated every other year. Unless it is in the exact right location it won't last once the soil is depleted.

Ginger is a tropical plant. It likes sheltered locations, filtered sunlight, warmth, humidity, rich soil. It hates direct sun and so on; basically it wants to be pampered and protected from the elements. It can't take freezing.

The root cuttings should be planted in late fall or early spring. No direct sun locations. Plant the cuttings 2 to 3 inches (5–10 cm) deep with the bud upward.

The plants need a lot of water, so don't let the soil dry out. Mulch them thickly. They hate dry air. The leaves die back in 8 to 10 months, and that is when the roots should be harvested. The roots will last a long time before they dry out.

Plant Chemistry

Several hundred constituents, including gingerols, zingiberol, zingiberene, shogaols, 3-dihydroshogaols, gingerdiols, mono- and diacetyl derivatives of gingerdiols, dihydrogingerdiones, labdadiene, and so on. The volatile oils such as the gingerols are very potent but much reduced in the dried roots. They are present at levels 6 to 15 times higher in fresh roots. Many constituents convert to shogaols as the root dries. The volatile constituents are the most antiviral.

Finding Ginger

Grocery stores everywhere (get organic if you can; if not, use what you can find).

Properties of Ginger

Actions

Analgesic
Anthelmintic
Antiarthritic
Antibacterial
Antidiarrheal
Antiemetic

Antifungal
Anti-inflammatory
Antispasmodic
Antitussive
Antiviral
Carminative

Circulatory stimulant
Diaphoretic
Elastase inhibitor
Hypotensive
Immune stimulant
Synergist

Active Against

Acinetobacter baumannii
Angiostrongylus cantonensis
Anisakis simplex
Aspergillus niger
Bacillus subtilis
Campylobacter jejuni
Candida albicans
Candida glabrata
Coliform bacilli
Dirofilaria immitis
Escherichia coli
Fusarium moniliforme

Haemonchus contortus
Haemophilus influenzae
Helicobacter pylori (cagA+ strains)
Hepatitis C
HIV-1
Human cytomegalovirus
Influenza A
Klebsiella pneumoniae
Listeria spp.
Porphyromonas endodontalis
Porphyromonas gingivalis

Prevotella intermedia
Proteus vulgaris
Pseudomonas aeruginosa
Rhinovirus spp. (especially 1B)
Salmonella typhimurium
Shigella dysentariae
Shigella flexneri
Staphylococcus aureus
Staphylococcus epidermidis
Viridans streptococci

Use to Treat

Ginger is a synergist, increasing the actions of other herbs and boosting their effectiveness by relaxing blood vessels and increasing circulation, thus carrying the active constituents of the other herbs more efficiently throughout the body. It is an effective circulatory stimulant, calms nausea, reduces diarrhea and stomach cramping, reduces fever (by stimulating sweating), reduces cold chills, reduces inflammation in bronchial passageways, thins mucus and helps it move out of the system, reduces coughing (as much as codeine cough syrups), ameliorates anxiety, and provides analgesic relief equal to or better than ibuprofen.

The herb can also be used in some bacterial diarrheal conditions, especially where there is cramping (cholera, dysentery, *E. coli*, etc.), for reduced circulation with coldness in the extremities, for migraine headache if accompanied by cold hands or feet, and for a sluggish constitution.

231

Traditional Uses of Ginger

It has been used every place it is grown as a medicine. *Everyone* not trapped in a technological culture uses it as a synergist for healing for colds and flu, nausea, poor circulation, and so on.

In Burma, fresh gingerroot is boiled in water (with palm sap as a sweetener) to get a hot infusion for treating colds and flu. In Congo, ginger is crushed and mixed with mango tree sap for colds and flu. In the Philippines fresh chopped ginger is boiled with water, and sugar added, to treat sore throat. It is used similarly in China and India. (There is a reason it is done this way.)

Ginger has a long historical tradition in warm climates as a food additive. Like many culinary spices it possesses strong antibacterial activity against a number of foodborne pathogens — especially against three of those now plaguing commercial foods: *Shigella, E. coli,* and *Salmonella.*

Two of the best ways to take ginger as food are the pickled ginger often served along with sushi in Japanese restaurants or candied gingerroot slices. Both make great snacks, can be eaten in large quantities, and are a healthy stimulant for the system.

AYURVEDA

Ginger has a very long history in Ayurveda, which calls it *srangavera* and about 50 other names depending on where you go. It is used for dyspepsia, flatulence, colic, vomiting, spasms of the stomach and bowels attended by fever, cold, cough, asthma, indigestion, lack of appetite, diarrhea, fever. The fresh juice (aha!), mixed with sugar and water, is a common form of preparation.

TRADITIONAL CHINESE MEDICINE

Fresh root: *sheng jiang.* (Dried root: *gan jiang* — a very different medicine.) Considered pungent and warm in traditional Chinese medicine (TCM), it is used as a diaphoretic, antiemetic, mucolytic, antitussive, detoxicant, anti-inflammatory. It is considered specific to warm the lungs, for pathogenic wind-cold conditions (i.e., severe intolerance to cold), slight fever, headache, general ache, nasal congestion, runny nose, cough, vomiting. It is usually prepared by decoction in water or pounded and the juice added to warm water. Ginger is generally combined with other herbs in TCM as it is considered to be a "guide" drug that carries the other herbs where they need to go. Ginger is also considered to be specific for ameliorating the toxic effects of other drugs or herbs. Estimates are that up to half of all Chinese herbal formulas contain it.

WESTERN BOTANIC PRACTICE

Everyone in the West has used ginger in much the same ways, though, historically, most of them tended to focus on its use for stomach and bowel complaints.

Scientific Research

The research on ginger has been problematic in that distinctions haven't been made (or looked for) between the actions of the fresh root and the dried root. (Common among scientists.) Nor has there been clarity about *how* the herb is prepared or what effect that might make on outcomes. (Common among scientists.) It is very rare that fresh preparations have been tested. (Ridiculous since that is the *primary* form of the medicine the world over.) Water extracts of the dried roots show very little antimicrobial activity — though they remain potently anti-inflammatory. If you don't understand the problems inherent in the journal papers, the outcomes found — which vary all over the place — are hard to understand. Sigh. Plants possess very different medicinal actions depending on: when they are harvested, how they are harvested, if they are dried or fresh, how they are prepared as medicines, how often they are taken, how much is taken, and if they are taken in isolation or in combination. Scientists coming from a reductionist orientation have a hard time understanding all that; they don't understand that herbal medicine really *is* rocket surgery.

As an overview: There have been some 30 clinical trials with 2,300 people using gingerroot. Following is just a sampling of a few of those and of a few in vivo and in vitro studies.

Anti-inflammatory action: Gingerol and its related compounds are potent inhibitors of lipopolysaccharide-induced PGE2 production in vitro. Inhibit both COX-1 and COX-2 in vitro through inhibiting several genes involved in the inflammatory response (acting on cytokines, chemokines, 5-lipoxygenase, and COX-2). Of 56 people (28 with rheumatoid arthritis, 18 with osteoarthritis, 10 with muscular discomfort) who took dried ginger, 75 percent reported relief from pain and swelling. In a double-blind, randomized, placebo-controlled clinical trial with 102 people with osteoarthritis, ginger was found to be as effective as ibuprofen in relieving pain and swelling. Numerous other in vivo studies have shown that ginger-root has both anti-inflammatory and analgesic actions; some used the essential oil massaged into the affected area — it works really well.

Antiemetic/antinausea: Various clinical studies have found that ginger-root is especially effective for treating severe morning sickness in pregnant women. The dried root was used, of course, and was found more effec-tive in severe cases. (The fresh root is better for nausea.)

Antiadhesion: In vivo, ginger-root interferes with the adhesion of enterobacterial disease organisms to the intestinal wall. This, in essence, reduces entero-infection of the GI tract, short-circuiting the disease process. Ginger is also an elastase inhibitor. Many bacteria use elastase to break down cellular tissue, helping their penetration of the body. (Ginger also reduces spasms in the intestinal tract, relaxing the intestinal wall at the same time.)

Antidiarrheal: Gingerroot inter-feres with the colonization of cells by enterogenic bacteria, thus reducing diarrhea, and reducing bacterial load. The root alters bacterial and host cell metabolism through a unique-to-ginger mechanism.

Cerebroprotective: In vivo studies found that gingerroot protects rats from brain damage and memory impairment.

Immunostimulant: In vivo studies with gingerroot have found that it increases immune markers across the board, pre- and post-infection.

Detoxification: In vivo rat studies found that ginger reduces cadmium levels and toxicity in rats, acting as a heavy metal detoxifier. And gingerroot in vivo reduces the effects of organo-phosphate insecticides.

Anthelmintic: Ginger was found to be effective in the treatment of endoparasites and stomach problems in ethnoveterinary practice in Paki-stan, killing all red stomach worms (*Haemonchus contortus*) in test ani-mals. It has been found active against a number of other endoparasites in other trials.

Other studies have found anti-ulcerative, antitumor, gastric anti-secretory, antifungal, antispasmodic, anticonvulsant, and antiallergenic actions in the plant.

SPECIFIC ACTIONS AS A SYNERGIST

Ginger increases the potency of herbs and pharmaceuticals if added to a protocol, inhibits bacterial resistance mechanisms in pathogens, stimu-lates circulation, and reduces the toxicity of endotoxins and pollutants. It dilates blood vessels and increases circulation, helping the blood, and the constituents in the blood from other herbs, to achieve faster and more effective distribution in the body.

Ginger is highly effective in reducing the ability of bacteria to extrude antibacterials out of their cells. (In consequence it increases the potency of a number of pharmaceuticals.)

Ginger potentiates the activity of aminoglycoside antibiotics (arbekacin, gentamicin, tobramycin, streptomycin) and other antibiotics such as bacitracin and polymyxin B, against vancomycin-resistant enterococci (which are Gram-positive) — essentially by increasing the permeability of the cell membrane; ginger is a strong p-glycoprotein inhibitor, as strong as the pharmaceutical verapamil. It also increases the effectiveness of daunomycin (used in the treatment of cancer), increasing the accumulation of the pharmaceutical three-fold and significantly reducing the P-gp-mediated efflux of the drug. This is common in P-gp inhibitors since cancer cells tend to use P-gp efflux mechanisms to get rid of pharmaceuticals.

Sublethal levels of tetracycline become lethal against staph organisms when ginger is added; compounds from ginger modify bacterial resistance in *Acinetobacter baumanii;* ginger potentiates the action of nifedipine on antiplatelet aggregation in normal human volunteers and the hypertensive; ginger potentiates the effectiveness of clarithromycin against *Helicobacter pylori* independent of whether the bacterial strain was susceptible to the pharmaceutical or not prior to the addition of ginger.

Ginger also has direct synergistic actions with other herbs. It potentiates their activity, increasing it substantially. For example, constituents in magnolia, but not in ginger, enhance sucrose intake in rats and reduce immobility time in swimming tests. But when ginger volatile oils are added to the mix, sucrose intake is increased exponentially; reduction time for immobility was also increased.

In other studies, when ginger oils are added to magnolia, they combine to produce a tremendously synergistic outcome in the treatment of depression. Serotonin in the brain and noradrenaline levels in the prefrontal cortex increase substantially after ginger is added to subclinical (inactive) doses of magnolia.

Ginger is also considered to be specific for ameliorating the toxic effects of other drugs or herbs used in TCM. In vivo studies found that ginger reduces cadmium levels and toxicity in rats, acting as a heavy metal detoxifier. It also reduces the effects of organophosphate insecticides in vivo.

Black Pepper/Piperine

Species Used: Piperine is a potent alkaloid found in two different peppers, black pepper (*Piper nigrum*) and long pepper (*Piper longum*). It is the primary constituent responsible (along with an isomer of piperine — chavicine) for the spicy pungency of pepper.

Piperine is the most common constituent in black pepper, running from 5 percent to 9 percent. Long pepper has much less, from 1 percent to 2 percent.

The pepper plant itself *can* be used as a synergist if you are so inclined; for a number of reasons I prefer the isolated constituent as a synergist, however. I will talk about both approaches in this section and the reasons why I am suggesting the constituent in this case.

Preparation and Dosage

Because this book is concentrating on the treatment of resistant bacterial organisms, many of which can have severe impacts if not treated effectively, it makes sense to me to use the isolated constituent piperine rather than the whole herb in this instance. The herb itself *can* be used; it is, however, about one-fifteenth as strong as piperine. Since piperine is, at this point, relatively easy to find, I would suggest having some on hand, just in case. If you don't have it or it becomes no longer available (see Finding Black Pepper and Piperine on opposite page) you can indeed use the pepper itself.

BLACK PEPPER TINCTURE

Both *Piper nigrum* and *Piper longum* are prepared as tinctures, 1:5, 65 percent alcohol. Dosage: 5–15 drops as needed. Piperine is not very water soluble; you need an alcohol tincture to extract it from the peppercorns. I would highly recommend using whole peppercorns, freshly ground, for making the tinctures. Previously ground pepper is much weaker.

Properties of Black Pepper/Piperine

Actions

Analgesic

Antibacterial

Anticonvulsant

Antidiarrheal

Antidysphagic (essential oil)

Antihyperlipidemic (reduces lipid levels in the blood)

Anti-inflammatory

Antimutagenic

Antioxidant

Antispasmodic

Antitumor inhibitor

CYP3A4 inhibitor

Free radical scavenger (potent)

Hepatoprotector

Immunostimulant

Increases oxygen uptake by red blood cells

Intestinal mucosa modulator

Melanocyte stimulant

Modulates thyroid hormone levels in the blood

Neural protector/ stimulant

P-glycoprotein inhibitor

Reduces blood glucose levels

Reduces erythrocyte fragility

Stimulates production and release of pancreatic enzymes, bile acids, and gastric acids

Stimulates the pituitary/adrenal axis

Synergist

Testosterone antagonist

Vasodilator

Finding Black Pepper and Piperine

Both black pepper and piperine are widely available. BioPerine by Source Naturals is a pretty good piperine product.

Potential future problems: Once again, the weight loss, muscle builder, and "herbal high" manufacturers are creating problems. All three are using piperine for their particular neuroses, to enhance either "fat burning" or bloodstream uptake of their particular products. This will, inevitably, be problematical down the road.

TRIKATU

You can also, if you wish, make trikatu, the traditional Ayurvedic combination that is added to herbs as a formulation synergist. It is prepared using *Piper nigrum* and *P. longum* and gingerroot in a ratio of 1:1:1; that is, equal parts of each herb or their tinctures. I prefer the tinctures. Use a tincture of fresh gingerroot, or, more preferably, the alcohol-stabilized fresh juice (as described in the ginger monograph) and tinctures of the two peppers as outlined above. Combine them in equal parts and then add that combined tincture to whatever formulation you are making. If you are making 4 ounces of an influenza formulation, then add an extra ounce of trikatu to make a total of 5 ounces. In other words, add 25 percent to any formulation you are making. It is going to be spicy.

PIPERINE

If you wish to use pure piperine, you will need to buy it, as it is a manufactured product. It is relatively inexpensive. Normal dosing, for instance to enhance the uptake of nutrients from food, is 20 mg daily.

Note: I would *not* use piperine as a regular supplement; in my opinion, it is indicated *only* for medical conditions that necessitate its use. If you have a systemic infection, especially if it is Gram-negative, piperine is a highly effective synergist for the herbs you will use to treat it and should be considered as a part of the treatment approach.

Dosage in acute conditions: Piperine should be taken prior to the herbal formulation you are using so that the intestinal wall has already been altered by the time your herbs get to the GI tract. Take 20 mg piperine 15–30 minutes prior to your herbs and then again 4–6 hours later, 30 minutes before taking your herbs again. Piperine will stay strongly present in the body for about 6 hours.

So . . . take piperine twice daily, 20 mg each time, in acute conditions to a max of 40 mg daily. Generally, not to exceed 7 days. If you are taking your herbs six times daily, you still only need to take piperine twice, once before the first dose, and then again 4–6 hours later.

Side Effects and Contraindications

Black pepper can exacerbate gastric reflux problems, but its major side effects occur on the reproductive system. In traditional medicine it is considered a mild contraceptive. The whole herb, however, is generally pretty safe along these lines unless taken in huge doses for extended periods of time. Studies on piperine, on the other hand, have found that it does interfere with egg implantation if taken long term in high doses.

However, the impacts on the male reproductive system are more severe. When taken as a supplement continued oral intake of piperine decreases the weight of the testes, lowers sperm production, decreases intracellular testosterone, and decreases the fertilizing capacity of sperm. Constant piperine intake has deleterious effects on the Leydig cells, epididymis, and seminiferous tubes even at doses of 1 mg/kg of body weight (that is, roughly, 70 to 80 mg daily for an adult male).

Piperine should primarily be used for short-term treatment of acute conditions. Women who are trying to become pregnant should not use it. Men with low testosterone levels should be very cautious in its use and not use it for longer than 2 weeks.

Herb/Drug Interactions

Piperine will increase the bioavailability of scores of drugs. (It will decrease the bioavailability of a few others such as diclofenac sodium.) If you are taking pharmaceuticals, you should check for synergy (the list is too long for this book) or simply not take them together. It is highly likely that the supplement *will* increase bioavailability and thus the impacts of the pharmaceutical.

Plant Chemistry

Piper nigrum contains at least 200 identified constituents with more being discovered all the time. The most important is considered to be the alkaloid piperine, which is present at levels of up to 9 percent of the dried peppercorns in black pepper. It is the primary substance responsible for the peppery taste of the spice.

Other major compounds are chavicine, coumaperine, piperidine, numerous piperidine amides, piperettine, piperanine, piperolein A, B, and C, piperonal, and so on.

Traditional Uses of Black Pepper

Piper nigrum is native to southern India, where it is extensively culti-vated. The plant is a flowering vine that produces grape-like clusters of dark red berries, at the center of which is a large white seed. The seed, as is sometimes the case, comprises most of the berry; the pulp sur-rounding it is fairly thin, with the usual thinnish outer rind of the fruit covering that. Basically, it is not a very exciting berry.

The black peppercorns that we use for a spice, however, are pro-duced from the green, unripe berries. The berries are harvested and briefly immersed in hot water, thus slightly cooking them. This ruptures the cell walls in the berry and activates a number of enzymes that will cause the outer pulp and rind that surround the white seed to blacken during drying. The fruits are then spread in the sun to dry for several days. The outer pulp and rind wrinkle and turn black. Once dried the fruits are usually sold whole to preserve the strength of the corns, then ground into the powder that we call black pepper just before use.

White pepper is simply the pepper seeds themselves absent the pulp and rind. In this case the ripe berries are soaked in water for a week until the outer rind and pulp soften and slough off the inner seed. The seed is then dried, sold, and ground into a fine powder.

Black pepper has been used in India for at least four thousand years as both spice and medicine. It is probably the most common spice in the world after salt.

AYURVEDA

Black pepper has a primary place in Ayurveda, often combined with long pepper (*Piper longum*) and ginger to form a compound called *tri-katu* or the three acrids. This combination has been a primary element of Ayurvedic compounding since at least 600 BCE; most Ayurvedic formulations contain it.

Trikatu is considered specific for correcting imbalances in the three *doshas*, psychospiritual aspects of the human body that when out of balance lead to disease expressing itself physically. This formulation is (as are the three herbs individually) considered specific for "activating" the potency of the plants with which it is combined. This has been its main use for millennia.

As a single herb, black pepper (and long pepper) has been used for a variety of conditions (constipation, diarrhea, earache, gangrene, heart disease, hernia, hoarseness, indigestion, insect bites, insomnia, joint pain, liver problems, lung disease, oral abscesses, sunburn, tooth decay, and toothaches), but its main uses have been, internally, for disease conditions accompanied by fever and/or diarrhea, dysentery, GI tract disorders, and urinary problems, and externally for rheumatism and neuralgia.

TRADITIONAL CHINESE MEDICINE

Black pepper was incorporated into the Chinese materia medica during the Middle Ages. It is considered specific for warming the middle, dispersing cold, dispelling phlegm, for wind-cold, and for diarrhea, usually for conditions accompanied by vomiting, diarrhea, and abdominal pain. It is also considered specific for epilepsy. The synergistic actions of the plant are apparently unknown in this system.

Scientific Research

I am splitting this section into two parts: 1) nonsynergist actions and 2) synergist actions. Most of the studies have been on the isolated constituent piperine. (There are several hundred studies on piperine; this is just a sampling; most of the studies have been in these areas.)

NONSYNERGIST ACTIVITY OF BLACK PEPPER AND PIPERINE

Black pepper does have some antibacterial activity itself. In vitro studies of a number of its constituents (not piperine) found them active against *Bacillus subtilis, Bacillus sphaericus, Staphylococcus aureus, Klebsiella aerogenes*, and *Chromobacterium violaceum*. The essential oil of black pepper is effective against *Bacillus subtilis, Pseudomonas aeruginosa, Candida albicans, Trichoderma* spp., and *Aspergillus niger.* An aqueous solution of black pepper was tested against 12 genera of oral bacteria isolated from 200 individuals and was found to be effective against 75 percent of them (unfortunately the abstract does not list the bacteria; the full paper is regrettably elusive). Piperine itself is active against *Leishmania* spp. and *Trypanosoma cruzi.*

Here is a look at some of the studies.

In vitro: Black pepper is a strong antioxidant, more potent than alpha-tocopherol when used at similar concentrations. One of pepper's constituents is as potent as the synthetic antioxidants BHA and BHT.

In vitro: Black pepper inhibits cholesterol esterification in HepG2 cells; it potently inhibits binding between slCAM-1 and LFA-1 of THP-1 cells, dose dependently.

In vivo, guinea pig and rabbits: Crude extracts of black pepper, at low doses, have a mild laxative effect in constipation. However, in larger doses they are antispasmodic, reducing contractions in the intestine, and are antisecretory and antidiarrheal. Piperine, at lower doses than the pepper extract, acts identically.

In vivo, diarrhea, mice: Piperine inhibits castor oil and arachidonic acid–induced diarrhea.

In vivo, inflammation, mice: 1) Piperine reduces inflammation in both chronic and acute models; 2) inhibits monosodium urate crystal–induced inflammation (specific for gouty arthritis); 3) significantly reduces inflammation around joints in arthritic mice studies. It produces anti-inflammatory, antinociceptive, and antiarthritic actions. It inhibits expression of IL6 and MMP13 and production of PGE2.

In vivo, cancer, animal models: Numerous studies have found that piperine protects animals from induced cancer, reduces tumor incidence in others, and increases life span in terminal cases.

In vivo, neuroprotection, mice/rats: 1) Piperine significantly improves memory and protects the hippocampus from neurodegeneration; 2) blocks convulsions induced by intracerebroventricular injection of kainate; 3) inhibits synchronized oscillation of intracellular calcium in rat hippocampal networks, represses spontaneous synaptic activities, and protects hippocampal neurons from apoptosis.

Human clinical trial, epilepsy in children: Clinical trials (randomized, crossover, placebo-controlled, double-blind) with a piperine derivative in China in the treatment of epilepsy found that it reduced the number of seizures in a majority of the children who used it.

Human clinical trial, dysphagia in elderly: Inhalation of black pepper essential oil by elderly persons suffering from difficulty or inability to swallow (dysphagia) showed remarkable effects in restoring swallowing ability.

SYNERGISTIC ACTIVITY OF BLACK PEPPER AND PIPERINE

The synergistic actions of black pepper and piperine are primarily generated by three things: 1) the circulatory actions of the plant or its isolated constituent; 2) their effects on P-gp and CYP3A4; 3) their impacts on efflux pumps in bacteria.

Pepper and piperine expand blood vessel diameter and increase circulation. Piperine is strongly present in the blood (it binds to albumin for transport) and easily crosses internal organism barriers (organs and systems both: blood-brain barrier and so on). It reaches every part of the body.

Piperine and pepper have specific effects on blood constituents. In my opinion the actions of the plant and its constituent on red blood cells (reducing their fragility and increasing their oxygen uptake) play an important part in their synergistic actions. Pepper and piperine also appear to have specific actions on white blood cells. They do have some immune-stimulating actions, but more importantly they seem to be highly protective of white blood cells, being active against leishmanial and tryposomal parasites of the macrophages. They seem to produce the same effects on white blood cells as they do on red, that is, reducing their fragility and enhancing their normal actions. Although no one has tested for this, it seems as if piperine may play a particular role as a hematoprotector and hematoregenerator not only of red blood cells but also white, though

differently than the other plants I have discussed so far.

A smaller role in the plant's synergism is played by the general medicinal actions of the plant — that is, it is to some extent antibacterial, which will give additive effects (at the least) to the antibacterial actions of the other herbs used with it; it is analgesic, helping with pain; it is anti-inflammatory; if you are treating inflammatory infections, its specific actions there will help immensely; and if you are treating CNS problems, it will, in addition to helping other herbs get to the affected area, add its own neuroprotective actions to the mix.

Black pepper and piperine also possess a number of efflux inhibition actions. Piperine inhibits the NorA efflux pump in *Staphylococcus aureus*. It also inhibits ethidium bromide efflux. Ethidium bromide is a substrate for all the efflux pumps in *Staphylococcus aureus* (except NorC). Ethidium bromide is also a substrate in a number of efflux pumps in some Gram-negative bacteria — those that possess the SMR efflux pumps, and in *Mycobacterium* spp. Specifically, piperine has been found to be an inhibitor of the RV1258c efflux pump in *Mycobacterium tuberculosis*.

But perhaps the major strength of the plant and its constituent piperine is the effects they have on permeability glycoprotein (P-glycoprotein or P-gp) and CYP3A4. Black pepper and piperine are potent inhibitors of both.

P-GP AND CYP3A4

All living organisms have to deal with one primary survival reality:

determining what is me and not me and then identifying whether or not the "not-me" is going to be harmful to the "me." There are a great many mechanisms that all organisms have to do this and they have a lot of options available for dealing with unsafe substances that "not-mes" can generate. Basically, they control access to their cells. In general, they all have four mechanisms for this: 1) assisted exclusion; 2) metabolic conversion; 3) solubilizer attachment; 4) reduction in assisted absorption. What this means in practical terms is this: When a substance is taken into the body and touches the GI tract membrane, an immediate identification process occurs. What is this thing? And is it safe? If the intestinal wall identifies it as harmful, then it can:

Exclude it; that is, use what is called an efflux pump or an efflux transporter to move the thing out, making sure it does not affect the cell/organism.

Metabolize it; that is, chemically turn it into something else that is not harmful, which is then either used or excreted from the cell/organism. The chemical substances that are thus created are called metabolites.

Attach it; that is, link the substance chemically to a highly water-soluble substance, often glucuronic acid. This creates a new compound that is unable to diffuse through cell membranes. It is then excreted in either urine or feces.

Reduce assisted absorption; that is, inhibit influx transporters. Assisted absorption involves the use of transporter proteins, a.k.a. influx transporters, in the lining of the intestinal wall. These proteins transfer useful substances into the cells of the intestinal wall and from there they are transported to the blood. Influx transporters are strongly active in moving such things as amino acids across the intestinal membrane. One of the most potent is gamma-glutamyltransferase (GGT). It is present in the cell membranes of the intestines, kidneys, bile duct, liver, spleen, heart, brain, and seminal vesicles.

All these responses make it harder for substances to get into the body and affect it. Many pharmaceuticals are considered to be foreign substances and, when these actions take place, up to 85 percent of a pharmaceutical may be inactivated, which is part of the reason doses are so high with some drugs.

Piperine affects all four of those mechanisms that control access to cells. It has particularly strong effects on efflux pumping, metabolization, glucuronic acid attachment, and GGT.

There are a number of efflux transporters. P-gp, or permeability glycoprotein, is one of the more prominent. P-gp is found mainly in the intestinal wall, kidneys, liver, brain, testes, adrenal gland, and uterus. It is also common in cancer cells and a few bacteria. You can visualize P-gp as a barrier lining the intestinal wall and choosing which substances to let into the body and, if so, how much (it also does this at the blood-brain barrier). Piperine significantly reduces the ability of P-gp to block incoming substances. As a result, if you take piperine or black pepper (or the traditional Ayurvedic blend trikatu), more of the medicinal will pass through the intestinal wall and into the bloodstream. Sometimes, the amount getting into the blood is substantially higher, up to 32 times its levels without piperine. This is why particular care needs to be taken if you are using piperine and are also taking pharmaceuticals. It is also why you should never take piperine with severe infections of the intestinal wall such as *E. coli* and cholera. Piperine would allow the bacteria to more easily infiltrate the intestinal wall and get deeper into your system.

CYP3A4 is one of the more important metabolizers in the human body. It affects the broadest range of substances (or substrates as they are called) of any of the CYP family of enzymes, affecting thousands if not hundreds of thousands of substances. It is a main metabolizer in the intestinal wall and liver. Generally, it does one of two things: converts a substance to another that has lower biological activity or makes substances more water soluble, which reduces their ability to move into cells. Inhibition of CYP3A4 means that the substance is left in its original, highly bioactive form when it gets into the body. Piperine strongly inhibits CYP3A4. (It has also been found to inhibit CYP1A2, CYP1A1, and CYP2D6.)

Piperine/black pepper also inhibits AHH or aryl hydrocarbon hydroxylase, which metabolizes aromatic hydrocarbons. (This makes piperine useful for enhancing the impact of herbs like juniper berry, which is high in aromatic hydrocarbons, in the treatment of UTI.)

Piperine/black pepper also strongly inhibits UDP-glucuronyltransferase (a.k.a. UGT). UGT is the enzyme that attaches glucuronic acid to xenobiotics to facilitate their removal from the body. This action

by piperine increases the time that foreign substances, e.g., herbs or pharmaceuticals, remain in the body/bloodstream prior to elimination, from 2 to 4 hours longer.

Piperine/black pepper also significantly stimulates the activity of the influx transporter GGT, increasing the movement of substances across the intestinal membrane.

Piperine, and black pepper, thus increase the amount of any substance going into the body, keep it in its most potent form (unmetabolized), and keep it in the body longer. Piperine/black pepper also, for similar reasons, facilitates the movement of substances into the brain and CNS, uterus, testes, adrenals, kidneys, and liver. If any of those systems are being treated for disease, for example, bacterial meningitis or hepatitis C, piperine will increase the amount of herb getting to the meninges or the liver.

At the same time piperine/black pepper stimulates circulation and increases blood vessel size so that the substances are widely circulated throughout the body very rapidly.

A number of studies have looked at the actions of black pepper and piperine along these lines. Most studies have occurred with piperine. However, there has been some work with trikatu, the traditional Ayurvedic blend of the two peppers and gingerroot.

In vivo, goats, pharmaceuticals: If trikatu was preadministered to mountain goats before their treatment with pefloxacin (a fluoroquinolone antibiotic used in India in veterinary practice), the drug levels in the body and its penetration into various parts of the body were substantially increased. Other studies have found that trikatu increases the bioavailability of vasicine and indomethacin.

Human clinical study, pharmaceuticals: Trikatu increased the concentrations of vasicine by over 200 percent and sparteine by over 100 percent in the blood plasma of human volunteers.

In vivo, mice/rats, pharmaceuticals: Piperine increased the effects of pentobarbital-induced hypnosis in mice. Blood and brain pentobarbital levels were higher in treated animals; piperine also prolonged hexobarbital sleeping time and zoxazolamine paralysis; enhanced the bioavailability of aflatoxin B1; enhanced the bioavailability of etoposide; increased the bioavailability of nimesulide, thus allowing the use of reduced, and safer, doses; and delayed elimination of phenytoin.

In vivo, mice/rats, herbs: Piperine increases the movement of radio-labeled L-leucine, L-isoleucine, and L-valine across the intestinal wall, enhancing uptake; increases the uptake of curcumin and its presence in serum; and increases plasma levels of epigallocatechin gallate from green tea.

Human clinical study/trial, pharmaceuticals: A single oral dose of propranolol (40 mg) or theophylline (150 mg) alone or in combination with piperine (20 mg) was given each day for 7 days. Increased oral bioavailability was found in the piperine group. A single dose of piperine (20 mg) administered with phenytoin significantly increased the mean plasma concentration of phenytoin; a crossover, placebo-controlled study found that piperine increased the bioavailability of nevirapine, increased its mean plasma concentrations, and reduced its elimination from the body; another study found it increased the bioavailability of vasicine and sparteine.

Human clinical trial/study, herbs: A crossover study with volunteers given 2 grams curcumin found that its serum levels were either undetectable or very low. When piperine was administered with the curcumin, serum levels were 2,000 percent higher. Piperine enhanced bioavailability, serum concentration, and extent of absorption; a double-blind study found that piperine (5 mg) increased plasma concentrations of CoQ10 by 30 percent.

7

THE FIRST LINE OF DEFENSE: STRENGTHENING THE IMMUNE SYSTEM

The man is not sick because he has an illness; he has an illness because he is sick.

— Chinese proverb

A basic truism of antibiotic treatment is that it just will not work under most circumstances unless the body can mount its own attack against invading bacteria.

— Marc Lappé, *When Antibiotics Fail*

No matter the virulence of a disease, and this includes fierce diseases such as Ebola, some people remain healthy in spite of being exposed. In fact, medical studies have consistently shown the presence of virulent bacteria in most peoples' systems though they never become ill.

Countless studies have found that the healthier your immune system, the less likely you are to get a disease and the more likely you are, if you do get sick, to have a milder episode. This is especially true in diseases such as Lyme. Researchers have consistently noted that the higher certain immune markers are, the less likely that infection will occur and, if it does, the disease will be less severe than if the immune markers are low.

Our immune system is in fact our first line of defense. Its job is to protect us from disease and, if disease occurs, to cure it. A healthy immune system is therefore the first and most important part of health and healing.

The Basic Elements of the Immune System

Some of the specific elements of our immune system are the thymus, spleen, liver, lymph system, lymph nodes, tonsils, appendix (basically a large lymph node), and bone marrow. The thymus coordinates immune activity, the spleen processes worn-out red blood cells and platelets and provides a location to engulf and destroy invading bacteria. The liver cleans toxins from the blood and produces most of the body's lymph. Lymph is the liquid that flows in the lymph system, somewhat similar to a city's sewer system. The lymph system runs parallel to the blood vessels and stores, filters, and circulates waste, especially dead bacteria and the massive numbers of white blood cells produced during active infections. Lymph nodes are large intersections of lymph channels and store or warehouse the waste products being processed through the lymph system. When the lymph nodes are processing a lot of waste they tend to swell, clog up, and become painful to the touch. When they do, the processing of waste slows down. Keeping the nodes clear helps the body process infections much more quickly. The lymph nodes also produce unique white blood cells called lymphocytes (as does the thymus gland) that are particularly strong elements of the immune system.

Eight Herbs for the Immune System

Ashwagandha | Eleuthero
Astragalus | Red root
Boneset | Reishi
Echinacea | Rhodiola

The bone marrow, and to some extent the thymus, manufactures other types of white blood cells that fight infections. Two of the most important are phagocytes and neutrophils. Phagocytes exist in three forms (monocytes, macrophages, and granulocytes). As macrophages they rove the body looking for foreign bodies, engulf invading bacteria, and help clean up residues of white blood cells and bacteria during and after infections. They also alert the neutrophils, which attack and destroy bacteria and viruses, of the presence of disease organisms.

All these various parts of the immune complex can be supported and kept healthy. A strong immune system means that infections are less frequent and healing is quicker.

Herbs for the Immune System

A number of herbs stand out when it comes to strengthening, rehabilitating, or enhancing the immune system. All of them can be used long term; few have any side effects. Though some of these herbs are active against specific disease organisms, their strength lies in enhancing various aspects of the immune system, offering protective activity against toxins or disease for specific organs in the body, antitumor activity, and/or tonic and restorative activity for general debility in the body or immune system. Many of these plant medicines are also considered to be antistressors and adaptogens. They protect the body from the effects of stress and stimulate the body, and especially the immune system, to more effectively deal with adverse events — internal or external.

Ashwagandha

Family: Solanaceae

Common Names: *Ashwagandha* • *Indian ginseng* • *winter cherry*

Species Used: After intense fisticuffs it was decided that there are six species in this genus. *Withania somnifera* is the species most commonly known as an immune herb. However, two other *Withania* species, *Withania obtusifolia* and *W. coagulans,* are used in much the same manner. *W. obtusifolia* has a long history of use in the Sudan while *W. coagulans* (especially the fruit) has long been used in Pakistan and India. *W. coagulans* is so termed because it is a powerful coagulating agent and is used in place of rennet by Indians to make cheese. (*Obtusifolia* is so named because its leaves are obtuse, that is, "lacking in insight or discernment," and is used in place of aware perception by taxonomists.)

Parts Used

The root is almost exclusively used in Western practice (a few people are starting to use the berry), the whole plant in the rest of the world.

Preparation and Dosage

TINCTURE

Dry root: 1:5, 70% alcohol, 30–40 drops up to 3x daily.

Fresh leaf: 1:2, 95% alcohol, 10–30 drops up to 3x daily.

Dry seed: 1:5, 65% alcohol, 15–30 drops up to 3x daily.

Fresh fruit: 1:2 (grind the whole mess well), 95% alcohol, 15–30 drops up to 3x daily.

CAPSULES

Take 500–1,000 mg daily, though in Ayurvedic practice 3–6 grams are used daily.

Some people, sigh, are standardizing the root capsules to 1.5 percent withanolides. Others are producing both 1:4 and 1:2 tinctures. All may be stronger than the whole, not-altered root and root tinctures … but maybe not.

Side Effects and Contraindications

Avoid high doses in pregnancy, as it may be abortifacient in large doses. May cause drowsiness. Take the herb after dinner to find out just how sleepy it makes you before using it during the day. In rare instances: diarrhea, GI tract upset, vomiting at large doses.

Herb/Drug Interactions

May potentiate barbiturates (anecdotal); don't use with sedatives and anxiolytics.

Habitat and Appearance

Ashwagandha is native to the dry regions of India and is now fairly prolific throughout northern Africa and the Mediterranean, essentially your warm, semi-arid climates that get some good rain during the rainy season. It's a small, perennial, bushy, woody shrub to about 2 feet tall, though with a lot of care, water, and fertilizer it can grow to 6 feet. The plant produces orange-red fruits looking much like cherries (hence that common name) that are enclosed in a papery husk. Ashwagandha is similar in appearance to both ground cherry and Chinese lantern. The roots are long, tuberous, and brown.

Cultivation and Collection

The plant is little grown (or known) in the United States but is a rather common agricultural plant in its region. It does well in warm, semi-arid to arid climates as long as it gets some water now and then. Perfect for parts of Arizona and Southern California — good in zones 8 and warmer. It is a hardy evergreen perennial to temperatures to just above freezing (and can survive occasional drops to as low as 15°F) but does well as an annual pretty much anyplace it is warm enough.

Properties of Ashwagandha

Actions

Root
Alterative
Amphoteric
Antibacterial
Antifatigue
Anti-inflammatory
Antioxidant
Antipyretic
Antistressor
Antitumor
Anxiolytic
Astringent
Chondroprotective
Collagenase inhibitor
Diuretic

Hematopoietic
Immune tonic
Immunomodulant
Insomnia reliever
  (especially stress- or
  disease-induced)
Nervine
Neuroprotective

Leaf and stem
Antibacterial
Antimicrobial
Antipyretic
Antitumor
Astringent

Bitter
Diuretic
Febrifuge
Nervine

Seed
Coagulant
Diuretic
Hypnotic

Fruit
Alterative
Antibacterial
Astringent
Immune tonic

Finding Ashwagandha

Herb stores everywhere, the Internet. Excellent seed stock can be purchased from Horizon Herbs. The plant is very easy to grow.

It needs at least a 200-day growing season to reach maturity but will produce a decent root system in 100 days if that's all you've got.

Ashwagandha is propagated by seed and it grows easily. Sow in early spring indoors. Germination is in about 15 days. Plants really like full sun and fast-draining soil with some limestone in it (alkaline soil lover). The plants are intolerant of wet soils. Harvest the roots just after the cherries become ripe. Dry the cherries for use the next year as new seed stock. Cut the roots into smallish pieces, and dry out of the sun. Store in plastic bags when well dried, in plastic tubs in a cool, dark location. The leaves can be harvested at any time.

Plant Chemistry

The major constituents are steroidal alkaloids and steroidal lactones: withanine, somniferine, somnine, somniferinine, withaninine, pseudo-withanine, tropine, pseudo-tropine, ashwagandhanolide, cuscohygrine, anferine, anhydryine, sitoindoside 7 and 8, a lot of other stuff, and a bunch of steroidal lactones in the leaves called withanolides. Withaferin A in the leaves has tremendous antitumor activity.

Traditional Uses of Ashwagandha

The primary traditional uses of the herb have all been in the Ayurveda system in India.

AYURVEDA

A major plant in India for at least three thousand years, ashwagandha is considered to be tonic, alterative, astringent, aphrodisiac, and a nervine sedative. It has been used for TB, emaciation in children, senile debility, rheumatism, general debility, nervous exhaustion, brain fog, loss of memory, loss of muscular energy, and spermatorrhea. Its primary use is to restore vigor and energy in a body worn out by long-term constitutional disease or old age.

TRADITIONAL CHINESE MEDICINE

Unknown as far as I can determine.

WESTERN BOTANIC PRACTICE

A recent plant to the West, almost an herb-of-the-day.

Scientific Research

There have been an increasing number of studies on ashwagandha since 2000; there are about 400 of them on pubmed as of 2011. Here's a sampling:

Clinical trial, antistressor activity: 100 men and women in a double-blind, placebo-controlled, randomized trial. The herb significantly reduced stress in all who took the herb.

Clinical trial, hemoglobin effects: A double-blind study with 60 healthy children age 8 to 12 years. There was a marked increase in level of hemoglobin at the end of 30 days and in packed cell volume, mean corpuscular volume, serum iron, and hand grip at the end of 60 days.

Clinical trial, hemoglobin effects: A double-blind study with 101 healthy men age 50 to 59 years. Each took 3 grams per day of ashwagandha for 1 year. All showed significantly increased hemoglobin and RBC count, improvement in melanin, and decreased SED rate, and three-quarters of them reported increased sexual performance.

In vitro, antibacterial action: Ashwagandha does have some antibacterial actions; whole-plant extracts have been found active against *Staphylococcus aureus, Pseudomonas aeruginosa, Salmonella* spp., *E. coli,* and *Bacillus subtilis.*

In vitro/in vivo, rats/mice, antineoplastic activity: There have been over 50 studies on the antineoplastic actions of the plant, primarily using the leaves. Tumor growth is retarded, tumor cell proliferation is reduced, side effects of radiation and chemotherapy are reduced, and life expectancy is increased.

In vivo, mice, pain relief: Withaferin A, a constituent of ashwagandha, has been shown to be analgesic and antipyretic.

In vitro studies, cartilage effects: Found the root extract to be highly chondroprotective of damaged human osteoarthritis cartilage matrix. It also was significantly inhibitive of the gelatinase activity of collagenase type 2 enzyme.

In vivo, rats, central nervous system effects: Showed the herb to have anxiolytic and antidepressant actions. Strong antioxidant.

In vivo, mice, central nervous system effects: Showed the herb to correct scopolamine-induced memory loss in mice.

In vitro, central nervous system effects: Root extracts induce neurite extension and outgrowth in human neuroblastoma SH-SY5Y. Stimulate neuritic regeneration and synaptic reconstruction in damaged cortical neurons. Completely inhibit dendritic atrophy.

In vivo, rats, central nervous system effects: Treatment for 14 days significantly improved nitropropionic-acid-induced cognitive dysfunction and oxidative damage in rats. (Note: There have been at least 30 studies finding cognitive improvements in various animal species from the use of the root.)

In vivo, rats, anti-inflammatory: Strongly anti-inflammatory in various rheumatological conditions.

In vivo, dogs, cardiac effects: Hypotensive, bradycardic, respiratory stimulant actions.

In vivo, mice, white blood cells: Ashwagandha significantly reduced induced leukopenia in mice. White blood cell count significantly increased.

In vivo, mice, thyroid enhancement: Significantly increased thyroid production of T3 and T4.

Astragalus

Family: Leguminosae

Common Names: *Astragalus (English)* • *huang-qi (Chinese)*

Species Used: This is a huge genus of some three thousand species, prevalent throughout the world. The primary species used is *Astragalus membranaceus*, a.k.a. *A. membranaceus* var. *mongholicus*, a.k.a. *A. mongholicus*. Sigh . . . now that the number of species in this genus has been, almost, settled, the number of variants is in question. (*Yes*, this one is *Astragalus membranaceus*, but it looks funny. I found it in Mongolia; therefore . . .)

There is not much information on whether any of the other species in the genus can be used similarly.

Note: *Astragalus propinquus* is, in some circles, a synonym for *A. membranaceus*. However, a number of sources now insist (cue shocked expression) that *this* is the correct name for the plant. And of course, *Astragalus mongholicus* is just a rose by any other name.

Parts Used

The plant is a perennial with a long fibrous rootstock. The root, which is the part used for medicine, is often found thinly sliced and dried (a traditional preparation in Chinese medicine) and most closely resembles a yellow (medical) tongue depressor. Bulk quantities of the powdered or coarsely ground organic root are commonly available through herbal suppliers to Western botanic practitioners.

Properties of Astragalus

Actions

Adaptogen	Cardioprotective	Hypotensive
Antibacterial	Diuretic	Immune enhancer,
Antihepatotoxic	Enhances function in	modulator, stimulant,
Antiviral	lungs, spleen, and	and restorative
	GI tract	Tonic

Astragalus is an immune potentiator and modulator. Increases interferon-gamma and interleukin-2 levels. Enhances CD4+ counts and balances the CD4:CD8 ratio. Astragalus is specific for immune atrophy and enhances function in the spleen and thymus.

Finding Astragalus

Herb stores everywhere and the Internet.

Preparation and Dosage

Many astragalus formulations are standardized, though I'm not sure that the literature really supports standardization with this herb.

The root is usually standardized for either 0.4 percent or 0.5 percent 4'-hydroxy-3'-methoxyisoflavone 7-sug, but the reasons are not entirely clear for doing so. No literature exists that I can find that lays out why in fact this particular constituent was singled out and not the astragalosides. (Astragaloside IV, for instance, is one of the primary active ingredients of the plant in heart disease. It increases exercise tolerance and reduces chest distress and dyspnea and optimizes left ventricular function.) The methoxyisoflavone constituent for which the plant is standardized is an anabolic-type compound that enhances strength and muscle formation and may have some protective actions in upper respiratory infections and on digestive function. Data on its functions are somewhat unclear and hard to come by; I have been unable to locate any clinical or laboratory studies on the constituent — though they must exist somewhere. Their rarity stimulates speculation.

The whole root contains constituents that are essential for carditis and enhanced immune function. And, indeed, the majority of the Chinese studies — clinical and laboratory — were with the whole herb.

The herb may be taken as tea, powder, capsules, or tincture or in food.

TEA

Use 2–3 ounces of herb per pot of tea; drink throughout the day.

TINCTURE

1:5, 60 percent alcohol, 30–60 drops up to 4x daily

POWDER

In chronic conditions: Take up to 3 tablespoons per day.
In acute conditions: Take up to 6 tablespoons per day.

FOOD

Astragalus has been used for centuries as an additive to meal preparation. The sliced root is placed in soups and removed before eating or a strong infusion of the root is made and used to cook rice and as a stock for soups.

Side Effects and Contraindications

No toxicity has ever been shown from the regular, daily use of the herb nor from the use of large doses. The Chinese report consistent use for millennia in the treatment of colds and flu and suppressed immune function without side effects.

Astragalus is contraindicated, however, in late-stage Lyme disease because it can exacerbate autoimmune responses in that particular disease.

Herb/Drug Interactions

Synergistic actions: Use of the herb with interferon and acyclovir may increase their effects. The herb has been used in clinical trials with interferon in the treatment of hepatitis B; outcomes were better than with interferon alone. It has also shown synergistic effects when used with interferon in the treatment of cervical erosion; antiviral activity is enhanced.

Drug inhibition: Use of the herb with cyclophosphamide may decrease the effectiveness of the drug. Not for use in people with transplanted organs.

Herb/Herb Interactions

Synergistic with echinacea and licorice in the stimulation of immune function.

Habitat and Appearance

Of the more than three thousand species of astragalus in the world, 16 grow in the United States. The leaf structure looks like a typical member of the pea family. It is a short-lived, sprawling perennial and grows up to 4 feet in size.

The medicinal astragalus is native to northeast China though it has been planted a great many other places, including the United States. Wild populations are still rare in the West though it is under wide cultivation as a medicinal in the United States and escape to the wild is imminent.

Cultivation and Collection

Astragalus is started from seeds in the early spring indoors. The seed coat needs to be scored with something like sandpaper prior to planting. Growers (e.g., Elixir Farm in Missouri) have found that it prefers a sunny location with, as the Elixir Farm website notes, "deep, sandy, well-drained, somewhat alkaline soil. It does not like mulch or deep cultivation. The crowns of the emerging plants are very sensitive to compost and respond well after they have gained some momentum in the spring." Not surprisingly, given the plant's medicinal actions, it is highly resistant to insect damage, crown rot, mildew, and drought.

The plant grows larger and more woody each year, with the roots harvested beginning the fall of the third year or spring of the fourth. Spring and fall harvests occur in China.

Plant Chemistry

Astragalosides 1-7, astraisoflavan, astramembranagenin, astraptero-carpan, beta-sitosterol, betaine, formononetin, GABA, isoastraga-loside 1, 2, and 4, isoliquiritigenin, linoleic acid, linolenic acid, soyasaponin I, kumatakenin, choline, glucuronic acid, 4'-hydroxy-3'-methoxyisoflavone 7-sug, a couple of dihydroxy-7, 4-dimethyl-isoflavones, 3'-hydroxyformonontin, calcium, folic acid, choline, copper, iron, magnesium, manganese, potassium, sodium, zinc.

Traditional Uses of Astragalus

Astragalus, first mentioned in the two-thousand-year-old Chinese text *Shen Nong Cao Jing*, is one of the 50 fundamental herbs in Chinese medicine and is considered to be one of the superior tonic herbs. The plant has developed into one of the primary immune herbs used world-wide over the past four decades.

AYURVEDA

Five species of astragalus are used in the materia medica of India, none of them this species. They are minor herbs, used primarily as emollients.

TRADITIONAL CHINESE MEDICINE

Astragalus has been a major herb in Chinese medicine for between two thousand and four thousand years. Its traditional uses are for spleen deficiency with lack of appetite, fatigue, and diarrhea. It is specific for disease conditions accompanied by weakness and sweating, stabilizes and protects the vital energy (qi), and is used for wasting diseases, numbness of the limbs, and paralysis. Other uses are: for tonifying the lungs, for shortness of breath, for frequent colds and flus; as a diuretic and for reduction of edema; for tonifying the blood and for blood loss, especially postpartum; for diabetes; for promoting the discharge of pus, for chronic ulcerations, including of the stomach, and sores that have not drained or healed well.

WESTERN BOTANIC PRACTICE

The herb was not used in Western botanic practice until the tremendous East/West herbal blending that began during the 1960s. It is now one of the primary immune tonic herbs in the Western pharmacopeia.

Scientific Research

A considerable amount of scientific testing has occurred with astragalus, including clinical trials and both in vivo and in vitro studies. Medline lists 799 citations for studies with astragalus and this does not include the many Chinese studies that have never been indexed for Medline. Two U.S. patents have been granted for the use of astragalus for immunostimulation. What follows is merely a sampling.

IMMUNE FUNCTION

Most of the clinical studies and trials regarding immunostimulation have been focused on the use of astragalus in the treatment of cancer and/or as an adjunct to chemotherapy to help stimulate chemo-depressed immune function. A number of other studies have examined its immune effects with a range of different conditions.

The herb has been used with children suffering tetralogy of Fallot after a radical operation to correct the condition. Tetralogy of Fallot is a complex of four heart abnormalities that occur together, generally at birth. Surgery is used to correct it. Astragalus was found to decrease abnormal levels of IgG, Igm, C3, C4, CD8+, and CD19+ while increasing levels of CD4+ and CD56+. The ratios of CD4:CD8, CD3:HLA-DR, and CD3:CD16 normalized between the second and third week of use. IL-6 and TNF-alpha both began decreasing in the first week and by week 4 were in the normal range.

When astragalus was used in the treatment of herpes simplex keratitis, levels of Th1, including IL-2 and IFN-gamma, increased and Th2 levels, including IL-4 ad IL-10, decreased, showing that the herb modulated Th1 and Th2 levels. This same kind of effect has been found in the treatment of numerous cancers. For example, in a study of 37 lung cancer patients astragalus was found to reverse the Th2 status normally present in that condition. Th1 cytokines (IFN-gamma and IL-2) and its transcript factor (T-bet) were enhanced and Th2 cytokines were decreased.

A clinical study with 63 people suffering serious abdominal traumatic injury found that the addition of astragalus to the treatment regimen significantly increased cellular immunity.

In clinical trials with a number of different cancers and congestive heart conditions, astragalus has been found to increase CD4+ levels, reduce CD8+ levels, and significantly increase the CD4:CD8 ratio. The plant has been found to have a broad immunostimulatory effect. Use of the herb with cancer patients undergoing chemotherapy found that white blood cell counts improved significantly (normalizing). The herb has been found to be specifically useful in preventing or reversing immunosuppression from any source: age-related, bacterial, viral, or chemical. It enhances phagocytosis and increases superoxide dismutase production from macrophages.

HEART DISEASE

There have been numerous clinical trials with the herb for treating heart disease. The herb has been found specific for inhibiting Coxsackie B infections, both as an antiviral and as a heart protector. It will reverse damage to the heart in a number of conditions. With respect to Lyme carditis probably the most important are its impacts on left ventricular function, angina, and shortness of breath. While it is not completely protective for atrioventricular (AV) block, it does improve electrophysiological parameters and ameliorates AV block to some extent.

In a trial of astragalus for 2 weeks with 19 people with congestive heart failure, 15 people experienced alleviation of symptoms of chest distress and dyspnea, and their exercise tolerance increased substantially. Radionuclide ventriculography showed that left ventricular modeling and ejection function improved, and heart rate slowed from 88.21 to 54.66 beats/minute.

In another trial, 43 people suffering from myocardial infarction were tested with astragalus. Left ventricular function strengthened. Superoxide dismutase activity or red blood cell levels increased, and lipid peroxidation of plasma was reduced.

In a study with 366 cardiac patients astragalus was found to be effective when compared to lidocaine and mexiletine (which were not found effective). With astragalus the duration of ventricular late potentials shortened significantly.

In the treatment of 92 patients suffering ischemic heart disease, astragalus was more successful than nifedipine. Patients were "markedly relieved" from angina pectoris. EKG test results improved 82.6 percent.

ANTI-INFLAMMATORY ACTIVITY

Astragalus has been found to possess anti-inflammatory activity by inhibiting the NF-kB pathway and blocking the effect of interleukin-1 beta in leukotriene C production in human amnions. The constituent astragaloside IV inhibits increases in microvascular permeability induced by histamine. The whole-herb decoction has been found to reduce capillary hyperpermeability.

NEUROLOGICAL ACTIONS

Astragalus has been found to improve anisodine-induced impairment of memory acquisition and alcohol-elicited deficit of memory retrieval. After use of the herb the number of errors was reduced. The plant has been found to exert potent antioxidant effects on the brain, helping to prevent senility.

FATIGUE

Astragalus has been found effective in alleviating fatigue in heart patients and in athletes. In one trial, 12 athletes were randomly separated into two groups, and six were given astragalus. Astragalus was found to positively influence anaerobic threshold, enhance recovery from fatigue, and increase fatigue threshold.

A double-blind, randomized, controlled trial with 36 adults with chronic fatigue found that a mixture of astragalus and Salviae Radix significantly decreased fatigue scores.

HEPATITIS

A number of trials have found the herb effective in the clinical treatment of hepatitis B and liver disease. Liver function is improved, the liver is protected from damage, and regeneration is stimulated.

IMMUNE-ENHANCING BROTH

Robyn Landis and K. P. S. Khalsa share a tasty recipe for an immune-enhancing astragalus broth in their book, *Herbal Defense* (Warner Books, 1997).

Immune-Enhancing Broth

INGREDIENTS

3 cups water or vegetable broth

1 ounce astragalus (five "tongue depressor" lengths of the sliced root)

1 bulb (5 to 10 cloves) fresh garlic, sliced or whole

Salt and pepper to taste

Combine the water, astragalus, and garlic and simmer for several hours, until the garlic is soft. Season with salt and pepper to taste. Consume all the broth if you feel an infection coming on, or take a cup or two several times during the week to prevent infection. Consume the garlic separately, leave in the broth, or use as a spread on toast.

Immune-Enhancing Rice

INGREDIENTS

1½ ounces sliced astragalus root

4 cups water, plus more as needed

2 cups (uncooked) brown rice

Add the astragalus to the water, bring to boil, and simmer, covered, for 2 hours. Remove from the heat and let stand overnight. Remove the astragalus, and add enough water to bring the broth volume back up to 4 cups. Add the rice, bring to a boil, then reduce the heat and simmer, covered, until the rice is done, approximately 1 hour. Use this rice as you would any rice, as a base for meals throughout the week.

Properties of Boneset

Actions

Antibacterial (mild)
Anti-inflammatory
Cytotoxic (strongly anticancer)
Diaphoretic
Emetic (mild)

Febrifuge
Gastric bitter
Immunostimulant (increases phagocytosis four times better than echinacea)

Mucous membrane tonic
Peripheral circulatory stimulant
Smooth muscle relaxant

Finding Boneset

Fields and streams in the eastern United States, the Internet, herb stores here and there. Horizon Herbs (see Resources) sells the seeds.

Boneset

Family: Compositae

Common Names: *Boneset, common boneset, throughwort, agueweed, feverwort, sweating plant — but no one has used those last three names since 1885. (And it's pronounced A-gyew-weed, not aaagh-weed, big fella.)*

Species Used: There are 36, or 60, or pi? numbers of species in the *Eupatorium* genus; taxonomists being troublesome again. Nearly all are native to the Americas, *Eupatorium cannabinum* being an exception. Many of the species in the genus are medicinal; however, for our purposes here, *Eupatorium perfoliatum* is the plant to use. The others do other things. For immune action, we want this one.

Parts Used

Aerial parts, in flower or just before flowering, depending.

Preparation and Dosage

May be taken as tea or tincture.

TEA

Cold tea: 1 ounce herb in 1 quart boiling water, let steep overnight, strain, and drink throughout the day. The cold infusion is better for the mucous membrane system and as a liver tonic.

Hot tea: 1 tsp herb in 8 ounces hot water, steep 15 minutes. Drink 4–6 ounces up to 4x per day. Boneset is only diaphoretic when hot and should be consumed hot for active infections or for recurring chills and fevers.

TINCTURE

Fresh herb in flower: 1:2, 95 percent alcohol, 20–40 drops in hot water up to 3x daily.

Dry herb: 1:5, 60 percent alcohol, 30–50 drops in hot water up to
3x daily.

In acute viral or bacterial upper respiratory infections, take
10 drops of tincture in hot water every half hour up to 6x daily. In
conditions where the acute stage has passed but there is continued
chronic fatigue and relapse, take 10 drops of tincture in hot water
4x daily.

Side Effects and Contraindications

The hot infusion in quantity can cause vomiting, and in moderate
doses mild nausea sometimes occurs. The cooler the tea the less
nausea. Otherwise, no side effects or contraindications. However,
boneset *may* be contraindicated in pregnancy.

Herb/Drug Interactions

None noted.

Habitat and Appearance

The plant is pervasive in the eastern half of the United States and
Canada, from Texas, Oklahoma, North Dakota, et cetera on eastward.
However, every place I've seen it grow has been wettish, humid, with
good soil.

Boneset grows up to 3 feet tall, they say, but I've never seen it get
that big; however, most of my experience of the plant has been in the
tiny state of Vermont. Two feet seemed about average, just like with
hominids. The plant grows in a straight stalk, the leaves going north/
south, then east/west, then north/south again. The leaves continue on
through the stalk, hence throughwort; it basically looks like the leaves
were glued together at the wide end and the stalk just punched through
them. Once seen, never forgotten.

Cultivation and Collection

The plant is a perennial and likes full or partial sun in moist to wet
conditions, on the edges of swamps, along streams, in wet meadows,

in marshlands, basically any place mosquitos like to breed except maybe old tires. It spreads by seed; there are a lot of sources on the Internet.

If collected at flowering and allowed to dry, the plant will usually go to seed as it dries. It should be collected only in flower (August or September) if being tinctured fresh and *right now*. If you are going to use it as a tea, it should be picked just prior to flowering, hung upside down in a shaded place, and allowed to thoroughly air-dry.

Plant Chemistry

Methylglucuronoxylan, astragalin, eufoliatin, eufoliatorin, eupatorin, euperfolin, euperfolitin, euperfolide, euccannabinolide, eupatorio-picrin, hyperoside, rutin, polysaccharides, and a bunch of other stuff. Many of those are sesquiterpene lactones, common in the eupatoriums.

Traditional Uses of Boneset

AYURVEDA
Nope.

TRADITIONAL CHINESE MEDICINE
Not hardly.

WESTERN BOTANIC PRACTICE
Oh, yes, used. The plant, indigenous to North America, has been used by Native American peoples for millennia, specifically for intermittent fevers and chills, with pain in the bones, weakness, and debility. The American Eclectics used it for intermittent (e.g., malarial), typhoid, and remittent fevers, and for general debility, pneumonia, cough, epidemic influenza, colds, catarrh, and pains accompanying those conditions. It was one of their primary remedies.

Scientific Research

The sesquiterpene lactones in boneset have a large range of actions. They are highly immunostimulatory and very active against cancers. They also possess antiplasmodial actions. The action is mild, but if the plant is added to a traditional antimalarial that is strong, such as cryptolepis, the effects are mutually supportive. A homeopathic formulation of boneset was found to significantly inhibit plasmodial replication (60 percent inhibition).

Clinical trials have shown that boneset stimulates phagocytosis better than echinacea, is analgesic (at least as effective as aspirin), and reduces cold and flu symptoms. In mice it has shown strong immuno-stimulant activity and cytotoxic action against cancer cells.

Despite boneset's long use and potent reputation, little research has occurred with the plant. In clinical practice, however, it is one of the most potent herbs for enhancing immune function, especially in periodic diseases like bartonellosis. It will reliably counter bacterial or viral immune suppression in diseases that present as periodics.

Echinacea

Family: Compositae

Common Names: *These days "echinacea" pretty much is the name, though "purple coneflower" is exceptionally common among gardeners who don't know about the medicinal actions of plants.*

Species Used: All nine members of the genus can be used; however, the most common are *Echinacea angustifolia* and *E. purpurea.* I don't particularly think that *purpurea* is all that strong in comparison. I really haven't found it all that effective, in spite of what everyone says, and I avoid it if possible. I would strongly suggest the use of *angustifolia* if you can get it. (There is some evidence that *Echinacea pallida* is more potent than *angustifolia,* but I haven't worked with it personally.)

Parts Used

Root primarily, but the flower heads in seed are also potent. The Germans, however, use the *juice* of *purpurea* as their primary medicinal.

Properties of Echinacea

Actions

Analgesic	Antiviral	Immune stimulant
Antibacterial	Hyaluronidase inhibitor	Sialagogue
Anti-inflammatory	Immune modulator	Stimulates antibody production

Finding Echinacea

E. purpurea is everywhere. I strongly advise against using it, ever, unless you are juicing the fresh plant yourself — which you should if it is growing in the garden; there's no need to kill the plant by digging it up. *Angustifolia* is harder to find; few herb shops carry it in tincture form. You can, however, find *angustifolia* tinctures here and there on the Internet. Try Sage Woman Herbs. Pacific Botanicals carries *angustifolia* root in bulk. Excellent quality. See Resources.

Preparation and Dosage

The most potent medicinal forms of the plant are tincture of the root and the fresh juice of the aerial plant.

Note: Echinacea extracts standardized for phenolic acid or echinocaside content have been found to be inactive as immunostimulants but do still retain their anti-inflammatory actions.

FRESH JUICE

Juice the aerial parts of the plant, when in flower if possible. Take immediately or stabilize with 20–25 percent alcohol (see page 227). Take 1–3 teaspoons per day, or up to 6x daily in acute episodes.

TINCTURE

E. angustifolia dry root, 1:5, 70 percent alcohol. (Or fresh flower heads of *purpurea* if you must, 1:2, 95 percent alcohol.)

Note: *The tincture's effectiveness is much reduced if taken in water* (unless you are taking large doses for septicemia or collagen support) and I would strongly recommend against doing so, especially in the treatment of strep infections of the throat.

For strep throat/tonsillitis: Direct contact with the tissue at the back of the throat with a tincture of echinacea (30 drops each hour minimum) liberally mixed with saliva is certain in these kinds of conditions. Echinacea actively stimulates saliva and numbs the tissue it comes into contact with, making it perfect for this (or any sore, swollen throat infections). I have found this reliably effective, again if treatment is assertive and consistent. In a number of cases (including a doubting physician who was ill himself) the throat had been positively cultured for strep; healing generally occurs within 24 hours.

As a mouth/gum wash for sores and ulcers: The tincture, 30 drops, hold in mouth until saliva is well stimulated, swish it around to cover all surfaces well, hold for 30 seconds, swallow. Repeat 3x or 4x daily.

For onset of colds and flus: Not less than 1 dropperful (30 drops) of tincture each hour until symptoms cease. (Note: Echinacea is more effective for cold and flu onset in combination with licorice root and red root.)

For septicemia, typhoid, diphtheria, and so on: 1 tsp *E. angustifolia* root tincture in very little water every half hour until the situation normalizes. If the tincture is held in the mouth for a minute or so, it will enter the bloodstream quite rapidly. Better outcomes will be achieved this way. If taken 30 minutes after piperine, its movement into the bloodstream will be very rapid.

For collagen tissue protection and repair: 1/4–1 tsp tincture, 3x daily for extended periods (weeks).

For external wounds: Because of its capacity to correct tissue abnormality, echinacea is perfect for this application. Its anti-inflammatory, antibacterial, and cell-normalizing actions all come into powerful play for any external wounds. In the case of infected wounds, take the tincture, frequently, diluted in a bit of water. In severe cases take 1/2–1 teaspoon of *angustifolia* root tincture each half hour to hour.

For venomous stings and bites: Mix the tincture with an equal amount of water and wash the affected area liberally every 30 minutes, and take 30 drops to 1 teaspoon of the tincture each half hour to hour depending on the type of bite/sting. For infected bites or stings, more; for venomous bites/stings, more; for simple bee or wasp stings, less. (You can also use a wash for this purpose: Boil 2 ounces ground flower heads or root in 8 ounces water for 15 minutes, let steep 1 hour, strain, and use to wash wounds and venomous bites and stings liberally, as often as needed.)

POWDER

As a wound powder: Powder the dried root (or seed heads) as finely as possible and sprinkle liberally over new or infected wounds. Best in combination with other herbs such as goldenseal, usnea, oak, and wormwood.

Poultice: Mix powder with water until thick and place on
affected area.

For abnormal Pap smear: Echinacea can easily correct even stage
three dysplasia. Whenever echinacea is placed directly on cells
that are displaying abnormal properties, the cells tend to return to
normal relatively quickly as long as the treatment is assertive and
consistent. I have seen no other herb that comes even close to echinacea's reliability in this regard. Use as a suppository; see page 355
for details.

Side Effects and Contraindications

Rarely: Joint pain may occur with large doses taken for extended
periods of time. Increased shoe size may occur from large doses
for extended periods. Current collagenosis? Don't take a lot for a
long time.

Echinacea is not an immune tonic; it is an immune stimulant. Continued immune stimulation in instances of immune depletion to avoid
necessary rest or more healthy lifestyle choices will always result in
a more severe illness than if the original colds and flus were allowed
to progress. Echinacea should not be used if you are getting sick a lot
and are only using echinacea to stave off illness without using the time
gained to heal the immune system itself through deep healing and
recuperation.

Herb/Drug Interactions

None have been noted; however, echinacea decreases the action of the
influx transporter OATP-B by 50 percent. It may decrease the absorption of OATP-B substrates. Phenobarbital, chloral hydrate, and mepro-
bamate can inhibit the anti-inflammatory actions of echinacea.

Herb/Herb Interactions

Synergistic with astragalus and licorice in the stimulation of immune
function.

Habitat and Appearance

The echinaceas are perennials, indigenous to eastern and central
North America, usually in moist or dry prairies and open woodlands.
E. purpurea is a major garden plant pretty much everyplace that has
gardens. It is also a major agricultural crop everywhere on Earth,
including China, so this member of the genus, even if no others, has
colonized numerous countries around the globe.

The plants are unbranched, erect, with wide-bladed leaves and
grow 3 to 5 feet tall. Writers often describe the plant leaves as hairy
with a rough texture. To me the experience is more like touching
Velcro; the plant doesn't mess around. The stems are strong, the plants
vigorous, intense. They are not *ooooooh* love/mushy plants and have no
resemblance to puppies or kittens.

All the species except *purpurea* have strong taproots, brown,
vigorous, intense. *Purpurea*'s roots are some sort of strange, glumpy,
fibrous sort of paleish-tannish thing. I never have been attracted to
that species and besides I don't think it is all that good medicinally so
I am prejudiced; the rootish things it produces just look wimpy to me,
sort of like a bag of earthworms curled around an irregular sort of tannish lump. But, you know, go ahead and use *purpurea* if you want.

Cultivation and Collection

The reason why so many people use *purpurea* for medicine rather than
angustifolia (which I think much stronger) is that it is easier to grow.
(Ah hah!) Throw the seeds in the ground in the fall and up they come
in the spring. Like all the echinaceas they prefer a period of cold before
germinating, but I have talked to people who just planted seeds in the
spring and found them to be decent if not spectacular germinators.
You can also separate the *purpurea* root thingies into chunks and propagate them that way. From personal experience, and from everyone I
have talked to, the other species of echinacea are decidedly cranky; you
have to work at it to get them to grow. *Angustifolia* is a poor germinator
until you figure out just what it likes; stratification is essential for the

plant — however, soaking the seeds in ethephon for 10 minutes will help germination tremendously, much more than stratification.

At one time it was almost impossible to get anything other than *purpurea* to put in a garden, but that has changed — many people now have seedlings available of most of the echinacea species. Horizon Herbs (see Resources) has one of the best selections. The plants self-seed once established, so beginning with seedlings and tending them carefully until they take is a good route to go if you want this medicinal as a permanent member of your herb garden.

Fall-harvest the roots — after 3 years or so in the ground — after the leaves turn brown. Harvest the seed heads just after the seeds mature. I prefer my root tincture to be from dried roots rather than fresh, but then I use *angustifolia* and am in a minority in this; most people use the fresh *purpurea* roots. In any event, let the (*angustifolia*) roots dry whole, then store them in plastic bags in the dark in a cool location. They will last for years if properly stored. (Studies on years-old dried roots found them just as effective as the fresh roots in their actions.)

You can harvest the fresh plants for juicing anytime, the German approach, and that won't kill the plant as taking the roots does. The plants are most potent if you take them in full flower, then run them through a juicer, and stabilize the juice with 20 percent alcohol by volume (see page 227).

Plant Chemistry

Echinacoside, echinacin, echinoline, echinacein, polyacetylenes, hydrocinnamic acid, betaine, alkylamides, caffeic acid glycosides, inulin, isobutyl amides, isobutylalkamines, sesquiterpene esters, and so on.

Traditional Uses of Echinacea

AYURVEDA
Nope.

TRADITIONAL CHINESE MEDICINE

Nein.

WESTERN BOTANIC PRACTICE

The various echinacea species were used for a very long time by the indigenous cultures of North America, who then passed on the knowledge to the nascent American medical movements (who really went with it). The native cultures used the plants, most often the roots, for wounds and sores; as a poultice for swellings; for septic wounds, sores in the mouth or gums, respiratory infections, sore throat, tonsillitis, enlarged glands, fevers, mumps and measles; as a wash for the pain of burns; for toothache and cavities; for snakebites and poisonous bites from insects and spiders; stomach cramps, GI tract distress, arthritis, rheumatism. They took large frequent doses.

The Eclectics were first alerted to the plant by its usefulness for snakebite treatment but went on to use it as one of their primary medicines. Generally, they used it much like the native cultures. They, however, felt the herb specific for septicemia, infected blood, severely infected wounds (with blood infection), generally infected mucous membrane systems of the throat, tongue, mouth, lungs, and stomach, tonsillitis, respiratory infections with foul smell, diphtheria, infected insect bites, and on and on and on. They used large frequent doses — every half hour to hour. The Eclectics *only* used *angustifolia*; they did not consider *purpurea* a legitimate substitute for it nor a very good herb in and of itself.

The use of *Echinacea purpurea* came about not only because of ease of growth but due to intense German interest in the plant; it is part of their standard-practice medicine. (They used *purpurea* because it was easy to grow and was already present in the country.) Most, if not all, of the German studies and use, however, have been with the expressed juice of the plant — which they often use parenterally (by injection) rather than taken by mouth; they don't use the root of *purpurea*. *Hello* — they don't use the root of *purpurea*. They do use the root of *E. pallida* as an ethanolic extract taken by mouth. *Purpurea* root

CONTINUED ON PAGE 278

Time for a Rant

Like goldenseal, echinacea is a North American plant and, as such, most of the studies in the United States are still arguing about whether it works or not (just as with goldenseal). The Germans are under no such illusions; it is part of their standard-practice medicine. Most of the early research occurred in Germany; the rest of the world is just starting to catch up. Unfortunately a great deal of the research has devoted itself to deciding whether the herb works or not (generally not) and way too many of the studies look at the use of the herb as a preventive for colds — in adults and children. Very few of them have looked at the traditional uses and dosages of the herb and oriented their studies around that, so that they are discovering it useless for what they are testing it for. What a shock. Basically, they are giving capsules of *purpurea* in small doses a few times a day to help prevent colds — some good double-blind studies, too. (That's where they poke out *both* of the researchers' eyes and . . .)

If I had a nickel for every person who has told me they had a cold and had taken some echinacea — usually *purpurea* — (dropperful 3x daily) and didn't notice any difference, I would be rich.

To be clear: The herb is very good, *if you are using it properly for the right things.* It is relatively useless for preventing colds. The overuse of the herb for that (especially combined with goldenseal — what a waste) is due entirely to marketing ploys by the larger herb companies. Echinacea *can* help at the onset of a cold or flu *if used in large doses every half hour or hour exactly at the onset of the cold or flu.* If the infection gets established, use lomatium, because echinacea just ain't gonna cut it. I have also found that echinacea is much less effective as a flu and cold treatment for people past the middle age shift. It is, however, very good for younger people *if used properly.*

Nevertheless, I don't consider that the main strength of the plant. In general, it is very good for exactly what the native peoples and Eclectics used it for: *severe* infections of the throat, infected wounds that stink, insect bites, snakebites, nastily infected mucous membranes especially if accompanied by foul smell, septicemia, wounds and sores, sores in the mouth and gums, and so on. If your condition is similar and you treat it aggressively, the plant can save your life.

The herb does enhance immune function, but most people think of it as an immune tonic. It isn't. Rhodiola and ashwagandha are tonics but not echinacea. Echinacea is an immune *stimulant.*

I have found the herb to be excellent for raising immune function in *active* infections if taken internally in the right doses and to be very specific for correcting problems in the skin or mucous membranes if used topically — basically anyplace the herb can touch the affected part. But the doses have to be high and frequent or else forget it. And again, if you have any kind of circulating infection, especially if there is bacteria in the blood (septicemia), the herb is very potent if taken properly.

The herb also has some good specific actions on the mucous membranes and collagen tissues of the body, but you really have to know what you are doing to get good outcomes. And again, I just haven't found *purpurea* to be as reliable as *angustifolia* for serious conditions. Some of the herbalists I know in Europe insist that they have, but I have personally tried really large doses of *purpurea*, for myself and others, and it just isn't up to snuff. The native cultures almost always used *angustifolia* for serious conditions (so did the Eclectics); *purpurea* had a very small profile in indigenous medicine in the United States. I tend to think they were on to something, as I have, as they apparently did, found *purpurea* weak.

> If I had a nickel for every person who has told me they had a cold and had taken some echinacea and didn't notice any difference, I would be rich.

Does *purpurea* work at all? Well, yes, but we are talking pretty good doses of the fresh plant juice here (6 to 15 ml, i.e., 1 to 3 teaspoons daily) and using it in specific ways for specific conditions and still — for colds and influenza even the Germans consider it to be only *supportive*. Its real strength in their system is as a topical treatment for wounds and sores.

There are very few if any commercial products in the United States that use the fresh juice or suggest the right dosing strategies and amounts. The main thing is . . . *angustifolia* (and the others) are just better. Much better.

came into vogue in the United States during the herbal renaissance of the late twentieth century *because* of the German use of the expressed juice of the aerial parts of the plant in flower (an invalid generalization to the root from the actions of the fresh juice) *and* because it was easily available in the eastern United States. It is native to the eastern United States and is widely grown there in gardens.

E. purpurea is used in Germany as a *supportive* therapy for colds, for chronic infections of the respiratory and lower urinary tract, or externally for poorly healing wounds and chronic ulceration. The tincture of *E. pallida* root is used as supportive therapy for influenza-like infections. Supportive, not primary.

Scientific Research

Most of the usable studies on echinacea have used the fresh juice of *Echinacea purpurea*. Unless otherwise noted, that is what these studies are referring to. There have been hundreds of papers published on the plant; this is just a sampling.

But first . . . echinacea (all species) really has two primary actions: it stimulates the immune system and it is a very potent hyaluronidase inhibitor. Many of its most potent medicinal actions come from these two things.

Hyaluronidase (HYL) is an enzyme that breaks down hyaluronic acid (HA), a glycosaminoglycan that is widely distributed throughout connective, epithelial, and neural tissues. It is, as well, a major part of the extracellular matrix. Inhibition of hyaluronidase has a number of beneficial actions: 1) In inflammatory diseases such as various forms of arthritis, the use of a hyaluronidase inhibitor stops the normal (and abnormal) breakdown of cartilage (and synovial fluid), which increases the amount of cartilage (and fluid) in and around the joints, helping counteract, even reverse, the condition. Combined with the anti-inflammatory actions of the herb, this means that large doses can be highly useful for reversing various forms of arthritis and rheumatism. 2) Hyaluronic acid is a major component of the skin and is highly involved in skin repair. HA contributes to tissue dynamics, cell movement and proliferation, and the generation of new cellular tissues. HA is strongly present in new wounds and enhances cellular filtration. It is an essential element of granulation; that is, the new cellular tissue that slowly takes the place of the clotted blood (scab) that first forms over a wound. This tissue forms from the bottom of the wound upward. The more HA, the faster and better it forms. Hyaluronidase inhibition means that more HA is present in the skin/wound area and skin repair is significantly enhanced. 3) With many types of cancer, hyaluronidase plays a major role in metastasis. It degrades the extracellular matrix and allows cancer cells to escape the main tumor mass. HYL also degrades other cellular structures, allowing the cancer cells to penetrate them as well. It also plays a role in the formation of the new blood vessels that cancerous tumors need to survive. HYL inhibition, then, produces a particular kind of anticancer, or antitumor, action. 4) Some bacteria (*Staphylococcus aureus*, *Streptococcus* spp., *Clostridium* spp., *Enterococcus* spp., *Mycobacterium* spp., etc.) create and release hyaluronidase in order to loosen the connective tissue matrix and facilitate their penetration into new areas of the body. Part of what echinacea does is to strengthen the structure of the mucous and skin membranes of the body by stopping their structural breakdown through HYL inhibition while at the same time counteracting the HYL release by bacteria. This stops the bacterial movement into the body. A number of viruses also use HYL to help them penetrate the body; this is especially true of cancer viruses. 5) Hyaluronidase is also found in some snake venoms. It increases the lethality of the venom, in part by allowing it to penetrate more easily into the body.

ANTIVIRAL ACTIVITY

Echinacea is antiviral; it's been found active against HIV and influenza H5N1, H7N7, and H1N1 (swine origin). However, in order to inactivate the influenza strains, it needs *direct contact* just prior to or right at the moment of infection. Echinacea inhibits receptor cell binding activity of the virus, interfering with its entry into the cells while at the same time strengthening the protective power of the mucous membranes through HYL inhibition.

ANTIBACTERIAL ACTIVITY

Echinacea is antibacterial; it inactivates *Streptococcus pyogenes*, *Haemophilus influenzae*, *Propionbacterium acnes*, and *Legionella pneumophila*. It also completely reverses the inflammatory processes that are initiated by those organisms. Echinacea is less active against *Staphylococcus aureus* and *Mycobacterium smegmatis* but also completely reverses the inflamation that they cause. Again, *direct contact* is necessary.

Echinacea is also active against *Leishmania major* promastigotes and *Leishmania enrietti*. *E. angustifolia* is active against *Pseudomonas aeruginosa*.

Echinacea is also active against numerous species of *Candida*. In vitro research found that a hexane extract of echinacea inhibited *Candida shehata*, *C. kefyr*, *C. albicans*, *C. steatulytica*, and *C. tropicalis*. In other studies echinacea increased the proliferation of phagocytes in spleen and bone marrow and the migration of granulocytes to peripheral blood. These studies found that echinacea was specifically active against systemic candida in the blood. In fact, mice were then protected from lethal injections of the yeast directly into the blood. In mice whose levels of leukocytes in the peripheral blood had been reduced through injection of cyclophosphamide, echinacea initiated an influx of neutrophil granulocytes that protected the mice from candida infection.

In a study of recurrent candida vaginal yeast infections, half the women were treated with econazole nitrate (EN) alone, the other half were treated with EN and echinacea. Those using EN alone had a 60 percent recurrence rate, while those using EN and echinacea had only a 17 percent recurrence rate.

WOUND-HEALING ACTIVITY

The alcoholic extract of *E. pallida* reverses stress-delayed wound healing in mice. *E. purpurea* enhances wound healing in vocal fold wounds in pigs. Echinacea (type not stated but probably *purpurea*) enhances fibrin formation in skin grafts, increases wound healing time, stimulates the formation of new connective tissue, and reduces leukocytic infiltration.

ANTI-INFLAMMATORY ACTIONS

Angustifolia, purpurea, and *pallida* are all potent inhibitors of nitric oxide. *Pallida* is the strongest. Arginase activity is significantly increased by all three, but only *pallida* inhibits inducible nitric oxide synthase.

Most echinacea species strongly inhibit PGE production; *sanguinea* is strongest, followed by *angustifolia* and *pallida.*

Constituents of echinacea (echinacoside, etc.) protect collagen from free-radical-induced degradation.

PAIN RELIEF

Angustifolia is 10 times more potent a pain reliever than capsaicin. It acts by desensitizing the TRPV1 channel.

ANTICANCER/RADIATION PROTECTION

Echinacea reversed the system effects of gamma-irradiated mice: Red blood cell parameters, white blood cell parameters, and bone marrow cell parameters were all ameliorated. Echinacea (type not stated) was found to significantly abate leukemia and extend the life span of leukemic mice.

IMMUNE ACTIVITY

Echinacea increases the expression of CD69 and CD25 immune cells in vitro.

In vitro studies on the effects of seven species of echinacea on peripheral blood mononuclear cells (PBMC) found that tinctures from four (*angustifolia, pallida, paradoxa,* and *tennesseensis*) stimulated proliferation of PBMCs and increased interleukin-2 (IL-2). Two tinctures (*sanguinea* and *simulata*) stimulated proliferation only. *E. purpurea* stimulated IL-2 only.

None of the extracts affected IL-4 or tumor necrosis factor-alpha (TNF-alpha). However, if volunteers were first immunized against influenza and *that* blood tested, tinctures from four (*pallida, paradoxa, sanguinea,* and *simulata*) diminished influenza-specific IL-2. None affected influenza-specific IL-10 or interferon-gamma (IFN-gamma). With blood drawn 6 months postvaccination, four tinctures (50 percent alcohol, *angustifolia, purpurea, simulata,* and *tennesseensis)* augmented IL-10 production and diminished IL-2, with no effect on IFN-gamma. Two *(paradoxa* and *sanguinea)* were similar though weaker. *E. pallida* suppressed all cytokines. The authors note that the various species have different immune-modulating actions.

Three echinacea species were tested for in vivo (mice) enhancement of innate and adaptive immune functions. All three *(angustifolia, purpurea,* and *pallida)* significantly increased antibody response, altered cytokine expression by splenic cells, significantly increased interferon-alpha production, and inhibited the release of TNF-alpha and IL-1 beta. Only two *(angustifolia* and *pallida)* strongly enhanced T cell proliferation, significantly stimulated IL-4 production, and decreased IL-10.

Alkamides from echinacea (type not stated) were found to potently inhibit inflammation in human blood and to exert modulatory effects on various cytokine expression (up-regulating IL-6 and inhibiting TNF-alpha, IL-1 beta, IL-12p70).

A butanol fraction from *purpurea* stems and leaves significantly up-regulated specific genes for IL-8, IL-1 beta, IL-18, and the chemokines CXCL2, CCL5, and CCL2 within 4 hours after treatment of immature dendritic cells.

In vivo studies on mice vaccinated with killed *Salmonella typhimurium* vaccine or an inactivated pertussis vaccine consisting of diphtheria/tetanus toxoids and inactivated virulence factors of *Bordetella pertussis* found that *E. angustifolia* and *purpurea* significantly increased antibody production and proliferation as well as IL-12 levels.

A rather large number of studies found that echinacea activates cellular immunity and stimulates phagocytosis of neutrophils in vitro, in vivo, and, in one case, after rinsing of the mouth cavity. In numerous studies echinacea increases interferon-gamma production, stimulates T helper cell production and proliferation, and strongly enhances CD4 and CD8 subsets.

Echinacea has a wide range of actions on the immune system and is both highly stimulatory and modulatory. It is an effective modulator of macrophage immune responses. It enhances antibody responses to infection. It is 30 percent more effective, for example, than sodium alginate in the stimulation of antivenom (snake) antibodies. It stimulates the production of neutrophils, macrophages, and T and B cells.

Eleuthero

Family: Araliaceae

Common Names: *(English) eleuthero • Siberian ginseng • touch-me-not • devil's shrub*

Species Used: There are 25 or maybe 38 species (thanks, guys) in the genus, and while the primary one used is *Eleutherococcus senticosus,* there is emerging evidence that a number of the species are also medicinally active in similar ways. *Eleutherococcus sessiflorus* is used in Korea, identically to eleuthero. *Eleutherococcus cissifolius* is used in Tibet, fresh juice for eczema.

Eleutherococcus spinosus (a.k.a. *E. pentaphyllus*, fiveleaf aralia) is an invasive in the United States in Connecticut, Indiana, Kentucky, Massachusetts, Utah, and West Virginia, and, as well, Ontario, Canada. It is used similarly to eleuthero as a tonic adaptogen for general debility, rheumatic pains, and weakness. Its use should be explored as a now locally established, important immune plant and adaptogen.

Note: *Acanthopanax senticosus* is sometimes given as a synonym for *E. senticosus.*

Parts Used

The root is the most commonly used part of the plant, but the bark from the woody stems is actually higher in what is considered to be the most active constituent of the plant (eleutheroside B). The fruits are also usable and the leaves have some activity as well. The Chinese use every part of the plant in various ways for this and that.

Preparation and Dosage

There are, in general, three primary forms of eleuthero that are used:
1) the Russian high-concentration formulations, generally 2:1, 1:1, or 1:2;
2) lower-strength 1:5 tincture formulations; and, finally,
3) capsules, usually standardized in some way or another (though I prefer the powdered herb myself).

If you are growing the plant and making your own extracts, the eleutheroside B content in the bark of woody stems is about four times that of the roots, so use that rather than kill the plant to get the roots.

Properties of Eleuthero

Actions

Adaptogen (a substance that increases non-specific resistance to adverse influences)

Adrenal tonic

Antidepressant

Antifatigue

Antistressor

Helps restore task endurance

Immune potentiator

Immune tonic

Immunoadjuvant

MAO inhibitor

Mental clarity stimulant

Finding Eleuthero

Herb stores everywhere; the Internet. But really, if you are in a region in which the plant will grow easily, buy a few seedlings and plant them. Once established, the plant will spread and provide medicine for you forever.

RUSSIAN/HIGH-STRENGTH FORMULATIONS

Most of the Russian studies were conducted using a 1:1 tincture in 30 percent to 33 percent alcohol. The dosage ranged from 2 to 20 ml per day (the smaller dose is a smidgeon under ½ teaspoon). This means people were taking from ¹⁄₁₆ to ⅔ ounce (and in some instances up to 1½ ounces) of tincture per day. At an average cost of $7 to $12 per ounce of tincture (in the United States) this can be prohibitively expensive at the upper dosage ranges.

The Russians generally dosed 2 to 16 ml, one to three times daily for 60 days with a 2- to 3-week rest period in between. Russian researchers, at these kinds of dosages, saw responses within a few days or even hours of administration.

In this concentration, and at those doses, eleuthero is an immune *stimulant*, not a tonic. Using it at those doses in this concentrated a form is, in my opinion, specific for debilitating diseases accompanied by severe fatigue, brain fog, depression, muscle weakness, tendency to start getting better with inevitable relapse, and chronically depressed immune function.

You can, of course, take lower doses of the concentrated extracts, which would indeed make the tincture more tonic in nature.

Dosage of the Russian formulation in treating chronic, debilitating disease: *Please read carefully.* In chronic, highly debilitated conditions, the stronger Russian formulation is the only type of tincture that should be used — at least initially. I suggest the product sold by Herb Pharm, which is the only company I know of that actually exceeds the Russian specifications. Their formula is a 2:1 rather than a 1:1 (i.e., 2 parts herb to 1 part liquid rather than 1 and 1).

For the first 30–60 days: 1 tsp, 3x daily, the last dose occurring no later than 4 P.M. This dose can be increased if necessary.

After 60 days: Discontinue the herb for 2 weeks.

Then: Repeat if necessary.

If symptoms decrease after using the Russian formulation for a while and immune function seems better, you can change to either an encapsulated form or a 1:5 alcohol/water tincture (see below). Both of these are weaker, but more tonic, in their actions.

If symptoms and overall health are better on the stronger extract but worsen once you stop it, or if the presenting symptoms are severe, then the extract may be a better choice for continual use instead. Continue the dosage of the stronger extract: 30–60 days on, 2–3 weeks off, 30–60 days on, and so on.

TONIC FORMULATIONS AND DOSAGES

I have generally used, and prefer in conditions other than persistent chronic disease (e.g., Lyme disease) or severe chronic fatigue, a weaker tincture, as do many American herbalists and herbal companies: 1:5, 60 percent alcohol, 1 dropperful (⅓ tsp) of the tincture, 1–3x daily for up to a year.

In my experience this dosage and pattern of use is less stimulating to the system and the long-term effects are better. The body gradually uses the herb to build itself up over time, the herb acting more as a long-term tonic and rejuvenative than an active stimulant. With this type of tincture it is not necessary to stop every 1 to 2 months, nor have I seen any of the side effects that can occur with the stronger Russian formula. The Chinese, much less given to tincturing anyway, use 4.5–27 grams, often as a decoction or powder.

This weaker American tincture in my clinical experience takes 6 months to become really effective and should be used at least that long; a year is better. It is great for long-term, mild chronic conditions that won't resolve and that present, in Caucasians, with a pallid face, poor elasticity in the skin, mild skin eruptions, weak energy, monotonic voice, and general passivity.

ENCAPSULATED HERB

As an encapsulated form I suggest 1,200 mg minimum daily. In acute conditions 3x that amount. Some manufacturers used to standardize the herb to 0.8 percent eleutherosides B&E, but that is becoming less common as the herb is understood better. I am not sure it is necessary.

POWDERED HERB

I like this form of the root and, in conditions such as severe, long-term chronic fatigue, blend it with some other powdered herbs that I buy by the pound (Pacific Botanicals — see Resources — is good for this): 2 parts each eleuthero, astragalus, milk thistle seed, and spirulina, and 1 part each licorice, chlorella, turmeric, and ashwagandha. Take it for a year, ¼ cup of the blend, every night just before bed, mixed in 8 to 12 ounces juice or water in a blender. It will turn the condition around.

I also use it by itself sometimes, a tablespoon in a bit of water or juice.

Side Effects and Contraindications

Insomnia and hyperactivity can occur with use of the stronger Russian formulation, especially when taken in large doses. *Do not take after 4 P.M.,* just an FYI on that one.

Eleutherococcus is, in general, completely nontoxic and the Russians have reported the use of exceptionally large doses for up to 20 years with no adverse reactions. It is especially indicated for people with pale unhealthy skin, lassitude, and depression.

For almost all people no side effects have been noted. A very small number of people have experienced transient diarrhea. It may temporarily increase blood pressure in some people. This tends to drop to normal within a few weeks. Caution should be exercised for people with very high blood pressure (180/90) especially if eleuthero is combined with other hypertensives such as licorice.

With extreme overuse: tension and insomnia.

Herb/Drug Interactions

Increases the effects of hexobarbital, monomycin, kanamycin.

Habitat and Appearance

Siberian ginseng, a persistent, aggressive shrub from 3 to 15 feet in height, grows throughout parts of China, Russia, Korea, and even a bit in the northern islands of Japan. The plant is native to, as Richo

Cech at Horizon Herbs puts it, "cold northern lakeshores and woods of China and Siberia." Essentially, it likes mixed and coniferous mountain forests that have good soils and get a bit cold. I have found related aralias growing to 9,500 feet (2,900 m) in the Colorado mountains in similar terrain. The American ginseng grows in similar, though wetter, and not nearly so high, terrain in the Midwest and northeastern United States, often among oaks or oak/pine mixed forest. Eleuthero will apparently grow wherever other aralias have established themselves — similar-terrain sort of thing.

Eleuthero's stem is covered with spines and the plant, when mature, presents an aggressive, intimidating presence that has given rise to some of its common Russian names: touch-me-not and devil's shrub. After flowering, it produces clusters of blue-black berries a bit similar to blueberries in appearance. Typical aralia/ginseng family leaves.

Due to its popularity as a medicinal, it is undergoing heavy planting in the United States and has begun to escape captivity. Soon it will be, like a number of important medicinals (among them Japanese knotweed and about half of the antibacterials discussed in this book), a naturalized, aggressive weed with qualities unknown to those it irritates. (It is currently considered invasive in Ohio and Tennessee.)

Cultivation and Collection

The plant is generally cultivated from seeds, but it will, so they say, apparently sprout easily from stem and root cuttings as well — strip or prune off the lower leaves from the stems, stick into moist potting soil or well-drained garden soil — in autumn. Keep moist until well rooted. Eleuthero, according to gardeners whom I trust, likes rich soil, lots of water, and deep woods. However, some other sources indicate the plant is hardy to zone 3 and can grow in sandy, loamy, or clay soils, even if they are nutritionally poor, even in full or partial sun. I don't know, I haven't seen an aralia or ginseng grow in those kind of soils or conditions. Nice, though, if true.

Horizon Herbs (see Resources) sells stratified seeds in hydrated coir, pretty much guaranteed to germinate. Once established, the plant never goes away. It takes about 4 years before the plant is mature enough to produce flowers and seeds. The eleutheroside content is much higher by the fourth year. Don't harvest before then.

The roots and stem bark are harvested in the fall. Cut the larger roots into smaller pieces, peel the stem bark off in strips. Leave in a drying tray until antihydration is completed. Store as usual — plastic bags, in plastic bins, out of the light in a cool location. I would strongly suggest harvesting the fruit and drying it for later use in syrups.

Commercially purchased root in bulk will already be cut and sifted or powdered to industry standards.

Plant Chemistry

Eleutherosides A through M, ciwujianosides, eleutherans, isofraxidin, friedelin, beta-sitosterol, daucosterol, ethylgalactoside, chlorogenic acid, rosmarinic acid, and so on. A lot of people think the eleutherosides are the important adaptogenic and immune constituents, especially eleutheroside B and perhaps E.

Chlorogenic acid is a fairly strong antioxidant and antihyperglycemic with antiviral, antibacterial, and antifungal actions. It slows the movement of glucose into the blood. Rosmarinic acid is also potently antioxidant and anti-inflammatory, with antiviral and antibacterial actions as well.

Eleutheroside B content in the bark of the woody stems (400 mg/100 gm) is nearly four times that of the roots; eleutheroside E content, however (30 mg/100 gm), is only about one-third that of the roots. The fruits have about the same eleutheroside E content as the stem bark but only about one-tenth the eleutheroside B content. The stem bark (850 mg/100 gm) has 50 percent more chlorogenic acid than the roots but half the rosmarinic acid (11 mg/100 gm). The fruits have half as much chlorogenic acid but eight times the rosmarinic acid as the stem bark. The fruits are high in rutoside (150 mg/100 gm), the stem bark not so much (66 mg/100 gm).

Traditional Uses of Eleuthero

Though used in China for several thousand years, *Eleutherococcus* was brought to prominence by intensive Russian research in the latter half of the twentieth century. Then the emerging herbal renaissance in the United States caught wind of it, retitled the plant Siberian ginseng, and the boom was born. It became a major herb-of-the-day for a while, then was supplanted by rhodiola — the new kid on the block.

AYURVEDA

No record of it in my library or anyplace else I can find.

TRADITIONAL CHINESE MEDICINE

Acanthopanax gracilistylus and *A. senticosus* (a.k.a. *Eleutherococcus senticosus*) are both used in Chinese medicine. The former plant goes by *wu jia pi* and is used for relieving rheumatic conditions, for strengthening the tendons and bones, and for rheumatic arthralgia, weakness in the legs, retarded walking in children (striking image), general weakness and debility. It does have some of the same eleutherosides in it.

Eleutherococcus senticosus goes by *ciwujia* in the Chinese system and does have a fairly strong presence in Chinese medicine. The Chinese use the root but also consider the stems, leaves, and fruit to be effective medicinals. Eleuthero is, in their system, vital-energy tonifying, spleen invigorating, kidney tonifying, and tranquilizing. It is used primarily for asthenia of the spleen and kidney, weakness and soreness of the lower back and knees, physical weakness, insomnia, frequent dreaming, and anorexia.

The Chinese have done some pretty good research on it as well.

WESTERN BOTANIC PRACTICE

Unknown in the West (unless you count Russia) until the herbal boom in the latter half of the twentieth century.

Scientific Research

Eleutherococcus has a number of complex effects on the body; there are four important ones: 1) on the hypothalamus/pituitary/adrenal system; 2) on the immune system; 3) on the liver and pancreas; and 4) on the heart and circulatory system. All these actions combine to produce the plant's unique adaptogenic actions.

The hypothalamus/pituitary/ adrenal system: *Eleutherococcus* maintains the functioning of the hypothalamus/pituitary/adrenal system at optimum levels, altering its function in response to external factors. (As well, the herb appears to act as an adrenal tonic, helping restore function and health in both overworked and damaged adrenals.) If a person is under severe stress, the system ramps up; if the stress is less, the system activity lowers — in essence, the definition of an adaptogen. It helps the body adapt to external stressors, no matter what they are. The result of this is more energy, greater endurance, and enhanced response capacity to demands on the system.

The immune system: The herb has the same effects on the immune system; in other words, it maintains its functioning at optimum levels in response to outside stressors. In this instance, the stressors are disease organisms entering the body. Studies have found that *how* the immune system responds depends on what kind of disease stressor is affecting it. The different parts of the immune system are activated to match the particular type of stressor affecting the organism. Eleuthero has particularly strong effects on the spleen and spleen functioning.

The liver and pancreas: *Eleutherococcus* strongly affects the way the body deals with glucose in both the liver and pancreas, essentially optimizing how both organs affect glucose and then optimizing the actions of glucose in the body. This substantially increases energy levels. Essentially, it is fuel optimization.

The heart and circulatory system: The herb affects heart and vessel function, optimizing oxygen uptake, availability, and use in the body, thus increasing energy and endurance. Tendency toward hypoxia is reduced, no matter the cause.

Pharmacokinetic studies have found that the constituents from *Eleutherococcus* are first concentrated in the liver, kidneys, spleen, and pancreas. Within 2 to 4 hours they concentrate in the pituitary, heart, and adrenals. There are lesser concentrations in the thymus, testes, and brain. The concentration in the adrenals is three times that of the other organs. The constituents, once they reach the organs, begin exerting specific effects.

In the pancreas, the constituents concentrate in the islets of Langerhans, which are responsible for insulin synthesis. *Eleutherococcus* stimulates more efficient functioning of the islets, protects them from damage, and can both reverse and prevent alloxan-induced injury to them. This is part of the way the plant exerts effects on glucose metabolism. The resynthesis of glycogen is enhanced in the liver and throughout the body. Thus, as glycogen levels fall during exertion, they are resynthesized very rapidly so that energy levels remain high.

In the spleen, eleuthero stimulates the production of antibodies and facilitates the removal of antibody-coated bacteria. The production of monocytes is increased and their movement to injured tissues is facilitated, as is their transformation into macrophages. This increases phagocytosis, macrophage activity, and both innate and adaptive immune responses. Dendritic cell numbers and function are also increased. Dendritic cells are highly present in tissues that contact the external environment — skin, nose, lungs, stomach, intestines — as well as in the blood. They interact with T and B cells to initiate and shape adaptive immune responses. They are a crucial and major part of the immune system, and they are highly activated by *Eleutherococcus*; in essence, they become more potently adaptable in their immune responses.

Again, *Eleutherococcus*'s effects on the immune system are both stimulatory and modulatory; that is, the potency and sensitivity of the system is increased but how it behaves after that depends on the stressors the body is experiencing. Numerous studies, in vivo, show that *Eleutherococcus* significantly increases the survival time and number of survivors of mice injected with lethal microbes, irrespective of the disease organism used. It is highly stimulatory of the adaptive immune response to disease. The plant also helps the body more effectively deal with pollutants and toxic overload.

Additionally, *Eleutherococcus* does have some antiviral action. It inhibits human rhinovirus, respiratory syncytial virus, and influenza A virus in vitro. This, combined with its immune actions, makes it a perfect herb in helping prevent viral infections. One Russian study on young men using the herb found a significantly reduced incidence of influenza infection compared to those who did not use the herb. Another Russian study of 13,000 auto workers found that those who took the herb developed 40 percent fewer respiratory infections than was normal for their group. And in yet another one, conducted from 1973–1975, 1,200 auto workers were given the herb with tea annually for 2 months each time; disease incidence decreased by 20 percent to 30 percent, depending on the year.

A number of clinical trials have shown significant immune-enhancing activity, including significant increases in immunocompetent cells, specifically T lymphocytes (helper/inducers, cytotoxic, and natural killer cells). Tests of the herb have repeatedly shown that it increases the ability of human beings to withstand adverse conditions, increases mental alertness, and improves performance. People taking the herb consistently report fewer illnesses than those who do not take the herb. Part of its power is its ability to act as a tonic stimulant on the adrenal glands. It normalizes adrenal activity and moves adrenal action away from a cortisol/catabolic dynamic to a DHEA/anabolic orientation. Basically, this reduces stress and normalizes physiological functioning throughout the body.

In another Russian clinical trial, 2,100 healthy adults were given the herb and found to better handle stressful conditions. They showed increased ability to perform physical labor, withstand motion sickness, and work with speed and precision despite loud surroundings. Their ability to accurately proofread documents increased and they more readily adapted to diverse physical stresses: high altitudes, heat, and low-oxygen environments.

Other studies have found that the herb heightens mental alertness, improves concentration, and boosts the transmission of nerve impulses in the brain.

There are scores of Russian studies; this just touches on them. A number of other studies have been conducted in the United States and Europe, most often on athlete endurance — which the herb helps.

The Chinese have done a number of studies on the plant. In vivo studies have found the plant to have significant calming actions in the CNS, to be highly regulatory of the body's response to nonspecific stimuli, to increase tolerance to hypoxia, to be protective from radiation exposure, to be actively detoxicant, to be a potent antistressor, to rectify endocrine disorders, to modulate both red and white blood cell levels and blood pressure levels, to have a wide range of immune modulation actions, to be antineoplastic and anti-inflammatory, to optimize heart function, to be gonadotrophic, and to stimulate tissue regeneration.

Chinese clinical studies found the herb useful in treating physical symptoms due to anxiety (insomnia, palpitations, anxiety, dizziness, and so on), to reverse leukopenia due to radiation, to be highly effective in treating coronary diseases of various etiology, and to be effective in acute obstructive cerebral thrombosis, chronic bronchitis in elderly patients, altitude sickness, arthritis, and chronic fatigue.

Eleutherococcus senticosus is strongly antihepatotoxic and hepatoprotective in vivo against CCL4-induced hepatotoxicity and is a hepatoregenerator, significantly stimulating liver regeneration in animals with portions of their liver surgically removed. Other studies have found the plant to have anticancer, antioxidant, and anti-inflammatory activity, to be of value in ischemic stroke, and to be fairly neuroprotective, while at the same time increasing mental alertness and acuity.

There is a fairly good reading list on the plant in the bibliography.

Red Root

Family: Rhamnaceae

Common Names: *In the old days it was supposedly called "New Jersey tea," but I never heard anyone use that phrase, at least when referring to a plant.*

Species Used: *Homo dissertationus* has determined that there are 50 or 60 or 4 to the third power species of *Ceanothus* in the Americas, from Canada to Guatemala. The genus doesn't grow anyplace else. (However, it has been widely planted as an ornamental in Europe. Take a flashlight and go late at night.) Most species can be used medicinally; the most common are *C. velutinus, C. cuneatus, C. integerrimus, C. greggii,* and *C. americanus.* All species are apparently identical in their medicinal actions. My personal favorite is *Ceanothus fendleri,* a.k.a. Fendler's ceanothus, which grows in my region and which I have been using for over 25 years. The important part is the color of the bark — see Cultivation and Collection on page 295.

Parts Used

The root or inner bark of the root.

Preparation and Dosage

Red root can be used as a tincture, tea, strong decoction, gargle, or capsules.

TINCTURE

Dry root, 1:5, 50 percent alcohol, 30–90 drops, up to 4x daily.

TEA

1 tsp powdered root in 8 ounces water, simmer 15 minutes, strain. Drink up to 6 cups daily.

STRONG DECOCTION

1 ounce herb in 16 ounces water, simmer slowly 30 minutes, strain. Take 1 tablespoon 3x or 4x per day.

Gargle for tonsillitis or throat inflammations: Gargle with strong decoction 4–6 times per day.

CAPSULES

Take 10–30 "00" capsules per day.

Properties of Red Root

Actions

First and foremost a lymph system stimulant and tonic. Red root is anti-inflammatory for both the liver and spleen. It is also an astringent, mucous membrane tonic, alterative, antiseptic, expectorant, antispasmodic, and exceptionally strong blood coagulant.

Finding Red Root

North and Central America, the Internet, herb shops, gardens throughout Europe.

Alternatives: Poke root (*Phytolacca*) is an excellent alternative; however, dosage should be one-third that of red root. Cleavers (*Galium*) will have some of the same effects, but the dosage should be four times that of red root. The fresh juice of the plant is best. Cleavers, additionally, strongly inhibits elastase (by about 60 percent) and is useful for bacteria that use elastase as part of their infection strategy.

Side Effects and Contraindications

No side effects have been noted; however, it is contraindicated in pregnancy.

Herb/Drug Interactions

Should not be used with pharmaceutical coagulants or anticoagulants.

Habitat and Appearance

The various species in this genus seemingly grow everywhere in North and Central America, from Canada to Guatemala, from sea-level coastal scrublands to pine forests at 9,000 feet (2,750 m) or higher. They can grow in hot, humid locations and semi-arid desert areas. They are widely divergent in appearance, too, from tiny deciduous ground covers (up to 12 inches tall) to large evergreen bushes (to 9 feet tall) to "small" trees to 25 feet in height. Their foliage ranges from tiny leathery leaves to large broad softies. Some species' branches have "spines," some don't. They do all have leaves, though, so identification should not be a problem.

The flowers grows in tufted clusters and are intensely fragrant. (Yummy to my nose — at least with *C. fendleri.*) The seed capsules are identical on all species I have seen, three-lobed triangular things that, again in all species I have seen, turn a reddish color, the exact color of the root bark (and tincture), when mature. That and the flowers, once you have seen them, are the easiest ways to identify the genus.

Cultivation and Collection

This genus has been intensively cultivated and there are scores if not hundreds of cultivars and hybrids. Adding to the confusion, the plants mix with abandon in the wild and . . . well, basically they just have sex whenever and with whomever they wish and the result is a very variable genus. In any event, you can get a large number of types if you wish to grow the species yourself. The genus should grow in just about any geographical location and I would be surprised if it had not already made a home in other places than the Americas by first masquerading as an ornamental (ahh, it has!). If so, it will soon escape into the wild, where it will be found to be invasive, for, in ceanothus habitat, there are some two million seeds produced per acre once the plants establish themselves. They are propelled under great force out of the capsules (to extend their range) and can remain viable for centuries. I love these guys.

The plants are propagated by seed or cuttings. The seeds need to be scarified first (show them horror films?) and then stratified. They are usually soaked in water for 12 hours followed by chilling for 3 months — mimicking winter.

The roots/inner root bark should be harvested in the fall or early spring — whenever the root has already had a good frost. The inner bark of the root should be a bright red and this color should extend through the white woody root as a pink tinge after a freeze. The root must look like this to be actively medicinal. If you get the roots in the late spring, summer, or early fall, they will be white throughout with just a hint of pink in the inner bark. They just will not work like that. It takes that cold snap to stimulate the production of the chemical constituents that you need the plant for.

Caution: The root is extremely tough when it dries. It should be cut into small 1- or 2-inch pieces with plant snips while still fresh or you will regret it. Really. Trust me on this one thing.

Store the cut and dried roots in plastic bags in large plastic bins in a cool place and they will last you for years.

Plant Chemistry

Betulin, betulinic acid, bacteriohopanetetrol, ceanothic acid, ceanothenic acid, ceanothine, ceanothamine, ceanothane, americine, integerressine, integerrenine, integerrine, methyl salycilate, a lot of tannins, flavonoids, flavonol glycosides, flavonones, dihydroflavonols. The leaves have a somewhat different profile, but I won't include it here as the root is what we are dealing with. The plant is fairly high in protein, iron, copper, zinc, and magnesium and very high in calcium. The roots are nitrogen fixers and possess nitrogen-filled nodules.

Traditional Uses of Red Root

Red root is an important herb in many disease conditions in that it helps facilitate clearing of dead cellular tissue from the lymph system. When the immune system is responding to acute conditions or the onset of disease, as white blood cells kill bacterial and viral pathogens, they are taken to the lymph system for disposal. If the lymph system clears out dead cellular material rapidly, the healing process is enhanced, sometimes dramatically. The herb shows especially strong action whenever any portion of the lymph system is swollen, infected, or inflamed. This includes the lymph nodes, tonsils (entire back of throat), spleen, appendix, and liver.

AYURVEDA

Nope.

TRADITIONAL CHINESE MEDICINE

Not remotely.

WESTERN BOTANIC PRACTICE

Red root has a very long history in the Americas. The indigenous cultures used the plant for a wide range of complaints from arthritis to influenza, primarily as an astringent. The early American herbalists picked it up and the Eclectics then developed the use of the plant considerably, using it as an astringent, expectorant, sedative, antispasmodic, and antisyphilitic. It was used specifically for gonorrhea, dysentery, asthma, chronic bronchitis, whooping cough, general pulmonary problems, and oral ulcerations due to fever and infection. Its primary use, however, was for enlarged spleen and, to some extent, enlarged liver.

Scientific Research

There hasn't been much study on the plant, however, and really nothing looking in depth at its actions on the lymph system, including the spleen, though there are some nice hints here and there.

In recent years there has been a minor amount of exploration on the antimicrobial actions of red root. Several of the root compounds have been found active against various oral pathogens including *Streptococcus mutans, Actinomyces viscosus, Porphyromonas gingivalis*, and *Prevotella intermedia*. The flowers are active against *Staphylococcus aureus* and a couple of candida species; the roots probably are, too.

Betulin and betulinic acid, which are fairly prominent in the root, have a broad range of actions, both in vivo and in vitro: antiplasmodial, anti-HIV, anti-inflammatory, anthelmintic, antioxidant, antitumor, immunomodulatory. Ceonothane is fairly strongly antistaphylococcal, antiplasmodial, and antimycobacterial. These various actions are going to have some effect on bacterial diseases, but exactly what and how much is not clear.

There is some evidence that red root's activity in the lymph nodes also enhances the lymph nodes' production of lymphocytes, specifically the formation of T cells. Clinicians working with AIDS patients, who historically have low levels of T cells, have noted increases after the use of red root. It is especially effective in reducing inflammations in the spleen and liver from such things as excessive bacterial garbage, white blood cell detritus

in the lymph, and red blood cell fragments in the blood in diseases like babesiosis. There is evidence, clinical, that it has broad action throughout the lymph system and helps reduce not only the spleen but also the appendix when inflamed and that it stimulates lymph drainage as well in the intestinal walls.

A number of human trials have used the herb as a tincture extract (usually 10 to 15 ml per person). The trials focused on heavy bleeding, including excessive menstruation, and the plant was found to be a powerful coagulant and hemostatic in all studies. A marked reduction of clotting time was noted.

In one study, a single oral administration of 3.5 to 7.0 ml of a hydro-alcoholic (tincture) extract of *Ceanothus* (*americanus*) resulted in an interesting effect: At low doses accelerated blood clotting occurred within 10 to 20 minutes after administration. However, at higher doses coagulation *decreased* 1 hour after administration. This raises interesting speculations about the herb's range of actions.

In vivo studies have shown marked hemostatic activity and hypotensive action. In vitro studies have also found a strong reverse transcriptase inhibition and a broad antifungal activity.

Reishi

Family: Ganodermataceae

Common Names: *Reishi, which is the Japanese name for the plant, has become the most common name for the herb in the West.*

Properties of Reishi

Actions

Analgesic	Cholagogue
Antiallergenic	Choleretic
Antibacterial	Coronary vasodilator
Antihepatotoxic	Cytotoxic
Antihyperbilirubinemic	Hepatoregenerator
Antihyperlipemic	Hypocholesterolemic
Antihypertriglyceridemic	Hypotensive
Anti-inflammatory	Immunomodulator
Antinephrotoxic	Immunostimulant
Antitumor	Spleen and thymus tonic
Antiviral	

As an immune stimulant, reishi stimulates interleukin 1 and 2, phagocytosis, and lymphocyte proliferation, enhances natural killer cells, activates macrophages, enhances polymorphonuclear leukocytes, protects and enhances T cells, enhances thymus weight and functioning, stimulates gamma-interferon production. As an antitumor agent, it also reduces the proliferation of tumor cells and inhibits tumor necrosis factor. And as an antiviral, it's been shown to be active against numerous viruses, including HBV and HIV.

Finding Reishi

Herb shops everywhere, the Internet, or you can grow your own fairly easily — try Fungi Perfecti (*www.fungi.com*), which sells easy-to-use starter kits.

Species Used: There are 80 or maybe 250 species of ganoderma (taxonomy is a science?). A number of them are used medicinally. The primary medicinal is considered to be *Ganoderma lucidum* but *G. luteum*, *G. tsugae*, *G. applanatum*, *G. australe*, *G. capense*, *G. tropicum*, *G. tenue*, and *G. sinense* are also used.

In the Chinese system all are considered to possess slightly different effects. The mushrooms are grouped, medicinally, by their color. Blue (sour) is considered to improve eyesight and liver function and calm the nerves; red (bitter) is considered the most medicinally potent, and aids internal organs, improves memory, enhances vitality; yellow (sweet) strengthens spleen function, calms the spirit; white (hot) improves lung function, gives courage and strong will; black (salty) protects the kidneys; and purple (sweet) enhances function of the ears, joints, muscles, and helps the complexion.

Part Used
Generally the fruiting body, i.e., the mushroom itself, and sometimes the mycelium.

Preparation and Dosage
May be taken as tablets, tincture, syrup decoction, or powder, or even used as a soup base.

TABLETS
Take three 1-gram tablets (bought retail) up to 3x daily.

TINCTURE
1:5, 20 percent alcohol, 10–20 ml (2–4 tsp), up to 3x daily.

The tincture is best made by first making a decoction of the herb; this will extract the polysaccharides most efficiently. If you have 16 ounces of powdered reishi, you would then use 80 ounces of liquid, 64 ounces of which would be water, and 16 alcohol. Add the powdered or chopped-up reishi to the water, bring to a boil, cover, and slow-boil for 30 minutes. Allow to cool with the lid on. When cool, pour into large jar, add 16 ounces pure grain alcohol, cover, and allow to steep for 2 weeks. Decant, press, and store.

SYRUP DECOCTION

Use 2–5 grams of reishi per quart of water depending on strength desired. Slowly bring to boil and simmer at lowest boil obtainable for 2 hours, uncovered, until the volume of water is reduced by two-thirds. Cool and strain. Consume in the evening before bed or in three equal amounts over the course of the day. In acute conditions the amount consumed can be increased as much as desired.

POWDER

Take 3–6 grams a day in chronic disease, 9–15 grams a day in acute conditions, equally divided in three doses. Stir into water and drink or encapsulate (6–12 "00" capsules in chronic disease, 18–30 in acute conditions).

For mushroom poisoning: Take 120–200 grams of dried powdered reishi in water, 3–5x daily.

Side Effects and Contraindications

Contraindicated in cases of obstructed bile duct. Occasionally, skin rash, loose stool, dry mouth, sleepiness, bloating, frequent urination, sweating, nausea may occur. Adverse reactions cease upon discontinuance of the herb. In the case of nausea take with meals.

Herb/Drug Interactions

Reishi is synergistic with cefazolin, interferon-alpha, and to some extent interferon-gamma, and potently so with acyclovir. Caution should be exercised if you are on immunosuppresive drugs. There may be an additive effect with blood-thinning medications such as aspirin or warfarin.

Habitat and Appearance

Reishi is a hard, tough, woody mushroom that has a shiny or varnished appearance to the cap. The Latin word for the primary medicinal species, *lucidum*, means "shiny" or "brilliant." Essentially, so does the genus name *Ganoderma*, from the Greek, *gano* meaning "sheen" or "brightness," *derma* meaning "skin." So . . . the Latinate term for the plant, created by botanists, means "shiny skin shiny." (Latin terminology is not all that philosophically deep. The sonorous sound of the words just makes us think so.)

The various species range in cap color from yellow to black, but the most common one found wild in the United States, *G. lucidum*, is red.

Reishi mushrooms grow on a wide variety of trees, often dead or dying, especially deciduous trees such as oak, elm, maple, willow, sweet gum, magnolia, plum, and locust. They will sometimes grow on coniferous trees such as pine, larch, and spruce. They tend to grow in temperate regions.

Cultivation and Collection

The fruiting mushroom bodies can be harvested at any time. They don't need any special treatment. Just let them sit out and dry thoroughly, then store in plastic bags in plastic tubs out of the light. They will last for years.

Reishi can be easily cultivated through the use of inoculated wooden dowels or plugs. It does best in nonaromatic hardwoods. Cut a log into sections, let it sit out for a few months, then drill and insert the plugs, generally in early spring after the last frost. The mycelium will spread through the log the first year and begin producing mushrooms the second year. Try Fungi Perfecti (*www.fungi.com*) for inoculated plugs and much more information.

Plant Chemistry

Over 400 different bioactive constituents have been identified in reishi so far. One hundred forty of them are triterpenes, primarily ganodermic acids, though there are 10 specific groups. Over 100 additional compounds are polysaccharides, which produce many of the plant's immune actions. There are numerous other compounds, one of which — the LZ-8 protein — has fairly strong immune-stimulating actions in the spleen and on peripheral lymphocytes.

Traditional Uses of Reishi

AYURVEDA

Apparently unknown, though there is a similar mushroom recorded in Indian lore, a mysterious *chih* fungus considered to be an herb of immortality. Versions of the Indian legends of the fungus are rife in ancient Chinese literature and are considered, by many historical figures, to be *ling chih,* or reishi. I can't find any reference to reishi in Ayurvedic practice in my library, however.

TRADITIONAL CHINESE MEDICINE

Ganoderma is known as *ling chih* or *ling zhi* (mushroom of immortality) in China and *reishi* (ten-thousand-year mushroom) in Japan, under which name it is now commonly known in the West. The reputation of the herb is as a longevity and vitality-enhancing tonic.

Reishi has been used in China and Japan for at least four thousand years in the treatment of debility from prolonged illness, for "deficiency" fatigue, as an antiaging herb, and for coronary heart disease, hepatitis, kidney disease, arthritis, hypertension, sleep disorders, asthma and bronchitis, ulcer, and nerve pain.

In TCM it is considered warming, tonic, nourishing, antitoxic, astringent, and dispersing of accumulations. At least five species of *Ganoderma* are used in traditional medicine in China and Japan, each for different disorders. *Ganoderma lucidum,* in many respects, is considered to be the most potent.

WESTERN BOTANIC PRACTICE

Apparently unknown until its introduction by traditional Chinese practitioners in the mid-to-late twentieth century. Western use has been stimulated by the extensive studies carried out in Japan (for the most part).

Scientific Research

The best overviews of *Ganoderma*, I think, are S. Bhagwan et al., *"Ganoderma lucidum:* A Potent Pharmacological Macrofungus," and R. Russel and M. Paterson, *"Ganoderma*: A Therapeutic Fungal Biofactory."[1] They cover about everything, however . . . a brief look:

In vivo and in vitro studies have found reishi to be liver regenerative, liver protective, choleretic, liver enzyme normalizing, analgesic, antiallergenic, anti-inflammatory, antibacterial, antiviral, antioxidant, antitumor (inhibiting or regressing tumors), hypotensive, a bronchial relaxant, immunostimulant, immunomodulating, cardiotonic, expectorant, and antitussive.

Human trials have found effectiveness for neurasthenia, insomnia, dizziness, duodenal ulcers, liver pain, rhinitis, muscular dystrophy, stress, Alzheimer's disease, hyperlipidemia, liver failure, diabetes, cancer, immune enhancement, and hepatitis.

Although not primarily thought of as such, reishi is antibacterial, antifungal, and a fairly potent antiviral against a number of pathogens.

Reishi is antibacterial against *Helicobacter pylori, Pseudomonas syringae, P. aeruginosa, E. coli, Bacillus subtilis, Staphylococcus aureus, Klebsiella pneumoniae, Salmonella typhi, Micrococcus flavus*, and *Micrococcus luteus*.

Reishi is a strong antiviral, especially against hepatitis viruses. It is active against influenza A viruses, potently so against herpes simplex virus 1 and 2 (it also inhibits their attachment and penetration into cells), and strongly so against vesicular stomatitis virus, Epstein-Barr virus, and HIV.

Reishi is active against *Candida* spp., *Microsporum canis, Trichophyton mentagrophytes*. It is also active against plasmodial parasites.

Like eleuthero, reishi has profound effects on the immune system, especially the spleen, stimulating its immune responses considerably. Reishi is strongly mitogenic, especially on splenocytes, stimulating the generation of highly active immune cells. It activates immune effector cells such as T cells, macrophages, and natural killer cells and increases the production of cytokines, including interleukins, tumor necrosis factor-alpha, and interferons. Reishi potently stimulates macrophages and their activity in the body against pathogens. The primary clinical studies on the enhancement of immune function have occurred with cancer patients; most immune studies have been in vivo or in vitro.

Reishi has a number of fairly potent anticancer actions, which are generating a lot of interest. It reduces angiogenesis, the formation of new blood cells by tumors, is antiproliferative, has direct anticancer effects on a number of cancer cell lines, including prostate, colon, leukemia, lymphoma, and myeloma cells, strongly inhibits intracellular signaling and invasive behavior of cancer cells, protects the body from radiation damage during cancer treatment, and mediates cancer cell growth through enhancement of host immune defenses.

Here is a sampling of a few clinical trials: In one human trial of 355 people with hepatitis B, with a combination formula containing reishi, 92.4 percent of patients showed improvement. Another trial found that patients with hepatitis B experienced the alleviation of hepatitis symptoms and lowering of

SGOT and SGPT levels. Other trials showed reduction in blood pressure in all patients with hypertension who took reishi over a 6-month period. In trials with over 2,000 patients with chronic bronchitis, 60 percent to 90 percent experienced alleviation of symptoms, marked improvement, and weight gain. Studies with people with high blood pressure have consistently showed improvement in blood pressure levels and people with impaired memory or thinking have shown increased mental clarity and memory.

Reishi has a long history of folk and historical clinical use in protecting the liver against *Amanita phalloides* poisoning, though I could locate no specific trials.

Rhodiola

Family: Crassulaceae

Common Names: *Rhodiola • golden root • roseroot • stonecrop • arctic root. The fresh roots smell a bit like roses, hence the origin of that name. They are golden in color, thus golden root.*

Species Used: There is, as usual, confusion among those with advanced degrees in plant science as to just how many species of rhodiola there are: 36, or maybe 60, or probably 90. It's like stamp collectors ("No, look at that tiny ink spot on the edge"); I just want to scream.

The primary medicinal that most people use is *Rhodiola rosea,* but many of the related species are used medicinally in the regions in which they grow. Because of the interest in *R. rosea,* the genus is being intensively studied for activity: I have found medicinal studies of one sort or another on *R. crenulata, R. quadrifida, R. heterodonta, R. semenovii, R. sachalinensis, R. sacra, R. fastigiata, R. kirilowii, R. bupleuroides, R. imbricata, R. rhodantha,* and *R. integrifolia.*

Properties of Rhodiola

Actions

Adaptogen	Cardiotonic (potent)	Immune tonic
Adrenal protectant	Endocrine tonic	Mental stimulant
Anticancer	Ergogenic	Mitochondrial tonic
Antidepressant	Hippocampal	and protectant
Antifatigue	protectant and tonic	Muscular stimulant
Antioxidant (strong)	Hypoxia antagonist	Nervous system tonic
Antistressor	(potent)	Neural protectant

Possibly a synergist, the plant is a strong inhibitor of CYP3A4 and P-glycoprotein. See the piperine monograph (page 236) for specifics.

Use to Treat

Brain fog	Chronic fatigue	Low immune function
Chronic disease	syndrome	Nervous exhaustion
conditions with	Chronic, long-term	Recurrent infections
depression	fatigue	

Rhodiola can also be used to accelerate recovery from debilitating conditions and long-term illness and infections.

Other Uses

The leaves of most species can be eaten, chopped finely and added to salads, or cooked as a pot herb. The plants are very high in vitamin C, with 33 mg per gram of fresh plant.

Finding Rhodiola

You can buy it pretty much everywhere. If you live in the right climate you can probably find it wild or grow it yourself.

There have been some extravagant claims (easily found on the Internet) that *only* Russian *Rhodiola rosea*, harvested near the Arctic Circle (presumably by fasting virgins as the northern lights first emerge over the rim of Earth), contains the necessary active constituents for the herb to be useful. However, *all* the *Rhodiola rosea* plants, irrespective of where they grow or in what country, have nearly identical chemistry. They are all perfectly usable as medicine.

But please note: The exact chemical profile of the *R. rosea* plants themselves differs depending on time of year, time of day, and geographical location (this valley in Russia or *that* one) irrespective of whether they are harvested at the Arctic Circle in Russia by fasting virgins or not. In other words, you can pick *R. rosea* from this location in May and again in September and the chemical profile of the plant *won't* be the same. The same is true of every species in the genus — and of every medicinal plant on Earth. Part of the art of herbalism is being able to determine medicinal potency of the plants you are harvesting by using the most sophisticated scientific instrument ever discovered — the focused power of human awareness. Machines just aren't a reliable substitute for the capacity to reason *and* feel simultaneously. Furthermore . . . oops! Sorry. Got carried away again.

Studies on 14 other species in the genus have found the same constituents in them as in *R. rosea*. They can all be used medicinally, they all do pretty much the same things, they all work identically to the usual commercial-variety *R. rosea* — see Scientific Research (page 312) for more. *Rhodiola integrifolia*, by the way, is considered to be a natural hybrid between *Rhodiola rhodantha* and *R. rosea*; you can consider it pretty much identical to *R. rosea*.

Note: The rhodiolas look much like sedums and were once included in that genus, so you will see rosea sometimes listed as *Sedum rosea* and so on.

Parts Used

The root.

Preparation and Dosage

Generally used as capsules or tincture.

TINCTURE

Dried root, 1:5, 50 percent alcohol. Some people use a 1:3 formulation.
I am not sure it is necessary.

Tonic dose: 30–40 drops, 3x or 4x daily, usually in water.

In acute conditions: ½–1 tsp, 3x daily for 20–30 days, then back to
the tonic dose.

CAPSULES

The root is most often used in capsule form, 100 mg each. Usual dose
is 1 or 2 capsules per day. In acute conditions up to 1,000 mg a day can
be taken. The capsules are often standardized to contain 2–3 percent
rosavins and 0.8–1 percent salidroside. They are usually taken just
before meals.

Side Effects and Contraindications

Some people experience jitteriness from the herb; you should not take
it at night until you know if you are one of them.

Herb/Drug Interactions

None noted.

Habitat and Appearance

Rhodiolas are plants that like high altitude and cold, either will do.
They are a circumpolar genus of the subarctic and cool, mountainous
regions of the northern hemisphere and are common in eastern
Russia, parts of China, Tibet (which has many species), the mountains
and northern climes of Europe, Canada, and the mountainous and
colder regions of the United States. The United States, Europe, and
Tibet appear to have the largest populations, with Tibet having the
most species.

The rhodiolas are typical succulents with fleshy, moisture-filled, grayish-green leaves. The plants grow to about 12 inches and they will have, depending on the species, a cluster of yellow, pink, red, or orange flowers at the top of the stalk. *R. rosea*'s flowers are yellow.

The root system is fairly large if the plants grow in a nutrient-rich environment. The farther north they grow, and the poorer the soils, the smaller the root.

There are three species of rhodiola in North America: *Rhodiola rosea* grows in the mountains of North Carolina, and in Pennsylvania through New England, into Canada, and all the way to the Arctic Circle. *R. rhodantha* grows in the Rocky Mountain states from New Mexico and Arizona up to the Canadian border. *R. integrifolia* has the widest distribution in North America. It ranges from the Rocky Mountain spine (New Mexico, et cetera, westward) up into Canada and into the Arctic. There are populations as well in Minnesota and New York State. Most of the eastern rhodiolas are considered to be endangered.

If you are in the western United States and wanting to wild-harvest your own roots, look for *R. integrifolia*; it is just as useful as *R. rosea* medicinally *and* it is not endangered as many of the eastern United States *R. rosea* populations are.

Cultivation and Collection

Due to the popularizing of the plant as an antiaging and chronic fatigue medicinal, wild populations of *R. rosea* are becoming endangered; the Russians have put them on their red list of threatened plants. The largest populations of the plant were formerly in the Altai region of southern Siberia. However, over 45 companies have been harvesting the plant for export ("*Real* Russian rhodiola") and those plant populations have been severely reduced.

If you live in a region in which rhodiola grows, you can harvest your own roots; you won't need to harvest much for yourself and your family. Commercial harvesting, except for very limited amounts in abundant areas, is highly discouraged.

If you find the plant in your area, harvest the roots in the fall after seeding or in the spring just as it is coming up. The roots will be bigger and, in my opinion, more potent in the spring. Slice the bigger roots; the interior of the root will change from white to a brown or reddish color as it begins to dry.

Due to the heavy worldwide demand for the plant, there are increasing efforts to make the plant an agricultural staple in regions where it will grow; Bulgaria, Canada, and Finland are early innovators in growing the crop. The yields are low, only about 3 tons per hectare, and they are labor intensive. Since the roots are taken, and only after 5 years, agricultural growing of the plant demands a minimum of five fields, planted in rotation so they can be harvested in successive years in order to keep up continual production.

The seeds are tiny; a thousand of them weigh only 0.2 gram. The germination rates are low, 2 percent to 36 percent; they are happier with a little stratification. Thirty days at −5°C (23°F) will increase germination rates to 50 percent to 75 percent. Soak the seeds in water overnight, mix into moist soil, store for 1 month at a temperature of 2° to 4°C (36° to 39°F). You will then get about a 75 percent germination rate.

In Finland they get 95 percent to 100 percent germination if they sow the seeds on the surface of a sand/peat mix and keep the trays outside all winter under the snow. In April/May the boxes are brought into a greenhouse at a temperature of 18° to 22°C (64° to 72°F). Germination begins in 3 days to a week.

If you keep the seedlings inside for a year before transplanting, yields are significantly higher. They like sandy, loamy soil, neutral or slightly acidic. NPK: 50/50/70. They don't need additional fertilizer after the first year. The easiest method, however, is to divide the roots of an established plant and plant the root cuttings, much like potatoes.

The plant takes a minimum of 3 years to mature, but the roots should not be harvested for 5 years. Dig in the fall, slice, let dry out of the sun. Store in plastic bags, inside plastic containers, in the dark.

Plant Chemistry

Most people think that salidroside (a.k.a. rhodioloside) is the most
important compound in the root, others insist it is the rosavin. Others
say, yeah, those and . . . rosin, rosarin, and tyrosol. Studies have found,
as usual, that saldroside is much more effective when combined with
rosavin, rosin, and rosarin. So I'm guessing, just a wild shot here, that
it's the whole root that is most active.

There are, of course, a great many other compounds in the root, at
least 85 essential oils and another 50 water-soluble nonvolatiles. Many
of the usual plant compounds are present.

Traditional Uses of Rhodiola

Rhodiola, as far as I can tell, and in spite of assertions that it is a long-
standing medicinal in traditional Chinese medicine (TCM), was a
contribution to the medicinal plant world by the Russians due to their
interest in adaptogens. This is pretty much a Russian-introduced
category of medicinal herb — a plant that enhances general overall
functioning, somewhat like a tonic but one that increases the ability of
the organism to respond to outside stressors of whatever sort, diseases
included. It enhances an organism's general resistance to multiple
adverse influences or conditions. Rhodiola, like the stronger preparations of *Eleutherococcus*, is considered to be not just adaptogenic but
an adaptogenic stimulant — part of the reason it can cause jitteriness
and wakefulness in some.

AYURVEDA AND TCM

Rhodiolas have been used in TCM, Tibetan medicine, and Ayurveda
for a very long time — according to many reports. But my library,
extensive, doesn't list the genus in any of my source books for those
systems of healing.

However, a few other, obscure sources reveal that the plants were
used in traditional Russian folk medicine to increase physical endurance, work productivity, longevity, resistance to altitude sickness and

for fatigue, depression, anemia, impotence, GI tract ailments, infections, and nervous afflictions.

In central Asia the tea has been used for a long time as the most
effective local treatment for colds and flu. Mongolian physicians use it
for TB and cancer. The plant is a part of traditional Tibetan medicine
for promoting blood circulation and relieving cough.

WESTERN BOTANIC PRACTICE

The plant never was a huge medicinal even though there are traces
of its use as far back as the seventeenth century in the Scandinavian
countries. *Rhodiola rosea* and *R. integrifolia* were used by the indigenous tribes of Alaska as a food, the root eaten for sores in the mouth,
for TB, stomachache, GI tract troubles. A couple of the sedums were
recognized by the Eclectics but none of the rhodiolas before their
name change.

Scientific Research

There is a lot of research on this plant right now, and more studies are occurring daily. There have been, unlike the case for many other newish medicinal plants, a lot of human clinical trials with this herb. I am primarily going to look at the neuroprotective/neurore-generative, immune, and antistress/antifatigue actions of the plant — they are strongly interrelated. The potent antioxidant actions of the plant are deeply interrelated with those as well. A comprehensive bibliography for the plant is in the reference section.

ANTIVIRAL/ANTIBACTERIAL

A number of the rhodiolas have been found to have antiviral and antibac-terial actions. *Rhodiola kirilowii* is active against the hepatitis C virus and *Mycobacterium tuberculosis, Rhodiola rosea* is active against H1N1 and H9N2 viral influenza strains as well as Cox-sackie virus B3.

NEUROPROTECTIVE/NEUROREGENERATIVE

Numerous rhodiola species have been found to be highly neuroprotective.

In vitro: Compounds in both *Rhodiola sacra* and *R. sachalinensis* protect neurons against beta-amyloid-induced, stauporine-induced, and H2O2-induced death. Salidroside, a common compound in many rho-diolas, protects cultured neurons from injury from hypoxia and hypoglycemia; protects neuronal PC12 cells and SH-SY5Y neuroblas-toma cells against cytotoxicity from beta-amyloid and against hypoglycemia and serum limitation; and protects neurons against H_2O_2-induced death. It does so by inducing the antioxidant enzymes thioredoxin, heme oxygenase-1, and peroxiredoxin-1, down-regulating the pro-apoptotic gene Bax, and up-regulating the anti-apoptotic genes Bcl-2 and Bcl-X(L). It also restores mitochondrial membrane potential negatively affected by H_2O_2 and restores intracellular calcium levels.

In vivo: *Rhodiola rosea* enhances the level of 5-hydroxytryptamine in the hippocampus, promotes the proliferation and differentiation of neural stem cells in the hippocampus, and protects hippocampal neurons from injury. *R. rosea* protects against cognitive deficits, neuronal injury, and oxidative stress induced by intracerebroventricular injection of streptozotocin. Salidroside protects rat hippocampal neurons against H_2O_2-induced apoptosis. A combination of rhodiola/astragalus protects rats against simulated plateau hypoxia (8,000 m/26,000 feet). It inhibits the accumulation of lactic acid in brain tissue and serum.

Human clinical trial: A double-blind, placebo-controlled, randomized study with 40 women, ages 20 to 68, who were highly stressed, found that a *Rhodiola rosea* extract increased attention, speed, and accuracy during stressful cognitive tasks. *Rhodiola rosea* was used with 120 adults with both physical and cognitive deficiencies: exhaustion, decreased motivation, daytime sleepiness, decreased libido, sleep disturbances, concentration deficiencies, forgetfulness, decreased memory, susceptibility to stress, irritability; after 12 weeks, 80 percent of patients showed improvements. A combination formula (Xinnaoxin capsule) of *Rhodiola rosea, Lycium chinense* berry, and fresh *Hippophae rhomnoides* fruit juice was given to 30 patients with chronic cerebral circulatory insufficiency; after 4 weeks the condition was significantly improved. A double-blind, crossover 3-week study on stress-induced fatigue on the mental performance of healthy physicians during night duty found that *Rhodiola rosea* extract decreased mental fatigue and increased cognitive functions such as associative thinking, short-term memory, calculation and concentration, and speed of audio-visual perception.

ANTIFATIGUE/ANTISTRESS

In vitro: Salidroside stimulates glucose uptake by rat muscle cells; *Rhodiola rosea* extract stimulates the synthesis or resynthesis of ATP and stimulates reparative processes in mitochondria.

In vivo: *Rhodiola rosea* extracts increased the life span of *Drosophila melanogaster*, lowered mitochondrial superoxide levels, and increased protection against the superoxide generator paraquat. Four weeks' supplementation with *R. rosea* extract significantly increased swimming time in exhausted mice — it significantly increased liver glycogen levels; SREBP-1, FAS, and heat shock protein 70 expression; Bcl-2/Bax ratios; and oxygen content in blood. Salidroside protected the hypothalamic/pituitary/gonad axis of male rats under intense stress — testosterone levels remained normal rather than dropping, secretary granules of the pituitary gland increased, and mitochondrial cells were strongly protected. *R. rosea* extract completely reversed the effects of chronic mild stress in female rats — that is, decreased sucrose intake, decreased movement, weight loss, and dysregulation of menstrual cycle. Rhodiola suppressed increased enzyme activity in rats subjected to noise stress — glutamic pyruvic transaminase, alkaline phosphatase, and creatine kinase levels all returned to normal, and glycogen, lactic acid, and cholesterol levels in the liver also returned to normal. *R. rosea* reduced stress and CRF-induced anorexia in rats. And so on.

Human clinical trial: Twenty-four men who had lived at high altitude for a year were tested to see the effects of rhodiola on blood oxygen saturation and sleep disorders. Rhodiola increased blood oxygen saturation significantly and increased both sleeping time and quality. In a double-blind, placebo-controlled study of the effects of *R. rosea* on fatigue in students caused by stress, physical fitness, mental fatigue, and neuro-motoric indices all increased (other studies found similar outcomes). *R. rosea* intake in a group of healthy volunteers reduced inflammatory C-reactive protein and creatinine kinase levels in the blood and protected muscle tissue during exercise. *Rhodiola rosea* in a placebo-controlled, double-blind, randomized study was found to increase physical capacity, muscle strength, speed of limb movement, reaction time, and attention — in other words it improved exercise endurance performance. A similarly structured study found that 1 week of rhodiola supplementation decreased fatigue and stress levels but more interestingly decreased photon emissions on the dorsal side of the hand. In another study *Rhodiola rosea* increased the efficiency of the cardio-vascular and respiratory systems and prevented fatigue during an hour of continuous physical exercise. A phase three clinical trial found that rhodiola exerts an antifatigue effect that increases mental performance and concentration and decreases cortisol response in burnout patients with fatigue syndrome; other studies have found similar outcomes, including the amelioration of depression and anxiety.

IMMUNE ACTIONS

In vitro: *Rhodiola imbricata* protects macrophages against tert-butyl hydroperoxide injury and up-regulates the immune response. Additionally it potently stimulates the innate immune pathway and initiates strong immunostimulatory actions, increasing Toll-like receptor 4, granzyme B, and Th1 cytokines. *Rhodiola sachalinensis* extract enhances the expression of inducible nitric oxide synthase in macrophages. *Rhodiola quadrifida* stimulates granulocyte activity and increases lymphocyte response to mitogens. *Rhodiola algida* stimulates human peripheral blood lymphocytes and up-regulates IL-2 in Th1 cells and IL-4, 6, and 10 in Th2 cells.

In vivo: *Rhodiola kirolowii* enhances cellular immunity — stimulating the activity of lymphocytes, increasing phagocytosis in response to microbial organisms. *Rhodiola imbricata* enhances specific immunoglobulin levels in response to tetanus toxoid and ovalbumin in rats — the plant has adjuvant/immunopotentiating activity in both humoral and cell-mediated immune response.

Human clinical use: *Rhodiola rosea* (in combination with schizandra, eleuthero, and leuzea) significantly increased both cell-mediated and humoral immune response in ovarian cancer patients. Rhodiola significantly reduced problems and infection after the treatment of acute lung injury caused by massive trauma/infection and thoracic-cardio operations. A combination formula of rhodiola, eleuthero, and schizandra significantly enhanced positive outcomes in the treatment of acute nonspecific pneumonia. *Rhodiola rosea* increased the parameters of leukocyte integrins and T-cell immunity in bladder cancer patients.

OTHER ACTIONS

Rhodiola, various species, has been found effective in the treatment of breast cancer. It inhibits the tumorigenic properties of invasive mammary epithelial cells, inhibits superficial bladder cancer, suppresses T241 fibrosarcoma tumor cell proliferation, and reduces angiogenesis in various tumor lines. *Rhodiola imbricata* is highly protective in mice against whole-body lethal radiation.

The plant has also been found highly antioxidant in numerous studies, to be liver protective, and to be highly protective of the cardiovascular system.

The plant is adaptogenic; that is, it increases the function of the organism to meet whatever adverse influences are affecting it, whether stress or illness. Most of the attention has been paid to its ability to increase endurance and mental acuity, but its effects on the immune system, though less studied than eleuthero's, are similar.

8

A HANDBOOK OF HERBAL MEDICINE MAKING

[Our bodies] are not distinct from the bodies of plants and animals, with which we are involved in the cycles of feeding and the intricate companionships of ecological systems and of the spirit. They are not distinct from the earth, the sun and moon, and the other heavenly bodies. It is therefore absurd to approach the subject of health piecemeal with a departmentalized band of specialists. A medical doctor uninterested in nutrition, in agriculture, in the wholesomeness of mind and spirit is as absurd as a farmer who is uninterested in health. Our fragmentation of this subject cannot be our cure, because it is our disease.

— **Wendell Berry,** *The Unsettling of America*

Tremendous empowerment comes from learning to recognize the medicinal plants that surround us, even more in learning how to make them into medicines for healing. And though it takes time, as your knowledge increases, as you learn how to tend to your illnesses and those of your family, the sense of helplessness that so many of us have experienced when we become ill, often ingrained since birth, begins to dissipate.

We have been trained to place our health in the hands of outside specialists who, very often, know neither ourselves nor our families, not the fabric of our lives, nor the communities in which we live. They have no understanding of, and often no interest in, the complexity in which we live and from which our illnesses emerge. But for most of us, those specialists are the *only* place we know to go when we are ill, uncertain, and afraid, to seek help — for ourselves or our loved ones.

The world, however, is a great deal more complex than that frame allows and there are many more options to healing than that system acknowledges. All of us live, all the time, in the midst of a living pharmacy that covers the surface of this planet. And that living pharmacy is there for you, or anyone, to use — anytime you wish. Once you *know* that, once you have been healed by the plants in that living pharmacy, often of something that physicians said could not be healed, things are never the same again. You begin to break the cycle of dependence on which the health care system depends.

Taking back control over personal health and healing is one of the greatest forms of personal empowerment that I know. It does take time and effort, this kind of learning, but the learning goes quickly. Harder, perhaps, is learning to trust the plants with your life. It is a truly frightening moment, that moment of decision, when trust is extended in that way, for, before it occurs, there is no way to experientially *know* what the outcome will be. Most people on this planet, though, people who do not live in the Western, industrialized nations, make that decision every day of their lives. It is a trust they extend every moment of every day. Trusting the healing capacities of the plants is not a new experience to the human species.

The next step in the journey is learning how to turn the plants you are learning about into medicines for yourself and your family. It isn't that hard — people all over the globe have been doing it for a hundred thousand years. At least.

To Begin With . . .

The first thing to understand is that there are no mistakes. You are learning a new skill and *everyone* learns what works by learning what doesn't. That is how human beings do it; we all learn to cook well by first cooking badly. So . . . enjoy the process, give yourself permission to make mistakes, to learn as you go.

If you are wildcrafting your medicines, the first step, of course, is getting to know the plants themselves, learning to recognize them in the wild, getting to know them where they live. I prefer finding a local plant person to help me with this; I like to be introduced to plants by someone who already knows them. It just seems more polite than learning about them from a book. An important part of this is increasing the acuteness of your *seeing*; you have to learn to see what is right in front of you. That is often hard with plants, as most of us have relegated them to the background as a sort of insentient and colorful backdrop to our city life.

One of the most common experiences herbalists have is going into the wild, looking diligently for a plant, not finding it, then giving up and sitting on a rock to rest and discovering they are in a field full of the very plant they are looking for.

As you increase your noticing, you will begin to see the plants sharply defined, as individuals, and you will find the ones you know everywhere. And as your experience of this new world opens up, you will find that plants are living beings and just like people they have their quirks, oddities, differences — plants of the same species don't always look the same. Where they live changes them (just as it does us).

If you learn them in the high mountains of Colorado and then seek them in eastern Washington State, they will look entirely different. Plants such as red root hug the ground at 9,000 feet (2,750 m) above sea level but will stand 6 feet tall at lower elevations. Plants that are pulled into themselves, conserving water resources, in semi-arid and arid regions will plump out in the humid tropics, grow fat and big with all the abundance of an easy life. They will often change so much from eco-range to eco-range that they don't appear to be the same plants — and, of course, their medicinal actions will change as well. They don't need to make the same chemicals in the Olympic Peninsula as they do in the south of Spain.

Plants, just like people, live in neighborhoods, in certain regions and habitats. Part of the journey is learning those neighborhoods and habitats, learning where they like to grow, learning how they appear in different regions, different continents, altitudes, climates, and how their medicine changes in each of those climates as well. It also means learning how they appear at different times of the year.

Plants go through cycles, and these cycles are more pronounced if there is a cold winter where they live. Once you make the acquaintance of a plant, learn where it lives, you can visit it in all seasons of the year, learn how it looks as the seasons progress, learn the differences in its medicine in each of those seasons. Illness comes at any time; if you wildcraft you will need to know your medicines no matter the time of year. If you live in a climate that is very cold with deep snow, then it becomes important to learn the trees, for they can be found and made into

> **Trusting the healing capacities of the plants is not a new experience to the human species.**

medicines in any season. It is important, too, to make enough medicine of the plants that sleep through the winter so that you have them on hand if you need them. All of the *vegetalistas* — plant people — that I know have an herb room, a place where they keep their medicines and store the plants they have harvested but not yet made into medicines.

As you learn the plants, you will come to know how they *look* but also how they feel to the hand, how they smell, how they taste, even how they *sound*. Aspens make a sound completely unlike any other tree as the wind moves among them. You also learn, over time, how a plant subtly changes your body the moment you take it inside you. *All* plants have different effects and this becomes part of the knowledge as well.

Learn, also, to pay attention to how the plant *feels* to your non-physical sensing. You have learned to pay attention to how a restaurant or someone's home *feels* to you when you first walk in the door, to notice whether it feels welcoming or not, emotionally warm or not, safe or not. This kind of sensing can be extended to the plants you use for your medicines. Pay attention to whether or not the plant you are harvesting feels healthy and vital to you. Your medicines will only be as good as the plants you use to make them.

And ... thank the plants as you harvest them. This is a form of saying grace for food, only now you are doing it for your medicines. This may not be a regular part of your life, this kind of thankfulness, but after 25 years of this work, I can tell you, it does make a difference to the quality of the medicines you make and of the relationship you will ultimately have with the plants you use for healing.

Harvesting

Making plant medicines is a full-immersion, full-sensory experience; it's very physical. Harvesting plants often means walking miles to find the ones you are looking for. If you are working with roots, you will be digging, of course, and some plants are very difficult to dig. You will need a shovel, sometimes a pick. Other plants, such as nettles or devil's club, have stinging hairs or thorns; you will need gloves. And despite their use, you will get bitten by the plant — *everybody* does. It's part of the journey.

Take an easy-to-carry bag, with a fold-up shovel, plant cutters, a knife, and plastic bags to put the plants in. Big plastic bags. Paper is relatively useless; it won't hold up to walking miles in the field and it is much bulkier than plastic. You can use a woven basket instead of a bag, but it's better to keep the herbs you are harvesting in their own bags, not roughly mixed together in a basket. Take Band-Aids and tweezers and comfortable walking shoes and a staff, a hat and water and a lunch to eat. Also: Don't walk any farther than half the distance you have the energy for. (Just an FYI on that one.)

Preparing Medicinal Plants

Once you have harvested the plants, take them home and begin preparing them as medicine right away; they will rot if you leave them in the plastic bags, or dry badly if you just dump them in a pile on the table and leave them too long. Never, never, never leave them in the truck overnight. (*Everyone* puts plant preparation off sooner or later and then has to throw the plants away. It *only* takes once . . . usually.)

Roots should be shaken and brushed to get the dirt off. Washing them is generally a bad idea unless, due to the nature of the root (e.g., coral root), they have to be washed. (Washing removes essential oils and the outer bark — things you don't want to lose.) Some roots are as tough as steel once they dry (e.g., red root), so cut them into small pieces while they are fresh. (*Everyone* fails to do this once.)

DRYING TRAYS

Get a good drying tray for seeds, roots, bark, and so on. Flattish trays that are fairly shallow are best. I like woven ones that let the air circulate or high-impact plastic trays. You will always drop and break a glass one. (Eventually.) Metal has too many reactions with plant chemicals and moisture and can contaminate the herb.

Leafy plants can be tied together — you will need some good twine — and hung from the rafters to dry unless you are making medicine from the fresh leaves. They dry well that way.

Storing Supplies and Medicines

Label *everything*. Everyone, and I mean *everyone*, thinks they will never forget the plant they just harvested, but everyone, and I mean *everyone*, does if it is not labeled. Then you will find yourself with a lot of unidentifiable plant matter on your hands that you can't use (and no, using them for illnesses you can't identify either won't work). And . . . label *all* your medicines once you've made them as well. You *will* forget what is in that bottle.

You will need bottles, of course, to store your finished medicines in. Tiny ones are nice for salves. Brown ones are nice for tinctures; they keep the light out and minimize degradation. Everything is best if kept in the dark; light has a strongly negative impact on the life of your medicines. (You will need droppers too — they are ridiculously expensive compared to the bottles they go with.)

The Different Kinds of Herbal Medicines

Herbal medicines, in general, fall into two groups: 1) those for internal use, and 2) those for external use.

The main forms of herbal medicines for internal use are:
- Water extracts (infusions and decoctions)
- Alcohol extracts (tinctures)
- Percolations (water or alcohol)
- Fluid extracts
- Syrups/oxymels/electuaries
- Glycerites
- Fermentations
- Vinegars
- Fresh juice (stabilized or not)
- Powders (plain or encapsulated)
- Food
- Suppositories/boluses
- Douches
- Essential oils
- Steams
- Smokes

The main forms of herbal medicines for external use are:
- Oil infusions
- Salves
- Evaporative concentrates
- Washes
- Liniments
- Lotions
- Compresses/poultices
- Essential oils
- Smudges

Most of these you can make yourself. Essential oils need special distilling equipment and I won't spend much time on them in this chapter — just a bit about using them as medicine.

If you are making tinctures, you will need Ball jars or something similar for the herbs to macerate in. I often get old olive or pickle jars, the *big* ones, from restaurants to use for larger batches. Make sure they are clean — the smell does get into the tincture if you don't. There are other things you will find you need as you go along. I will mention a number of them when I talk about the particular kinds of medicines you can make.

In general, there are only a few kinds of herbal medicines: salves, infusions, tinctures, and powders. The list I am going to give you will appear more complicated than that, but that is pretty much all it comes down to. There are just a number of different *forms* to those four types of medicines. Most of them you will never need; still, I'm going to tell you about them. You never know what might come in handy.

Remember: Have fun. This is an art as much as a science and art always, *always*, has a depth of feeling and intuition to it that can never be captured and quantified. Trust your *feelings* and understand that your heart is as important to listen to as your head. Life without heart, you know, is not much of a life at all.

A Comment on Solvents

Unless you are using the plant itself in some form — as powder, food, juice, or so on — what you will be doing when you make your medicines is extracting the chemical constituents of the plant in some kind of liquid solvent. (When you take the whole herb internally, the stomach acids, bile salts, and so on *are* the solvent media. They leach out the active constituents of the plants for you.)

Every solvent has its own properties and people use different ones for many different reasons, some of which I will go into in this chapter. Generally, a solvent is referred to as a *menstruum*. It comes from *menstruus*, a Latin word meaning "month." It was felt, in the old days, that the moon and its cycle of 28 days had an influence on liquids, just as it does on the tides. So, herbs were placed in liquids — on particular days by the fanatical — and left in there for one cycle of the moon. Hence *menstruum*. Though derided as superstition by scientists, there is some legitimacy to this kind of thinking. Plants really are stronger when harvested on certain days, the moon does affect the underground aquifers of the earth, just as it does the oceans (causing the ground to breathe out moisture-laden air), leeches really are useful (surgeons use them regularly now), maggots really do clean gangrenous wounds better than anything else, and . . . oops, sorry, got carried away again.

Anyway, the solvent is called the *menstruum*, herbs are placed in the menstruum, and once there they begin to *macerate*. Maceration is the soaking of something — usually a plant of some sort — in a solvent until the cell walls begin to break down so the compounds in the herb will leach into the solvent, where they are held in suspension. When you later separate the liquid (now containing the medicinal compounds) from the solids, the solids that are left are called the *marc*. The liquid is called whatever kind of medicine you were making: tincture, infusion, or so on.

Water is considered to be *the* universal solvent; it works for most things to some extent. For most of human history, it has been the primary solvent people have used. Alcohol is the next most effective solvent. Combining them will give you the most comprehensive solvent medium that exists.

Just as with the plants you harvest, use the best-quality solvents you can get. Your water, especially, should be well, spring, or rain water — if you can get it. If you use tap water, have a filter on the water line if you are at all able to do so. Or else buy a good-quality water. The better the water, the better the medicine. (Tap water is, as well, filled with minute quantities of pharmaceuticals — you really don't want to ingest them. They are highly bioactive.)

Another thing to understand is that the more finely powdered your herb, the more surface area that is exposed to the solvent. This allows more of the chemical constituents to leach into the solvent.

When you are making extracts, part of what you learn, and develop in your practice, is knowledge of just what kinds of solvents are right for which herbs and in what combinations. The goal is to get as many of the medicinal compounds as possible into the extractive medium. Each herb is different and needs different combinations of water and alcohol — that is, a different formula for preparation. Some do better in pure alcohol, some in pure water. Some need oils to extract the active constituents (*Artemisia annua* is an example of this; artemisinin is more easily soluble in fats than in either alcohol or water). Some need boiling, some prefer cold liquids.

Pharmacists, prior to World War II (before pharmaceuticals began to dominate medicine), were extensively trained in very sophisticated forms of herbal medicine making — many of which are beyond the scope of this book (and of most pharmacists these days). This is why pharmacists are still called "chemists" in England and the drugstores there the "chemist's" shops. Distressingly, that kind of training no longer occurs; it is now a lost art. I doubt there is a medicinal pharmacist in practice anywhere in the Western world who can prepare a tincture of *Colchicum officinale* and determine, exactly, the amount of colchicine in it — as all pharmacists could do in 1920.

In becoming an herbal medicine maker, you are learning how to be a practical dispensing pharmacist. Part of what that means is discovering how to best prepare the herbs and with which solvents. Chapter 9 is an herbal formulary that will give you the ratio of alcohol and water for several hundred plant tinctures.

Water Extractions

The two most common forms of water extractions are infusions and decoctions. Two lesser-known forms are evaporative concentrates and percolations.

Infusions

Teas are, at heart, weak infusions. When making medicine, however, you are usually working with what would formally be called an infusion. Infusions are stronger than teas since the herbs sit, *infuse*, in the water for a much longer period.

An infusion is made by immersing an herb in either cold or hot, not boiling, water for an extended time. Again, the water you use should be the purest you can find, *not* tap water. Water from rain, a healthy well, or a spring is best.

The weakness of infusions, cold or hot, is that they do not keep well; they tend to spoil very quickly. Refrigeration will only slow the process a little. Infusions, unless you stabilize them with something like alcohol, need to be used shortly after you make them. Their strength is that nearly everyone has access to enough water to make them without resorting to the expense of buying alcohol.

HOT INFUSIONS

Although the guidelines below call for short timelines for hot infusions, I often make my infusions at night just before bed and let them infuse overnight. I usually make enough for one day, then drink the infusions throughout the next day.

Most *hot* infusions are consumed, confusingly, not hot but warm or at room temperature; the infusion periods are too long for the water to stay hot. *Hot* infusion, in this sense, is a description of the extraction process, not of its temperature when used.

Some herbs, however, are best consumed while still hot, such as diaphoretics that stimulate sweating. For example, yarrow, if being used to help break a fever, is best consumed hot (steeped 15 minutes, covered). If being used for GI tract distress or to stimulate menstruation, though, it is best prepared as a hot infusion but consumed hours later at room temperature.

To prepare a hot infusion, bring water to a boil, then combine it with the herb in the following manner:

- **For leaves:** 1 ounce per quart of hot water, let steep 4 hours, tightly covered. Tougher leaves require longer steeping. The more powdered the leaves (if dried), the stronger the infusion. If you are using fresh leaves, cut them finely with scissors or chop them as finely as possible with a sharp knife.

- **For flowers:** 1 ounce per quart of hot water, let steep 2 hours, tightly covered. More fragile flowers require less time. Most flowers can be infused whole.
- **For seeds:** 1 ounce per pint of hot water, let steep 30 minutes, tightly covered. More fragrant seeds such as fennel need less time (15 minutes), rose hips longer (3 to 4 hours). Most seeds possess very strong seed coats to protect them from the world until they sprout. You will need to break the seed coat in order for the solvent to work; the seeds should be powdered as finely as possible.
- **For barks and roots:** 1 ounce per pint of hot water, let steep 8 hours, tightly covered. Some barks, such as slippery elm, need less

Infusion Tools

There are many kinds of infusion pitchers and mugs that are available to buy; they are pretty common. Most of them have some form of basket in which to place the herbs (and a lid to cover them). The basket is suspended at the top of the mug or pitcher so that the herbs and the liquid do not mix together. It does make it a bit easier. (Avoid plastic if you can; use stainless steel, glass, or pottery infusers.) You can also buy (or make) small cloth bags to hold the herbs, which you then suspend in whatever container you are using. A tea ball will also work, but I don't find them as effective; they don't usually hold enough herb.

The best infusers work by holding the herb in the upper part of the pot, so that only the upper portion of the liquid is in contact with the herb. As the water at the top of the infuser becomes saturated with the herbal constituents, it gets heavier and sinks to the bottom. This creates a circulating current in the water that brings the unsaturated water to the top of the jar where it can then infuse as well. This will make the strongest infusion. You can just put the herb in a jar with hot water and cover it; it will work fine, but it won't be quite as strong as this method. (See Percolations on page 336 for more on the dynamics of this.)

time (1 to 2 hours). Most barks and roots are infused after being dried; powder them as finely as possible. If you are using fresh roots, mince them as finely as possible.

If you keep the containers tightly covered, the volatile components in the herb will remain in the liquid rather than evaporating into the air. The heat will vaporize the volatiles and they will rise up in the steam, then collect on the underside of the lid. As the mixture cools, the volatiles will condense and drip from the lid back into the infusion. This ensures that the essential oils, which are very volatile, will remain. You can easily identify an herb that has a high volatiles content; it will have a strong essential oil or perfumey smell to it. These must always be covered when making a hot infusion.

When you are ready to use the infusion, pour off the water and squeeze out the marc as much as possible. The liquid in the saturated herbs is often much stronger than the infused liquid, so keep it if you can.

COLD INFUSIONS

Cold infusions are preferable for some herbs. The bitter components of herbs tend to be less soluble in cold water. Yarrow, for instance, is much less bitter when prepared in cold water. Usually cold infusions need to steep for much longer periods of time; each herb is different. The necessity for a cold infusion rarely arises; nevertheless, it may. If so, place the herb in room-temperature water, cover, and let steep overnight.

A Hot Infusion for Parasites

INGREDIENTS:

2 ounces dried alchornea leaf

2 ounces fresh gingerroot, chopped finely

2 ounces dried sida leaf

2 ounces dried wormwood leaf (*Artemisia absinthium*)

2 quarts water

Place herbs in container, pour near-boiling water on top, cover tightly, and let sit overnight. Strain and press the marc to extract as much liquid as possible. Drink 1 cup four times per day. This amount will last 2 days. Make it again every 2 days until you have been using it for 8 days. This is a good infusion for treating intestinal worms (you can just use the wormwood and ginger if you wish). It will be very bitter, though the ginger will help that a bit.

Decoctions

Decoctions are much stronger than infusions. Basically, they are boiled infusions. There are two forms of decoctions: 1) simple decoctions, and 2) concentrated decoctions. A simple decoction is any water extract that is boiled for a short length of time. Concentrated decoctions are boiled until the water is reduced to some extent. Normally, herbs that are highly resinous or filled with volatile oils are not decocted. Only herbs whose constituents are not damaged by heat are boiled.

It is important to begin with cold water, not warm or hot, add the herbs, and bring to a boil. The extraction will be more efficient if you begin with cold water as different constituents extract better at different temperatures.

Some herbs, such as isatis, are stronger if they are boiled for a few minutes simply because the higher heat is a better extractant. Herbs high in polysaccharides such as reishi are also often helped by boiling; polysaccharides tend to extract more efficiently when decocted. In essence, anytime an herb is boiled, no matter how short a time, it is considered to be a decoction. If you are just boiling the herb to better extract the constituents, you are making a simple decoction.

Recipe for a Simple Decoction

INGREDIENTS:

1 ounce herb   1 pint cold water

> Combine herb and water. Bring to boil. Boil at least 15 minutes (some herbs will need longer). Let cool enough that you can handle it. Strain the decoction to remove the herb. Press the herb to extract all liquid. Add enough water to bring the liquid back to 1 pint. Take as directed.

In a concentrated decoction, which is more common than simple decoctions, the herb is boiled in water long enough that the amount of water you began with is reduced to some extent, often by half, sometimes more. This acts to concentrate the constituents in less liquid, making the medicine stronger. Concentrated decoctions are not often drunk as a tea (reishi is an exception). However, they are sometimes used in smaller doses similarly to a tincture. Once the decoction is made it is allowed to cool, the liquid strained, then dispensed a tablespoon at a time — usually three or four times a day depending on the

As an Aside

Oxymels, which I won't discuss more than this, have been used for thousands of years. The basic form is 40 ounces of honey to which is added 5 fluid ounces of water and 5 fluid ounces of vinegar. Oxymels were often used for colds, flu, and sore throats. However, a more medicinal form of an oxymel is made using a concentrated decoction for the water part of the recipe. Electuaries, on the other hand, are medicinal pastes (the core of which can be a concentrated decoction to which powdered herbs are added) that are made palatable by the addition of sweeteners such as honey or syrups. Marsh mallows, originally, were not candy but a particular kind of electuary that made the medicine more palatable. This is still a good way to take powdered herbs: mix the powdered herbs you wish to take very well, then add enough honey to make a ball only slightly sticky to the hand, then eat it.

herb and the disease. The usual dosage range for concentrated decoctions, depending on the herb, is 1 to 4 fluid ounces a day.

The most common form of medicine made from concentrated decoctions is a cough syrup. They are also used to make a fomentation — that is, a very condensed water extract that is soaked into a cloth and applied to the surface of the body (to treat pain and inflammation in a joint, for example). Decoctions are also used as enemas — should the need arise, which everyone hopes it won't. This gets a very strong concentrate into the bowel where it will, usually, rather easily move across the membranes of the colon into the bloodstream.

When you are making your concentrated decoctions, use porcelain, glass, or stainless steel pots if you can; iron and aluminum will often contaminate the mix. When the decoction is cool, prepare it as needed for whatever you are going to use it for. Concentrated decoctions will last longer than infusions, especially if kept cold. Syrups will often last a year in a refrigerator just fine.

A Concentrated Decoction for Colds and Flu

INGREDIENTS:

1 ounce dried white or culinary sage leaf
Pinch of cayenne

3 cups cold water
Wildflower honey
Juice of one lemon

Combine sage and cayenne with water. Bring to boil, then reduce heat and simmer, uncovered, until liquid is reduced by half. Let cool enough that you can work with it. Strain the liquid and press sage to extract as much liquid as possible. Add wildflower honey to taste. Add juice of one lemon. Store in refrigerator. Take 1 tablespoon or more as often as needed at the onset of throat or upper respiratory infection.

Cough Syrup Recipe

INGREDIENTS:

3 ounces horehound leaves/stems

2 ounces cherry bark

2 ounces elder berries

2 ounces elecampane root

2 ounces licorice root

2 ounces mallow root

1 ounce slippery elm bark

1 ounce vervain leaf

1 ounce lomatium (or osha) root

7 pints water

3 ounces glycerine

Wildflower honey

2 ounces mullein tincture

1 ounce grindelia tincture

Combine the horehound, cherry bark, elder berries, elecampane, licorice, mallow, slippery elm bark, and vervain, along with half the lomatium, in the water in a large pot. Bring to a boil. Stir frequently as it heats to prevent sticking. Once it boils, reduce heat a bit and, stirring constantly, cook until the liquid is reduced by half. Let cool. (You can put the pot in a bath of cold water to cool it faster. Don't let it tip over.) Strain the liquid, and press the marc through a cloth to extract as much liquid as you can.

(The mucilaginous herbs — the licorice and mallow — can make it hard for the liquid to pass through the weave of the cloth you are using to press the marc. So, conversely, you can keep the licorice and mallow out of the mix and, once the marc is pressed, reheat the liquid, adding the licorice and mallow to the pot in a muslin bag. Bring to a boil and let simmer, stirring constantly, for 30 minutes. Remove the bag, let it cool, then squeeze it out as best you can.)

Warm the liquid again, just enough that it will dissolve the honey and glycerine. Add the glycerine, then the honey to taste. Powder the remaining lomatium to a fine powder — a nut or coffee grinder or mortar and pestle is good for this — then add it to the liquid. Let the mix cool, then add the mullein and grindelia tinctures.

The honey, glycerine, and two tinctures help stabilize the syrup, keeping it from going bad. I do keep the whole thing in the refrigerator, though. It will last a year very easily. Generally, it is best to make this kind of a syrup in the fall, after the berries are ripe and ready for harvest, and just before flu season. (You can substitute similar herbs for any used in this recipe.) Use as needed — I just drink it from the bottle — it is very effective.

Washes

Washes are simply infusions or decoctions that are used directly on the skin. If you have hurt your skin, an abrasion or sunburn for example, any wash that contains a tannin herb such as oak or acacia or older pine needles and soothing herbs such as mallow or chamomile will facilitate healing immensely — prickly pear (a soothing mucilaginous herb) is immensely good for this.

If you have a skin infection or a wound that you want to keep from becoming infected, use a wash of the applicable herbs from this book. If you don't know what kind of infection it is, use the antibacterial wash described below.

General Antibacterial Wash

INGREDIENTS:

2 ounces antibacterial herbs, such as artemisia (the *absinthium* species is very good), cryptolepis, or sida

2 ounces echinacea

2 ounces evergreen needles (any kind)

1 quart water

Combine the herbs with the water. Cover, bring to boil, and simmer uncovered for 30 minutes. Let cool and strain. Then wash the affected skin liberally with the decoction four times daily.

Steams

Steams are excellent for upper respiratory infections. They can be used as often as desired or needed. Wonderful steams can be made from most of the artemisias, any of the evergreens, any of the sages, and many other aromatic plants. You can also make them with essential oils.

The process involves putting a highly aromatic, antibacterial herb in water, boiling it, and breathing the steam.

A Steam for Upper Respiratory Infections

Though this steam recipe calls for dried herbs, it can be prepared with fresh herbs if desired.

INGREDIENTS:

2 ounces young eucalyptus leaves, dried

1 ounce sage leaf, dried

1 ounce juniper leaf or berry, dried

1 gallon water

Place herbs in water (in glass, stainless steel, or ceramic-coated pot) and bring to roiling boil. Remove from heat, hold head over steam, and cover head and steaming pot with large towel. Breathe steam deep into lungs. Bring herbs to boil and repeat as often as necessary. Replace herbs when their strong smell begins to noticeably diminish.

Essential oil steam: This steam method can also be undertaken with essential oils. Use 30 drops each of the essential oil of rosemary, sage, juniper, eucalyptus, and bergamot in 1 quart of water.

Wound wash: This recipe can also be prepared as a wash for infected or weeping wounds. Rather than boiling, bring the mixture to the edge of boiling, remove from heat, and let steep until lukewarm. Strain, use it to wash the wound thoroughly, then apply a wound powder.

Evaporative Concentrates

Evaporative concentrates are remarkable medicines but are rarely used in herbal practice and are poorly understood. The most common evaporative concentrate in the United States is made from chaparral leaf and is used for treating mastitis in women. However, the primary reason to use evaporative concentrates — in my opinion — is that this is the one process I know of to create a topical corticosteroid cream as potent as those made by pharmaceutical companies.

An evaporative concentrate is made by making a very, *very* slow-cooking decoction. A slow cooker (or Crock-Pot) is necessary; I don't know of another way to do it. You need a cooking pot where you can keep the heat at the slowest simmer possible, very slightly below boiling or very slightly over it.

To make a corticosteroid herbal cream, you need to begin with an anti-inflammatory herb. There are many of these and it is worth exploring different plants to find which ones work best for you. I tend to use the ones that contain a lot of salicylates, like aspen or willow, and are water soluble. When the decoction is finished, it will be very thick — the consistency of a hand cream. When used on the skin, for rashes, varicose veins, skin eruptions, and inflammations, it is as potent as pharmaceutical corticosteroids. The only drawback — not solvable — is that the concentrates are nearly black in color. It's very visible on the skin. Difficult if it is your face you are treating.

I usually refrigerate these concentrates, but when I haven't, even after months, they have never gone bad. The chemical concentration is apparently too high for bacteria to deal with. Needless to say, these concentrates are *not* for internal use.

Herbal Corticosteroid Evaporative Concentrate

INGREDIENTS:

32 ounces water

6 ounces powdered willow (or aspen) bark

Put the water in a slow cooker, and add the herb. Cover and turn the cooker on high. As the water warms, stir the mix well. When the water has come to a boil, reduce the heat to just under or just slightly over a simmer. Leave the cooker on that setting, covered, for 2 days.

Turn off the cooker, let the mix cool, and strain out the herb, squeezing the marc through a cloth to extract as much as possible. Clean the slow cooker and then put the liquid back in it. Turn on high and bring to a boil. Reduce immediately to just under or just slightly over a simmer. Keep it covered. Cook until the liquid is reduced to nearly nothing, essentially 1 to 2 ounces. This will take up to a week.

As the liquid begins to approach 1 to 2 ounces, watch it carefully. At this point it can lose the remaining water very quickly and it will burn once it does. *Once the liquid is this low, the remainder will go very fast.* It helps to stir it regularly at this point to get an idea of how much liquid is left. Once it has reduced enough, turn off the cooker, let it cool, and then place the concentrate in a jar. Label well. *Not* for internal use.

Percolations

Percolations are just the same as drip-grind coffee. You are letting liquid drip slowly through the herb — which is held in filter paper — into a container.

Percolations are handy to know about in case you run short of a tincture and need some in a hurry. They take a few hours rather than a few weeks. They are also the best way to make a cold-process water extract, much better than letting the herb steep in cold water. The main strength of a percolation, however, is its potency. This is due to the nature of solvents.

In essence, a solvent is a pure liquid; it doesn't have anything in it but itself. As a solvent leaches chemical constituents into itself, it begins filling up, or getting saturated as they say. Once it is saturated it can't take any more into itself. A good way to visualize this is to see, in your imagination, the liquid on one side, the herb on the other. The herb is full, the liquid is empty. As the two combine, the constituents in the herb begin to flow into the liquid. However, once the amount of constituents in the liquid are in equilibrium with those in the herb — like a weight scale where equal weights are on each side of the scale — it is very difficult for the constituents to keep flowing into the liquid. A saturation point is being reached.

The way a percolator works, however, means that the liquid never becomes saturated, the liquid that is touching the herb is always pure. So, the extract becomes very strong. You will see how this works when I describe how the percolator works in practice.

To make a percolation, however, you will need a percolator — this is why so few people make them. It is a bit more complex than using a jar to make a tincture or a coffee cone to make coffee. Some people do make their own percolators (it can be done fairly simply), or you can buy one from a scientific glass supplier.

Most scientific percolators are several feet long and look somewhat like a giant glass ice cream cone, wider at the top (big enough to easily put your hand and arm into) and narrowing to a point at the bottom. There is a narrow opening at the bottom that flows into an integral glass tube with a control knob on it, a spigot essentially, that you turn to control the flow of liquid out of the percolator.

(You can make your own percolator by cutting the bottom off a glass water bottle — don't use plastic — such as a mid-sized Perrier container. *Sand the edges well.* Until they are smooth. Keep the cap; you will need it.)

To use a percolator, you first determine what kind of percolation you are going to make, water or an alcohol and water mix. Make up the liquid mixture you are going to need and keep it close. Then take the dried herb and grind it as finely as possible. Percolation will not work with fresh herbs; they have to be dried. For a percolation to work well, the herb really does need to be as close to a powder as possible. You need as much plant surface area exposed to the liquid as possible. Once the herb is powdered, and before you start percolating, put the herb in a large bowl and add enough alcohol to the herb to moisten it — not wet, just moist. This will begin breaking down the cell walls of the plant and make the extraction more efficient.

Let the moist herb sit a couple of hours, but if you are impatient, at least 30 minutes. Then take some filter paper — I use the same coffee filters as are used for drip-grind coffee cones — and place it in the bottom of the percolator. It helps if the inside of the percolator is slightly dampened first so that the paper will adhere to the glass and fit snugly. Press the paper into place, being sure to not punch a hole in it with your fingers. Once that is done, carefully put the moistened herb in the cone, making sure you don't get any between the filter paper and the glass. Press it lightly into place — you don't want it compacted though, since liquid has to flow through it.

Depending on the amount of herb you use, the percolator can be filled nearly to the top with plant matter. When all the plant material is in the percolator, put a circular piece of filter paper on top of the herb and put something heavy on that to keep the paper, and the herb, from floating up — a small stone works well. (Not scientific, I know, but very aesthetic.)

Then, slowly, begin pouring the liquid into the percolator. Do it slowly so that you don't stir up the powdered herb. The liquid will slowly percolate down into the plant matter, and air bubbles will come up. (You may not be able to get all the liquid into the percolator in one go. If so you will have to add the rest as the liquid level drops.) When the herb is fully saturated, put a container under the spigot and very slowly open the spigot. (Some people run a plastic hose from the spigot into a container — needless to say, the percolator has to be held in the air on a stand of some sort in order to work.) You want to get one drop per second coming out of the spigot, so adjust the spigot until you get just that rate of drip.

The reason this makes such a good tincture (or cold water infusion) is that *only* clean liquid is flowing over the herb. This means that the liquid is completely unsaturated; its extraction capacity remains very high. So as the liquid flows over the herb, it pulls chemical compounds out of the plant, then more clean liquid comes behind and pulls more out. It's very elegant.

If you are using a homemade percolator, prepare it the same way, but when you are ready to percolate, very slightly open the bottle cap — just enough that a very slow drip comes out. Again, one drip per second is very effective.

Alcohol Extractions

Because alcohol extractions, i.e., tinctures, keep so well over time and because they are so easily dispensed, many herbalists prefer them over infusions. They are made by immersing a fresh plant in full-strength alcohol or a dried plant in an alcohol and water mixture.

I am a fan of using pure grain alcohol for tinctures. What that means in practice, however, is using an alcohol that is 190 proof, or 95 percent alcohol. (There is such a thing as 100 percent or 200-proof alcohol, but the only people who generally use it are scientists or large commercial enterprises; you will probably never see it.) Most people buy their 190-proof alcohol at their local liquor store; the most common brand in the United States is called Everclear.

Some states — some countries — will not allow their citizens to buy 190-proof alcohol (for their own good, of course). If you live in such a place, you will have to cross state (or country) lines and buy your alcohol from a more enlightened place or else make do with what they allow you to buy. In such places, most people use a 40 percent to 50 percent alcohol-content vodka; that is, 80 to 100 proof. Get the highest proof you can — you will see why this is important as we go on.

In the United States, the amount you pay for liquor, regardless of what you are buying, is directly proportional to its alcohol content. The actual cost of a gallon of 190-proof alcohol is about $1.00. The rest of the cost is federal and state taxes — which are then taxed again by sales tax when you buy the thing. So you may be tempted to buy a lower-proof vodka because it is cheaper. That is a bad idea. Your tinctures will be weak.

Fresh Plant Tinctures

Fresh herb tinctures, again, are made by putting the fresh herb in pure grain alcohol. These tinctures are nearly always made in a one-to-two ratio, which is written 1:2. (There are a few exceptions.) This ratio means you are using 1 part herb (dry weight measurement) to 2 parts liquid (liquid measurement). The amount of herb in such ratios is

The Origin of "Proof"

As an aside: In the eighteenth century the English navy paid sailors partly in rum. The watering of drinks has always been a problem. So to test their rum before accepting it as pay, the sailors would soak gunpowder with it. If the gunpowder would still burn, the rum was "proved." Hence 100 proof. The rum had to be a minimum of 57.5 percent alcohol for the gunpowder to burn, but that has been watered down to a simple rule of thumb: 50 percent alcohol = 100 proof.

always indicated by the first number, the amount of liquid by the second number.

So, for example, if you have 3 ounces (dry weight measure) of fresh echinacea flower heads, you would place them in a jar with 6 ounces (liquid measure) of 190-proof alcohol. I generally use well-sealed Mason or Ball jars, stored out of the sun and shaken daily. At the end of 2 weeks the herb is decanted and squeezed through a cloth until as dry as possible (an herb or wine press is good for this), and the resulting liquid is then stored in labeled, amber bottles.

Fresh plants naturally contain a certain percentage of water and alcohol is a very good extractor of water. (One of the main symptoms of a hangover comes from the alcohol extracting the water from your body — you get the same kind of headache from too much alcohol as you do from dehydration.) Alcohol will pull not only the medicinal constituents out of the plant but the plant's water as well.

The water in the fresh plant dilutes the alcohol, how much depends on the kind of plant it is. Peppermint has a lot of water in it, 50 percent or more by weight. So what you get when you tincture fresh peppermint leaves is a tincture that is about 50 percent alcohol and 50 percent water. Myrrh gum has virtually no water in it, so you end up with a tincture that is 95 percent alcohol and 5 percent water — and all that water was already in the alcohol, assuming you began with 95 percent alcohol.

Fresh leafy plants may be chopped or left whole before placing them into the alcohol or pureed with the alcohol in a blender. Fresh roots should be ground with the alcohol in a blender into a pulpy mush. (I generally think it better to make root tinctures from dried roots, but there are a few exceptions; coral root is one.)

Dried Plant Tinctures

Plants, as they dry, lose their natural moisture content (the amount of water you combine with alcohol to make a tincture is the amount of water that the plant loses when it dries). Tables detailing the moisture content of many medicinal plants are available. When making a tincture of a dried plant, you always add back the amount of water that was present in the plant when it was fresh. This enables the extraction of the water-soluble constituents to occur.

Dried plants are usually tinctured at a one-to-five ratio, which is written 1:5. (There are, as always, exceptions.) That means 1 part dried herb to 5 parts liquid. Fresh *Echinacea angustifolia* root, for example, contains 30 percent water by weight. If you have 10 ounces of powdered root (dry weight) you would then add to it 50 ounces of liquid (liquid measurement). This gives you your 1:5 ratio. The tricky part for many people comes in figuring out how much of that liquid should be water and how much alcohol. In this instance you are wanting your liquid to be 30 percent water (fresh echinacea root's water content); that is, 30 percent of 50 ounces, which would be 15 ounces water. The rest of the liquid will be alcohol; that is, 35 ounces.

A formula for this particular plant tincture would look something like this:

> *Echinacea angustifolia:* fresh root tincture 1:2; dried root tincture 1:5, 70 percent alcohol. Dosage: 30–60 drops as needed. In acute conditions: 30 drops minimum each hour.

Pressing Herbal Tinctures

When your tinctures are done, and you pour off the liquid, the marc will still have some, often a great deal of, liquid in it. The marc needs to be pressed to remove the remaining tincture. Most people do this by hand. The best thing to use is a good-quality cloth with a close weave to it — I use the same surgical cloths hospitals do; they hold up really well. An herb press facilitates this immensely, though a cider press, depending on the style, will work very well, too. You will get a lot more out of a press than when doing it by hand, but they do tend to be expensive.

With fresh plants you can generally get out about as much liquid as you put in; with dried material, especially roots, you get out as much as you can. Sometimes this isn't much.

It is just *assumed* that you already know that all fresh plant tinc-tures at 1:2 will be using 95 percent alcohol. (Note: Everyone I know just assumes that the 95 percent alcohol they are using is 100 percent; no one I know takes that 5 percent into account in figuring this stuff out. Life is too short.)

Again, don't use tap water if you can avoid it. Powder the herbs you are tincturing as finely as possible — many people in the United States use a Vitamix for this. It is a pretty indestructible mixer/grinder, especially if you get a commercial-grade unit. (The demo video shows them grinding 2×4s into sawdust.) I have had mine for 25 years and have replaced the blades only twice in spite of the heavy use I've subjected it to.

Unless the herbs become tremendously hard when dried (as red root does), it is best to store herbs as whole as possible until they are needed. This reduces the cell surface area that is exposed to air. Oxygen degrades plant matter fairly quickly.

Dry plant tinctures, like fresh, are left to macerate for 2 weeks, out of the light, before decanting.

Combination Tincture Formulas

In spite of our aversion in the United States toward the metric system, all scientific glassware in the United States is metric. Most herbalists use a *graduated cylinder* to measure the amount of tincture they are pouring out (available from any scientific glassware company). Most herbal bottles, of course, are in ounces, while the measuring cylinders are in milliliters. Roughly, 30 milliliters is equal to 1 ounce.

As an example, if you were going to make a combination tincture formula for the early onset of colds and flu, a good mix would be 10 milliliters each of echinacea, red root, and licorice tinctures mixed together. This would give you 1 fluid ounce total.

You can mix something like this in the graduated cylinder, as long as your hand is steady, then pour the mixture into a 1-ounce amber bottle with a dropper lid. Dosage would be one full dropper at least each hour during the onset of upper respiratory infections. This will

How Long Will Tinctures Last?

Tinctures should be kept out of the sun — a dark, cool room is good. Keeping them in dark or amber-colored glass jars is even better — though if they are in the dark you can leave them in clear jars as many of us do with our larger quantities of tinctures. Tinctures will, in general, last many years. However, you should know about precipitation, a very neglected area of herbal medicine.

The constituents that you have extracted from the herbs are held in suspension in a liquid medium. Over time, some of these constituents will precipitate out and settle on the bottom of the tincture bottle. Some herbs such as *Echinacea angustifolia* root are heavy precipitators, while others, like elder flower, are such light precipitators that you will almost never see a precipitate in the bottle. Unfortunately, there has been little study on this, nor has a chart of herbal precipitation rates ever been prepared (as far as I know; intent searching has never turned one up). Technically, we need one that shows both the rate of precipitation and the amount of precipitation for each plant.

Some herbalists will add 1 to 2 ounces of glycerine to every 16 ounces of tincture (10 percent to 15 percent of the total liquid) to help slow down or eliminate precipitation. It does help retard the precipitation of tannins; I am not sure how well it works for other constituents or over time but you might try it and see how it works if precipitation becomes a concern for you.

You will find that some herbs will produce an ever larger precipitate on the bottom of your storage bottles as time goes by. It is not possible to get that precipitate back into solution. Most herbalists simply shake the bottle prior to dispensing and suggest the user do the same before ingesting it. I do it this way and it seems to work fine, medicinally speaking.

There is, as yet, no data on whether the efficacy of a tincture is affected by precipitation. Certainly the ones that do not precipitate are good for decades if kept in a dark, cool location in well-sealed bottles.

usually prevent the onset of colds and flu if your immune system is relatively healthy.

Glycerites

Glycerine can also be used for making extracts; it has become a popular alternative for children's tinctures and for people who don't like alcohol.

Glycerine is technically a kind of alcohol, though most people don't know it (and when told they don't seem to think it evil). It is formed through the hydrolysis of oils or fats, usually animal or vegetable. It is a common by-product of the industrial production of soap. Glycerine is a relatively new substance (to people), discovered in 1789 and used medicinally only since the mid-1800s.

Glycerine is fairly viscous and very sweet; I've never had any undiluted glycerine go bad, even after years of being unrefrigerated. It is very stable, like alcohol, and possesses its own antimicrobial properties. It is not as efficient an extractive as water or alcohol; it won't extract gums, resins, or volatile or fixed oils, so its range of use is limited.

If you do dilute the glycerine, as you will have to do in making an extract, it won't hold up as well as an alcohol tincture. Most people add 10 percent to 15 percent alcohol to glycerites to ensure stability.

One of the very good things about glycerine is that it is moisturizing, demulcent, emollient, and soothing to the skin. I have found it to be exceptional for making extractions to be used for ear infections. Unlike alcohol, it won't irritate the inside of the ear but will soothe it instead while still carrying antimicrobial constituents to the place they need to go.

Glycerine is only about 60 percent as extractive as water or alcohol; glycerites will be 40 percent less strong than those other extractions. Glycerites should be dosed at one and a half to two times the dosage for tinctures. If you would normally dose with ½ dropperful (15 drops) of tincture, you would, with a glycerite, give ¾ dropperful (22 drops) to 1 full dropper (30 drops).

MAKING GLYCERITES FROM DRIED HERBS

The ratio is the same as for alcohol tinctures, 1:5. The liquid, however, to better preserve the glycerine and to help the extraction be more effective, should contain at least 10 percent 190-proof alcohol, then 60 percent glycerine, and finally 30 percent water.

As an example: If you are starting with 5 ounces of powdered echinacea root, then you would need 25 ounces of liquid, of which 2.5 ounces would be alcohol, 15 ounces would be glycerine, and 7.5 ounces would be water.

It is more effective if you add the alcohol to the powdered herbs first and let it sit for 24 hours, then add the glycerine and water, mix well, and leave in a jar with the lid on for 2 weeks. Decant and store as with alcohol tinctures.

Ear Infection Glycerite

INGREDIENTS:

1 ounce berberine plant

1 ounce cryptolepis (or sida or alchornea)

1 ounce echinacea

1 ounce juniper (or other evergreen needles)

1 ounce usnea lichen

2.5 ounces grain alcohol

15 ounces glycerine

7.5 ounces water

Powder herbs well, place in jar, add alcohol, mix thoroughly, and let sit for 24 hours. Mix glycerine and water together, and add to powdered herbs in jar. Let macerate 2 weeks, then decant and strain. Store in amber jar. Use 1–3 drops in the ear up to six times daily for ear infections.

MAKING GLYCERITES FROM FRESH HERBS

This is made with the usual 1:2 ratio for fresh herbs. In this instance, however, use 15 percent pure alcohol and 85 percent glycerine. So if you have 5 ounces fresh herb, you would want 10 ounces of liquid, of which 1.5 ounces would be 95 percent alcohol and 8.5 ounces would be glycerine.

A Comment on Alcohol

There has been a tremendous resurgence of puritanitis in the United States and a few other parts of the globe (notably the United Kingdom) over the past 20 years or so. One object of attention of this spasming of the puritan reflex has been the evils of alcohol. Many on the right and on the left seem to think it is some sort of inherently evil substance that is going to destroy Western civilization or at least make God really, really mad.

Alcohol existed long before human beings emerged out of the ecological matrix of this planet. It is a highly natural substance, both inside and outside of our bodies. *All* living beings partake of it, including trees, bees, and elephants. (Not kidding.) All of them enjoy it. It facilitates the functioning of the body, enhances organ function in many respects, and reduces the incidence of many diseases. It is not an evil substance.

One of the continual queries about tinctures concerns the alcohol content. Many people are afraid to take tinctures because of the evil alcohol in them.

To be really specific: The amount of alcohol in tinctures is incredibly tiny. Less than you will get from eating a few pieces of bread (yes, bread does have alcohol in it, enough to produce a breathalyzer reading of 0.05 just by itself). If you are taking 20 drops of a 60 percent alcohol tincture *every* hour for an acute condition, you will get about $1/17$ of an ounce of alcohol over the course of a day (less than 2 milliliters). If you are taking a general dose (20 drops three times daily) you will be getting about $1/30$ of an ounce over a day. Again, this is less than you will get from eating two slices of bread.

If this truly is a problem for you, you can make infusions or use glycerites — though the glycerites really aren't as effective and the water extractions won't extract some of the more important alcohol-soluble constituents. Some people heat their tinctures to remove the alcohol; it doesn't work very well and I suspect the heat alters the quality of the tincture. I don't recommend it.

Herbal Honeys

Honey can be used just like glycerine, following the same directions for making a glycerite. Make sure to use a good wildflower honey.

Nasal Sprays

Nasal sprays are excellent for helping with the onset of upper respiratory or sinus infections. Simply take an herbal tincture and place up to 10 drops or so in a 1-ounce nasal spray bottle (available from pharmacies). Add pure water and spray up nostrils as often as needed.

Nasal Spray Formula for Sinus Infections

INGREDIENTS:

5 drops cryptolepis tincture	5 drops juniper berry tincture
5 drops bidens tincture	5 drops usnea tincture

Combine the tinctures in a 1-ounce nasal spray bottle, add enough pure water to make 1 ounce, replace cap, and spray into nostrils as often as desired. (You could substitute 2 drops each of the essential oils of eucalyptus, sage, rosemary, and juniper for the tinctures if you wish.)

Vinegar Tinctures

I don't use these much, but they have a long history of use in many different cultures. One of their strengths is that vinegar itself is a highly medicinal substance; another is that they don't go bad, no matter how long you keep them. Natural vinegars should be used; most people use an unpasteurized, organic apple cider vinegar. Make your tinctures at a 1:2 ratio if using fresh herbs, or 1:5 if using dried. You don't need to add any water to vinegar tinctures.

Fluid Extracts

Not many people make their own fluid extracts any more, though a few herbal companies sell them. Herb Pharm's *Eleutherococcus* tincture is one of the better known. Essentially, 1 gram of fluid extract is supposed to be equivalent to 1 gram of the herb. They are very concentrated alcohol tinctures. In the nineteenth century they generally contained other substances such as vinegar or sugar. *All* trained pharmacists could make fluid extracts in the nineteenth and early twentieth centuries. They would make them in their pharmacies, in the lab in back, and keep them on hand for when needed. Most companies that make fluid extracts these days use specialized equipment to do so.

Here are the directions for a fluid extract of ipecac, from an early U.S. pharmacopeia.

> Moisten 16 Troy ounces ipecacuanha in fine powder with 6 fluid ounces alcohol; press it firmly into a conical percolator, and displace 3 pints of tincture, or until the ipecacuanha is exhausted. Distill the tincture over a water-bath until the residue is of a syrupy consistence. Mix with 1 fluid ounce acetic acid and 10 fluid ounces water; boil until reduced to ½ pint, and the resinous matter has separated. Filter when cold, and add water through the filter to make the filtrate up to ½ pint. Mix with ½ pint alcohol.

An alternate form of a fluid extract would be an evaporative concentrate. For example, make up a willow bark concentrate as described earlier but save the marc. Add to the marc 5 ounces of 190-proof alcohol and let it macerate as you reduce your decoction in the slow cooker. Once the decoction is reduced to 1 ounce of a very thick liquid, press out the alcohol from the marc and combine it with the concentrate. This will give you approximately 6 ounces of a fluid extract, essentially a 1:1 ratio. The dosage for internal use would be tiny, 1 to 3 drops. It is much stronger than a regular tincture.

This form of a fluid extract will work only with plants that have primarily water-soluble constituents. A percolator really is necessary for those that need alcohol extraction.

Here is Michael Moore's recipe for a fluid extract using a percolator:

> Briefly, take 8 ounces of Tabebuia (Pau D'Arco), grind it, make up an arbitrary amount of menstruum (let's say four times as much, or 32 ounces). The tincture lists a 50% strength; make your fluidextract menstruum 20 percent higher in alcohol content (i.e. 70%). Mix 22.4 ounces of alcohol with 9.6 ounces of water to get a quart of 70 percent alcohol menstruum. Take

the Tabebuia, moisten it, digest it for TWO days, pack a larger [percolator] cone with it, and drip (very slowly) a first batch of tincture that is only 75% of the volume as the original dried herb weighed. This means after you have dripped 6 fluid ounces, take it away, and continue dripping everything else into a second jar. As the rest of the menstruum finally starts to sink below the top of the herb column, start adding water into the cone. This second drip can be any amount you wish . . . a quart, two quarts, whatever. You will need to evaporate it all in a double boiler until it is reduced to 25% in volume of the herb weight . . . 2 ounces in this case. Add the vile remnant of the second percolation to the 6 ounces from the first percolation, and you now have 8 ounces of fluidextract, made from 8 ounces of Tabebuia Bark. A fluidextract is by definition 1:1 in strength.[1]

Douches

The easiest way to make a douche is to add ½ ounce of tincture to 1 pint of water. This is especially effective in the treatment of vaginal infections. Usnea is particularly valuable as a douche, as are the berberines. In general, douching twice a day for 3 days is sufficient.

You can also make a strong infusion or decoction and, when cooled, douche with that. Sida and cryptolepis would be good as either an infusion or a decoction.

Liniments

Liniments are generally made with rubbing alcohol. Use a 1:2 ratio with fresh plants, 1:5 with dried. You don't need to add any additional water. I use these for topical use, generally for arthritis and sore muscles. Cayenne is a very good liniment herb for both: 3 ounces powdered cayenne in 15 ounces rubbing alcohol, macerate for 2 weeks, decant, and press. I just pour a bit in my hand and rub the affected area as often as needed. **Caution:** Wash your hands afterward and *never, ever, ever* touch *any* mucous membranes before you do. Cuts are nearly as bad. And for sure, never, never go to the bathroom and then wipe yourself after using one of these unless you have washed your hands really, really well first. Just an FYI on that one.

Oil Infusions

Oil infusions are exceptionally useful for burns, sunburn, chapped and dry skin, skin infections; as ear drops; and for use on wounds as salves. With oil infusions the medicinal properties of the plant are transferred to an oil base rather than water or alcohol. A salve is just an oil infusion thickened by the addition of beeswax.

Oil Infusions with Dried Herbs

To make an oil infusion of *dried* herbs, grind the herbs you wish to use into as fine a powder as possible. Place the herbs in a glass baking dish, and pour enough oil on top of them to soak them well. Stir the powdered herbs to make sure they are well saturated with oil; add just enough extra oil to cover them by ¼ inch or so. I generally use olive oil because it is very stable; it doesn't go rancid easily and is, itself, strongly antimicrobial.

Some people just leave the mix, covered, in a sunny location for a few weeks. That will work fine as long as they do get sun and are warmed well every day. I prefer using the oven. I cover the container, put it in the oven on low heat just before bed, and leave it overnight. Some herbalists prefer to cook the herbs for as many as 10 days at 100°F in a slow cooker. (Most of us are too impatient for that.) However you do it, when the mix is done, let it cool, then strain the oil out of the herbs by pressing through a strong cloth with a good weave.

Herbal Oil for Skin Infections

INGREDIENTS:

- 1 ounce dried artemisia leaf (any species)
- 1 ounce dried berberine plant (any species; root, bark, or leaf as the case may be)
- 1 ounce dried cryptolepis (or sida or bidens or alchornea leaf)
- 1 ounce dried echinacea root or seed
- 1 ounce dried evergreen needles (any species)
- 1 ounce dried usnea
- 1 quart olive oil

Grind all the herbs as finely as you can, then place them in a glass or ceramic pot — do not use metal. Pour in enough oil to saturate the herbs, stir the mix well, then add enough extra oil to cover the herbs by ¼ inch. Heat the mixture, covered, overnight in the oven with the setting on low (150° to 200°F) or on low in a slow cooker for 7 days. Let the mixture cool. Press the oily herb mixture through a cloth to extract the oil. Store the oil in a sealed glass container out of the sun. It does not need to be refrigerated.

Oil Infusions with Fresh Herbs

To make an oil infusion from *fresh* herbs, place the herbs in a clear glass jar and cover them with just enough oil to make sure no part of the plant is exposed to air. Let the jar sit in the sun for 2 weeks (or cook in a slow cooker for 5 days at low setting). Then press the herbs through a cloth. Let the decanted oil sit. After a day the water that is naturally present in fresh herbs will settle to the bottom; carefully pour off the oil and discard the water. Note: You may have to do this two or three times to get all the water out. If any water remains in the oil, it will spoil.

Some herbalists prefer to start the oil infusion by pouring just a bit of alcohol over the herb and letting it sit in the alcohol for 24 hours. This begins breaking down the cell walls of the plant, making the oil extraction stronger.

Salves

To make a salve all you do is take the oil you have made (the recipe on the preceding page is a good one) and add beeswax to it. *Only* beeswax should be used, not petroleum waxes. For a variety of reasons beeswax is better, among them: beeswax itself has antimicrobial properties.

So . . . after pressing out the oil from your cooled oil infusion, put it in a glass, ceramic, or stainless steel pot and slowly reheat it. It needs to be reheated just enough to melt the beeswax.

It usually takes somewhere around 2 ounces of beeswax per cup of infused oil to make a salve. It goes a lot faster if the beeswax is in the form of beads or is as finely chopped as you can get it.

When the beeswax is melted and stirred in, place a few drops from the pot on a small plate and let it cool. Touch it; if it is too soft add more wax, if too hard add a bit more oil. A perfect salve should stay hard for a few seconds as you press your fingertip on it and then suddenly soften from your body heat. If you do make up your salve and it is too soft, you can just reheat it slowly and add a bit more beeswax. If too hard, you can add a bit more oil.

I used to make my salves and put them into scores of tiny salve jars. Now, I just put them into a larger container such as a Ball or Mason jar, slowly reheat it if I need some to use, and then pour that into a smaller container to carry with me.

Lotions

Contrary to popular belief, oil and water do mix. It's called a lotion. You can make water infusions of herbs, then blend them with oil (and an emulsifier) to make a lotion for the skin. Many herbs that are good for the skin can be blended into these kinds of lotions. Some of the best information on this (not my thing really) can be found online.

Using Whole Herbs

Herbs don't have to be made into tinctures or infusions; they can be taken directly in various forms: as powders, as food, as juice. They are very effective in these forms for a variety of ailments.

Wound Powders

Some wounds do not respond well to a wet dressing like a salve. However, dried herbs placed directly on the wound are exceptional in such cases. Herbal combinations, when powdered well, will stop bleeding and facilitate rapid healing while preventing infection. After the wound has begun healing, you can switch to a salve or even honey directly on the wound.

(As an aside, I once accidently shot a 16d nail through the first joint of the index finger on my left hand — a complicated misfire by a compressed air nail gun. After I used a hammer to remove my finger from the board it was nailed to, I poured some cryptolepis tincture on the nail, then pulled it out of the finger. I used a wound powder, much like the one in this book, on the wound for 2 days, then switched to pure honey dressings for a week. It worked fine; full function restored.)

There is probably no more powerful way to treat wound infections than with powdered herbs. I have yet to find an infection that will not respond to one.

The herbs need to be powdered as fine as possible. I usually begin with a Vitamix, which will give me a semi-small grind, then switch to a nut or coffee grinder for further powdering. This will get the herbs about as fine as you can get them. A mortar and pestle will do very well, but they are time consuming.

After the herbs are powdered, they should be sifted through a fine-mesh sieve, so make sure you are getting only the finest powder possible. (Discard any pieces that refuse to reduce to a powder or save them for use in an oil infusion later.) Once it has been sieved, put the powder in a tightly sealed container and keep it in a freezer or in a cool location away from sunlight. Powdered herbs lose their potency fairly quickly unless protected. Replace the powder every 6 months, unless you are keeping it frozen, which will allow it to last several years.

When needed sprinkle the powder liberally on wet wounds. It will stop the bleeding, prevent infection, and stimulate cell wall binding. Infected, oozing, pus-filled wounds should be opened up, cleaned with an antibacterial herbal wash, then liberally sprinkled with the powder as often as needed. Once the wound is healing cleanly it should not be disturbed (i.e., by scrubbing or trying to open it up again) — just add more wound powder, or switch to honey, as needed.

A Good Wound Powder

INGREDIENTS:

1 ounce berberine plant (root or bark, as the case may be)

1 ounce cryptolepis root or sida, bidens, or alchornea leaf

1 ounce echinacea root or seed

1 ounce juniper leaf

1 ounce lomatium root

1 ounce usnea lichen

Powder all herbs as finely as possible, and strain through a sieve. Use as needed. This same formula can be sprinkled onto feet or into shoes and socks for athlete's foot fungal infections. It may also be used on babies for diaper rash.

Herbal Powders for Internal Use

Herbs are often powdered and then pressed into tablets or put into capsules for internal use, generally by commercial companies. You can get a simple herbal capsule machine if you wish. Packing a lot of capsules by hand is tremendously tedious. These days, I usually just take the herbs internally in their powdered form. Many people don't like to do it this way because of the flavor of the herbs — they are often bitter. (I just use juice or honey; I am very lazy.)

Although many herbs are available as capsules or tablets, for some conditions the herbs really do need to be taken as powders; they shouldn't be encapsulated. This is especially true in cases of severe stomach ulceration. The herbs should be powdered, then mixed with liquid and consumed. This allows the herb to make contact with the entire affected area.

If the ulceration is in the duodenum, which lies just below the stomach, then capsules *should* be used. The capsules tend to sit at the bottom of the stomach and then drop through into the duodenum where they are needed. Duodenal ulcers are often accompanied by painful cramping or spasming. This can be alleviated by the addition of a few drops of peppermint essential oil to the herbal mixture before encapsulating it.

Herbal Regimen for an Ulcerated Stomach

INGREDIENTS:

4 ounces dried licorice root

4 ounces dried marsh mallow root

4 ounces dried comfrey root

2 ounces berberine plant tincture

1 quart wildflower honey

Powder licorice, marsh mallow, and comfrey roots (as finely as possible) and mix together in equal parts. Take 2 tablespoons, twice a day (morning and evening), mixed in any liquid (e.g., apple juice), for 30 days. For the next 60 days use just powdered licorice and marsh mallow roots (omitting the comfrey), again mixed in equal parts; take 1 tablespoon in the morning only. The herbs should not be in capsules in order to allow them to fully coat the stomach lining. (For duodenal ulcers, you would take them in capsules.)

At the same time, as you first begin the treatment with the powder, take 1 teaspoon of the berberine plant tincture three times daily for 15 days. And . . . take 1 tablespoon honey six times daily for 30 days.

Suppositories

Suppositories can be made from powdered herbs to treat things such as vaginal infections and hemorrhoids. I have recommended the use of echinacea suppositories for abnormal Pap smears for many years; they work very well. The powdered herbs are combined with enough liquid to make them hold together, be shaped properly, and be inserted.

Suppository for an Abnormal Pap Smear

INGREDIENTS:

Echinacea angustifolia root

Vegetable glycerine

Flour

Usnea tincture

Calendula tincture

Powder the echinacea root as finely as you can, then mix it with enough vegetable glycerine to bring it to the consistency of cookie dough. At this point it will still be a bit sticky, so mix it with enough flour (any kind — chlorella or spirulina can also be used) to bring it to the consistency of bread dough. Once you have, take a bit of the mix and press it into the shape of a suppository, about the size of your thumb. Repeat until you've used up all the mixture. Place the suppositories on a tray and put them in the freezer. They won't freeze; they will remain pliable but manageable.

Each evening, after you are in bed, place one suppository up against the cervix. The next morning, use a douche made from a mix of equal parts usnea and calendula tinctures, ½ ounce in 1 pint water (otherwise the remains of the suppository will drip out throughout the day — messy). Repeat every day for 14 days.

Using Fresh Herbs

Some herbs are particularly potent if used fresh and taken internally. The most obvious form of this is food. Our ancestors ate several hundred plants over the course of the year, most of them wildcrafted. Our bodies are used to it and in many respects a number of our diseases come from the lack of wild plants in our diets. Nearly all plants can be eaten for food and their medicinal constituents then become a part of the regular diet. I won't go into that in any depth here but do want to mention a few herbs that really are best if used fresh, primarily when juiced.

Medicinal Plant Juices

Ginger, of course, is only strongly effective if used fresh and the best way to do that is to juice the plant. (See the ginger monograph on page 227 for more.) The fresh leaf juices from bidens and *Artemisia annua* are also much more potent than using the plants in their dried form. And, of course, the fresh juice of *Echinacea purpurea* is part of standard-practice medicine in Germany. Some of the other plants that possess particularly potent medicinal juices are cabbage and plantain.

Cabbage is particularly high in S-methylmethionine (SMM) — it used to be called vitamin U. (This substance is also strongly present in malted barley.) SMM is exceptionally effective in healing and protecting the GI tract from ulceration and inflammation. It is present in its most active form, and at the highest concentrations, in fresh cabbage juice. One of the best combinations for treating irritable bowel syndrom, Crohn's disease, or ulceration in the GI tract is the juice from one piece of cabbage about the size of a carrot and six leaves of plantain. (I prefer to also add the juice of two carrots, one beet, and four stalks of celery.)

Although the juicing of fruits and vegetables has a long history, there are few people exploring the use of medicinal plant juices in any depth. It is a very open field with a lot of potential for development. Many of the plants are much stronger if their fresh juice is used.

You can juice the plants, then stabilize the juice with the addition of 20 percent alcohol by volume. That is, if you have 5 ounces of juice, you would add 1 ounce of pure grain alcohol to keep the juice from spoiling. The juice can then be dispensed much like a tincture, though in somewhat larger doses.

Essential Oils

Essential oils are made by distilling volatile oils from plants. From 0.5 percent to 5 percent of a plant's weight is composed of volatiles, or what we call essential oils. Most plants tend toward the lower end of that scale. To get an idea of how much plant it takes to make an essential oil: If a plant has 1 percent essential oil, it will take 100 ounces of the plant (a little over 6 pounds) to get 1 ounce of essential oil.

To make essential oils, distillation is necessary. In recent years a number of herbalists have begun to reclaim home distilling in order to make their own essential oils, but most of us just buy them already made.

Essential oils are used as medicine, mainly, in three ways: 1) placed directly on the skin, sometimes diluted, sometimes not; 2) inhaled (i.e., aromatherapy); and 3) in minute doses internally.

Essential oils move through the skin fairly easily. Lateral epicondylitis (a.k.a., tennis elbow) is a very painful and often debilitating inflammation of the nerve in the elbow, usually from repeated stress on the joint. Birch essential oil, rubbed on the area and about 5 inches around it, will usually reduce both the inflammation and the pain within 15 minutes. (It takes months for it to heal, but this does help immensely.)

Essential oils can be added to hot water and inhaled as steams or added to water and used as nasal sprays, for instance.

It *is* possible to take essential oils internally, but great caution should be exercised. Because so much plant matter is used to make an essential oil, these oils are incredibly potent. If you were foolish enough to take a whole ounce of essential oil by mouth — a very, very bad idea — you would be consuming 6 pounds of a medicinal plant in a form that would

Measuring Herbal Medicines

It seems nearly everyone uses a different way to describe how much to take; some say milliliters (ml), some say drops, some say dropperful, some say teaspoon or tablespoon, so here is a conversion table for you. It may help.

A drop: A drop is not always a drop (see why there's confusion?). A drop of water and a drop of alcohol are about the same, but a drop of glycerine is bigger — about five times bigger than a drop of water — because it is so viscous. Nevertheless, pretty much everyone treats a drop as a drop. Now, is that clear or what?

Dropperful: A 1-ounce glass tincture bottle has a standard glass dropper that fits in it and when the dropper is full of tincture, that is what I call a dropperful. It generally holds around 30 drops, so I consider a dropperful to be 30 drops, or 1.5 ml. Normally, a glass dropper will fill only halfway with one squeeze, so it takes two to get a full dropper.

A milliliter is, for water or alcohol, 20 drops or two-thirds of a dropper.

A teaspoon is 5 ml or 100 drops or three and one-third dropperfuls.

A tablespoon is ½ ounce, 15 ml, 3 teaspoons, 300 drops.

An ounce is in the neighborhood of 600 drops.

go into the bloodstream almost instantly. This is why essential oils are greatly diluted when put into formulations, used in diffusers, or taken internally in tiny, tiny doses (from one to five drops at a time). Generally, for internal use, I stick to things like peppermint oil, one drop at a time, for severe indigestion.

Treatment of Children

Children's bodies are much smaller than adults' and if you are using herbal medicines with them, you need to adjust the dosages. You can determine the dosages for children through one of three approaches:

Clark's Rule: Divide the weight in pounds by 150 to give an approximate fraction of an adult's dose. For a 75-pound child the dose would be 75 divided by 150, or half the adult dose. (This is the one I find most useful.)

Cowling's Rule: The age of a child at his or her next birthday divided by 24. For a child coming 8 years of age, the dose would be 8 divided by 24, or one-third the adult dose.

Young's Rule: The child's age divided by (12 + age of child). For a 3-year-old it would be 3 divided by (12 + 3; that is, 15) for a dose of one-fifth the adult dose.

Childhood Ear Infections

Most childhood ear infections can be treated successfully with herbs. Tinctures, glycerites, honeys, teas, and herbal steams are all effective approaches.

Children are most susceptible to ear infections from antibiotic-resistant strains of *Haemophilus influenzae*, *Staphylococcus aureus*, *Streptococcus pneumoniae*, and *Branhamella catarrhalis*. These kinds of treatment plans have been found highly effective for treating them, individually or together.

Children's Ear Oil

INGREDIENTS:

5 cloves garlic

4 ounces olive oil

20 drops eucalyptus essential oil

Chop garlic finely, place in small baking dish with olive oil, cook over low heat overnight, and strain, pressing cloves well. Add essential oil of eucalyptus to garlic oil and mix well. Place in amber bottle for storage. To use: Hold glass eyedropper under hot water for 1 minute, dry well (quickly), and suction up ear oil from bottle. Place 2 drops in both ears every half hour or as often as needed for 2 to 7 days.

Brigitte Mars's Herbal Tea for Ear Infections

INGREDIENTS:

1 ounce elder flower (*Sambucus* spp.)

1 ounce licorice root

1 ounce Mormon tea (*Ephedra viridis*)

1 ounce peppermint leaf

1 ounce rose hips

1 quart water

Wildflower honey (optional)

Roughly crush all herbs. Bring water to a near boil, then pour over the herbs and allow to steep until cooled enough to drink. Consume as hot as is comfortable for drinking. Sweeten with honey if desired. As much as is wanted can be consumed. The Mormon tea is a decongestant, the rose hips are slightly astringent and anti-inflammatory and high in vitamin C, the elder flowers are slightly sedative and reduce fevers, the licorice root is anti-inflammatory and tastes good and is antiviral and antibacterial, and the peppermint helps reduce fevers and decongests and is calming. Catnip can be added to help lower fever.

Ear Infection Tincture Combination

INGREDIENTS:

1 ounce echinacea tincture   1 ounce licorice tincture

1 ounce ginger tincture   1 ounce red root tincture

Mix together the tinctures. Give one full dropper (30 drops) of the mixture each hour per 150 pounds of body weight until symptoms cease. Best administered in juice. Dosage should be altered for the child's weight. Eucalyptus and sage tinctures can also be used. You can also prepare this as a glycerite or a medicinal honey.

Children's Diarrheal Diseases

Children are also susceptible to diarrheal infections from *E. coli* O157:H7 bacteria and antibiotic-resistant strains of *Shigella dysentariae*. When they get extremely ill with these bacteria, they may also experience high fever and diarrhea. The berberine plants are the best for this.

To Lower a Fever in a Child

The best herb for lowering seriously high fevers is coral root (*Corallorhiza maculata*), as either a tea or tincture. One teaspoon of the root steeped in 8 ounces hot water for 30 minutes and drunk or up to 30 drops tincture for a child of 60 pounds. Brigitte Mars's herbal tea for ear infections (page 360), with the addition of catnip, is also exceptionally effective in lowering fevers. Finally, bathing with cool water will also work very well.

Treating Diarrhea in Children

The use of a tea and tincture combination together is usually effective.

Rosemary Gladstar's Tea for Diarrhea

INGREDIENTS:

3 parts blackberry root

2 parts slippery elm bark

Mix the herbs together (for example, 3 ounces blackberry root and 2 ounces slippery elm bark). Simmer 1 teaspoon of the herb mixture in 1 cup water for 20 minutes. Strain and cool. Take 2 to 4 tablespoons every hour or as often as needed.

Tincture Combination for Diarrhea

INGREDIENTS:

1 ounce acacia tincture

1 ounce berberine plant tincture

1 ounce cryptolepis tincture

1 ounce evergreen needle tincture

Combine the tinctures, and shake well. Give 1 full dropper (30 drops) for every 150 pounds of body weight every 1 to 2 hours in water or orange juice until symptoms cease.

A Final Note

You, more than anyone else ever will, know how you are feeling in your body. Pay close attention to how you respond to any medicines you take. If you don't feel right when you take an herbal medicine, stop taking it.

9

AN HERBAL FORMULARY

All the technical information has been stolen from reliable sources and I am happy to stand behind it.

— **Edward Abbey**

When making herbal tinctures you need to know the proportion of water to alcohol — among other things. *Everyone* needs a handy list of medicinal plants and their tincture requirements. This list won't have every plant you will ever need on it, but it does have many of them.

By the way, this list was compiled from a number of sources: Michael Moore, King's Eclectic Dispensatory, several Chinese materia medicas, various lists I have received over the years, and my own work with a number of plants that either were on no lists at all or whose formulations in the literature I found to be ineffective. Michael Moore's work is the most comprehensive and valuable, and you can access it on the website for his school, the Southwest School of Botanical Medicine. **Note:** Plants are listed here by botanical name. If you're searching by common name, check the index to cross-reference.

Abies (**the firs**). Tincture, fresh needles (must include spring growth), 1:2; dried needles, 1:5, 50 percent alcohol. Dosage: 5–20 drops. Infusion: internal, 1–3 fluid ounces; external, as needed.

Acacia greggii (**catclaw acacia**). Standard infusion, pod/leaf: 2–4 fluid ounces.

Achillea (**yarrow**). Tincture, fresh plant in flower, 1:2; dried plant, 1:5, 50 percent alcohol (note: not preferred, as the volatiles are lost). Dosage: 10–30 drops up to 4x daily. Infusion: 3–6 cups daily as needed.

Acorus calamus (**calamus, sweet flag**). Tincture, fresh root, 1:2; dried root, 1:5, 60 percent alcohol. Dosage: 15–45 drops up to 4x daily.

***Actaea rubra* (baneberry, red cohosh).** Tincture, fresh root, 1:2; dried root, 1:5, 80 percent alcohol. Dosage: 10–20 drops up to 3x daily.

***Adiantum* (maidenhair fern).** Infusion, dried herb: 1–3 fluid ounces.

***Aesculus hippocastanum* (horse chestnut).** Tincture, dried bark or nut, 1:5, 50 percent alcohol. Dosage: 3–10 drops daily.

***Agave* (century plant).** Tincture, fresh leaf, 1:2; dried root, 1:5, 50 percent alcohol. Dosage: 30–60 drops up to 4x daily.

***Agrimonia* (agrimony).** Tincture, fresh leaf, 1:2; dried leaf, 1:5, 50 percent alcohol. Dosage: 1/4–1 tsp up to 4x daily.

***Agropyron repens* (couchgrass).** Tincture, dried root, 1:5, 50 percent alcohol. Dosage: 30–60 drops up to 6x daily. Cold infusion: 2–4 fluid ounces.

***Ailanthus altissima* (tree of heaven).** Tincture, dried inner bark, 1:5, 50 percent alcohol. Dosage: 1/2–1 tsp up to 6x daily for acute diarrheal conditions, 1/2–1 tsp up to 3x daily for giardia, 30–90 drops up to 3x daily for everything else. Cold infusion: 1–2 ounces up to 5x daily.

***Alchemilla* (lady's mantle).** Tincture, fresh plant, 1:2. Dosage: 30–90 drops up to 3x daily. Infusion: as needed.

***Alchornea* (alchornea).** Tincture, dried leaf or bark, 1:5, 50 percent alcohol. Dosage: 1/4 tsp every 4 hours.

***Allium sativum* (garlic).** Fresh juice of the bulb: 1/4–1 tsp. Tincture, fresh bulb, 1:2. Dosage: 15–40 drops. Caution: Fresh juice is emetic in larger doses.

***Alnus serrulata* (tag alder).** Decoction, bark (fresh or recently harvested only): internal use, 1/2–2 tbl up to 3x daily; external use (as a wash), as needed.

***Alpinia* (galangal).** Tincture, dried root, 1:5, 65 percent alcohol. Dosage: 30–90 drops as needed.

***Althaea* (marsh mallow or hollyhock).** Tincture, fresh root, 1:2; dried root (the fresher the better), 1:5, 50 percent alcohol. Dosage: as needed.

***Ambrosia* (ragweed).** Tincture, fresh or recently dried plant only, 1:2. Dosage: 20–40 drops up to 4x daily.

***Ammi visnaga* (khella, bishop's weed).** Tincture, seed, 1:5, 60 percent alcohol. Dosage: 60–120 drops up to 4x daily.

***Anemone hirsutissima* (pulsatilla ludoviciana, pulsatilla patens, anemone patens, pulsatilla hirsutissima, pasque flower, eastern pasque flower).** Tincture, fresh plant in flower, 1:2. Dosage: 10–15 drops, as needed, not more often than each hour. May cause vomiting in large doses.

***Anemone tuberosa* (desert anemone, desert pasque flower).** Same as for *A. hirsutissima*.

***Anemopsis* (yerba mansa).** Tincture, fresh root, 1:2; dried root, 1:5, 60 percent alcohol. Dosage: 20–60 drops up to 5x daily. Cold water percolation: 2–4 fluid ounces up to 5x daily — if you can stand it.

Angelica (angelica). Tincture, fresh root, 1:2; dried root, 1:5, 65 percent alcohol. Dosage: 30–60 drops up to 4x daily. Tincture, seed, 1:2. Dosage : 10–30 drops up to 4x daily.

Angelica sinensis (dong quai). Tincture, cured Asian root, 1:5, 70 percent alcohol. Dosage: 15–30 drops up to 3x daily.

Anisum (anise). Tincture, seed, 1:5, 60 percent alcohol. Dosage: 3–15 drops on the tongue as needed. Infusion: 2–4 fluid ounces as needed.

Antennaria (cat's paw, pussy toes, mountain everlasting). Standard infusion, whole plant: 3–6 fluid ounces up to 4x a day.

Anthemis nobilis (Roman chamomile). Tincture, fresh flowering herb, 1:2, 50 percent alcohol. Dosage: 30 drops in water as needed. Infusion: 2–4 fluid ounces.

Apium (celery). Tincture, fresh seed, 1:2. Dosage: 15–80 drops in water up to 3x daily. Infusion, dried seed: 1/2–1 tsp seeds in 1 cup hot water up to 4x daily.

Aralia californica (California spikenard, elk clover). Tincture, fresh root, 1:2; dried root 1:5, 50 percent alcohol. Dosage: 10–30 drops up to 3x daily.

Aralia hispida (bristly sarsaparilla). Tincture, dried root or bark, 1:5, 50 percent alcohol. Dosage: 5–25 drops up to 3x daily.

Aralia nudicaulis (sarsaparilla). Tincture, dried root, 1:5, 60 percent alcohol. Dosage: 15–30 drops up to 6x daily.

Aralia racemosa (spikenard). Tincture, fresh root, 1:2; dried root, 1:5, 50 percent alcohol. Dosage: 10–30 drops up to 3x daily.

Aralia spinosa (devil's walking stick). Tincture, dried root or bark, 1:5, 50 percent alcohol. Dosage: 5–25 drops up to 3x daily.

Arctium (burdock). Tincture, dried root, 1:5, 60 percent alcohol. Dosage: 30–90 drops up to 3x daily. Tincture, seed, 1:5, 60 percent alcohol. Dosage: 10–25 drops up to 3x daily.

Arctostaphylos (uva ursi, bearberry). Tincture, dried leaf, 1:5, 50 percent alcohol. Dosage: 30–60 drops in 8 ounces water up to 3x a day.

Argemone corymbosa (prickly poppy, Mojave prickly poppy). Tincture, fresh herb in seed, 1:2. Dosage: 5–15 drops as needed.

Argemone mexicana (prickly poppy, Mojave prickly poppy). Same as for *A. corymbosa.*

Arnica (arnica). Tincture for external use, fresh plant in flower, 1:2, 70 percent rubbing alcohol; apply as needed to affected area. Tincture for internal use, fresh plant in flower or fresh root, 1:2. Dosage: 1–5 drops up to 3x daily. Do not exceed recommended dosage.

Artemisia absinthium (wormwood). Tincture, fresh plant in flower, 1:2; dried plant, 1:5, 60 percent alcohol. Dosage: 30–90 drops up to 6x daily. Cold infusion, fresh plant in flower: 1–3 fluid ounces up to 3x daily.

Artemisia annua (**sweet Annie**).
Tincture, fresh plant in flower, 1:2.
Dosage: 30–90 drops up to 6x daily.

Artemisia tridentata (**sagebrush**).
Same as for *A. absinthium*.

Artemisia vulgaris (**mugwort,
California mugwort**). Tincture, fresh
plant, 1:2; dried plant, 1:5, 50 percent
alcohol. Dosage: 15–30 drops up to 3x
daily.

Asarum (**wild ginger**). Tincture,
fresh root, 1:2; dried root, 1:5, 60 percent alcohol. Dosage: 20–50 drops in
water up to 3x daily.

Asclepias asperula (**immortal root**).
Tincture, dried root, 1:5, 50 percent
alcohol. Dosage: 5–30 drops up to
3x daily. Best if used in combination
tinctures.

Asclepias cornuta (**common milk-
weed**). Same as for *A. asperula*.

Asclepias incarnata (**swamp milk-
weed**). Same as for *A. asperula*.

Asclepias subulata (**desert milk-
weed**). Tincture, dried root, 1:5, 50
percent alcohol. Dosage: 10–20 drops
in water up to 3x daily.

Asclepias tuberosa (**pleurisy
root**). Tincture, fresh root, 1:2; dried
root, 1:5, 50 percent alcohol. Dosage:
30–90 drops up to 3x daily.

Asparagus officinale (**asparagus**).
Tincture, fresh root, 1:2; dried root,
1:5, 50 percent alcohol. Dosage:
30–60 drops up to 3x daily.

Aspidosperma (**quebrache bark**).
Tincture, dried bark, 1:5, 50 percent
alcohol. Dosage: 15–30 drops up to 3x
daily.

Astragalus membranaceus (**astragalus**). Tincture, dried sliced root, 1:5,
60 percent alcohol. Dosage: 30–60
drops up to 4x daily. Cold water percolation: 2–3 fluid ounces up to 3x daily.

Avena (**wild oats**). Tincture, fresh
milky seed top, 1:2. Dosage: 10–30
drops up to 4x daily. Infusion, dried
plant: 4–8 fluid ounces daily.

Balsamorhiza (**balsam root**).
Tincture, fresh root, 1:2; dried root,
1:5, 65 percent alcohol. Dosage:
25–45 drops up to 4x daily. Note: Cut
the root well before grinding it as it
contains tough threads that will wrap
around your blender blades and freeze
them up.

Baptisia tinctoria (**wild indigo
root**). Tincture, dried root, 1:5, 65 percent alcohol. Dosage: 10–25 drops up
to 3x daily.

Berberis vulgaris (**common barberry**). Tincture, dried root, 1:5, 50 percent alcohol. Dosage: 10–60 drops up to
3x daily. Infusion or cold water percolation: 1–3 fluid ounces to 3x daily. More
in acute GI tract conditions.

Bidens (**same insulting names as
for *B. pilosa***). Same as for *B. pilosa*
except most species will be weaker.
B. pinnata dosage should be 50 percent
more than that of *pilosa*.

Bidens pilosa (**beggar's ticks,
Spanish needles**). Best if fresh.
Tincture, fresh herb, 1:2. Dosage:
45–90 drops in water up to 2x daily,
or in acute conditions ¼–1 tsp on up
to 1 tbl in water up to 6x daily. Fresh
juice: dosage is same as for tincture;
stabilize with 20–25 percent alcohol if
you intend on storing it.

***Brickellia grandiflora* (brickellia).** Tincture, dried herb, 1:5, 50 percent alcohol. Dosage: 30–60 drops up to 3x daily. Infusion: 2–4 fluid ounces, to 2x daily.

***Bursera microphylla* (elephant tree).** Tincture, small twigs and dried leaves (such as they are), 1:5, 70 percent alcohol. Dosage: 10–30 drops daily. Best if used in combination formulas. Tincture, gum, 1:5, 80 percent alcohol. Dosage: 5–20 drops daily.

***Calendula officinalis* (marigold).** Tincture, fresh flower, 1:2; dried flower (must be brilliant orange/yellow), 1:5, 70 percent alcohol. Dosage: 5–30 drops up to 4x daily.

***Capsella bursa-pastoris* (shepherd's purse).** Tincture, fresh whole plant, 1:2; very recently dried plant (would not recommend unless desperate), 1:5, 50 percent alcohol. Dosage: 10–30 drops up to 2x daily.

***Capsicum* (cayenne).** Tincture, dried seed pod, 1:5, 95 percent alcohol. Dosage: 5–15 drops, normally in hot tea of some sort.

***Cardamomum* (cardamom).** Tincture, seed, 1:5, 50 percent alcohol. Dosage: 5–10 drops.

***Carum* (caraway seed).** Tincture, seed, 1:5, 50 percent alcohol. Dosage: 10–20 drops in liquid of one sort or another.

***Castela emoryi* (holacantha emoryi, chaparro amargosa).** Tincture, dried plant, 1:5, 50 percent alcohol. Dosage: 20–50 drops up to 2x daily.

***Caulophyllum* (blue cohosh).** Tincture, dried root, 1:5, 60 percent alcohol. Dosage: 5–20 drops. Rarely used alone; best in combination formulas.

***Ceanothus* (red root).** Tincture, dried root, 1:5, 50 percent alcohol. Dosage: 30–90 drops up to 4x daily. Best if used in combination unless you are using it specifically for lymph problems. Cold water percolation: 2–4 fluid ounces daily.

***Centaurium* (centaury).** Tincture, fresh plant, 1:2. Dosage: 10–20 drops before meals.

***Centella asiatica* (gotu kola).** Tincture, fresh plant, 1:2. Dosage: 15–30 drops up to 3x daily. Tincture, dried plant, 1:5, 50 percent alcohol. Dosage: 20–40 drops up to 4x daily.

***Cercocarpus* (mountain mahogany).** Tincture, twigs/stems, 1:5, 50 percent alcohol. Dosage: 15–45 drops in water up to 3x daily. Decoction: 2–3 fluid ounces to 3x daily.

***Cereus grandiflorus* (night-blooming cereus).** Tincture, fresh plant, 1:2. Dosage: 5–25 drops up to 4x daily.

***Chamaecyparis lawsoniana* (Lawson's cypress).** Tincture, fresh needles/stems, 1:2, 5 percent glycerine. Tincture, recently dried needles, 1:5, 60 percent alcohol, 5 percent glycerine. Dosage: for diarrhea, 20 drops as necessary, usually not for more than 3 days; for gum infections, 5 drops in water, used to wash mouth. Not for long-term use internally. Infusion, dried needles/twigs: 2–4 fluid ounces, generally for GI tract problems.

Chamaecyparis nootkatensis **(yellow cedar).** Same as for *C. lawsoniana.*

Chamaelirium **(helonias, unicorn root).** Tincture, dried root, 1:5, 50 percent alcohol. Dosage: 10–40 drops daily. Best if used in combination formulas.

Chelidonium **(greater celandine).** Tincture, fresh plant, 1:2. Dosage: 10–25 drops. Short-term use.

Chelone **(balmony).** Tincture, fresh herb, 1:2. Dosage: 10–20 drops up to 3x daily.

Chilopsis linearis **(desert willow).** Tincture, dried bark and twigs, 1:5, 50 percent alcohol. Dosage: $1/4$–1 tsp up to 3x daily for systemic candida. Decoction or cold water percolation: 3–6 fluid ounces up to 3x daily.

Chimaphila **(pipsissewa).** Tincture, fresh herb, 1:2; dried herb, 1:5, 50 percent alcohol. Dosage: 20–50 drops up to 4x daily.

Chionanthus **(fringetree).** Tincture, fresh bark, 1:2; dried bark, 1:5, 65 percent alcohol. Dosage: 30 drops up to 2x daily. Cold water percolation, bark or leaf: 2–4 fluid ounces.

Cimicifuga racemosa **(black cohosh).** Tincture, dried root, 1:5, 80 percent alcohol. Dosage: 10–25 drops up to 3x daily.

Cinchona **(quinine bark).** Tincture, dried bark, 1:3, 45 percent alcohol. Dosage: 15–30 drops up to 3x daily; for malaria, $1/4$–1 tsp up to 3x daily, not to exceed 7 days, and repeat in 2 days. Cold water percolation: 2–3 fluid ounces up to 3x a day, not to exceed 7 days.

Cinnamomum **(cinnamon).** Tincture, dried powdered bark, 1:5, 60 percent alcohol, 5 percent glycerine. Dosage: 20–60 drops up to 4x daily.

Clematis **(virgin's bower).** Tincture, freshly dried herb, 1:5, 50 percent alcohol. Dosage: 10–40 drops up to 3x daily.

Cnicus benedictus **(blessed thistle).** Tincture, fresh herb in flower, 1:2; dried herb, 1:5, 60 percent alcohol. Dosage: 20–40 drops in hot water up to 3x daily.

Collinsonia **(stone root).** Tincture, dried root, 1:5, 60 percent alcohol. Dosage: 45–60 drops up to 4x daily. Michael Moore considers the tincture of the fresh plant to be far superior to that of the dried root. Tincture, fresh plant, 1:2, 20–40 drops up to 4x daily.

Commiphora **(myrrh).** Tincture, dried resin, 1:5, 95 percent alcohol. Dosage: 5–20 drops up to 3x daily.

Conyza canadensis **(Canadian fleabane).** Tincture, fresh flowering herb, 1:2. Dosage: 15–20 drops up to 3x daily. Infusion, dried flowering herb: 2–4 fluid ounces up to 4x daily.

Coptis **(goldthread).** Tincture, dried root, 1:5, 50 percent alcohol. Dosage: 30–60 drops up to 3x daily.

Corallorhiza **(coral root).** Tincture, fresh root, 1:2. Dosage: for acute conditions, 15–30 drops no more than each hour, as needed; as a tonic, 30–90 drops up to 3x daily. I don't think the dried root is a good choice for this herb, however — tincture, dried root, 1:5, 60 percent alcohol.

Coriandrum (**coriander**). Tincture, dried seed, 1:5, 65 percent alcohol. Dosage: 10–20 drops as needed.

Cornus sericea (**red osier dogwood**). Cold water percolation or infusion, dried root or bark: 3–6 fluid ounces up to 3x daily.

Corydalis aurea (**goldensmoke**). Tincture, dried herb, 1:5, 50 percent alcohol. Dosage: 10–15 drops up to 4x daily.

Crataegus (**hawthorn**). Tincture, dried berries, 1:5, 60 percent alcohol; fresh flowering branches, 1:2. Dosage: 10–30 drops up to 3x a day.

Crocus (**saffron**). Tincture, dried stigmas (expensive), 1:5, 95 percent alcohol. Dosage: 5–20 drops.

Cubeba (**cubeb berries**). Tincture, unripe fruit, 1:5, 80 percent alcohol. Dosage: 10–30 drops up to 3x daily. Not for long-term use.

Cupressus (**true cypress**). Tincture, fresh needles/stems, 1:2, 5 percent glycerine; recently dried needles, 1:5, 60 percent alcohol, 5 percent glycerine. Dosage: for diarrhea, 20 drops as necessary, usually not for more than 3 days; for gum infections, 5 drops in water, used to wash mouth. Not for long-term use internally. Infusion, dried needles/twigs: 2–4 fluid ounces, generally for GI tract problems.

Curcuma (**turmeric**). Tincture, dried root, 1:5, 50 percent alcohol. Dosage: 10–30 drops up to 2x daily.

Datura (**jimsonweed**). Tincture, fresh or dried leaf, 1:3, 70 percent rubbing alcohol. For external use.

Daucus carota (**wild carrot**). Tincture, dried seed, 1:5, 60 percent alcohol. Dosage: 20–60 drops up to 2x daily.

Dicentra formosa (**bleeding heart**). Tincture, fresh root, 1:2. Dosage: 10–20 drops up to 3x daily. Tincture, dried root, 1:5, 50 percent alcohol. Dosage: 15–30 drops up to 3x daily.

Dioscorea villosa (**wild yam**). Tincture, dried root: 1:5, 60 percent alcohol. Dosage: 30–100 drops up to 4x daily.

Dipsacus (**teasel**). Tincture, freshly dried autumn first-year root or spring second-year root, 1:3, 45 percent alcohol. Dosage: 1–30 drops up to 3x daily depending on whether you are a homeopathic herbalist or a regular one.

Dracontium (**symplocarpus, skunk cabbage**). Tincture, freshly dried root, 1:5, 50 percent alcohol. Dosage: 20–60 drops up to 3x daily.

Echinacea angustifolia (**purple coneflower**). Tincture, fresh flower heads in seed, 1:2; dried root, 1:5, 70 percent alcohol. Dosage: acute, 30 drops each hour; tonic, 30–100 drops up to 3x daily.

Echinacea pallida (**purple coneflower**). Same as for *E. angustifolia*.

Echinacea purpurea (**purple coneflower**). Same as for *E. angustifolia*, except I consider the plant to be much less effective, so dosage needs to be much higher, 1–2 tsp up to 5x daily.

Eleutherococcus (**eleuthero, Siberian ginseng**). Tincture, dried root, 1:5, 60 percent alcohol. Dosage: as long-term tonic, 20–60 drops daily.

Fluid extract: dried root, 1:1, 60 per-cent alcohol. Dosage: as a tonic, 10–15 drops up to 3x daily; for acute conditions with severe fatigue, ½–1 tsp 2x daily, 20 days on, 10 days off, then repeat.

Ephedra viridis (Mormon tea, American ephedra). Tincture, dried herb, 1:5, 50 percent alcohol. Dosage: 15–30 drops. Best if used in combina-tion formulas.

Ephedra vulgaris (ma huang). Tincture, dried herb, 1:5, 50 percent alcohol. Dosage: 10–15 drops. In my opinion, should only be used in com-bination formulas. Note: now illegal in the United States.

Epipactis gigantea (stream orchid). Tincture, fresh plant, 1:2; dried root, 1:5, 60 percent alcohol. Dosage: 30–90 drops. A very nice nervine.

Equisetum arvense (horsetail). Tincture, fresh spring plant, 1:2. Dosage: 15 drops to ½ tsp up to 5x daily. Infusion, dried spring or early summer herb: 2–4 fluid ounces daily.

Equisetum hyemale (scouring rush). Same as for *E. arvense.*

Eriodictyon (yerba santa). Tincture, fresh leaf, 1:2; dried, 1:5, 75 percent alcohol. Dosage: 15–30 drops up to 5x daily. I prefer this tincture in com-bination formulas. Infusion: 2–4 fluid ounces as needed.

Eschscholtzia californica (Cali-fornia poppy). Tincture, fresh flow-ering plant, 1:2. Dosage: 15–25 drops up to 3x daily.

Eucalyptus (eucalyptus). Tincture, dried leaf, 1:5, 65 percent alcohol.

Dosage: 5–15 drops in hot water up to 5x daily. Infusion: 2–4 fluid ounces up to 4x daily.

Eupatorium perfoliatum (boneset). Tincture, fresh flowering herb, 1:2. Dosage: 20–40 drops in hot water up to 3x daily. Infusion, dried herb: 6–8 fluid ounces up to 3x daily.

Eupatorium purpureum (gravel root, queen of the meadow, joe-pye weed). Tincture, fresh root, 1:2; dried root, 1:5, 60 percent alcohol. Dosage: 30–90 drops in hot water up to 3x daily. Decoction, dried root: 2–4 fluid ounces up to 4x daily.

Euphrasia (eyebright). Tincture, dried herb, 1:5, 50 percent alcohol. Dosage: 30–90 drops, orally, up to 4x daily. I prefer this tincture in combina-tion formulas. Decoction, dried herb: 2–4 fluid ounces up to 4x daily.

Filipendula (meadowsweet). Tincture, fresh flowering herb, 1:2. Dosage: 60–90 drops up to 4x daily. Tincture, dried flowering herb, 1:5, 50 percent alcohol, 90–120 drops up to 4x daily. Infusion, dried herb in flower: 3–6 fluid ounces up to 4x daily.

Foeniculum (fennel seed). Tincture, dried seed, 1:5, 60 percent alcohol. Dosage: 10–15 drops directly on the tongue or 30–60 drops in warm water as needed. Infusion: as needed.

Fouquieria splendens (ocotillo). Tincture, fresh bark, 1:2. Dosage: 10–30 drops up to 4x daily.

Fragaria (strawberry): Infusion, dried herb: as needed.

Galium aparine (**cleavers, bed-straw**). Tincture, fresh plant, 1:2. Dosage: 1–2 tsp up to 4x daily. Fresh plant juice: up to ¼ ounce daily. Or plant juice stabilized with 25 percent alcohol: same dosage as tincture. Infusion: as needed.

Ganoderma (**reishi**). Tincture, fruiting body, 1:5, 20 percent alcohol. Dosage: 10–20 ml (2–4 tsp) 3x daily. Note: Prepare a decoction of the herb in the amount of water to be used in tincturing. Add to cold water, bring to boil, cover, slow-boil for 30 minutes. Turn off heat, allow to cool. Pour into jar, add alcohol, put on lid, and let sit 2 weeks. Decant and store. You can also use a slow cooker to slow-cook it, covered, for 24–72 hours.

Garrya (**silk tassel**). Tincture, fresh leaf, 1:2; dried leaf, 1:5, 50 percent alcohol. Dosage: 45–60 drops up to 5x daily. Tincture, root bark, 1:5, 50 percent alcohol. Dosage: 10–20 drops up to 5x daily.

Gentiana (**gentian**). Tincture, dried root, 1:5, 50 percent alcohol. Dosage: 5–20 drops before meals, if you can take it.

Geranium (**cranesbill**). Tincture, dried root, 1:5, 50 percent alcohol, 10 percent glycerin. Dosage: 30 drops–1 tsp up to 4x daily. Decoction: 1–4 fluid ounces up to 4x daily.

Glycyrrhiza glabra (**licorice**). Tincture, dried root, 1:5, 50 percent alcohol. Dosage: 10 drops up to 3x daily. Best if used in formula combinations. I do not recommend this herb singly.

Glycyrrhiza lepidota (**American licorice**): Same as for *G. glabra.*

Gossypium (**cotton**). Tincture, fresh root bark, 1:2. Dosage: 30–60 drops up to 3x daily. Tincture, freshly dried root bark, 1:5, 50 percent alcohol. Dosage: 1–2 tsp up to 4x daily. Try to avoid commercial cotton; it's highly chemicalized.

Grindelia (**gumweed**). Tincture, fresh flowering top, 1:2; freshly dried flowering herb, 1:5, 70 percent alcohol. Dosage: 15–40 drops up to 5x daily.

Guaiacum officinale (**lignum vitae**). Tincture, dried bark or wood, 1:5, 95 percent alcohol. Dosage: 5–15 drops in water, frequently.

Hamamelis (**witch hazel**). Tincture, fresh twigs and leaves, 1:2. Dosage: 10–60 drops as needed.

Harpagophytum procumbens (**devil's claw**). Tincture, dried root, 1:2, 60 percent alcohol. Dosage: up to 1 tsp 2x daily. Cold water percolation: 4–6 fluid ounces daily.

Heracleum (**cow parsnip**). Tincture, fresh seed, 1:2. Dosage: 5–10 drops as needed for hiatus hernia. Tincture: fresh root, 1:2. Dosage: 5–10 drops as needed as oral antimicrobial for gums.

Heterotheca (**camphor weed**). Tincture for external use, fresh flowering herb, 1:2, 70 percent rubbing alcohol; recently dried, 1:5, 70 percent rubbing alcohol. Topically as liniment. Powdered dried root as antifungal for athlete's foot.

Humulus (**hops**). Tincture, fresh strobiles (i.e., flowery things on the vine), 1:2; dried strobiles, 1:5, 65 percent alcohol. Dosage: 30–90 drops up to 3x daily.

Hydrangea arborescens (seven barks). Tincture, fresh root, 1:2; dried root, 1:5, 50 percent alcohol. Dosage: ½–1 tsp in water up to 4x daily.

Hydrastis (goldenseal). Tincture, dried root, 1:5, 70 percent alcohol. Dosage: 20–50 drops up to 4x daily. Would highly recommend berberine alternatives.

Hyoscyamus niger (henbane). Tincture, fresh flowering top, 1:2. Dosage: 3–10 drops up to 3x daily. Caution is advised.

Hypericum (St. John's wort). Tincture: fresh flowering top, 1:2. Dosage: 20–30 drops up to 3x daily. Dried plant is useless.

Illicium (star anise). Tincture, dried seed, 1:5, 50 percent alcohol. Dosage: 5–10 drops as needed.

Impatiens (jewelweed). Juice of fresh plant, stabilized with 20 percent alcohol. Topical use for poison ivy and other itchy rashes as needed. (Fresh plant tincture not quite as good.)

Inula (elecampane). Tincture, fresh root, 1:2; dried root, 1:5, 60 percent alcohol. Dosage: 10–30 drops up to 4x daily.

Iris missouriensis (blue flag). Tincture, dried root only, 1:5, 80 percent alcohol. Dosage: 5–20 drops up to 3x daily. Not for long-term use.

Iris versicolor (blue flag). Same as for *I. missouriensis*.

Isatis (woad). Tincture, dried leaf or root, 1:5, 25 percent alcohol. Both leaves and root should be heated in the water to be used for the tincture, to a boil, and left to steep until cool; then add alcohol. Dosage: as a tonic, 30 drops up to 6x day; for acute conditions, 1 tsp up to 10 times day. Decoction, root: 10–30 grams (⅓–1 ounce) of the root boiled for 30 minutes. Dosage: 1 cup 3x daily for a max of 3 weeks. Decoction, leaf: 9–15 grams of the leaf as a tonic, 60–120 grams in acute conditions, boiled for 30 minutes. Dosage: 1 cup 3x daily.

Juglans major (black walnut). Tincture: fresh leaf, 1:2; dried leaf, 1:5, 50 percent alcohol. Dosage: 30–90 drops up to 3x daily. Tincture, dried hull, 1:5, 50 percent alcohol. Dosage: 20–50 drops up to 4x daily.

Juniperus (juniper). Tincture, dryish berries, 1:5, 75 percent alcohol. Dosage: 10–20 drops up to 3x daily. Tincture, fresh needles, 1:2. Dosage: 30–50 drops up to 4x daily.

Krameria (rhatany). Tincture, dried root, 1:5, 50 percent alcohol, 10 percent glycerin (or not; I haven't noticed a problem without glycerin). Dosage: 20–50 drops up to 3x daily. World-class astringent.

Lactuca (wild lettuce). Tincture, fresh herb in seed, 1:2. Dosage: ½–1 tsp up to 3x daily.

Larrea (chaparral). Tincture, leaves and small twigs, 1:5, 75 percent alcohol. Dosage: 20–60 drops up to 3x daily.

Leonurus cardiaca (motherwort). Tincture, fresh flowering herb, 1:2. (Would not suggest using the dried plant at all.) Dosage: 30–60 drops up to 4x daily. Up to ¼ fluid ounce at a time, in water. Exceptional if combined with *Pedicularis*, equal parts.

Leptandra **(Culver's root).** Tincture, dried root, 1:5, 65 percent alcohol. Dosage: 10–30 drops up to 3x daily. I prefer this herb in combination formulas. Nice herb but very strong.

Ligusticum porteri **(osha).** Tincture, dried root, 1:5, 70 percent alcohol. Dosage: 20–60 drops up to 5x daily. Very intense.

Lobelia inflata **(lobelia).** Tincture, fresh flowering plant, 1:4, pure grain alcohol. Dosage: 5–20 drops up to 4x daily. Skip the dried plant; it's relatively useless. Tincture, fresh seed, 1:5, 65 percent alcohol. Dosage: 3–10 drops.

Lomatium dissectum **(lomatium).** Tincture, fresh root, 1:2; tincture, dried root, 1:5, 70 percent alcohol. Dosage: 10–30 drops up to 4x daily.

Lycium pallidum **(wolfberry).** Tincture, fresh herb, 1:2. Dosage: 15–40 drops up to 4x daily.

Lycopus **(bugleweed, water horehound).** Tincture, fresh herb, 1:2. Dosage: 15–40 drops up to 3x daily.

Lysichiton americanum **(western skunk cabbage), my favorite.** Tincture, freshly dried root, 1:5, 50 percent alcohol. Dosage: 20–60 drops up to 3x daily.

Mahonia **(Oregon grape).** Tincture, dried root, 1:5, 50 percent alcohol. Dosage: 10–60 drops up to 3x daily. Infusion or cold water percolation: 1–3 fluid ounces up to 3x daily. More in acute GI tract conditions.

Malva neglecta **(mallow).** Infusion: 2–6 fluid ounces as needed. Highly useful as part of decoction mix for cough syrups.

Marrubium **(horehound).** Tincture, fresh flowering herb, 1:2; dried plant, 1:5, 50 percent alcohol. Dosage: 30–90 drops up to 4x daily. (Yuck, talk about bitter.) Exceptionally useful as part of a combination decoction for cough syrups.

Matricaria **(chamomile).** Tincture, fresh flower, 1:2; dried flower, 1:5, 45 percent alcohol. Dosage: 100–150 drops up to 3x daily.

Matricaria matricarioides, **a.k.a.** *discoidea* **(pineapple weed).** Same as for *Matricaria*.

Medicago sativa **(alfalfa).** Infusion, dried flowering plant: usually in the morning, or as needed. Exceptionally good blended with red clover and wild oat straw, equal parts.

Melissa officinalis **(lemon balm).** Tincture, fresh flowering herb, 1:2; recently dried flowering herb, 1:5, 50 percent alcohol. Dosage: $1/2$–1 tsp in warm water up to 4x daily. Tincture for external use: 1:3, 25 percent alcohol, 30 percent glycerine, 45 percent water; use topically for itching skin blisters/shingles.

Mentha arvensis **(poleo mint).** Tincture, fresh herb (in flower if possible just for the added mass), 1:2. Dosage: 1 drop on up.

Mentha piperita **(peppermint).** Same as for *M. arvensis*.

Mentha spicata **(spearmint, yerba buena).** Same as for *M. arvensis*.

Menyanthes **(buckbean, bogbean).** Tincture, whole fresh plant, 1:2; dried plant, 1:5, 50 percent alcohol. Dosage: 10–30 drops up to 3x daily.

***Mitchella repens* (squaw vine).**
Tincture, fresh plant, 1:2; dried plant,
1:5, 50 percent alcohol. Dosage: 1/2–
1 tsp up to 3x daily.

***Myrica* (bayberry).** Tincture, fresh
root bark, 1:2; dried root bark, 1:5, 60
percent alcohol. Dosage: 20–60 drops
up to 3x daily; in acute conditions 1/2–
1 tsp up to 4x daily. Cold water percolation: 2–4 fluid ounces up to 3x daily;
in acute conditions up to 6x daily.

***Nepeta cataria* (catnip).** Tincture,
fresh flowering herb, 1:2; recently
dried herb if you must, 1:5, 50 percent
alcohol. Dosage: 1/2–1 tsp up to 4x daily.

***Nuphar* (yellow pond lily).** Tincture,
fresh root, 1:2. Dosage: 10–20 drops up
to 3x daily.

***Oenothera* (evening primrose).**
Tincture, fresh flowering herb stalk,
1:2. Dosage: 30 drops up to 1 tsp as
needed. Tincture, seed, 1:5, 60 percent
alcohol, 10 percent glycerine. Dosage:
3–10 drops up to 6x daily.

***Olea europaea* (olive).** Tincture,
fresh leaf, 1:2; dried leaf, 1:5, 60 percent
alcohol. Dosage: 20–40 drops up to
3x daily.

***Oplopanax horridus* (devil's club).**
Tincture, dried root bark, 1:5, 60 percent alcohol. Dosage: 10–40 drops up
to 3x daily.

***Opuntia* (prickly pear).** Fresh pad
juice, stabilized with 25 percent
alcohol: 1–3 fluid ounces up to 2x daily.

***Osmorhiza occidentalis* (western
sweet cicely).** Tincture, dried root,
1:5, 65 percent alcohol. Dosage: 45–
60 drops up to 3x daily.

***Paeonia* (peony).** Tincture, dried
root, 1:5, 60 percent alcohol. Dosage:
10–25 drops up to 4x daily.

***Panax ginseng* (Asian ginseng).**
Tincture, cured (red) root, 1:5, 70 percent alcohol. Dosage: 5–30 drops up
to 3x daily. Tincture, uncured (white)
root, 1:5, 70 percent alcohol. Dosage:
20–40 drops.

***Panax quinquefolium* (American
ginseng).** Tincture, all forms of dried
roots, 1:5, 70 percent alcohol. Woods-
grown dosage: 10–20 drops 3x daily.
Field-cultivated dosage: 20–40 drops
3x daily.

***Parietaria* (pellitory-of-the-wall).**
Tincture, flowering herb, 1:5, 50 percent alcohol. Dosage: 60–90 drops up
to 5x daily.

***Passiflora* (passionflower).** Tinc-
ture, fresh flowering herb (if you can
get it in flower; otherwise, just the
whole herb), 1:2; dried, 1:5, 50 percent
alcohol. Dosage: 1/2–1 1/2 tsp up to
4x daily.

***Paullinia cupana* (guarana).** Take
this one as a powder of the seed, 1 tsp
in a little water. Makes the mind *clear*
and the self energetic. Very unlike
caffeine. Tincture the dried seed if you
want, 1:5, 65 percent alcohol. Dosage:
1/4–1 tsp.

***Pausinystalia* (yohimbe).** Tincture,
dried bark, 1:5, 65 percent alcohol.
Dosage: 5–30 drops. Careful with
this one.

***Pedicularis* and *P. groenlandica*
in particular (lousewort, elephant
head).** Same as for *P. bracteosa*
below. A lot of people use the species

interchangeably, but *groenlandica* and fernleaf lousewort (*P. bracteosa*) are the only two I have tried, and I think *groenlandica* tastes dreadful. Michael Moore notes the pediculari are semi-parasitic and pick up stuff from their hosts. I generally harvest the fernleaf lousewort that grows among aspen groves and haven't noticed a problem. Moore suggests that you avoid species growing in close proximity to *Senecio* species or toxic legumes. I think the dried herb is useless.

Pediculari bracteosa (betony, fernleaf lousewort). Tincture, fresh plant, 1:2. Dosage: 30 drops up to $\frac{1}{2}$ fluid ounce in water as needed. My favorite of the pediculari. Very nice as a general muscle relaxant, especially if combined in equal parts with motherwort tincture.

Petasites (western coltsfoot). Tincture, fresh herb, 1:2. Dosage: 30–60 drops up to 3x daily.

Petroselinum (parsley). Tincture, dried root, 1:5, 60 percent alcohol. Dosage: 30–60 drops up to 3x daily; I'd mix the tincture in water with this one.

Phytolacca (poke). Tincture, dried root, 1:5, 50 percent alcohol. Dosage: 5–15 drops up to 3x daily. Not nearly as unsafe as portrayed; nevertheless, use with awareness and be careful with that dose.

Picraena (quassia). Tincture, dried bark, 1:5, 50 percent alcohol. Dosage: 30–60 drops up to 3x daily.

Pilocarpus (jaborandi). Tincture, dried leaf, 1:5, 60 percent alcohol. Dosage: 15–30 drops in warm water.

Pinus (pine). Tincture, needles, 1:5, 60 percent alcohol. Dosage: 10–30 drops up to 3x daily. Powdered: topically as needed.

Pinus pollen (pollen pini). Tincture, 1:5, 60 percent alcohol. Dosage: as a tonic, 10 drops up to 3x daily; as a treatment for specific conditions, 30 drops 3x daily. Not for men under 45 without a specific medical condition. Not generally for women except in certain medical conditions. Not for muscle builders. Contains high amounts of testosterone. Large doses ($\frac{1}{2}$ fluid ounce a day or more) will shrink testes and reduce normal testosterone production.

Piper methysticum (kava kava). Tincture, dried root, 1:5, 60 percent alcohol. Dosage: 30–90 drops up to 4x daily. The fresher the root, the better.

Piper nigrum (black pepper). Tincture, dried fruit (i.e., peppercorns), 1:5, 65 percent alcohol. Dosage: 5–15 drops.

Plantago major (plantain). Fresh leaf juice, really the only good way to use this plant: 1–2 tbl up to 4x daily. Can be frozen or stabilized with 20–25 percent alcohol. Specific for Crohn's, IBS, intestinal ulceration. Topical poultice of the fresh leaf for splinters, basically, embedded things in the skin. Magic.

Polygonatum (Solomon's seal). Tincture, fresh root, 1:2. Dosage: 10–30 drops up to 3x daily.

Polygonum bistorta (bistort root). Tincture, dried root, 1:5, 50 percent alcohol, 10 percent glycerin. Dosage: 30–90 drops up to 3x daily.

Polypodium glycyrrhiza (**licorice fern**). Tincture, dried root, 1:5, 50 percent alcohol. Dosage: 10–30 drops up to 3x daily.

Populus balsamifera (**balsam poplar**). Tincture, fresh early-spring leaf buds, 1:2; very recently dried early-spring leaf buds, 1:5, 75 percent alcohol. Dosage: 15–30 drops up to 3x daily. You can also infuse the early-spring leaf buds in oil for topical use. Yum.

Populus tremuloides (**quaking aspen**). Tincture, freshly dried bark, 1:5, 50 percent alcohol. Dosage: 10–30 drops up to 3x daily.

Prinos (**black alder**). Tincture, freshly dried bark, 1:5, 65 percent alcohol. Dosage: 10–30 drops up to 2x daily.

Propolis (from the hive). Tincture, 1:5, 95 percent alcohol. Dosage: 5–15 drops in a little honey or straight if you can take it. Doesn't mix well with others.

Prunella (**self-heal, heal-all**). Tincture, fresh plant, 1:2. Dosage: as needed. A highly underrated plant.

Prunus (**choke cherry**). Tincture, late summer or fall bark, 1:5, 60 percent alcohol, 10 percent glycerin. Dosage: 30–90 drops up to 4x daily. I prefer the small, high-mountain varieties, especially in syrups. They really are better. The berries should be dried and added to the syrup decoction as it is cooking.

Prunus persica (**peach tree**). Tincture, recently dried leaf, 1:5, 50 percent alcohol. Dosage: 10–60 drops up to 3x daily.

Ptelea (**wafer ash, hop tree**). Tincture, bark, seed, or leaf, 1:5, 65 percent alcohol. Dosage: 10–30 drops up to 3x daily.

Ptychopetalum (**muira puama, potency wood**). Tincture, dried bark, 1:5, 70 percent alcohol. Dosage: 30–60 drops. Careful, this one does have an effect on the male organs of reproduction.

Pulmonaria (**lungwort**). Tincture, fresh flowering herb, 1:2. Dosage: 30–90 drops as needed.

Pygeum africanum (**African prune**). Tincture, dried bark, 1:5, 50 percent alcohol. Dosage: 40–80 drops up to 3x daily.

Pyrola (**false wintergreen**). Tincture, 1:5, 60 percent alcohol. Dosage: 20–40 drops up to 3x daily.

Quercus (**oak**). Tincture, dried root, 1:5, 50 percent alcohol, 10 percent glycerin. Dosage: 30 drops to 1 tsp up to 4x daily. Decoction: 1–4 fluid ounces up to 4x daily.

Rhamnus californica (**California buckthorn, coffeeberry**). Tincture, well-dried bark, 1:5, 50 percent alcohol. Dosage: 1–2 tsp.

Rheum officinale (**rhubarb**). Tincture, dried root, 1:5, 50 percent alcohol, 10 percent glycerin. Dosage: 15–30 drops up to 4x daily. Note: Vitamin C powder is a much better solution for constipation.

Rhodiola rosea, R. integrifolia (**rhodiola, golden root, rose root**). Tincture, dried root, 1:5, 50 percent alcohol (some people use a 1:3). Dosage: as a tonic, 30–40 drops 3–4x daily; in acute conditions, $\frac{1}{2}$–1 tsp 3x daily for 20–30 days, then back to the tonic dose. The tincture is usually taken in water — the plant is extremely astringent.

Rhus aromatica (sweet sumac). Tincture, dried root bark, 1:5, 50 percent alcohol, 10 percent glycerin. Dosage: 20–40 drops up to 4x daily.

Rhus glabra (smooth sumac). Tincture, dried leaf or fruit, 1:5, 50 percent alcohol, 10 percent glycerin. Dosage: 20–40 drops up to 4x daily.

Rosmarinus (rosemary). Tincture, dryish leaf, 1:5, 60 percent alcohol. Dosage: 30–60 drops up to 3x daily.

Rubus idaeus (raspberry). Infusion, dried leaf: as often as needed. Excellent for diarrhea.

Rubus villosus (blackberry). Infusion or decoction, dried root bark: 2–4 fluid ounces. Really excellent for diarrhea. If it just won't quit, use this. I don't know why more people don't.

Rumex crispus (yellow dock). Tincture, dried root, 1:5, 50 percent alcohol. Dosage: 30–75 drops up to 3x daily.

Rumex hymenosepalus (canaigre, red dock). Decoction, dried root. Dosage: not a lot. World-class astringent; it will suck the moisture out of your body starting at your toes and then go all the way up. Great topically as either powder or cooled decoction for any kind of seeping wounds. Tincture, dried root, 1:5, 50 percent alcohol, 10 percent glycerin. Great in gum toner combinations.

Ruscus aculeatus (butcher's broom). Tincture, fresh root, 1:2. Dosage: 30–60 drops up to 3x daily.

Salix (willow). Decoction, dried bark: 2–4 fluid ounces to 4x daily. Evaporative concentrate for topical use.

Salvia (sage). Tincture, fresh herb (in flower), 1:2; dried herb, 1:5, 50 percent alcohol. Dosage: 30–60 drops as needed. Decoctions and infusions are also useful.

Sambucus (elder). Tincture, fresh flower, 1:2. Dosage: 30–90 drops up to 3x daily. Tincture, fresh leaf, 1:2. Dosage: 10 drops, not more than once per hour (good nervine). Tincture, dried berry, 1:5, 50 percent alcohol. Dosage: 20–40 drops up to 3x daily. If nausea occurs back off on the dose.

Scoparius (broom). Tincture, dried flowering top, 1:5, 50 percent alcohol. Dosage: 20–40 drops up to 4x daily.

Scrophularia (figwort). Tincture, fresh herb, 1:2. Dosage: 30–60 drops up to 3x daily.

Scutellaria (skullcap). Tincture, fresh plant, 1:2. Dosage: 20–60 drops or more to 3x daily. Some people are highly responsive to it, others — nothing. Would skip the dried herb unless very recently harvested; fairly useless otherwise: 1:5, 50 percent alcohol.

Serenoa (saw palmetto). Tincture, dried berry, 1:5, 80 percent alcohol. Dosage: 30–90 drops up to 3x daily. Yuck. Fetid soap.

Sida (sida). Tincture, fresh leaf, 1:2; dried leaf, 1:5, 60 percent alcohol. Dosage: 20–40 drops up to 4x day; in acute conditions, $\frac{1}{2}$ tsp–1 tbl, 3–6x daily, generally for less than 60 days.

***Silybum marianum* (milk thistle).**
Tincture, dried seed, 1:3, 70 percent
alcohol. Dosage: 30–60 drops up to 5x
daily minimum; or 1–2 tsp 3x daily in
liver disease. For liver disease, though,
the standardized capsules are much
better, 1,200 mg daily. In tonic liver
mixes, the powdered seeds are good in
larger doses.

***Smilacina racemosa* (false Solo-
mon's seal).** Tincture, fresh root, 1:2.
Dosage: 10–20 drops up to 3x daily.
The dried root is very good in syrups.

***Smilax* (sarsaparilla).** Tincture,
fresh root, 1:2; dried root, 1:5, 60 percent alcohol. Dosage: 30–90 drops up
to 3x daily.

***Solanum dulcamara* (bittersweet).**
Tincture, fresh stem, 1:2; dried stem,
1:5, 60 percent alcohol. Dosage: 10–
20 drops 1–2x daily. The plant is a lot
milder than its reputation.

***Solidago* (goldenrod).** Tincture,
fresh plant in flower, 1:2. Dosage:
20–60 drops up to 3x daily.

***Stachys officinalis* (European
betony).** Tincture, fresh flowering
herb, 1:2; dried herb, 1:5, 50 percent
alcohol. Dosage: 3 drops to 1 tsp up to
4x daily.

***Sticta* (lobaria pulmonaria,
lungwort moss).** Tincture, lichen,
1:5, 60 percent alcohol. Dosage:
20–30 drops up to 4x daily.

***Stillingia sylvatica* (queen's root).**
Tincture, fresh root, 1:2; recently dried
root, 1:5, 50 percent alcohol. Dosage:
10–30 drops daily.

***Swertia radiata,* a.k.a. *Frasera
speciosa* (green gentian, cebadilla).**
Powdered root, recently dried: mix
with petroleum jelly and place on skin
cancers, cover with bandage, leave
72 hours, remove.

***Symphytum* (comfrey).** Tincture,
dried root: 1:5, 50 percent alcohol.
Dosage: 30–60 drops up to 3x daily
for up to 30 days. Root powder for
ulceration in GI tract: 1 tsp 3x daily for
30 days.

***Tabebuia* (pau d'arco).** Tincture,
dried bark, 1:5, 50 percent alcohol.
Dosage: ½–1 tsp up to 4x daily.

***Tanacetum* (feverfew).** Tincture,
fresh plant, 1:2; dried plant, 1:5, 50 percent alcohol. Dosage: 30–60 drops up
to 4x daily. Cold infusion, fresh plant
in flower: 2–4 fluid ounces.

***Taraxacum* (dandelion).** Tincture,
fresh root, 1:2; fresh leaf, 1:2. Dosage:
½–1 tsp up to 4x daily. Don't take the
leaf before bed; it's a strong diuretic.

***Thuja* (arborvitæ, red or yellow
cedar).** Tincture, fresh herb, needle,
or leaf, 1:2. Dosage: 5–15 drops in water
up to 4x daily.

***Thymus* (thyme).** Tincture, fresh
herb, 1:2; dried herb, 1:5, 45 percent
alcohol. Dosage: 20–40 drops up to
3x daily.

***Tribulus* (puncture vine).** Tincture,
dried seed (and herb if you must), 1:5,
60 percent alcohol. Dosage: 30–40
drops up to 2x daily.

***Trifolium pratense* (red clover).**
Infusion or decoction, flowering herb:
4–6 fluid ounces daily.

***Trillium* (beth root).** Tincture, fresh plant, 1:2. Dosage: 15–25 drops up to 3x daily.

***Turnera diffusa* (damiana).** Tincture, fresh flowering herb, 1:2. Dosage: 20–30 drops up to 3x daily (yum). The dried plant isn't really worth it, but it would be 1:5, 60 percent alcohol. Fresh plant is the way to go.

***Ulmus pumila* (Siberian elm).** Cold infusion, powdered or shredded bark. Dosage: as needed for GI tract problems, debility. Note: *Ulmus fulva*, slippery elm, is endangered. Siberian elm is the primary elm that is an exact substitute for slippery elm. It is an invasive and should be used with abandon. It is really good, plus the fresh seeds are highly edible and tasty, especially if lightly cooked in butter. The dried seeds make a great flour.

***Umbellularia* (California bay, Oregon myrtle).** Tincture, fresh leaf, 1:2; recently dried leaf, 1:5, 65 percent alcohol. Dosage: 10–20 drops up to 3x daily.

***Uncaria tomentosa* (cat's claw).** Tincture, dried root bark or vine inner bark, 1:5, 60 percent alcohol. Dosage: 40–60 drops up to 3x daily.

***Urtica* (nettles).** Infusion, whole herb: as needed.

***Usnea* (old man's beard).** Tincture, dried herb, 1:5, 50 percent alcohol. Dosage: 30–60 drops up to 4x a day. Herb should be well ground, moistened with a little alcohol, then added to the proper amount of water to be used in the tincturing process, brought to a boil, slow-boiled, covered, for 30 minutes, then allowed to cool, still covered. Then the alcohol should be added, the whole mess put in a jar and allowed to macerate for 2 weeks, decanted, and bottled. A slow cooker can also be used instead of the boiling; let cook on the low setting for a couple of days.

***Valeriana* (valerian).** Tincture, dried root, 1:5, 70 percent alcohol. Dosage: 30–90 drops up to 3x daily. Old sock special.

***Verbascum* (mullein).** Tincture, fresh flowering head stalk, 1:2. Dosage: 20–40 drops up to 4x daily.

***Verbena* (blue vervain).** Tincture, fresh flowering herb, 1:2; dried flowering herb, 1:5, 60 percent alcohol. Dosage: 30–90 drops up to 4x daily.

***Viburnum* (cramp bark, black haw).** Tincture, root bark, and bark, 1:5, 50 percent alcohol. Dosage: 30–90 drops up to 4x daily.

***Vinca major* (periwinkle).** Tincture, fresh herb, 1:2; dried herb, 1:5, 50 percent alcohol. Dosage: 20–40 drops up to 2x daily.

***Vinca minor* (periwinkle).** Same as for *V. major*.

***Viola odorata* (violet).** Tincture, fresh plant in flower, 1:2. Dosage: 1–2 tsp up to 2x daily.

***Vitex agnus-castus* (chaste tree).** Tincture, dried berry, 1:5, 65 percent alcohol. Dosage: 30–60 drops in the morning. Michael Moore suggests using the tincture or the tea in the 2-week period before menses as it strengthens the progesterone phase of the cycle.

Withania somnifera **(ashwa-gandha).** Tincture, dried root, 1:5, 70 percent alcohol. Dosage: 30–40 drops up to 3x daily. Tincture, fresh leaf, 1:2. Dosage: 10–30 drops up to 3x daily. Tincture, dried seed, 1:5, 65 percent alcohol. Dosage: 15–30 drops up to 3x daily. Tincture, fresh fruit, 1:2 (grind the whole mess well). Dosage: 15–30 drops up to 3x daily.

Xanthoxylum **(prickly ash).** Tincture, bark/berry, 1:5, 65 percent alcohol. Dosage: 10–30 drops up to 3x daily.

Zea mays **(corn silk).** Tincture, fresh silk, 1:2. Dosage: $1/2$–$1^1/2$ tsp in water. Excellent in UTI combinations.

Zingiber **(ginger).** Fresh juice of the root, stabilized with 20–25 percent pure grain alcohol. Add $1/4$ cup fresh juice of gingerroot to 8 ounces hot water, and add 1 tbl wildflower honey, $1/8$ tsp cayenne, and a squeeze of $1/4$ lime (then drop the peel in). Drink up to 6 cups daily. Fresh root tincture, 1:2. Dosage: 10–60 drops in warm to hot water up to 6x daily.

EPILOGUE

Underestimating the evolutionary potential of living organisms is the single most important mistake made by those who use chemical means to subdue nature. . . . Such vehement antipathy toward any corner of the living world should have given us pause. Through our related mistakes in the world of higher animals, we should have gained the evolutionary wisdom to predict the outcome.

— Marc Lappé, PhD

One of the most important lessons from our ancient legends and myths is that the gods take a dim view of human arrogance.

Ancient versions of this message are to be found in the story of Arachne, a mortal weaver who boasted that she could weave better than Minerva, the goddess of wisdom and crafts. After losing the contest, she was turned into a spider for her presumption.

Another is the legend of Achilles, whose mother dipped him into water that made him invulnerable — except of course for the heel by which she held him. To this day an "Achilles' heel" serves to remind us of the foolishness of thinking ourselves invulnerable.

An even more recent warning to us is Mary Shelley's book *Frankenstein*. The message in her book is the same as that of the ancient legends and myths; in this instance, it specifically addresses the arrogance of medical science in thinking it can take upon itself the capacities of the gods.

In spite of all the accomplishments of our technological civilization, these ancient warnings are still relevant to our species. As Václav Havel once so eloquently put it, there are powers in the universe against which it is advisable not to blaspheme. Perhaps it is fitting that the lowly bacteria will be the ones to teach us humility.

Chymia egregia ancilla medicinae; non alia pejor domina.
(Chemistry makes an excellent handmaid but the worst possible mistress.)

ENDNOTES

Prologue

1. Sarah White, "The Empowered Patient," *Medhill Reports*, December 8, 2010.
2. Denis Campbell and Anushka Asthana, "The 'Catalogue of Errors' That Cost This Father His Life," *The Guardian*, November 27, 2010.
3. "'The NHS Failed My Mum,' Says Distraught Daughter," *Grantham Journal*, December 14, 2010.

Chapter 1 — The End of Antibiotics

1. W. J. Powell, "Molecular Mechanisms of Antimicrobial Resistance," technical report #14, Feb. 2000. Online at http://foodsafety.ksu.edu/articles/280/molecular_mechanisms_antimic_resist.pdf, page 2.
2. Stuart Levy, *The Antibiotic Paradox* (NY: Plenum Press, 1992), 94.
3. Ibid., 75.
4. Ibid., 3.
5. Ibid.
6. Quoted in Barbara Griggs, *Green Pharmacy* (Rochester, VT: Healing Arts Press, 1991), 261.
7. Brad Spellberg, *Rising Plague* (NY: Prometheus, 2009), 36–37.
8. R. L. Berkelman and J. M . Hughes, "The Conquest of Infectious Diseases: Who Are We Kidding?" *Annals of Internal Medicine* 119, no. 5 (1993): 426–27.
9. Marc Lappé, *When Antibiotics Fail* (Berkeley, CA: North Atlantic Books, 1995), 187.
10. Steven Projan, "Antibacteria Drug Discovery in the 21st Century," in Richard Wax et al., *Bacterial Resistance to Antimicrobials,* second edition (Boca Raton, FL: CRC Press, 2008), 413.
11. David Hooper, "Target Modification as a Mechanism of Antimicrobial Resistance," in Richard Wax et al., *Bacterial Resistance to Antimicrobials,* second edition (Boca Raton, FL: CRC Press, 2008), 134.
12. Harry Taber, "Antibiotic Permeability," in Richard Wax et al., *Bacterial Resistance to Antimicrobials,* second edition (Boca Raton, FL: CRC Press, 2008), 172.
13. Rob Stein, "New 'Superbugs' Raising Concerns Worldwide," *Washington Post*, October 11, 2010.
14. Olga Lomovskaya et al., "Multidrug Efflux Pumps: Structure, Mechanism, and Inhibition," in Richard Wax et al., *Bacterial Resistance to Antimicrobials,* second edition (Boca Raton, FL: CRC Press, 2008), 46.
15. C. Werry, "Contamination of Detergent Cleaning Solutions during Hospital Cleaning," *Journal of Hospital Infection* 11, no. 1 (1988): 44–49.
16. W. J. Powell, "Molecular Mechanisms of Antimicrobial Resistance," technical report #14, Feb. 2000. Online at http://foodsafety.ksu.edu/articles/280/molecular_mechanisms_antimic_resist.pdf.
17. Abigail Salyers et al., "Ecology of Antibiotic Resistant Genes," in Richard Wax et al., *Bacterial Resistance to Antimicrobials,* second edition (Boca Raton, FL: CRC Press, 2008), 11.
18. Stuart Levy, *The Antibiotic Paradox* (NY: Plenum Press, 1992), 101.
19. Ibid., 87.
20. Quoted in Philip Frappaolo, "Risks to Human Health from the Use of Antibiotics in Animal Feeds," in William Moats (ed.), *Agricultural Uses of Antibiotics* (American Chemical Society, 1986), 102.
21. Quoted in W. J. Powell, "Molecular Mechanisms of Antimicrobial Resistance," technical report #14, Feb. 2000. Online at http://foodsafety.ksu.edu/articles/280/molecular_mechanisms_antimic_resist.pdf.

22. W. J. Powell, "Molecular Mechanisms of Antimicrobial Resistance," technical report #14, Feb. 2000. Online at http://foodsafety.ksu.edu/articles/280/molecular_mechanisms_antimic_resist.pdf.

23. "Staph Bacteria: Blood-Sucking Superbug Prefers the Taste of Humans," *Science Daily*, December 22, 2010.

24. Infectious Diseases Society of America, "Facts about Antibiotic Resistance," April 2011, http://www.idsociety.org/AR_Facts/.

25. Quoted in Philip Hilts, "Gene Jumps to Spread a Toxin in Meat," *New York Times*, April 23, 1996.

26. Maggie Fox, "Modern Life Comes with Disease Price Tag," Reuters, AOL Online, September 20, 2000.

27. Brandon Keim, "Antibiotics Breed Superbugs Faster Than Expected," Wired.com, December 22, 2010.

28. Nicols Fox, *Spoiled: The Dangerous Truth about a Food Chain Gone Haywire* (NY: Penguin, 1998), 122.

29. Marissa Cevallos, "Meat Contaminated with Resistant Bacteria," LATimes.com, April 15, 2011.

30. Stuart Levy, *The Antibiotic Paradox* (NY: Plenum, 1992), 183.

31. Sarah Bosley, "Are You Ready for a World without Antibiotics?," *The Guardian*, August 12, 2010.

32. Jeffrey Fisher, *The Plague Makers* (NY: Simon and Schuster, 1994), 90.

33. C. G. Daughton and T. A. Ternes, "Pharmaceutical and Personal Care Products in the Environment: Agents of Subtle Change?" *Environmental Health Perspectives* 107, suppl. 6 (1999), 907–38; see also Janet Raloff, "Waterways Carry Antibiotic Resistance," *Science News Online* 155, no. 23 (June 5, 1999).

34. C. G. Daughton and T. A. Ternes, "Pharmaceutical and Personal Care Products in the Environment: Agents of Subtle Change?" *Environmental Health Perspectives* 107, suppl. 6 (1999), 907–38.

35. Stuart Levy, *The Antibiotic Paradox* (NY: Plenum Press, 1992), 175.

36. Lynn Margulis, *Symbiotic Planet* (NY: Basic Books, 1998), 75.

37. Marc Lappé, *When Antibiotics Fail* (Berkeley, CA: North Atlantic Books, 1995), xviii.

38. Ibid., 25–26.

39. Sarah Bosley, "Are You Ready for a World without Antibiotics?," *The Guardian*, August 12, 2010.

Chapter 2 — The Resistant Organisms, the Diseases They Cause and How to Treat Them

1. Brad Spellberg, *Rising Plague* (NY: Prometheus, 2009), 84.

2. "Experts List Dangerous 'Super Bugs': Doctors Warn of Antibiotic Overuse," WCVB-TV (Boston), March 1, 2006, http://www.thebostonchannel.com/r/7586367/detail.html.

3. Brad Spellberg, *Rising Plague* (NY: Prometheus, 2009), 63.

4. Molly Hennessy-Fiske, "Drug-Resistant 'Superbug' Mostly Limited to Southern California Nursing Homes, Health Officials Say," *Los Angeles Times*, L.A. Now blog, March 24, 2010.

5. "Drug-Resistant 'Superbug' Hits LA County Hospitals, Nursing Homes," CBSLosAngeles.com, March 24, 2011, http://losangeles.cbslocal.com/2011/03/24/drug-resistant-super-bug-hits-la-county-hospitals-nursing-homes/.

6. Steve Sternberg, "Superbug Spreading," *USA Today*, September 17, 2010.

7. Sarah Bosley, "Are You Ready for a World without Antibiotics?," *The Guardian*, August 12, 2010.

8. George Eliopoulos, "Antimicrobial Resistance in the Enterococcus," in Richard Wax et al., *Bacterial Resistance to Antimicrobials*, second edition (Boca Raton, FL: CRC Press, 2008), 256.

9. Brad Spellberg, *Rising Plague* (NY: Prometheus, 2009), 79.

10. Sue Fischer, personal communication, March 2011.

Chapter 3 — About Herbal Antibiotics

1. Z. K. Maskatia and K. Baker, "Hypereosinophilia Associated with Echinacea Use," *Southern Medical Journal* 103, no. 11 (2010): 1173–74.

2. M. A. Ekpo and P. C. Elim, "Antimicrobial Activity of Ethanolic and Aqueous Extracts of *Sida acuta* of Microorganisms from Skin Infections," *Journal of Medicinal Plants Research* 3, no. 9 (2009): 621–24.

3. Erich Fromm, as quoted by GoodReads, www.goodreads.com/quotes/show/233200 (accessed March 26, 2010).

Chapter 4 — Herbal Antibiotics: The Systemics

1. Nii-Ayi Ankrah, "Treatment of Falciparum Malaria with a Tea-Bag Formulation of Cryptolepis sanguinolenta root," *Ghana Medical Journal* 44, no. 1 (2010): 2.

2. Damintoti Karou et al., "Antibacterial Activity of Alkaloids from *Sida acuta*," *African Journal of Biotechnology* 5, no. 2 (2008): 195–200.

3. Michael Moore, *Medicinal Plants of the Pacific West* (Sante Fe, NM: Red Crane Books, 1993), 69.

4. Ibid., 71.

5. F. H. Jansen, "The Herbal Tea Approach for Artemisinin as a Therapy for Malaria?" *Transactions of the Royal Society of Tropical Medicine and Hygiene* 100, no. 3 (2006): 285–86.

6. J. Falquet et al., "Artemisia annua as a Herbal Tea for Malaria," *African Journal of Traditional, Complementary, and Alternative Medicines* 4, no. 1 (2007): 121–23.

Chapter 5 — Herbal Antibiotics: The Localized Nonsystemics

1. L. Iauk et al., "Activity of Berberis aetnensis Root Extracts on Candida Strains," *Fitoterapia* 78, no. 2 (2007): 159–61.

2. L. Slobodníková et al., "Antimicrobial Activity of Mahonia aquifolium Crude Extract and Its Major Isolated Alkaloids," *Phytotherapy Research* 18, no. 8 (2004): 674–76.

3. Ahmed Ali Sanaa et al., "Protective Role of *Juniperus phoenicea* and *Cupressus sempervirens* against CCl4," *World Journal of Gastrointestinal Pharmacology and Therapeutics* 1, no. 6 (2010): 123–131.

4. A. Schneider, "Tests Show Most Store Honey Isn't Honey," Food Safety News (online), November 7, 2011, www.foodsafetynews.com/2011/11/tests-show-most-store-honey-isnt-honey/.

Chapter 7 — The First Line of Defense

1. S. Bhagwan et al., "*Ganoderma lucidum:* A Potent Pharmacological Macrofungus," *Current Pharmaceutical Biotechnology* 10 (2009): 717–42, and R. Russel and M. Paterson, "*Ganoderma:* A Therapeutic Fungal Biofactory," *Phytochemistry* 67 (2006): 1985–2001.

Chapter 8 — A Handbook of Herbal Medicine Making

1. Michael Moore, *Herbal Materia Medica*, 5th ed. (Bisbee, AZ: Southwest School of Botanical Medicine, 1995).

RECOMMENDED READING

Aggarwal, Bhrat, et al. *Molecular Targets and Therapeutic Uses of Spices.* Singapore: World Scientific, 2009.

Bergner, Paul. *Medical Herbalism,* all issues.

Blumenthal, Mark, et al. *The Complete German Commission E Monographs.* Austin, TX: American Botanical Council, 1998.

Brinker, Francis. *Herb Contraindications and Drug Interactions.* Sandy, OR: Eclectic Publications, 1998.

Bryan, L. E. *Bacterial Resistance and Susceptibility to Chemotherapeutic Agents.* Cambridge: Cambridge University Press, 1982.

Buhner, Stephen. *Herbal Antibiotics,* 1st ed. North Adams, MA: Storey Publishing, 1999.

Cech, Richo. *Making Plant Medicine.* Williams, OR: Horizon Herbs Publication, 2000.

Duke, James. *The Green Pharmacy.* Emmaus, PA: Rodale, 1998.

Ellingwood, Finley. *American Materia Medica, Therapeutics, and Pharmacognosy.* Cincinnati: Eclectic Publications, 1919.

Farnsworth, Norman. "The Present and Future of Pharmacognosy." American Botanical Council reprint number 209, reprinted from *The American Journal of Pharmaceutical Education* 43 (1979): 239–243. Re: World Health Organization mandate on traditional medicines.

Felter, Harvey, and John Uri Lloyd. *King's American Dispensatory.* Cincinnati: Eclectic Publications, 1895.

Fisher, Jeffery. *The Plague Makers.* New York: Simon and Schuster, 1994.

Fox, Nicols. *Spoiled: The Dangerous Truth about a Food Chain Gone Haywire.* New York: Basic Books, 1998.

Green, James. *The Herbal Medicine-Maker's Handbook,* 4th ed. Forestville, CA: Wildlife and Green, 1990.

Harborne, Jeffrey, et al. *Phytochemical Dictionary: A Handbook of Bioactive Compounds from Plants,* 2nd ed. London: Taylor and Francis, 1999.

Hoffman, David. *The Herbal Handbook: A User's Guide to Medical Herbalism.* Rochester, VT: Healing Arts Press, 1988.

———. *Medical Herbalism.* Rochester, VT: Healing Arts Press, 2003.

———. *The New Holistic Herbal.* Rockport, MA: Element, 1992.

Hson-Mon Chang and Paul Pui-Hay But. *Pharmacology and Applications of Chinese Materia Medica,* 2 vols. Singapore: World Scientific, 2001.

Jing-Nuan Wu. *An Illustrated Chinese Materia Medica.* New York: Oxford University Press, 2005.

Khan, Ikhlas, and Ehab Abourashed. *Leung's Encyclopedia of Common Natural Ingredients Used in Food, Drugs, and Cosmetics.* Hoboken, NJ: Wiley, 2010.

Landis, Robyn, and K. P. Khalsa. *Herbal Defense.* New York: Warner Books, 1997.

Langenheim, Jean. *Plant Resins: Chemistry, Evolution, Ecology, Ethnobotany.* Portland, OR: Timber Press, 2003.

Lappé, Marc. *When Antibiotics Fail.* Berkeley, CA: North Atlantic Books, 1986.

Levy, Stuart. *The Antibiotic Paradox.* New York: Plenum, 1992.

Lieberman, P. B. *Protecting the Crown Jewels of Medicine: A Strategic Plan to Preserve the Effectiveness of Antibiotics.* Washington, DC: Center for Science in the Public Interest, 1998.

Mabey, Richard, ed. *The New Age Herbalist*. New York: Simon and Schuster, 1988.

Manandhar, Narayan. *Plants and People of Nepal*. Portland, OR: Timber Press, 2002.

Mitsuhashi, S. *Drug Action and Drug Resistance in Bacteria*. Tokyo, University of Tokyo Press, 1971.

Moerman, Daniel. *Native American Ethnobotany*. Portland, OR: Timber Press, 1998.

Moore, Michael. *Herbal Materia Medica*. Albuquerque, NM: Southwest School of Botanical Medicine, 1990.

——. *Herbal Repertory in Clinical Practice*. Albuquerque, NM: Southwest School of Botanical Medicine, 1990.

——. *Herbal Tinctures in Clinical Practice*. Albuquerque, NM: Southwest School of Botanical Medicine, 1990.

——. *Medicinal Plants of the Desert and Canyon West*. Sante Fe, NM: Museum of New Mexico Press, 1989.

——. *Medicinal Plants of the Mountain West*. Sante Fe: Museum of New Mexico Press, 1976.

——. *Medicinal Plants of the Pacific Northwest*. Sante Fe, NM: Red Crane Books, 1993.

Nadkarni, A. K. *Indian Materia Medica*, 2 vols. Bombay: Popular Frakashan, 1927.

NAPRALERT database of botanicals effective against human pathogenic bacteria as of December 1, 1998.

The Protocol Journal of Botanic Medicine, all issues.

Schmidt, Michael, et al. *Beyond Antibiotics*. Berkeley, CA: North Atlantic Books, 1994.

Science Magazine 257, no. 5073, American Association for the Advancement of Science, August 21, 1992. Entire volume focuses on antibiotic-resistant bacteria.

Scott, Timothy Lee. *Invasive Plant Medicine*. Rochester, VT: Healing Arts Press, 2010.

Shiu-Ying Hu. *An Enumeration of Chinese Materia Medica*. Hong Kong: Chinese University Press, 1980.

Spellberg, Brad. *Rising Plague*. Amherst, NY: Prometheus Books, 2009.

Stuart, G. A. *Chinese Materia Medica: Vegetable Kingdom*. Shanghai: American Presbyterian Mission Press, 1911.

Tillotson, Alan. *The One Earth Herbal Sourcebook*. New York: Kensington, 2001.

Van Wyck, Ben-Erik, and Michael Wink. *Medicinal Plants of the World*. Portland, OR: Timber Press, 2004.

Wax, Richard, et al., eds. *Bacterial Resistance to Antimicrobials*, 2nd ed. Boca Raton, FL: CRC Press, 2008.

Weiss, Rudolph. *Herbal Medicine*. Sweden: Beaconsfield, 1988.

Willcox, Merlin, et al., eds. *Traditional Medicinal Plants and Malaria*. Boca Raton, FL: CRC Press, 2004.

Williams, J. E. *Viral Immunity*. Charlottesville, VA: Hampton Roads, 2002.

Winston, David, and Steven Maimes. *Adaptogens*. Rochester, VT: Healing Arts Press, 2007.

You-Ping Zhu. *Chinese Materia Medica: Chemistry, Pharmacology and Applications*. Amsterdam: Harwood Academic Publishers, 1998.

Zhang Enqin. *Rare Chinese Materia Medica*. Shanghai: Shanghai University of Traditional Chinese Medicine, 1989.

RESOURCES

The Lord hath created medicines out of the earth; and he that is wise will not abhor them.

Ecclesiastes 38.4

Many of the herbs I have talked about in this book — and, of course, a great many others — grow wild. Even if you live in a city you can find many of them cohabitating with you or only a short drive away. Since many of these herbs are invasives, most people will be glad for you to take them away.

If you need to buy your herbs, the Internet is a good way to seek them. I suggest running a web search for the herbs you are looking for to find the cheapest prices; if you are persistent you can often save half off normal retail.

If you are going to be buying a lot of herbs and you live in the United States it makes sense to buy a resale license from your state. The price is often minimal and it will allow you to buy wholesale; most wholesalers will want a resale certificate before they will sell to you.

And, of course, you can grow them yourself. Once established most of the herbs in this book will provide medicine for you and your family forever.

Listed on the following page are some of the best sources I know of for the herbs in this book.

Elk Mountain Herbs

214 Ord Street
Laramie, WY 82070
307-742-0404
www.elkmountainherbs.com
Wonderful tinctures from local wild-crafted Western plants.

1st Chinese Herbs

5018 Viewridge Drive
Olympia, WA 98501
888-842-2049
360-923-0486
www.1stchineseherbs.com
Wonderful people with a very large selection of Chinese herbs, including most of those discussed in this book. Most herbs by the pound.

Healing Spirits Herb Farm

61247 Route 415
Avoca, NY 14809
607-566-2701
www.healingspiritsherbfarm.com
Matthias and Andrea Reisen have been growing wonderful medicinal plants for years. The plants just jump out of the bag and laugh when you open it up.

Horizon Herbs

P. O. Box 69
Williams, OR 97544
541-846-6704
wwww.horizonherbs.com
Richo Cech has spent much of his life learning how to grow common and rare medicinals. He has seeds or young stock for most of the plants in this book as well as great information on how to grow them.

Mountain Rose Herbs

P. O. Box 50220
Eugene, OR 97405
800-879-3337
541-741-7307
www.mountainroseherbs.com
A nice selection, sustainably produced.

Pacific Botanicals

4840 Fish Hatchery Road
Grants Pass, OR 97527
541-479-7777
www.pacificbotanicals.com
This is perhaps the best wholesaler (they also sell retail) in the United States. Their herbs are magnificent. Normally, all are sold by the pound.

Sage Woman Herbs

108 East Cheyenne Road
Colorado Springs, CO 80906
888-350-3911
719-473-9702
www.sagewomanherbs.com
They have some herbs that are otherwise hard to get (e.g., *Echinacea angustifolia*), and I like their quality.

Woodland Essence

392 Teacup Street
Cold Brook, NY 13324
315-845-1515
www.woodlandessence.com
Kate and Don make wonderful tinctures and medicines and can sell you many of the herbal tinctures that I discuss in this book; if they don't have them, they can probably point you in the right direction.

Zack Woods Herb Farm

278 Mead Road
Hyde Park, VT 05655
802-888-7278
www.zackwoodsherbs.com
Melanie and Jeff are wonderful people and grow tremendously beautiful medicinal plants. Very, very high-quality herbs. Usually sold by the pound.

BIBLIOGRAPHY

General: Resistant Bacteria

Abera, B., et al. Antimicrobial susceptibility of *V. cholerae* in north west Ethiopia. *Ethiop Med J* 48, no. 1 (2010): 23–28.

Adabi, M. Distribution of class I integron and sulfamethoxazole trimethoprim constin in *Vibrio cholerae* isolated from patients in Iran. *Microb Drug Resist* 15, no. 3 (2009): 179–84.

Aeschlimann, Jeffrey R., and the University of Connecticut Health Center Department of Pharmacology (Farmington, Conn.). The role of multidrug efflux pumps in antibiotic resistance: multidrug efflux pump-based resistance in Gram-negative bacteria. MedScape Today News. http://medscape.com/viewarticle/458871_2 (accessed March 20, 2011).

Agence France-Presse (AFP). WHO calls for monitoring of new superbug. PhysOrg. com, August 20, 2010. http://physorg.com/news201528869.html.

Anonymous. Antibiotic resistance. Wikipedia. http://en.wikipedia.org/wiki/Antibiotic_resistance (accessed December 22, 2010).

Anonymous. Beta-lactamase. Wikipedia. http://en.wikipedia.org/wiki/Beta-lactamase (accessed March 14, 2011).

Anonymous. *Drug-resistant salmonella.* World Health Organization fact sheet 139, revised April 2005. http://www.who.int/mediacentre/factsheets/fs139/en/.

Anonymous. Drug-resistant "super bug" hits LA county hospitals, nursing homes. CBS Local Media (Los Angeles), March 24, 2011. http://losangeles.cbslocal.com/2011/03/24/drug-resistant-super-bug-hits-la-county-hospitals-nursing-homes/.

Anonymous. Experts list dangerous "super bugs." TheBostonChannel.com (WCVBTV), March 1, 2006. http://www.thebostonchannel.com/r/7586367/detail.html.

Anonymous. Extended-spectrum beta-lactamases (ESBLs). UK Health Protection Agency. http://www.hpa.org.uk/Topics/InfectiousDiseases/InfectionsAZ/ESBLs/ (accessed January 24, 2011).

Anonymous. Facts about antibiotic resistance. Infectious Diseases Society of America, revised April 2011. http://www.idsociety.org/AR_Facts/.

Anonymous. Hospital continues to limit visitors as it fights superbugs. *Ottawa Citizen*, December 21, 2010.

Anonymous. Hospitals preparing for killer bug. AsiaOne Health, December 2, 2010. http://asiaone.com/Health/News/Story/A1Story20101202-250352.html.

Anonymous. New deadly superbug Steno an ever-increasing threat. News-Medical. Net, May 8, 2008. http://news-medical.net/news/2008/05/08/38189.aspx.

Anonymous. 'The NHS failed my mum' says distraught daughter, *Grantham Journal* (UK), December 14, 2010. http://granthamjournal.co.uk/community/local_services_2_1767/health-care-services/the_nhs_failed_my_mum_says_distraught_daughter_1_1919865.

Associated Press. Update: new drug-resistant superbugs found in 3 states. FoxNews.com, September 14, 2010. http://foxnews.com/health/2010/09/14/update-new-drug-resistant-superbugs-states/.

Borland, Sophie. Flu crisis hits cancer surgery: Hospitals struggle to cope as deaths rise and Britain teeters on the brink of an epidemic. Mail Online (UK), December 27, 2010. http://dailymail.co.uk/news/article-1341807/As-deaths-rise-Britain-teeters-brink-epidemic-Flu-crisis-hits-cancer-surgery.html.

——. 460 flu victims fighting for life as experts admit 24 deaths from swine strain may be only fraction of the true number. Mail Online (UK), December 24, 2010. http://www.dailymail.co.uk/health/article-1341300/460-flu-victims-fighting-life-experts-admit-24-deaths-swine-strain-fraction-true-number.html.

Boseley, Sarah. Are you ready for a world without antibiotics? *The Guardian*, August 11, 2010. http://www.guardian.co.uk/society/2010/aug/12/the-end-of-antibiotics-health-infections.

Caldwell, Emily. Pandemic flu, like seasonal H1N1, shows signs of resisting Tamiflu. Ohio State University Research Communications news release, March 1, 2010. http://researchnews.osu.edu/archive/tamiflu.htm.

Campbell, D., and Anushka Asthana. The "catalogue of errors" that cost this father his life. *The Observer*, November 27, 2010. http://www.guardian.co.uk/society/2010/nov/27/nhs-hospitals-dr-foster-report.

Chakraborty, S., et al. Concomitant infection of enterotoxigenic *Escherichia coli* in an outbreak of cholera caused by *Vibrio cholerae* O1 and O139 in Ahmedabad, India. *J Clin Microbiol* 39, no. 9 (2001): 3241–46.

Chamilos, G., et al. Update on antifungal drug resistance mechanisms of *Aspergillus fumigatus*. *Drug Resist Updates* 8 (2005): 344–58.

Chander, J., et al. Epidemiology & antibiograms of *Vibrio cholerae* isolates from a tertiary care hospital in Chandigarth, north India. *Indian J Med Res* 129, no. 5 (2009): 613–17.

Chandrasekar, P. H. Antifungal resistance in *Aspergillus*. *Med Mycol* 43, suppl. 1 (May 2005): S295–98.

Dalsgaard, D. A., et al. Is *Vibrio cholerae* serotype O139 a potential cause of a new pandemic? *Ugeskr Laeger* 157, no. 3 (1995): 280–83.

Das, S., et al. Trend of antibiotic resistance of *Vibrio cholerae* strains from east Delhi. *Indian J Med Res* 127, no. 5 (2008): 478–82.

Dickinson, Boonsri. The fight for life against superbugs. SmartPlanet *Science Scope* (blog), March 24, 2010. http://www.smartplanet.com/blog/science-scope/the-fight-for-life-against-superbugs/548.

———. Five superbug defenses that can keep you from dying in the hospital. SmartPlanet *Science Scope* (blog), December 22, 2010. http://smartplanet.com/blog/science-scope/five-superbug-defenses-that-can-keep-you-from-dying-in-the-hospital/5888.

Duke Medicine News and Communications. New superbug surpasses MRSA infection rates in community hospitals. News release, March 22, 2010. http://www.dukehealth.org/health_library/news/new_superbug_surpasses_mrsa_infection_rates_in_community_hospitals.

Engel, Mary. Deadly bacteria defy drugs, alarming doctors. *Los Angeles Times*, February 17, 2009. http://articles.latimes.com/2009/feb/17/science/sci-badbugs17.

Farkosh, Mary S. Extended-spectrum beta-lactamase producing Gram negative bacilli. Johns Hopkins Medicine: Hospital Epidemiology/Infection Control. http://hopkinsmedicine.org/heic/ID/esbl/ (accessed March 14, 2011).

Fernández-Delgado, M. *Vibrio cholerae* non-O1, non-O139 associated with seawater and plankton from coastal marine areas of the Caribbean Sea. *Int J Environ Helth Res* 19, no. 4 (2009): 279–89.

Ferreira, C., et al. *Candida albicans* virulence and drug-resistance requires the O-acyltransferase Gup1p. *BMC Microbiol* 10 (2010): 238–53.

Garg, P., et al. Expanding multiple antibiotic resistance among clinical strains of *Vibrio cholerae* isolated from 1992–7 in Calcutta, India. *Epidemiol Infect* 124, no. 3 (2000): 393–99.

Glass, R. I., et al. Emergence of multiple antibiotic-resistant *Vibrio cholerae* in Bangladesh. *J Infect Dis* 142, no. 6 (1980): 939–42.

Goel, A. K., et al. Genetic determinants of virulence, antibiogram and altered biotype among the *Vibrio cholerae* O1 isolates from different cholera outbreaks in India. *Infect Genet Evol* 10, no. 6 (2010): 815–19.

Goel, A. K., et al. Molecular characterization of *Vibrio cholerae* outbreak strains with altered El Tor biotype from southern India. *World J Microbiol Biotechnol* 26, no. 2 (2010): 281–87.

Hagemann, M., et al. The plant-associated bacterium *Stenotrophomonas rhizophila* expresses a new enzyme for the synthesis of the compatible solute glucosylglycerol. *J Bacteriol* 190, no. 7 (2008): 5898–906.

Haller, Brad. New superbug genes resist all antibiotics. OzarksFirst.com, December 15, 2010. http://ozarksfirst.com/fulltext?nxd_id=372146.

Hennessy-Fiske, Molly. Drug-resistant 'superbug' mostly limited to Southern California nursing homes, health officials say. *L.A. Now* (blog of the *Los Angeles Times*), March 24, 2011. http://latimesblogs.latimes.com/lanow/2011/03/superbug-in-southern-california.html.

Herper, Matthew. The most dangerous bacteria. Forbes.com, March 1, 2006. http://forbes.com/2006/03/01/antibiotics-pfizer-cubist-cx_mh_0301badbugs.html.

Hicks, L. A., et al. *Antimicrobial prescription data reveal wide geographic variability in antimicrobial use in the United States, 2009.* U.S. Centers for Disease Control, National Center for Immunization and Respiratory Diseases, Division of Bacterial Diseases. http://www.imshealth.com/deployedfiles/imshealth/global/content/staticfile/Antimicrobial_Prescription_Data_2009.pdf (accessed March 26, 2011).

Hirche, T. O., et al. Myeloperoxidase plays critical roles in killing *Klebsiella pneumoniae* and inactivating neutrophil elastase: effects on host defense. *J Immunol* 174, no. 3 (2005): 1557–65.

Hooper, David C. Efflux pumps and nosocomial antibiotic resistance: a primer for hospital epidemiologists. *Healthcare Epidem CID* 40 (2005): 1811–17.

Huff, E. New drug-resistant bacteria emerging in hospitals. NaturalNews.com, March 6, 2010. http://naturalnews.com/028313_drug-resistant_bacteria_hospitals.html.

Hutheesing, Nikhil. Eight deadly superbugs lurking in hospitals. DailyFinance, October 17, 2010. http://www.dailyfinance.com/2010/10/17/eight-deadly-superbugs-lurking-in-hospitals/.

Johns Hopkins Bloomberg School of Public Health News Center. Flies may spread drug-resistant bacteria from poultry operations. News release, March 16, 2009. http://www.jhsph.edu/publichealthnews/press_releases/2009/graham_flies.html.

Johnson, J. R., et al. *Escherichia coli* sequence type ST131 as the major cause of serious multidrug-resistant *E. coli* infections in the United States. *Clin Infect Dis* 51, no. 3 (2010): 286–94.

Keim, Brandon. Antibiotics breed superbugs faster than expected. *Wired Science* (blog), February 11, 2010. http://wired.com/wiredscience/2010/02/mutagen-antibiotics/.

———. Obama, farm industry clash over antibiotics. *Wired Science* (blog), July 21, 2009. http://wired.com/wiredscience/2009/07/farmantibiotic/.

———. Swine flu ancestor born on U.S. factory farms. *Wired Science* (blog), May 1, 2009. http://wired.com/wiredscience/2009/05/swineflufarm/.

———. Swine flu genes from pigs only, not human or birds. *Wired Science* (blog), April 28, 2009. http://wired.com/wiredscience/2009/04/swinefluupdate/.

Kelland, Kate, and Ben Hirschler. Scientists find new superbug spreading from India. Reuters, August 11, 2010. http://reuters.com/article/2010/08/11/us-infections-superbug-idUSTRE67A0YU20100811.

Khuntia, H. K., et al. An Ogawa cholera outbreak 6 months after the Inaba cholera outbreaks in India, 2006. *J Microbiol Immunol Infect* 43, no. 2 (2010): 133–37.

Kim, H. B., et al. Transferable quinolone resistance in *Vibrio cholerae. Antimicrob Agents Chemother* 54, no. 2 (2010): 799–803.

Klepser, Michael E. Antifungal resistance among *Candida* species. *Pharmacotherapy* 21, no. 8, part 2 (2001): 124S–132S.

Klevens, R. M., et al. Invasive methicillin-resistant *Staphylococcus aureus* infections in the United States. *JAMA* 298 (2007): 1763–71.

Knight, Danielle. US: Over-Use of Antibiotics Threatens Humans. TWN (Third World Network), October 11, 2009. http://twnside.org.sg/title/overuse-cn.htm.

Knorr, R., et al. Endocytosis of MHC molecules by distinct membrane rafts. *J Cell Sci* 122, part 10 (2009): 1584–94.

Koo, Ingrid. Superbugs on the rise. About.com, updated November 6, 2008. http://infectiousdiseases.about.com/od/rarediseases/a/rising_superbug.htm.

Kristof, Nicholas D. The spread of superbugs. Op-ed., *New York Times*, March 6, 2010. http://www.nytimes.com/2010/03/07/opinion/07kristof.html.

Kumar, P., et al. Characterization of an SXT variant *Vibrio cholerae* O1 Ogawa isolated from a patient in Trivandrum, India. *FEMS Microbiol Lett* 303, no. 2 (2010): 132–36.

Laurance, Jeremy. Doctors shocked by spread of swine flu—and its severity. *The Independent*, December 11, 2010. http://independent.co.uk/life-style/health-and-families/health-news/doctors-shocked-by-spread-of-swine-flu-ndash-and-its-severity-2157407.html.

Li, B. S., et al. Phenotypic and genotypic characterization *Vibrio cholerae* O139 of clinical and aquatic isolates in China. *Curr Microbiol* 62, no. 3 (2011): 950–955. E-pub (preprint) November 16, 2010.

Li-ting, Chen and Liu, Fanny. CDC to list new superbug NDM-1 as communicable disease. Focus Taiwan News Channel, September 7, 2010. http://focustaiwan.tw/ShowNews/WebNews_Detail.aspx?ID=201009070016&Type=aLIV.

Lloyd, Robin. Infectious superbug invades beaches. LiveScience, February 13, 2009. http://livescience.com/health/090213-beach-superbugs-mrsa.html.

Long, F., et al. Functional cloning and characterization of the multidrug efflux pumps NorM from *Neisseria gonorrhoeae* and YdhE from *Escherichia coli*. *Antimicrob Agents Chemother* 52, no. 9 (2008): 3052–60.

Loyola University Health System. Is re-emerging superbug the next MRSA? News release, September 15, 2008. http://www.eurekalert.org/pub_releases/2008-09/luhs-irs091508.php.

Lutz, B. D., et al. Outbreak of invasive aspergillus infection in surgical patients, associated with a contaminated air-handling system. *CID* 37 (2003): 786–87.

Manga, N. M., et al. Cholera in Senegal from 2004 to 2006: lessons learned from successive outbreaks. *Med Trop (Mars)* 68, no. 6 (2008): 589–92.

Martin, Daniel. Superbugs on the increase in care homes. Mail Online (UK), July 16, 2007. http://www.dailymail.co.uk/news/article-468837/Superbugs-increase-care-homes.html.

Meng, J., et al. Antibiotic resistance of *Escherichia coli* O157:H7 and O157:NM isolated from animals, food and humans. *J Food Prod* 61, no. 11 (1998): 1511–14.

Mora, A., et al. Antimicrobial resistance of Shiga toxin (verotoxin)-producing *Escherichia coli* O157:H7 and non-O157 strains isolated from humans, cattle, sheep and food in Spain. *Res Microbiol* 156, no. 7 (2005): 793–806.

Morse, J. Staph infection—a newly discovered STD? Yahoo! Voices, October 18, 2007. http://voices.yahoo.com/staph-infection-newly-discovered-std-604179.html.

Neergaard, Lauran. "C-diff" superbug on the rise: last-method at fighting intestinal bug. *Huffington Post* (blog), December 13, 2010. http://www.huffingtonpost.com/2010/12/13/cdiff-superbug_n_796156.html.

Nikaido, Hiroshi. Multidrug efflux pumps of Gram-negative bacteria. *J Bacteriol* 178, no. 20 (1996): 5853–59.

Nygren, E., et al. Establishment of an adult mouse model for direct evaluation of the efficacy of vaccines against *Vibrio cholerae*. *Infect Immun* 77, no. 8 (2009): 3475–84.

Osamor, V. S. The etiology of malaria scourge: a comparative study of endemic nations of Africa and Asia. *J Biol Sci* 10, no. 5 (2010): 440–47.

Paddock, Catharine. Polar bear droppings might help us understand superbugs. Medical News Today, January 15, 2010. http://medicalnewstoday.com/articles/176110.php?nfid=60100.

Pal, B. B., et al. Epidemics of severe cholera caused by El Tor *Vibrio cholerae* O1 Ogawa possessing the ctxB gene of the classical biotype in Orissa, India. *Int J Infect Dis* 14, no. 5 (2010): e384–89.

Perrone, Matthew. Congressman pushes FDA on chemical safety review. From the Associated Press, on the ABC News website, December 22, 2010. http://abcnews.go.com/Business/wireStory?id=12458030.

Powell, W. J. *Molecular mechanisms of antimicrobial resistance*. Technical report #14. Food Safety Network, February 2000. http://foodsafety.k-state.edu/articles/280/molecular_mechanisms_antimic_resist.pdf.

Preidt, Robert. Hospital-acquired infections a serious threat to ICU patients: study. HealthDay News, on the Bloomberg Businessweek website, December 1, 2010. http://businessweek.com/lifestyle/content/healthday/646702.html.

Qiao, J., et al. Antifungal resistance mechanisms of Aspergillus. *Jpn J Med Mycol* 49 (2008): 157–63.

Qureshi, A., et al. *Stenotrophomonas maltophelia* in salad. *Emerg Infect Dis* 11, no. 7 (2005): 1157–58.

Rahim, N., et al. Antibacterial activity of *Psidium guajava* leaf and bark against multidrug-resistant *Vibrio cholerae*: implication for cholera control. *Jpn J Infect Dis* 63, no. 4 (2010): 271–74.

Raloff, Janet. Tamiflu in rivers could breed drug-resistant flu strains. *Wired Science* (blog), September 20, 2009. http://www.wired.com/wiredscience/2009/09/drug-resistant-influenza/.

Reig, S., et al. Resistance against antimicrobial peptides is independent of *Escherichia coli* AcrAB, *Pseudomonas aeruginosa* MexAB and *Staphylococcus aureus* NorA efflux pumps. *Int J Antimicrob Agents* 33, no. 2 (2009): 174–76.

Reuters. New superbug genes sure to spread in the U.S., expert says. FoxNews.com, December 16, 2010. http://foxnews.com/health/2010/12/16/new-superbug-genes-sure-to-spread-expert-says/.

Roberts, Michelle. Seagulls "may be spreading superbugs." BBC News, September 20, 2010. http://bbc.co.uk/news/health-11374536.

Rodriguez, C., et al. Diversity and antimicrobial susceptibility of oxytetracycline-resistant isolates of *Stenotrophomonas* sp. and *Serratia* sp. associated with Costa Rican crops. *J Appl Microbiol* 103, no. 6 (2007): 2550–60.

Rosenberg, Martha. 15 dangerous drugs big pharma shoves down our throats. AlterNet, November 19, 2010. http://alternet.org/story/148907/15_dangerous_drugs_big_pharma_shoves_down_our_throats?page=entire.

Roy, S., et al. Gut colonization by multidrug-resistant and carbapenem-resistant *Acinetobacter baumannii* in neonates. *Eur J Clin Microbiol Infect Dis* 29, no. 12 (2010): 1495–500.

Rubenstein, Adam. Colorado attacking IDSA superbug list. *Life Science Deal Flow* (blog), March 6, 2006. http://rnaventures.blogspot.com/2006/03/colorado-attacking-idsa-superbug-list.html.

Ryan, David B. List of drug-resistant bacteria. LiveStrong.com, March 28, 2011. http://livestrong.com/article/28797-list-drugresistant-bacteria.

Ryan, R. P., et al. Interspecies signaling via the *Stenotrophomonas maltophilia* diffusible signal factor influences biofilm formation and polymyxin tolerance in *Pseudomonas aeruginosa*. *Mol Microbiol* 68, no. 1 (2008): 75–86.

Sá, L. L., et al. Occurrence and composition of class 1 and class 2 integrons in clinical and environmental O1 and non-O1/non-O139 *Vibrio cholerae* strains from the Brazilian Amazon. *Mem Inst Oswaldo Cruz* 105, no. 2 (2010): 229–32.

Sakai, Jill. Virus hybridization could create pandemic bird flu. University of Wisconsin–Madison news release, February 22, 2010. http://www.news.wisc.edu/17698.

Savel'ev, V. N., et al. Antibacterial susceptibility/resistance of *Vibrio cholerae* eltor clinical strains isolated in the Caucasus during the seventh cholera pandemic. *Antibiot Khimioter* 55, no. 5–6 (2010): 8–13.

Saviola, B., et al. The genus *Mycobacterium*—medical. *Prokaryotes* 1, part B (2006): 919–33.

Schroeder, C. M., et al. Antimicrobial resistance of *Escherichia coli* O157 isolated from humans, cattle, swine, and food. *Appl Environ Microbiol* 68, no. 2 (2002): 576–81.

Shepherd, Tory. Hygiene hypothesis: let children eat dirt. The Punch (Australia), December 6, 2010. http://thepunch.com.au/articles/a-dirty-piece-on-cleanliness/.

Smith, Jennie. More seasonal flu strains show worrisome dual antiviral resistance. Internal Medicine News Digital Network, December 7, 2010. http://internalmedicinenews.com/specialty-focus/women-s-health/single-article-page/more-seasonal-flu-strains-show-worrisome-dual-antiviral-resistance/17f055c464.html.

Sohn, Emily. Superbug: neither super nor a bug. Discovery News, September 17, 2010. http://news.discovery.com/human/superbug-bacteria-gene-threat.html.

Stein, Rob. New "superbugs" raising concerns worldwide. Website of the *Washington Post*, October 11, 2010. http://www.washingtonpost.com/wp-dyn/content/article/2010/10/11/AR2010101104518.html.

Sternberg, Steve. Drug-resistant "superbugs" hit 35 states, spread worldwide. *USA Today*, September 16, 2010. http://www.usatoday.com/yourlife/health/medical/2010-09-17-1Asuperbug17_ST_N.htm.

Stoler, Steve. Woman who lost 428 lbs. faces new health battle. WFAA TV, on the website azfamily.com, December 1, 2010. http://www.azfamily.com/news/Woman-who-lost-428-lbsfaces-new-health-battle-111159229.html.

Trafton, Anne. Mutation identified that might allow H1N1 to spread more easily. PhysOrg.com, March 9, 2011. http://physorg.com/news/2011-03-mutation-h1n1-easily.html.

Tristram, S., et al. Antimicrobial resistance in *Hamophilus influenzae*. *Clin Microbiol Rev* 20, no. 2 (2007): 368–89.

United Press International (UPI). Report: superbugs killed record number. UPI.com, May 23, 2008. http://www.upi.com/Science_News/2008/05/23/Report-Superbugs-killed-record-number/UPI-57821211586105/.

University of Texas Southwestern Medical Center. "Superbug" breast infections controllable in nursing mothers, UT Southwestern researchers find. News release, September 3, 2008. http://www.utsouthwestern.edu/newsroom/news-releases/year-2008/superbug-breast-infections-controllable-in-nursing-mothers-researchers-find.html.

Vanderbilt University Medical Center. Staph bacteria: blood-sucking superbug prefers taste of humans. News release, December 15, 2010. http://www.eurekalert.org/pub_releases/2010-12/vumc-bsp121310.php.

Veselova, M., et al. Production of N-acylhomoserine lactone singal molecules by Gram-negative soil-borne and plant-associated bacteria. *Folia Microbiol* 48, no. 6 (2003): 794–98.

Wagner, H. Multitarget therapy—the future of treatment for more than just functional dyspepsia. *Phytomedicine* 13, suppl. 5 (2006): 122–29.

White, Sarah V. The empowered patient. Medill Reports, from the Medill School at Northwestern University, December 8, 2010. http://news.medill.northwestern.edu/chicago/news.aspx?id=175221.

Xu, X. J., et al. Molecular cloning and characterization of the HmrM multidrug efflux pump from *Haemophilus influenzae* Rd. *Microbiol Immunol* 47, no. 12 (2003): 937–43.

Yang, J. S., et al. A duplex vibriocidal assay to simultaneously measure bactericidal antibody titers against *Vibrio cholerae* O1 Inaba and Ogawa serotypes. *J Microbiol Methods* 79, no. 3 (2009): 289–94.

Yee, D. Gonorrhoea joins "superbugs" list. IOL (Independent Online, South Africa) SciTech, April 13, 2010. http://www.iol.co.za/scitech/technology/gonorrhoea-joins-superbugs-list-1.322949.

Zhang, C., et al. Redox signaling via lipid raft clustering in homocysteine-induced injury of podocytes. *Biochim Biophys Acta* 1803, no. 4 (2010): 482–91.

General: Medicinal Plants (Herbal Antibiotics)

Abeysinghe, P. D. Antibacterial activity of some medicinal mangroves against antibiotic resistant pathogenic bacteria. *Indian J Pharm Sci* 72, no. 2 (2010): 167–72.

Abo-Khatwa, A. N., et al. Lichen acids as uncouplers of oxidative phosphorylation of mouse-liver mitochondria. *Nat Toxins* 4, no. 2 (1996): 96–102.

Addy, Marian E. Western Africa Network of Natural Products Research Scientists (WANNPRES), First Scientific Meeting August 15–20, 2004. Accra, Ghana: A Report. Conference report published in *Afr J Tradit Complement Altern Med* 2, no. 2 (2005): 177–205.

Anonymous. Africa: turning to traditional medicines in fight against malaria. IRIN (news service of the U.N. Office for the Coordination of Humanitarian Affairs), November 4, 2009. http://irinnews.org/report.aspx?ReportId=86866.

Anonymous. *Report of the International Conference on Traditional Medicine in HIV/AIDS and Malaria* (December 5–7, 2000, Nicon Hilton Hotel, Abuja, Nigeria). International Centre for Ethnomedicine and Drug Development and the Bioresources Development and Conservation Programme, 2000. http://intercedd.com/downloads/bdcp-interceddconf.pdf.

Arias, M. E., et al. Antibacterial activity of ethanolic and aqueous extracts of *Acacia aroma* Gill. ex Hook et Arn. *Life Sci* 75, no. 2 (2004): 191–202.

Bačkorová M., et al. Variable responses of different human cancer cells to the lichen compounds parietin, atranorin, usnic acid and gyrophoric acid. *Toxicol In Vitro* 25, no. 1 (2011): 37–44. E-pub (preprint) September 17, 2010.

Batista, R., et al. Plant-derived antimalarial agents: new leads and efficient phytomedicines. Part II. Non-alkaloidal natural products. *Molecules* 14 (2009): 3037–72.

Bayir, Y., et al. The inhibition of gastric mucosal lesion, oxidative stress and neutrophil-infiltration in rats by the lichen constituent diffractaic acid. *Phytomedicine* 13, no. 8 (2006): 584–90.

Bazin, M. A., et al. Synthesis and cytotoxic activities of usnic acid derivatives. *Bioorg Med Chem* 16, no. 14 (2008): 6860–66.

Behera, B. C., et al. Antioxidant and antibacterial activities of lichen *Usnea ghattensis* in vitro. *Biotechnol Lett* 27, no. 14 (2005): 991–95.

Behera, B. C., et al. Antioxidant and antibacterial properties of some cultured lichens. *Bioresour Technol* 99, no. 4 (2008): 776–84.

Behera, B. C., et al. Evaluation of antioxidant potential of the cultured mycobiont of a lichen *Usnea ghattensis*. *Phytother Res* 19, no. 1 (2005): 58–64.

Behera, B. C., et al. Tissue culture of some lichens and screening of their antioxidant, antityrosinase and antibacterial properties. *Phytother Res* 21, no. 12 (2007): 1159–70.

Belofsky, G., et al. Metabolites of the "smoke tree," *Dalea spinosa*, potentiate antibiotic activity against multi-drug-resistant *Staphylococcus aureus*. *J Nat Prod* 69, no. 2 (2006): 261–64.

Belofsky, G., et al. Phenolic metabolites of *Dalea versicolor* that enhance antibiotic activity against model pathogenic bacteria. *J Nat Prod* 67, no. 3 (2004): 481–84.

Bian, X., et al. Study on the scavenging action of polysaccharide of *Usnea longissima* to oxygen radical and its anti-lipi peroxidation effects. *Zhong Yao Cai* 25, no. 3 (2002): 188–89.

Boehm, F. Lichens—photophysical studies of potential new sunscreens. *J Photochem Photobiol B* 95, no. 1 (2009): 40–45.

Brijesh, S., et al. Studies on *Pongamia pinnata* (L.) Pierre leaves: understanding the mechanism(s) of action in infectious diarrhea. *J Zhejiang Univ Sci B* 7, no. 8 (2006): 665–74.

Brijesh, S., et al. Studies on the antidiarrhoeal activity of *Aegle marmelos* unripe fruit: validating its traditional usage. *BMC Complement Altern Med* 9 (2009): 47.

Burlando, B., et al. Antiproliferative effects on tumour cells and promotion of keratinocyte wound healing by different lichen compounds. *Planta Med* 75, no. 6 (2009): 607–13.

Burt, S. Essential oils: their antibacterial properties and potential applications in food—a review. *Int J Food Microbiol* 94, no. 3 (2004): 223–53.

Campanella, L., et al. Molecular characterization and action of usnic acid: a drug that inhibits proliferation of mouse polyomavirus in vitro and whose main target is RNA transcription. *Biochimie* 84, no. 4 (2002): 329–34.

Cansaran, D., et al. Identification and quantitation of usnic acid from the lichen Usnea species of Anatolia and antimicrobial activity. *Z Naturforsch C* 61, no. 11–12 (2006): 773–76.

Cermelli, C., et al. Effect of eucalyptus essential oil on respiratory bacteria and viruses. *Curr Microbiol* 56, no. 1 (2008): 89–92.

Cheng, Y. B., et al. Oral acute toxicity of (+)-usnic acid in mice and its cytotoxicity in rat cardiac fibroblasts. *Nan Fang Yi Ke Da Xue Xue Bao* 29, no. 8 (2009): 1749–51.

Chérigo, L., et al. Bacterial resistance modifying tetrasaccharide agents from *Ipomoea murucoides*. *Phytochemistry* 70, no. 2 (2009): 222–27.

Chérigo, L., et al. Inhibitors of bacterial multidrug efflux pumps from the resin glycosides of *Ipomoea murucoides*. *J Nat Prod* 71, no. 6 (2008): 1037–45.

Chérigo, L., et al. Resin glycosides from the flowers of *Ipomoea murucoides*. *J Nat Prod* 69, no. 4 (2006): 595–99.

Cheruiyot, K. R., et al. In-vitro antibacterial activity of selected medicinal plants from Longisa region of Bomet district, Kenya. *Afr Health Sci* 9, suppl. 1 (2009): S42–46.

Choudhary, M. I., et al. Bioactive phenolic compounds from a medicinal lichen, *Usnea longissima*. *Phytochemistry* 66, no. 19 (2005): 2346–50.

Cloutier, M. M., et al. Tannin inhibits adenylate cyclase in airway epithelial cells. *Am J Physiol* 268, no. 5, part 1 (1995): L851–55.

Crutchley, R. D., et al. Crofelemer, a novel agent for treatment of secretory diarrhea. *Ann Pharmacother* 44, no. 5 (2010): 878–84.

da Silva, S. N. P. Nanoencapsulation of usnic acid: an attempt to improve antitumor activity and reduce hepatoxicity. *Eur J Pharm Biopharm* 64, no. 2 (2006): 154–60.

DalBó, S., et al. Activation of endothelial nitric oxide synthase by proanthocyanidin-rich fraction from *Croton celtidifolius* (Euphorbiaceae): involvement of extracellular calcium influx in rat thoracic aorta. *J Pharmacol Sci* 107, no. 2 (2008): 181–89.

De Carvalho, E. A., et al. Effect of usnic acid from the lichen *Cladonia substellata* on *Trypanosoma cruzi* in vitro: an ultrastructural study. *Micron* 36, no. 2 (2005): 155–61.

Dharmananda, Subhuti. Safety issues affecting herbs. Usnea: an herb used in Western and Chinese medicine. Institute for Traditional Medicine (Portland, Ore.). December 2003. http://itmonline.org/arts/usnea.htm.

Dobrescu, D. Contributions to the complex study of some lichens–*Usnea* genus. Pharmacological studies on *Usnea barbata* and *Usnea hirta* species. *Rom J Physiol* 30, no. 1–2 (1993): 101–7.

Dugour, M., et al. Development of a method to quantify in vitro the synergistic activity of "natural" antimicrobials. *Int J Food Microbiol* 85, no. 3 (2003): 249–58.

Durazo, F. A., et al. Fulminant liver failure due to usnic acid for weight loss. *Am J Gastroenterol* 99, no. 5 (2004): 950–52.

Einarsdóttir, E., et al. Cellular mechanisms of the anticancer effects of the lichen compound usnic acid. *Planta Med* 76, no. 10 (2010): 969–74.

Engel, K., et al. *Usnea barbata* extract prevents ultraviolet-B induced prostaglandin E2 synthesis and COX-2 expression in HaCaT keratinocytes. *J Photochem Photobiol* 89, no. 1 (2007): 9–14.

Faustova, N. M., et al. Antibacterial activity of aspen bark extracts against some pneumotropic microorganisms. *Zh Mikrobiol Epidemiol Immunobiol* 3 (2006): 3–7.

Feng, J., et al. New dibenzofuran and anthraquinone from *Usnea longissima*. *Zhongguo Zhong Yao Za Zhi* 34, no. 7 (2009): 852–53.

Feng, J., et al. Studies on chemical constituents from herbs of *Usnea longissima*. *Zhongguo Zhong Yao Za Zhi* 34, no. 6 (2009): 708–11.

Fisher, K., et al. The effect of lemon, orange and bergamot essential oils and their components on the survival of *Campylobacter jejuni*, *Escherichia coli* O157, *Listeria monocytogenes*, *Bacillus cereus* and *Staphylococcus aureus* in vitro and in food systems. *J Appl Microbiol* 101, no. 6 (2006): 1232–40.

Foti, R. S., et al. Metabolism and related human risk factors for hepatic damage by usnic acid containing nutritional supplements. *Xenobiotica* 38, no. 3 (2008): 264–80.

Francolini, I., et al. Usnic acid, a natural antimicrobial agent able to inhibit bacterial biofilm formation on polymer surfaces. *Antimicrob Agents Chemother* 48, no. 11 (2004): 4360–65.

Frankos, V. H. *NTP nomination for usnic acid and Usnea barbata herb.* U.S. Food and Drug Administration Division of Dietary Supplement Programs, January 2005. http://ntp.niehs.nih.gov/ntp/htdocs/Chem_Background/ExSumPdf/UsnicAcid.pdf.

Frederich, M., et al. Potential antimalarial activity of indole alkaloids. *Trans Royal Soc Trop Med Hyg* 102 (2008): 11–19.

Gangoué-Piéboji, J., et al. The in-vitro antimicrobial activity of some medicinal plants against beta-lactam-resistant bacteria. *J Infect Dev Ctries* 3, no. 9 (2009): 671–80.

Gauslaa, Y., et al. Size-dependent growth of two old-growth associated macrolichen species. *New Phytol* 181, no. 3 (2009): 683–92.

Gibbons, S. Phytochemicals for bacterial resistance—strengths, weaknesses and opportunities. *Planta Med* 74, no. 6 (2008): 594–602.

Gonçalves, F. A., et al. Antibacterial activity of guava, *Psidium guajava* Linnaeus, leaf extracts on diarrhea-causing enteric bacteria isolated from Seabob shrimp, *Xiphopenaeus kroyeri* (Heller). *Rev Inst Med Trop Sao Paulo* 50, no. 1 (2008): 11–15.

Graz, B., et al. *Argemone mexicana* decoction versus artesunate-amodiaquine for the management of malaria in Mali: policy and public-health implications. *Trans R Soc Trop Med Hyg* 104, no. 1 (2010): 33–41.

Guevara, J. M., et al. The in vitro action of plants on *Vibrio cholerae*. *Rev Gastroenterol Peru* 14, no. 1 (1994): 27–31.

Guo, L., et al. Review of usnic acid and *Usnea barbata* toxicity. *J Environ Sci Health C Environ Carcinog Ecotoxicol Rev* 26, no. 4 (2008): 317–38.

Halici, M., et al. Effects of water extract of *Usnea longissima* on antioxidant enzyme activity and mucosal damage caused by indomethacin in rats. *Phytomedicine* 12, no. 9 (2005): 656–62.

Han, D., et al. Usnic acid-induced necrosis of cultured mouse hepatocytes: inhibition of mitochondrial function and oxidative stress. *Biochem Pharmacol* 67, no. 3 (2004): 439–51.

He, X., et al. Anti-mutagenic lichen extract has double-edged effect on azoxymethane-induced colorectal oncogenesis in C57BL/6J mice. *Toxicol Mech Methods* 20, no. 1 (2010): 31–35.

Honda, N. K., et al. Antimycobacterial activity of lichen substances. *Phytomedicine* 17, no. 5 (2010): 328–32.

Hör, M., et al. Inhibition of intestinal chloride secretion by proanthocyanidins from *Guazuma ulmifolia*. *Planta Med* 61, no. 3 (1995): 208–12.

Hsu, L. M., et al. "Fat burner" herb, usnic acid, induced acute hepatitis in a family. *J Gastroenterol Hepatol* 20, no. 7 (2005): 1138–39.

Ji, X. Quantitative determination of usnic acid in *Usnea* lichen and its products by reversed-phase liquid chromatography with photodiode array detector. *J AOAC* 88, no. 5 (2005): 1256–58.

Jin, J. Q., et al. Down-regulatory effect of usnic acid on nuclear factor-kappaB-dependent tumor necrosis factor-alpha and inducible nitric oxide synthase expression in lipopolysaccharide-stimulated macrophages. *Phytother Res* 22, no. 12 (2008): 1605–9.

Jin, J., et al. The study on skin wound healing promoting action of sodium usnic acid. *Zhong Yao Cai* 28, no. 2 (2005): 109–11.

Kathirgamanathar, S., et al. Beta-orcinol depsidones from the lichen *Usnea* sp. from Sri Lanka. *Nat Prod Res* 19, no. 7 (2005): 695–701.

Kaur, K., et al. Antimalarials from nature. *Bioorg Med Chem* 17, no. 9 (2009): 3229–56.

Knight, K. P., et al. Influence of cinnamon and clove essential oil on the D- and z-values of *Escherichia coli* O157:H7 in apple cider. *J Food Prod* 70, no. 9 (2007): 2089–94.

Koparal, A. T., et al. In vitro cytotoxic activities of (+)-usnic acid and (-)-usnic acid on V79, A549, and human lymphocyte cells and their non-genotoxicity on human lymphocytes. *Nat Prod Res* 20, no. 14 (2006): 1300–1307.

Kristinsson, K. G., et al. Effective treatment of experimental acute otitis media by application of volatile fluids into the ear canal. *J Infect Dis* 191, no. 11 (2005): 1876–80.

Lee, J. A., et al. Effect of (+)-usnic acid on mitochondrial functions as measured by mitochondria-specific oligonucleotide microarray in liver of B6CF1 mice. *Mitochondrion* 9, no. 2 (2009): 149–58.

Lee, K. A., et al. Antiplatelet and antithrombotic activities of methanol extract of *Usnea longissima*. *Phytother Res* 19, no. 12 (2005): 1061–64.

Léon, I., et al. Pentasaccharide glycosides from the roots of *Ipomoea murucoides*. *J Nat Prod* 68, no. 8 (2005): 1141–46.

Leonard, D. B. Medicine at your feet: plants and food: *Usnea* spp. On the website of Medicine at Your Feet, produced by David Bruce Leonard, L.Ac. http://medicineatyourfeet.com/usneaspp.html (accessed January 21, 2011).

Lewis, K. In search of natural substrates and inhibitors of MDR pumps. *J Mol Microbiol Biotechnol* 3, no. 2 (2001): 247–54.

Lohézic,-Le, D. F., et al. Stictic acid derivatives from the lichen *Usnea articulata* and their antioxidant activities. *J Nat Prod* 70, no. 7 (2007): 1218–20.

Lounasmaa, M., et al. Simple indole alkaloids and those with a nonrearranged monoterpenoid unit. *Nat Prod Rep* 17 (2000): 175–91.

Madamombe, I. T., et al. Evaluation of antimicrobial activity of extracts from South African *Usnea barbata*. *Pharm Bio* 41, no. 3 (2003): 199–202.

Marcano, V., et al. Occurrence of usnic acid in *Usnea laevis* Nylander (lichenized ascomycetes) from the Venezuelan Andes. *J Ethnopharmacol* 66, no. 3 (1999): 343–46.

Mathabe, M. C., et al. Antibacterial activities of medicinal plants used for the treatment of diarrhoea in Limpopo Province, South Africa. *J Ethnopharmacol* 105, no. 1–2 (2006): 286–93.

Mayer, M., et al. Usnic acid: a non-genotoxic compound with anti-cancer properties. *Anticancer Drugs* 16, no. 8 (2005): 805–9.

Morinaga, N., et al. Differential activities of plant polyphenols on the binding and internalization of cholera toxin in vero cells. *J Biol Chem* 280, no. 24 (2005): 23303–9.

Muñoz-Ochoa, M., et al. Screening of extracts of algae from Baja California sur, Mexico as reversers of the antibiotic resistance of some pathogenic bacteria. *Eur Rev Med Pharmacol Sci* 14, no. 9 (2010): 739–47.

Nagy, Maria M. Quorum sensing inhibitory activities of various folk-medicinal plants and the thyme-tetracycline effect. PhD diss., Georgia State University, December 14, 2010. http://digitalarchive.gsu.edu/biology_diss/90.

Neff, G. W., et al. Severe hepatotoxicity associated with the use of weight loss diet supplements containing ma huang or usnic acid. *J Hepatol* 41, no. 6 (2004): 1062–64.

Nishikawa, Y., et al. Studies on the water soluble constituents of lichens. II. Antitumor polysaccharides of *Lasallia, Usnea*, and *Cladonia* species. *Chem Pharm Bull* (Tokyo) 22, no. 11 (1974): 2692–702.

Nybakken, L., et al. Forest successional stage affects the cortical secondary chemistry of three old forest lichens. *J Chem Ecol* 33, no. 8 (2007): 1607–18.

O'Neill, M. A., et al. Does usnic acid affect microtubules in human cancer cells? *Braz J Biol* 70, no. 3 (2010): 659–64.

Odabasoglu, F., et al. Comparison of antioxidant activity and phenolic content of three lichen species. *Phytother Res* 18, no. 11 (2004): 938–41.

Odabasoglu, F., et al. Gastroprotective and antioxidant effects of usnic acid on indomethacin-induced gastric ulcer in rats. *J Ethnopharmacol* 103, no. 1 (2006): 59–65.

Ofuji, K., et al. Effects of an antidiarrhoeica containing an extract from geranium herb on astringent action and short-circuit current across jejunal mucosa. *Nippon Yakurigaku Zasshi* 111, no. 4 (1998): 265–75.

Oi, H., et al. Identification in traditional herbal medications and confirmation by synthesis of factors that inhibit cholera toxin-induced fluid accumulation. *Proc Natl Acad Sci USA* 99, no. 5 (2002): 3042–46.

Okuyama, E., et al. Usnic acid and diffractaic acid as analgesic and antipyretic components of *Usnea diffracta*. *Planta Med* 61, no. 2 (1995): 113–15.

Oliveira, A. B., et al. Plant-derived antimalarial agents: new leads and efficient phytomedicines. *An Acad Bras Cienc* 81, no. 4 (2009): 716–40.

Ordoñez, A. A., et al. Design and quality control of pharmaceutical formulation containing natural products with antibacterial, antifungal and antioxidant properties. *Int J Pharm* 378, no. 1–2 (2009): 51–58.

Otniukova, T. N., et al. Lichens on branches of Siberian fir (*Abies sibirica* Ladeb) as indicators of atmospheric pollution in forests. *Izv Akad Nauk Ser Biol* 4 (2008): 479–90.

Oussalah, M., et al. Mechanism of action of Spanish oregano, Chinese cinnamon, and savory essential oils against cell membranes and walls of *Escherichia coli* O157:H7 and *Listeria monocytogenes*. *J Food Prod* 69, no. 5 (2006): 1046–55.

Palaniappan, K., et al. Use of natural antimicrobials to increase antibiotic susceptibility of drug resistant bacteria. *Int J Food Microbiol* 140, no. 2–3 (2010): 164–68.

Paranagama, P. A., et al. Heptaketides from *Corynespora* sp. inhabitating the cavern beard lichen, *Usnea cavernosa*: first report of metabolites of an endolichenic fungus. *J Nat Prod* 70, no. 11 (2007): 1700–1705.

Pereda-Miranda, R., et al. Polyacylated oligosaccharides from medicinal Mexican morning glory species as antibacterials and inhibitors of multidrug resistance in *Staphylococcus aureus*. *J Nat Prod* 69, no. 3 (2006): 406–9.

Periera, E. C., et al. Analysis of *Usnea fasciata* crude extracts with antineoplastic activity. *Tokai J Exp Clin Med* 19, no. 1–2 (1994): 47–52.

Plouzek, C. A., et al. Inhibition of P-glycoprotein activity and reversal of multidrug resistance in vitro by rosemary extract. *Eur J Cancer* 35, no. 10 (1999): 1541–45.

Pramyothin, P., et al. Hepatotoxic effect of (+) usnic acid from *Usnea siamensis* Wainio in rats, isolated rat hepatocytes and isolated rat liver mitochondria. *J Ethnopharmacol* 90, no. 2–3 (2004): 381–87.

Preuss, H. G., et al. Minimum inhibitory concentrations of herbal essential oils and monolaurin for Gram-positive and Gram-negative bacteria. *Mol Cell Biochem* 272, no. 1–2 (2005): 29–34.

Rahim, N., et al. Antibacterial activity of *Psidium guajava* leaf and bark against multidrug-resistant *Vibrio cholerae*: implication for cholera control. *Jpn J Infect Dis* 63, no. 4 (2010): 271–74.

Rezanka, T., et al. Hirtusneanoside, an unsymmetrical dimeric tetrahydroxanthone from the lichen *Usnea hirta*. *J Nat Prod* 70, no. 9 (2007): 1487–91.

Ribeiro-Costa, R. M., et al. In vitro and in vivo properties of usnic acid encapsulated into PLGA-microspheres. *J Microencapsul* 21, no. 4 (2004): 371–84.

Rukayadi, Y., et al. Screening of Thai medicinal plants for anticandidal activity. *Mycoses* 51, no. 4 (2008): 308–12.

Saenz, M. T., et al. Antimicrobial activity and phytochemical studies of some lichens from south of Spain. *Fitoterapia* 77, no. 3 (2006): 156–59.

Safak, B., et al. In vitro anti-*Helicobacter pylori* activity of usnic acid. *Phytother Res* 23, no. 7 (2009): 955–57.

Salari, M. H., et al. Antibacterial effects of *Eucalyptus globulus* leaf extract on pathological bacteria isolated from specimens of patients with respiratory tract disorders. *Clin Microbiol Infect* 12, no. 2 (2006): 194–96.

Sánchez, E., et al. Extracts of edible and medicinal plants damage membranes of *Vibrio cholerae*. *Appl Environ Microbiol* 76, no. 20 (2010): 6888–94.

Sanchez, W., et al. Severe hepatotoxicity associated with use of a dietary supplement containing usnic acid. *Mayo Clin Proc* 81, no. 4 (2006): 541–44.

Santiesteban-López, A., et al. Susceptibility of food-borne bacteria to binary combinations of antimicrobials at selected a(w) and pH. *J Appl Microbiol* 102, no. 2 (2007): 486–97.

Sarac, N., et al. Antimicrobial activities of the essential oils of *Origanum onites* L., *Origanum vulgare* L. subspecies *hirtum* (Link) Ietswaart, *Satureja thymbra* L., and *Thymus cilicicus* Boiss. & Bal. growing wild in Turkey. *J Med Food* 11, no. 3 (2008): 568–73.

Saxena, S., et al. Antimalarial agents from plant sources. *Current Science* 85, no. 9 (2003): 1314–29.

Schmeda-Hirschmann, G., et al. A new antifungal and antiprotozoal depside from the Andean lichen *Protousnea poeppigii*. *Phytother Res* 22, no. 3 (2008): 349–55.

Sharma, A., et al. Antibacterial activity of medicinal plants against pathogens causing complicated urinary tract infections. *Indian J Pharm Sci* 71, no. 2 (2009): 136–39.

Sharma, A., et al. Vibriocidal activity of certain medicinal plants used in Indian folklore medicine by tribals of Mahakoshal region of central India. *Indian J Pharmacol* 41, no. 3 (2009): 129–33.

Spelman, K., et al. Modulation of cytokine expression by traditional medicines: a review of herbal immunomodulators. *Altern Med Rev* 11, no. 2 (2006): 128–50.

Stavri, M., et al. Bacterial efflux pump inhibitors from natural sources. *J Antimicrob Chemother* 59, no. 6 (2007): 1247–60.

Stermitz, F. R., et al. Polyacylated neohesperidosides from *Geranium caespitosum*: bacterial multidrug resistance pump inhibitors. *Bioorg Med Chem Lett* 13, no. 11 (2003): 1915–18.

Tay, T., et al. Evaluation of the antimicrobial activity of the acetone extract of the lichen *Ramalina farinacea* and its (+)-usnic acid, norstictic acid, and protocetraric acid constituents. *Z Naturforsch C* 59, no. 5–6 (2004): 384–88.

Tegos, G., et al. Multidrug pump inhibitors uncover remarkable activity of plant antimicrobials. *Antimicrob Agents Chemother* 46, no. 10 (2002): 3133–41.

Thakurta, P., et al. Antibacterial, antisecretory and antihemorrhagic activity of *Azadirachta indica* used to treat cholera and diarrhea in India. *J Ethnopharmacol* 111, no. 3 (2007): 607–12.

Velázquez, C., et al. Antisecretory activity of plants used to treat gastrointestinal disorders in Mexico. *J Ethnopharmacol* 103, no. 1 (2006): 66–70.

Vijayakumar, C. S., et al. Anti-inflammatory activity of (+)-usnic acid. *Fitoterapia* 71, no. 5 (2000): 564–66.

Voravuthikunchai, S. P., et al. Medicinal plant extracts as anti-*Escherichia coli* O157:H7 agents and their effects on bacterial cell aggregation. *J Food Prot* 69, no. 10 (2006): 2336–41.

Willcox, M. L., et al. Traditional herbal medicines for malaria. *BMJ* 329 (2004): 1156–59.

Wongsamitkul, N., et al. A plant-derived hydrolysable tannin inhibits CFTR chloride channel: a potential treatment of diarrhea. *Pharm Res* 27, no. 3 (2010): 490–97.

Yoshino, N., et al. Co-administration of cholera toxin and apple polyphenol extracts as a novel and safe mucosal adjuvant strategy. *Vaccine* 27, no. 35 (2009): 4808–17.

Zampini, I. C., et al. Antibacterial activity of *Zuccagnia* Cav. ethanolic extracts. *J Ethnopharmacol* 102, no. 3 (2005): 450–56.

Alchornea

Abo, K. A., et al. Antimicrobial screening of *Bridelia micrantha, Alchornea cordifolia* and *Boerhavia diffusa*. *Afr J Med Med Sci* 28, no. 3–4 (1999): 167–69.

Adedapo, A. A., et al. Effects of some plants of the spurge family on haematological and biochemical parameters in rats. *Vet Arhiv* 77, no. 1 (2007): 29–38.

Adeshina, G. O., et al. Pharmacognostic studies of the leaf of *Alchornea cordifolia* (Euphorbiaceae) found in Abuja. *Nigerian J Pharma Sci* 7, no. 1 (2008): 29–35.

Adeshina, G. O., et al. Phytochemical and antimicrobial studies of the ethyl acetate extract of *Alchornea cordifolia* leaf found in Abuja, Nigeria. *J Med Plants Res* 4, no. 8 (2010): 649–58.

Adewunmi, C. O., et al. Ethno-veterinary medicine: screenings of Nigerian medicinal plants for trypanocidal properties. *J Ethnopharmacol* 77, no. 1 (2001): 19–24.

Agbor, G. A., et al. Medicinal plants can be good source of antioxidants: case study in Cameroon. *Pakistan J Biol Sci* 10, no. 4 (2007): 537–44.

Agbor, K., et al. The antidiarrhoeal activity of *Alchornea cordifolia* leaf extract, *Phytother Res* 18, no. 11 (2004): 873–76.

Akoachere, J. F., et al. Antibacterial effect of *Zingiber officinale* and *Garcinia kola* on respiratory tract pathogens. *East Afr Med J* 79, no. 11 (2002): 588–92.

Al-Waili, N. S. Investigating the antimicrobial activity of natural honey and its effects on the pathogenic bacterial infections of surgical wounds and conjunctiva. *J Med Fosod* 7, no. 2 (2004): 210–22.

Anonymous. Agriculture ministry asked to review "hazardous" herb listing. MCOT.net (Thailand), February 18, 2009. http://enews.mcot.net/view.php?id=8668.

Anonymous. Falciparum malaria: New findings from University of Antwerp in the area of falciparum malaria published. *Malaria Weekly*, April 28, 2008. http://newsrx.com/newsletters/Malaria-Weekly/2008-04-28/26042820083MW.html.

Ayisi, N. K., et al. Comparative in vitro effects of AZT and extracts of *Ocimum gratissimum, Ficus polita, Clausena anistata, Alchornea cordifolia,* and *Elaeophorbia drupifera* against HIV-1 and HIV-2 infections. *Antiviral Res* 58, no. 1 (2003): 25–33.

Banzouzi, J. T., et al. In vitro antiplasmodial activity of extracts of *Alchornea cordifolia* and identification of an active constituent: ellagic acid. *J Ethnopharmacol* 81, no. 3 (2002): 399–401.

Bayor, M. T., et al. *Alchornea cordifolia* (Euphorbiaceae), the major constituent of antiasthmatic herbal formulations. *J Ghana Sci Assoc* 10, no. 2 (2008): 1.

Bum, E. N., et al. Validation of anticonvulsant and sedative activity of six medicinal plants. *Epilepsy Behav* 14, no. 3 (2009): 454–58.

Ebi, G. C. Antimicrobial activities of *Alchornea cordifolia*. *Filoterapia* 72, no. 1 (2001): 69–72.

Eliakim-Ikechukwu, C. F., et al. Histological changes in the pancreas following administration of ethanolic extract of *Alchornea cordifolia* leaf in alloxan-induced diabetic wistar rats. *Niger J Physiol Sci* 24, no. 2 (2009): 153–55.

Eliakim-Ikechukwu, C. F., et al. The effect of aqueous ethanolic extract of *Alchornea cordifolia* leaf on the histology of the aorta of Wistar rats. *Niger J Physiol Sci* 24, no. 2 (2009): 149–51.

Farombi, E. O. African indigenous plants with chemotherapeutic potentials and biotechnology approach to the production of bioactive prophylactic agents. *Afr J Biotechnol* 2, no. 12 (2003): 662–71.

Farombi, E. O., et al. Antioxidant properties of extracts from *Alchornea laxiflora* (Benth) Pax and Hoffman. *Phytother Res* 17, no. 7 (2003): 713–16.

Gatsing, D., et al. Antibacterial activity, bioavailability and acute toxicity evaluation of the leaf extract of *Alchornea cordifolia* (Euphorbiaceae). *Int J Pharmacol* 6, no. 3 (2010): 173–82.

Guédé, N. Z., et al. Ethnopharmacological study of plants used to treat malaria, in traditional medicine, by Bete populations of Issia (Côte d'Ivoire). *J Pharm Sci & Res* 2, no. 4 (2010): 216–27.

Igbeneghu, O. A., et al. A study of the in vivo activity of the leaf extract of *Alchornea cordifolia* against multiply antibiotic resistant *S. aureus* isolates in mice. *Phytother Res* 21, no. 1 (2007): 67–71.

Ismaila, O., et al. Evaluation of antistress potential and phytochemical constituents of aqueous root extract of *Alchornea cordifolia. Asian J Sci Res* 1, no. 4 (2008): 476–80.

Kleiman, R., et al. *Alchornea cordifolia* seed oil: a rich source of a new C20 epoxide, (+)cis-14, 15-epoxy-cis-11-eicosenoic acid. *Lipids* 12, no. 7 (1977): 610–12.

Kouakou-Siransy, G., et al. Effects of *Alchornea cordifolia* on elastase and superoxide anion produced by human neutrophils. *Pharm Biol* 48, no. 2 (2010): 128–33.

Manga, H. M., et al. In vivo anti-inflammatory activity of *Alchornea cordifolia* (Schumach. & Thonn.) Müll. Arg. (Euphorbiaceae). *J Ethnopharmacol* 92, no. 2–3 (2004): 209–14.

Mavar-Manga, H., et al. *Alchornea cordifolia* (Schumach. & Thonn.) Müll. Arg. *Prota* 11, no. 1 (2007): 1–10.

Mavar-Manga, H., et al. Anti-inflammatory compounds from leaves and root bark of *Alchornea cordifolia* (Schumach. & Thonn.) Müll. Arg. *J Ethnopharmacol* 115, no. 1 (2008): 25–29.

Mavar-Manga, H., et al. N1, N2, N3-trisisopentenyl guanidine and N1, N2-dilsopentenyl guanidine, two cytotoxic alkaloids from *Alchornea cordifolia* (Schumach. & Thonn.) Müll. Arg. (Euphorbiaceae) root barks. *Nat Prod Commun* 1, no. 12 (2006): 1097–100.

Mesia, G. K., et al. Antiprotozoal and cytotoxic screening of 45 plant extracts from Democratic Republic of Congo. *J Ethnopharmacol* 115, no. 3 (2008): 409–15.

Moshi, M. J., et al. The ethnomedicine of the Haya people of Bugabo Ward, Kagera Region, north western Tanzania. *J Ethnobiol Ethnomed* 5 (2009): 24.

Mpiana, P. T., et al. In vitro antidrepanocytary activity (anti-sickle cell anemia) of some Congolese plants. *Phytomedicine* 14, no. 2–3 (2007): 192–95.

Nworu, C. S., et al. Activation of murine lymphocytes and modulation of macrophage functions by fractions of *Alchornea cordifolia* (Euphorbiaceae) leaf extract. *Immunopharmacol Immunotoxicol* 32, no. 1 (2010): 28–36.

Ogundipe, O. O., et al. Bioactive chemical constituents from *Alchornea laxiflora* (Benth.) Pax and Hoffman. *J Ethnopharm* 74, no. 3 (2001): 275–80.

Ogundipe, O. O., et al. Biological activities of *Alchornea laxiflora* extractives. In *Standardization and utilization of herbal medicines: challenges of the 21st century*, 201–8. Proceedings of the 1st International Workshop on Herbal Medicine Products, Ibadan, Nigeria, November 22–24, 1998. Available from CAB Direct, http://cabdirect.org/abstracts/20043041503.html.

Okeke, I. N., et al. Antimicrobial spectrum of *Alchornea cordifolia* leaf extract. *Phytother Res* 13, no. 1 (1999): 67–69.

Okpuzor, J., et al. The potential of medicinal plants in sickle cell disease control: A review. *Int J Biomed Health Sci* 4, no. 2 (2008): 47.

Okwu, D. E., et al. Isolation, characterization and antibacterial activity screening of anthocyanidin glycosides from *Alchornea cordifolia* (Schumach. and Thonn.) Müll. Arg. leaves. *E-J Chem* 7, no. 1 (2010): 41–48.

Olaleye, M. T., et al. Acetaminophen-induced liver damage in mice: effects of some medicinal plants on the oxidative defense system. *Exp Toxicol Pathol* 59, no. 5 (2008): 319–27.

Olaleye, M. T., et al. Commonly used tropical medicinal plants exhibit distinct in vitro antioxidant activities against hepatotoxins in rat liver. *Exp Toxicol Pathol* 58, no. 6 (2007): 433–38.

Osadebe, P. O., et al. Anti-inflammatory effects of crude methanolic extract and fractions of *Alchornea cordifolia* leaves. *J Ethnopharmacol* 89, no. 1 (2003): 19–24.

Oyewale, A. O., et al. Cytotoxic correlation of some traditional medicinal plants using brine shrimp lethality test. *ChemClass J* 1 (2004): 110–12.

Pesewu, G. A., et al. Antibacterial activity of plants used in traditional medicines of Ghana with particular reference to MRSA. *J Ethnopharmacol* 116, no. 1 (2008): 102–11.

Soh, P. N., et al. In vitro and in vivo properties of ellagic acid in malaria treatment. *Antimicrob Agents Chemother* 53, no. 3 (2009): 1100–1106.

Tanaka, Y., et al. Antibacterial compounds of licorice against upper airway respiratory tract pathogens. *J Nutr Sci Vitaminol* (Tokyo) 47, no. 3 (2011): 270–73.

Tona, L., et al. Antiamoebic and phytochemical screening of some Congolese medicinal plants. *J Ethnopharmacol* 61, no. 1 (1998): 57–65.

Tona, L., et al. Antiamoebic and spasmolytic activities of extracts from some antidiarrhoeal traditional preparations used in Kinshasa, Congo. *Phytomedicine* 7, no. 1 (2000): 31–38.

Tona, L., et al. Biological screening of traditional preparations from some medicinal plants used as antidiarrhoeal in Kinshasa, Congo. *Phytomedicine* 6, no. 1 (1999): 59–66.

Umukoro, S., et al. Evaluation of the anti-stress and anticonvulsant activities of leaf extract of *Alchornea cordifolia* in mice. *J Ethnopharmacol* 127, no. 3 (2010): 768–70.

Artemisia

Abdul-Ghani, R., et al. Artemether shows promising female schizonticidal and ovicidal effects on the Egyptian strain of *Schistosoma mansoni* after maturity of infection. *Parasitol Res* 108, no. 5 (2011): 1199–205. E-pub (preprint) November 25, 2010.

Agarwal, S. P., et al. Determination of artemisinin in bulk and pharmaceutical dosage forms using HPTLC. *Indian J Pharm Sci* 71, no. 1 (2009): 98–100.

Aghajani, Z., et al. Composition and antimicrobial activity of the essential oil of *Artemisia kulbadica* from Iran. *Nat Prod Commun* 4, no. 9 (2009): 1261–66.

Ahameethunisa, A. R., et al. Antibacterial activity of *Artemisia nilagirica* leaf extracts against clinical and phytopathogenic bacteria. *BMC Complement Alt Medicine* 10, no. 6 (2010): 1–9.

Anamed. Artemesia annua *for the treatment of malaria.* A report for a workshop of the same name sponsored by Green Templeton College, anamed, and RITAM and organized by M. Willcox, et al., at Green Templeton College, Oxford, on March 13, 2010. http://www.anamed.net/world_anamed_groups/England_and_Scotland/Oxford_Artemisia_Workshop_Marc/oxford_artemisia_workshop_marc.html.

Anonymous. Artemisinin. Wikipedia. http://en.Wikipedia.org/wiki/Artemisinin (accessed January 16, 2011).

Anonymous. Research initiative on traditional antimalarial methods. Home page of the Research Initiative on Traditional Antimalarial Methods (RITAM). http://giftsofhealth.org/ritam/ (accessed January 17, 2011).

Anyasor, G. N., et al. Artesunate opens mitochondrial membrane permeability transition pore. *Annals Trop Med Pub Health* 2, no. 2 (2009): 37–41.

Arab, H. A., et al. Determination of artemisinin in *Artemisia sieberi* and anticoccidial effects of the plant extract in broiler chickens. *Trop Anim Health Prod* 38, no. 6 (2006): 497–503.

Arystan, L., et al. Experimental evaluation of the antibacterial and phagocytosis-stimulating properties of leucomisine. *Eksp Klin Farmakol* 72, no. 5 (2009): 35–37.

Ashton, M., et al. Artemisinin pharmacokinetics in healthy adults after 250, 500, and 100mg single oral doses. *Biopharm Drug Dispos* 19, no. 4 (1998): 245–50.

Ashton, M., et al. Artemisinin pharmacokinetics is time-dependent during repeated oral administrations in healthy male adults. *Drug Metab Dispos* 26, no. 1 (1998): 25–27.

Aydin-Schmift, B., et al. Carolus Linnaeus, the ash, worm-wood and other anti-malarial plants. *Scand J Infect Dis* 42, no. 11–12 (2010): 941–42.

Bavdekar, S. B., et al. Treatment of malaria in children. *J Postgrad Med* 42, no. 4 (1996): 115–20.

Berger, T. G., et al. Artesunate in the treatment of metastatic uveal melanoma—first experiences. *Oncol Rep* 14, no. 6 (2005): 1599–603.

Bhakuni, R. S., et al. Secondary metabolites of *Artemisia annua* and their biological activity. *Current Sci* 80, no. 1 (2001): 35–48.

Bilia, A. R., et al. Simple and rapid physico-chemical methods to examine action of antimalarial drugs with hemin: its application to *Artemesia annua* constituents. *Life Sci* 70, no. 7 (2002): 769–78.

Bilia, A. R., et al. Simultaneous analysis of artemisinin and flavonoids of several extracts of *Artemisia annua* L. obtained from a commercial sample and a selected cultivar. *Phytomedicine* 13, no. 7 (2006): 487–93.

Blanke, C. H., et al. Herba Artemisiae annuae tea preparation compared to sulfadoxine-pyrimethamine in the treatment of uncomplicated falciparum malaria in adults: a randomized double-blind clinical trial. *Trop Doct* 38, no. 2 (2008): 113–16.

Boareto, A. C., et al. Toxicity of artemisinin [*Artemisia annua* L.] in two different periods of pregnancy in Wistar rats. *Reprod Toxicol* 25, no. 2 (2008): 239–46.

Brown, G. D., et al. The biosynthesis of artemisinin (Qinghaosu) and the phytochemistry of *Artemisia annua* L. (Qinghao). *Molecules* 15, no. 11 (2010): 7603–98.

Castillo-Juarez, I., et al. Anti-*Helicobacter pylori* activity of plants used in Mexican traditional medicine for gastrointestinal disorders. *J Ethnopharmacol* 122, no. 2 (2009): 402–5.

Chang, H., et al. Antifungal activity of *Artemisia annua* endophyte cultures against phytopathogenic fungi. *J Biotechnol* 88, no. 3 (2001): 277–82.

Chen, C. P., et al. Screening of Taiwanese crude drugs for antibacterial activity against *Streptococcus mutans. J Ethnopharmacol* 27, no. 3 (1989): 285–95.

Cho, S. H., et al. Growth-inhibiting effects of seco-tanapartholides identified in *Artemisia princeps* var. *orientalis* whole plant on human intestinal bacteria. *J Appl Microbiol* 95, no. 1 (2003): 7–12.

Chung, E. Y., et al. Antibacterial effects of vulgarone B from *Artemisia iwayomogi* alone and in combination with oxacillin. *Arch Pharm Res* 32, no. 12 (2009): 1711–19.

Clark, R. L. Embryotoxicity of the artemisinin antimalarials and potential consequences for the use in women in the first trimester. *Reprod Toxicol* 28, no. 3 (2009): 285–96.

Connelly, Patrice. Horrible weed or miracle herb? A review of *Bidens pilosa. J Australian Trad Med* 15, no. 2 (2009): 77–79.

Darwish, R. M., et al. Effect of ethnomedicinal plants in folklore medicine in Jordan as antibiotic resistant inhibitors on *Escherichia coli. BMC Complement Altern Med* 10 (2010): 9.

de Ridder, S., et al. *Artemisia annua* as a self-reliant treatment for malaria in developing countries. *J Ethnopharmacol* 120, no. 3 (2008): 302–14.

De Vries, P. J., et al. The pharmacokinetics of a single dose of artemisinin in patients with uncomplicated falciparum malaria. *Am J Trop Med Hyg* 56, no. 5 (1997): 503–7.

Duc, D. D., et al. The pharmacokinetics of a single dose of artemisinin in healthy Vietnamese subjects. *Am J Trop Med Hyg* 51, no. 6 (1994): 785–90.

Efferth, T., et al. The antiviral activities of artemisinin and artesunate. *Clin Infect Dis* 47, no. 6 (2008): 804–11.

Efferth, T., et al. Toxicity of the antimalarial artemisinin and its derivitives. *Crit Rev Toxicol* 40, no. 5 (2010): 405–21.

Ene, A. C., et al. Antitrypanosomal effects of petroleum ether, chloroform and methanol extracts of *Artemisia maciverae* Linn. *Indian J Exp Biol* 47, no. 12 (2009): 981–86.

Ene, A. C., et al. Bioassay-guided fractionation and in vivo antiplasmodial effect of fractions of chloroform extract of *Artemisia maciverae* Linn. *Acta Trop* 112, no. 3 (2009): 288–94.

Esfandiari, B., et al. In vivo evaluation of anti-parasitic effects of *Artemisia absinthium* extracts on *Syphacia* parasite. *Internet J Parasit Dis* 2, no. 2 (2007) http://www.ispub.com/journal/the-internet-journal-of-parasitic-diseases/volume-2-number-2/in-vivo-evaluation-of-anti-parasitic-effects-of-artemisia-absinthium-extracts-on-syphacia-parasite.html.

Esimone, C. O., et al. In vitro antimicrobial interactions of arthemeter with some 4-quinolones. *Boll Chim Farm* 141, no. 5 (2002): 385–88.

Ferreira, J. F., et al. Drying affects artemisinin, dihydroartemisinic acid, and the antioxidant capacity of *Artemisia annua* L. leaves. *J Agric Food Chem* 58, no. 3 (2010): 1691–98.

Ferreira, J. F., et al. Flavonoids from *Artemisia annua* L. as antioxidants and their potential synergism with artemisinin against malaria and cancer. *Molecules* 15, no. 5 (2010): 3135–70.

Ferriera, Jorge F. S. Nutrient deficiency in the production of artemisinin, dihydroartemisinic acid, and artemisinic acid in *Artemisia annua* L. *J Agric Food Chem* 55, no. 5 (2007): 1686–94.

Gomes, M., et al. Rectal artemisinins for malaria: a review of efficacy and safety from individual patient data in clinical studies. *BMC Infect Dis* 8 (2008): 39.

Guonggrong, H., et al. Antioxidative and antibacterial activity of the methanol extract of *Artemisia anomala* S. Moore. *Afr J Biotechnol* 7, no. 9 (2008): 1335–38.

Gupta, P. C., et al. In vitro antibacterial activity of *Artemisia annua* Linn. growing in India. *Int J Green Pharm* 3, no. 3 (2009): 255–58.

Hayat, M. Q., et al. Palynological study of the genus *Artemisia* (Asteraceae) and its systematic implications. *P J Bot* 42, no. 2 (2010): 751–63.

Haynes, R. K., et al. Extraction of artemisinin and artemisinic acid: preparation of artemether and new analogues. *Trans R Soc Trop Med Hyg* 88, suppl. 1 (1994): S23–26.

Hong, J., et al. Suppression of the antigen-stimulated RBL-2H3 mast cell activation by artekeiskeanol A. *Planta Med* 75, no. 14 (2009): 1494–98.

Hsu, E. The history of qing hao in the Chinese material medica. *Trans R Soc Trop Med Hyg* 100, no. 6 (2006): 505–8.

Hussain, I., et al. Analysis of artemisinin in *Artemisia* species using high performance liquid chromatography. *World Applied Sci J* 10, no. 6 (2010): 632–36.

Juteau, F., et al. Antibacterial and antioxidant activities of *Artemisia annua* essential oil. *Fitoterapia* 73, no. 6 (2002): 532–35.

Kamchonwongpaisan, S., et al. Artemisian neurotoxicity: neuropathology in rats and mechanistic studies in vitro. *Am J Trop Med* 56, no. 1 (1997): 7–12.

Karunajeewa, H. A., et al. Artesunate suppositories versus intramuscular artemether for treatment of severe malaria in children in Papua New Guinea. *Antimicrob Agents Chemother* 50, no. 3 (2006): 968–74.

Kawazoe, K., et al. Sesquiterpenoids from *Artemisia gilvescens* and an anti-MRSA compound. *J Nat Prod* 66, no. 4 (2003): 538–39.

Kazemi, M., et al. Chemical composition and antimicrobial activity of *Artemisia tschernieviana* Besser from Iran. *Pharmacog Res* 1, no. 3 (2009): 120–24.

Keiser, J., et al. Effect of artemether, artesunate, OZ78, praziquantel, and tribendimidine alone or in combination chemotherapy on the tegument of *Clonorchis sinensis*. *Parasitol Int* 59, no. 3 (2010): 472–76.

Klayman, D. L. Qinghaosu (artemisinin): an antimalarial drug from China. *Science* 228, no. 4703 (1985): 1049–55.

Kordali, S., et al. Determination of the chemical composition and antioxidant activity of the essential oil of *Artemisia dracunculus* and of the antifungal and antibacterial activities of Turkish *Artemisia absinthium*, *A. dracunculus*, *Artemisia santonicum*, and *Artemisia spicigera* essential oils. *J Agric Food Chem* 53, no. 24 (2005): 9452–58.

Kurzhals, J. A., et al. Ineffective change of antimalaria prophylaxis to *Artemisia vulgaris* in a group travelling to West Africa. *Ugeskr Laeger* 167, no. 43 (2005): 4082–83.

Laciar, A., et al. Antibacterial and antioxidant activities of the essential oil of *Artemisia echegarayi* Hieron. (Asteraceae). *Revista argentina de microbiologia* (online) 41, no. 4 (2009): 226–31. http://www.scielo.org.ar/scielo.php?script=sci_arttext&pid=S0325-75412009000400006&lng=es&nrm=iso. ISSN 1851-7617.

Lee, S., et al. DA-9601 inhibits activation of the human mast cell line HMC-1 through inhibition of NF-kappaB. *Cell Biol Toxicol* 23, no. 2 (2007): 105–12.

Li, Q., et al. Toxicokinetic and toxicodynamic (TK/TD) evaluation to determine and predict the neurotoxicity of artemisinins. *Toxicology* 279, no. 1–3 (2011): 1–9.

Li, S., et al. Studies on prophylactic effect of artesunate on *Schistomiasis japonica*. *Chin Med J* (English) 109, no. 11 (1996): 848–53.

Lommen, W. J., et al. Artemisinin and sesquiterpene precursors in dead and green leaves of *Artemisia annua* L. crops. *Planta Med* 73, no. 10 (2007): 1133–39.

Lommen, W. J., et al. Trichome dynamics and artemisinin accumulation during development and senescence of *Artemisia annua* leaves. *Planta Med* 72, no. 4 (2006): 336–45.

Longo, M., et al. In vivo and in vitro investigations of the effects of the antimalarial drug dihydroartemisinin (DHA) on rat embryos. *Reprod Toxicol* 22, no. 4 (2006): 797–810.

Luo, H., et al. Antioxidant and antimicrobial capacity of Chinese medicinal herb extracts in raw sheep meat. *J Food Prot* 70, no. 6 (2007): 1440–45.

Mannan, A., et al. Hairy roots induction and artemisinin analysis in *Artemisia dubia* and *Artemisia indica*. *Afr J Biotechnol* 7, no. 18 (2008): 3288–92.

Mannan, A., et al. Survey of artemisinin production by diverse *Artemisia* species in northern Pakistan. *Malar J* 9 (2010): 310.

McGovern, P. E., et al. Anticancer activity of botanical compounds in ancient fermented beverages (review). *Int J Oncol* 37, no. 1 (2010): 5–14.

McGovern, P. E., et al. Fermented beverages of pre- and proto-historic China. *Proc Natl Acad Sci U.S.A* 101, no. 51 (2004): 17593–98.

Medhi, B., et al. Pharmacokinetics and toxicological profile of artemisinin compounds: an update. *Pharmacology* 84, no. 6 (2009): 323–32.

Min, S. W., et al. Inhibitory effect of eupatilin and jaceosidin from *Artemisia princeps* on carrageenan-induced inflammation in mice. *J Ethnopharmacol* 125, no. 3 (2009): 497–500.

Mueller, M. S., et al. The potential of *Artemisia annua* L. as a locally produced remedy for malaria in the tropics: agricultural, chemical and clinical aspects. *J Ethnopharmacol* 73, no. 3 (2000): 487–93.

Mueller, M. S., et al. Randomized controlled trial of a traditional preparation of *Artemesia annua* L. (annual wormwood) in the treatment of malaria. *Trans R Soc Trop Med Hyg* 98, no. 5 (2004): 318–21.

Nagai, A., et al. Growth-inhibitory effects of artesunate, pyrimethamine, and pamaquine against *Babesia equi* and *Babesia caballi* in in vitro cultures. *Antimicrob Agents Chemother* 47, no. 2 (2003): 800–803.

N'Goran, E. K., et al. Randomized, double-blind, placebo-controlled trial of oral artemether for the prevention of patent *Schistosoma haematobium* infections. *Am J Trop Med Hyg* 68, no. 1 (2003): 24–32.

Noedl, H., et al. Evidence of artemisinin-resistant malaria in western Cambodia. *N Eng J Med* 359, no. 24 (2008): 2619–20.

Ortet, R., et al. Sesquiterpene lactones from the endemic Cape Verdean *Artemisia gorgonum*. *Phytochemistry* 69, no. 17 (2008): 2961–65.

Panossian, L. A., et al. Toxic brainstem encephalopathy after artemisinin treatment for breast cancer. *Ann Neurolog* 59, no. 4 (2006): 725–26.

Phan, V. T., et al. Artemisinine and artesunate in the treatment of malaria in Vietnam (1984–1999). *Bull Soc Pathol Exot* 95, no. 2 (2002): 86–88.

Poiată, A., et al. Antibacterial activity of some *Artemisia* species extract. *Rev Med Chir Soc Med Nat Iasi* 113, no. 3 (2009): 911–14.

Rabe, T., et al. Antibacterial activity of South African plants used for medicinal purposes. *J Ethnopharmacol* 56, no. 1 (1997): 81–87.

Ramazani, A., et al. In vitro antiplasmodial and phytochemical study of five *Artemisia* species from Iran and in vivo activity of two species. *Parasitol Res* 107, no. 3 (2010): 593–99.

Ramirez, C. Antibacterial action of non-volatile substances extracted from *Artemisia tridentata* Nutt. ssp. *tridentata*. *Can J Microbiol* 15, no. 11 (1969): 1341.

Räth, K., et al. Pharmacokinetic study of artemisinin after oral intake of a traditional preparation of *Artemisia annua* L. (annual wormwood). *Am J Trop Med Hyg* 70, no. 2 (2004): 128–32.

Romero, M. R., et al. Antiviral effect of artemisinin from *Artemisia annua* against a model member of the Flaviviridae family, the bovine viral diarrhoea virus (BVDV). *Planta Med* 72, no. 13 (2006): 1169–74.

Romero, M. R., et al. Effect of artemisinin/ artesunate as inhibitors of hepatitis B virus production in an "in vitro" replicative system. *Antiviral Res* 68, no. 2 (2005): 75–83.

Rowen, Robert J. Artemisinin: from malaria to cancer treatment. *Townsend Letter* 91 (1995): 41–46.

Rustaiyan, Abdolhossein. A new antimalarial agent, effect of extracts of *Artemisia diffusa* against *Plasmodium berghei*. *Pharmacog Mag* 5, no. 17 (2009): 1–7.

Seddik, K., et al. Antioxidant and antibacterial activities of extracts from *Artemisia herba-alba* Asso. leaves and some phenolic compounds. *J Med Plants Res* 4, no. 13 (2010): 1273–80.

Shahverdi, A. R., et al. A TLC bioautographic assay for the detection of nitrofurantoin resistance reversal compound. *J Chromatograph B* 850, no. 1–2 (2007): 528–30.

Sherif, H., et al. Drugs, insecticides and other agents from *Artemisia*. *Med Hypotheses* 23, no. 2 (1987): 187–93.

Shin, T. Y., et al. *Artemisia iwayomogi* inhibits immediate-type allergic reaction and inflammatory cytokine secretion. *Immunopharmacol immunotoxicol* 28, no. 3 (2006): 421–30.

Squires, J. M., et al. Effects of artemisinin and *Artemisia* extracts on *Haemonchus contortus* in gerbils (*Meriones unguiculatus*). *Vet Parasitol* 175, no. 1–2: 103–8. E-pub (preprint) September 16, 2010.

Stavri, M., et al. Bioactive constituents of *Artemisia monosperma*. *Phytochemistry* 66, no. 2 (2005): 233–39.

Stermitz, F. R., et al. Two flavonoids from *Artemisia annua* which potentiate the activity of berberine and norfloxacin against a resistant strain of *Staphylococcus aureus*. *Planta Med* 68, no. 12 (2002): 1140–41.

Tallet, S. M., et al. Antifungal leaf-surface metabolites correlate with fungal abundance in sagebrush populations. *J Chem Ecol* 28, no. 11 (2002): 2141–68.

Tan, R. X., et al. Biologically active substances from the genus *Artemisia*. *Planta Med* 64, no. 4 (1998): 295–302.

Tawfik, A. F., et al. Effects of artemisinin, dihydroartemisinin and arteether on immune responses of normal mice. *Int J Immunopharmacol* 12, no. 4 (1990): 385–89.

Tuescher, F., et al. Artemisinin-induced dormancy in *Plasmodium falciparum*: duration, recovery rates, and implications in treatment failure. *J Infect Dis* 202, no. 9 (2010): 1362–68.

Umano, K., et al. Volatile chemicals identified in extracts from leaves of Japanese mugwort (*Artemisia princeps* Pamp.). *J Agric Food Chem* 48, no. 8 (2000): 3463–69.

Utzinger, J., et al. Oral artemether for prevention of *Schistosoma mansoni* infection: randomised controlled trial. *Lancet* 355, no. 9212 (2000): 1320–25.

Valdéz, A. F.-C., et al. In vitro anti-microbial activity of the Cuban medicinal plants *Simarouba glauca* DC, *Melaleuca leucadedron* L and *Artemisia absinthium* L. *Mem Inst Oswaldo Cruz* (Rio de Janeiro) 103, no. 6 (2008): 615–18.

Valecha, N., et al. Artemisinin: current status in malaria. *Indian J Pharmacol* 29, no. 2 (1997): 71–75.

Valentini, P., et al. *Fighting malaria in Africa and Artemisia annua L. infusion*. Pamphlet for the 2nd International Conference organized by (Istituto Cooperazione Economica Internazionale) and Piattaforma Artemesia, in Rome, Italy, April 23, 2010. http://icei.info/attachments/VIATM/Artemisia_Depli_Inglese_web.pdf.

van Agtmael, M. A., et al. Artemisinin drugs in the treatment of malaria: from medicinal herb to registered medication. *Trends Pharmacol Sci* 20, no. 5 (1999): 199–205.

Van de Meersch, H. Review of the use of artemisinin and its derivatives in the treatment of malaria. *J Pharm Belg* 60, no. 1 (2005): 23–9; 60, no. 3 (2005): 103.

Vega, E. A., et al. Antimicrobial activity of *Artemisia douglasiana* and dehydroleucodine against *Helicobacter pylori*. *J Ethnopharmacol* 124, no. 3 (2009): 653–55.

Verdian-rizi, M. R. Chemical composition and antimicrobial activity of the essential oil of *Artemisia annua* L. from Iran. *J Med Plant* 1, no. 1 (2009): 21–24.

Wallaart, T. E., et al. Seasonal variation of artemisinin and its biosynthetic precursors in plants of *Artemisia annua* of different geographical origin: proof for the existence of chemotypes. *Planta Med* 66, no. 1 (2000): 57–62.

Wan, Y. D., et al. Studies on the antimalarial action of gelatin capsules of *Artemisia annua*. *Zhongguo Ji Sheng Chong Xue Yu Ji Sheng Chong Bing Za Zhi* 10, no. 4 (1992): 290–94.

Wang, Y. C., et al. Screening of anti-*Helicobacter pylori* herbs deriving from Taiwanese folk medicinal plants. *FEMS Immunol Med Microbiol* 43, no. 2 (2005): 295–300.

Wesche, D. L., et al. Neurotoxicity of artemisinin analogs in vitro. *Antimicrob Agents Chemother* 38, no. 8 (1994): 1813–19.

Willcox, M., et al. *Artemesia annua* as a herbal tea for malaria. *Afr J Tradit Complement Altern Med* 4, no. 1 (2007): 121–23.

Willcox, M., et al. *Artemesia annua* as a traditional herbal antimalarial. Chapter 3 in *Traditional Medicinal Plants and Malaria*, ed. M. Willcox, et al. Vol. 4 of Traditional Herbal Medicines for Modern Times. Boca Raton, Fla.: CRC Press, 2004. Available online from the Istituto Cooperazione Economica Internazionale at http://icei.info/attachments/VIATM/A_annua_as_a_traditional_herbal_antimalarial.pdf.

Willcox, M. L., et al. Is parasite clearance clinically important after malaria treatment in a high transmission area? A 3-month follow-up of home-based management with herbal medicine or ACT. *Trans R Soc Trop Med Hyg* 105, no. 1 (2011): 23–31.

Wootton, D. G., et al. Open-label comparative clinical study of chlorproguanil-dapsone fixed dose combination (Lapdap) alone or with three different doses of artesunate for uncomplicated *Plasmodium falciparum* malaria. *PLoS One* 3, no. 3 (2008): e1779.

Wright, C. W., et al. Ancient Chinese methods are remarkably effective for the preparation of artemisinin-rich extracts of qing hao with potent antimalarial activity. *Molecules* 15, no. 2 (2010): 804–12.

Wu, T. X., et al. Systematic review of benefits and harms of artemisinin-type compounds for preventing schistosomiasis. *Zhonghua Yi Xue Za Zhi* 83, no. 14 (2003): 1219–24.

Xiao, S., et al. Field studies on preventative effect of artemether against infection with *Schistosoma japonicum*. *Zhongguo Ji Sheng Chong Xue Yu Ji Sheng Chong Bing Za Zhi* 13, no. 3 (1995): 170–73.

Xiao, S., et al. Recent investigations of artemether, a novel agent for the prevention of schistosomiasis japonica, mansoni amd haematobia. *Acta Trop* 82, no. 2 (2002): 175–81.

Yashphe, J., et al. Antibacterial activity of *Artemisia herba-alba*. *J Pharm Sci* 68, no. 7 (1979): 924–25, 1979.

Zafar, M. M., et al. Screening of *Artemisia absinthium* for antimalarial effects on *Plasmodium berghei* in mice: a preliminary report. *J Ethnopharmacol* 30, no. 2 (1990): 223–26.

Zhang, Q. H., et al. Artemisia Zhuolu antibacterial activity of different ways to extract more. Free Papers Download Center, December 26, 2008. http://eng.hi138.com/?i120926.

Zheng, W. F., et al. Two flavonoids from *Artemisia giraldii* and their antimicrobial activity, *Planta Med* 62, no. 2 (1996): 160–62.

Zia, M., et al. Effect of growth regulators and amino acids on artemisinin production in the callus of *Artemisia absinthium*. *Pak J Bot* 39, no. 2 (2007): 799–805.

Ashwagandha

Aalinkeel, R., et al. Genomic analysis highlights the role of the JAK-STAT signaling in the anti-proliferative effects of dietary flavonoid "ashwagandha" in prostate cancer cells. *Evid Based Complement Alternat Med* 7, no. 2 (2010): 177–87. E-pub (preprint) January 10, 2008.

Agarwal, R., et al. Studies on immunomodulatory activity of *Withania somnifera* (ashwagandha) extracts in experimental immune inflammation. *J Ethnopharmacol* 67, no. 1 (1999): 27–35.

Ahmad, M., et al. Neuroprotective effects of *Withania somnifera* on 6-hydroxydopamine induced Parkinsonism in rats. *Hum Exp Toxicol* 24, no. 3 (2005): 137–47.

Ahmad, M. K. *Withania somnifera* improves semen quality by regulating reproductive hormone levels and oxidative stress in seminal plasma of infertile males. *Fertil Steril* 94, no. 3 (2010): 989–96.

Anonymous. Monograph. *Withania somnifera*. *Altern Med Rev* 9, no. 2 (2004): 211–14.

Anonymous. Role of ashwagandha in human health. On the website of Well Corps International. http://wellcorps.com/RoleOfAshwagandhaInHumanHealth.html (accessed February 8, 2012).

Archana, R., et al. Antistressor effect of *Withania somnifera*. *J Ethnopharmacol* 64, no. 1 (1999): 91–93.

Auddy, B., et al. A standardized *Withania somnifera* extract significantly reduces stress-related parameters in chronically stressed humans: a double-blind, randomized, placebo-controlled study. *JANA* 11, no. 1 (2008): 51–57.

Bani, S., et al. Selective Th1 up-regulating activity of *Withania somnifera* aqueous extract in an experimental system using flow cytometry. *J Ethnopharmacol* 107, no. 1 (2006): 107–15.

Bhat, J., et al. In vivo enhancement of natural killer cell activity through tea fortified with Ayurvedic herbs. *Phytother Res* 24, no. 1 (2010): 129–35.

Bhatnager, M., et al. Neuroprotective effects of *Withania somnifera* Dunal.: a possible mechanism. *Neurochem Res* 34, no. 11 (2009): 1975–83.

Bhattacharya, S. K., et al. Adaptogenic activity of *Withania somnifera*: an experimental study using rat model of chronic stress. *Pharmacol Biochem Behav* 75, no. 3 (2003): 547–55.

Chaudhary, G., et al. Evaluation of *Withania somnifera* in a middle cerebral artery occlusion model of stroke in rats. *Clin Exp Pharmacol Physiol* 30, no. 5–6 (2003): 399–404.

Davis, L., et al. Effect of *Withania somnifera* on cell mediated immune responses in mice. *J Exp Clin Cancer Res* 21, no. 4 (2002): 585–90.

Davis, L., et al. Suppressive effect of cyclophosphamide-induced toxicity by *Withania somnifera* extract in mice. *J Ethnopharmacol* 62, no. 3 (1998): 209–14.

Grandhi, A., et al. A comprehensive pharmacological investigation of ashwagandha and ginseng. *J Ethnopharmacol* 44, no. 3 (1994): 131–35.

Guatam, M., et al. Immune response modulation to DPT vaccine by aqueous extract of *Withania somnifera* in experimental system. *Int Immunopharmacol* 4, no. 6 (2004): 841–49.

Immanuel, G., et al. Dietary medicinal plant extracts improve growth, immune activity and survival of tilapia *Oreochromis mossambicus*. *J Fish Biol* 74, no. 7 (2009): 1462–75.

Jain, S., et al. Neuroprotective effects of *Withania somnifera* Dunn. in hippocampal sub-regions of female albino rat. *Phytother Res* 15, no. 6 (2001): 544–48.

Jaleel, Cheruth A. Antioxidant profile changes in leaf and root tissues of *Withania somnifera* Dunal. *Plant Omics J* 2, no. 4 (2009): 163–68.

Kaileh, M., et al. Withaferin A strongly elicits IkappaB kinase beta hyperphosphorylation concomitant with potent inhibition of its kinase activity. *J Biol Chem* 282, no. 7 (2007): 4253–64.

Khan, B., et al. Augmentation and proliferation of T lymphocytes and Th-1 cytokines by *Withania somnifera* in stressed mice. *Int Immunopharmacol* 6, no. 9 (2006): 1394–403.

Khan, S., et al. Molecular insight into the immune up-regulatory properties of the leaf extract of ashwagandha and identification of Th1 immunostimulatory chemical entity. *Vaccine* 27, no. 43 (2009): 6080–87.

Kour, K., et al. Restoration of stress-induced altered T cell function and corresponding cytokines patterns by withanolide A. *Int Immunopharmacol* 9, no. 10 (2009): 1137–44.

Kumar, A., et al. Protective effect of *Withania somnifera* Dunal on the behavioral and biochemical alterations in sleep-disturbed mice (grid over water suspended method). *Indian J Exp Biol* 45, no. 6 (2007): 524–28.

Kumar, P., and A. Kumar. Effects of root extract of *Withania somnifera* in 3-nitropropionic acid-induced cognitive dysfunction and oxidative damage in rats. *Intrl J Health Res* 1, no. 3 (2008): 139–49.

Kumar, P., et al. Possible neuroprotective effect of *Withania somnifera* root extract against 3-nitropropionic acid-induced behavioral, biochemical, and mitochondrial dysfunction in an animal model of Huntington's disease. *J Med Food* 12, no. 3 (2009): 591–600.

Malik, F., et al. Immune modulation and apoptosis induction: Two sides of antitumoural activity of a standardised herbal formulation of *Withania somnifera*. *Eur J Cancer* 45, no. 8 (2009): 1494–509.

Malik, F., et al. A standardized root extract of *Withania somnifera* and its major constituent withanolide-A elicit humoral and cell-mediated immune responses by up regulation of Th1-dominant polarization in BALB/c mice. *Life Sci* 80, no. 16 (2007): 1525–38.

Mikolai, J., et al. In vivo effects of ashwagandha (*Withania somnifera*) extract on the activation of lymphocytes. *J Altern Complement Med* 15, no. 4 (2009): 423–30.

Mirjalili, M. H., et al. Steroidal lactones from *Withania somnifera*, an ancient plant for novel medicine. *Molecules* 14 (2009): 2373–93.

Mishra, L.-C., et al. Scientific basis for the therapeutic use of *Withania somnifera* (ashwagandha): a review. *Altern Med Rev* 5, no. 4 (2000): 334–46.

Muralikrishnan, G., et al. Immunomodulatory effects of *Withania somnifera* on azoxymethane induced experimental colon cancer in mice. *Immunol Invest* 39, no. 7 (2010): 688–98.

Naidu, P. S., et al. Effect of *Withania somnifera* root extract on reserpine-induced orofacial dyskinesia and cognitive dysfunction. *Phytother Res* 20, no. 2 (2006): 140–46.

Niaz, A., et al. Calcium channel blocking activities of *Withania coagulans*. *Afr J Pharm Pharmacol* 3, no. 9 (2009): 439–42.

Padmavathi, B., et al. Roots of *Withania somnifera* inhibit forestomach and skin carcinogenesis in mice. *Evid Based Complement Alternat Med* 2, no. 1 (2005): 99–105.

Pretorius, E., et al. Comparing the cytotoxic potential of *Withania somnifera* water and methanol extracts. *Afr J Tradit Complement Altern Med* 6, no. 3 (2009): 275–80.

Rajasankar, S., et al. Ashwagandha leaf extract: a potential agent in treating oxidative damage and physiological abnormalities seen in a mouse model of Parkinson's disease. *Neurosci Lett* 454, no. 1 (2009): 11–15.

Rajasankar, S., et al. *Withania somnifera* root extract improves catecholamines and physiological abnormalities seen in a Parkinson's disease model mouse. *J Ethnopharmacol* 125, no. 3 (2009): 369–73.

Rasool, M., et al. Immunomodulatory role of *Withania somnifera* root powder on experimental induced inflammation: an in vivo and in vitro study. *Vascul Pharmacol* 44, no. 6 (2006): 406–10.

Rege, N. N., et al. Adaptogenic properties of six rasayana herbs in Ayurvedic medicine. *Phytother Res* 13, no. 4 (1999): 275–91.

Sabina, E. P. Evaluation of analgesic, antipyretic and ulcerogenic effort of withaferin A. *Intl J Integr Biol* 6, no. 2 (2009): 52–56.

Senthilnathan, P., et al. Enhancement of antitumor effect of paclitaxel in combination with immunomodulatory *Withania somnifera* on benzo(a)pyrene induced experimental lung cancer. *Chem Biol Interact* 159, no. 3 (2006): 180–85.

Shukla, S. D., et al. Stress induced neuron degeneration and protective effects of *Semecarpus anacardium* Linn. and *Withania somnifera* Dunn. in hippocampus of albino rats: an ultrastructural study. *Indian J Exp Biol* 38, no. 10 (2000): 1007–13.

Singh, A., et al. Effect of natural and synthetic antioxidants in a mouse model of chronic fatigue syndrome. *J Med Food* 5, no. 4 (2002): 211–20.

Singh, B., et al. Adaptogenic activity of a novel, withanolide-free aqueous fraction from the roots of *Withania somnifera* Dun. *Phytother Res* 15, no. 4 (2001): 311–18.

Singh, B., et al. Adaptogenic activity of a novel withanolide-free aqueous fraction from the roots of *Withania somnifera* Dun. (Part II). *Phytother Res* 17, no. 5 (2003): 531–36.

Sumantran, V. N., et al. Chondroprotective potential of root extracts of *Withania somnifera* in osteoarthritis. *J Biosci* 32, no. 2 (2007): 299–307.

Sundaram, S., et al. In vitro evaluation of antibacterial activities of crude extracts of *Withania somnifera* (ashwagandha) to bacterial pathogens. *Asian J Biotech* 3, no. 2 (2011): 194–99.

Teixeira, S. T., et al. Prophylactic administration of *Withania somnifera* extract increases host resistence in *Listeria monocytogenes* infected mice. *Int Immunopharmacol* 6, no. 10 (2006): 1535–42.

Ven Murthy, M. R., et al. Scientific basis for the use of Indian ayurvedic medicinal plants in the treatment of neurodegenerative disorders: ashwagandha. *Cent Nerv Syst Agents Med Chem* 10, no. 3 (2010): 238–46.

Widodo, N., et al. Deceleration of senescence in normal human fibroblasts by withanone extracted from ashwagandha leaves. *J Gerontol A Biol Sci Med Sci* 64, no. 10 (2009): 1031–38.

Winters, M. Ancient medicine, modern use: *Withania somnifera* and its potential role in integrative oncology. *Altern Med Rev* 11, no. 4 (2006): 269–77.

Winters, Marie. Ancient medicine, modern use: *Withania somnifera* and its potential role in integrative oncology. *Altern Med Rev* 11, no. 4 (2006): 269–77.

Yadav, C. S., et al. Propoxur-induced acetylcholine esterase inhibition and impairment of cognitive function: attenuation by *Withania somnifera*. *Indian J Biochem Biophys* 47, no. 2 (2010): 117–20.

Ziauddin, M., et al. Studies on the immunomodulatory effects of ashwagandha. *J Ethnopharmacol* 50, no. 2 (1996): 69–76.

Astragalus

Ai, P., et al. Aqueous extract of astragali radix induces human natriuresis through enhancement of renal response to arterial natriuretic peptide. *J Ethnopharmacol* 116, no. 3 (2008): 413–21.

Anonymous. Astragalous. *Herbs at a Glance NCCAM* (updated 2008).

Anonymous. *Astragalus membranaceus.* Monograph. *Altern Med Rev* 8, no. 1 (2003): 72–77.

Brush, J., et al. The effect of *Echinacea purpurea, Astragalus membranaceus* and *Glycyrrhiza glabra* on CD69 expression and immune cell activation in humans. *Phytother Res* 20, no. 8 (2006): 687–95.

Cho, J. H., et al. Myelophil, an extract mix of astragali radix and salviae radix, ameliorates chronic fatigue: a randomized, double-blind, controlled pilot study. *Complement Ther Med* 17, no. 3 (2009): 141–46.

Dobrowolski, C., and K. Jackson. *In vitro* rate of phagocytosis in macrophages stimulated by *Astragalus membranaceus. Journal of Research Across the Disciplines* (Jackson University, Jacksonville, Fla.) 2009, no. 1. https://my.ju.edu/departments/AcademicAffairs/WritingAtJU/JRAD/Documents/Dobrowolski-AM_Research_Paper.pdf.

Duan, P., et al. Clinical study on effect of astragalus in efficacy enhancing and toxicity reducing of chemotherapy in patients of malignant tumor. *Zhongguo Zhong Xi Yi Jie He Za Zhi* 22, no. 7 (2002): 515–17.

Gao, X. P., et al. Effect of huangqi zengmian powder on interstitial response in patients with esophageal cancer at peri-operational period. *Zhongguo Zhong Xi Yi Jie He Za Zhi* 21, no. 3 (2001): 171–73.

Haixue, K., et al. Secocycloartane triterpenoidal saponins from the leaves of *Astragalus membranaceus* Bunge. *Helv Chim Acta* 92, no. 5 (2009): 950–58.

Huang, Z. Q., et al. Effect of *Astragalus membranaceus* on T-lymphocyte subsets in patients with viral myocarditis. *Zhongguo Zhong Xi Yi Jie He Za Zhi* 15, no. 6 (1995): 328–30.

Hyun-Jung, P., et al. The effects of *Astralagus Membranaceus* on repeated restraint stress-induced biochemical and behavioral responses. *Korean J Physiol Pharmacol* 13, no. 4 (2009): 315–19.

Ka-Shun Ko, J., et al. Amelioration of experimental colitis by *Astragalus membranaceus* through anti-oxidation and inhibition of adhesion molecule synthesis. *World J Gastroenterol* 11, no. 37 (2005): 5787–94.

Kemper, K. J., and R. Small. Astragalus (*Astragalus membranaceus*). Longwood Herbal Task Force, September 3, 1999. http://longwoodherbal.org/astragalus/astragalus.PDF.

Kong, X. F., et al. Chinese herbal ingredients are effective immune stimulators for chickens infected with the Newcastle disease virus. *Poult Sci* 85, no. 12 (2006): 2169–75.

Li, S. P., et al. Synergy of astragalus polysaccharides and probiotics (*Lactobacillus* and *Bacillus cerus*) on immunity and intestinal microbiota in chicks. *Poult Sci* 88, no. 3 (2009): 519–25.

Li, Z. P., et al. Effect of mikvetch injection on immune function of children with tetralogy of Fallot after radical operation. *Zhongguo Zhong Xi Yi Jie He Za Zhi* 24, no. 7 (2004): 596–600.

Liu, K. Z., et al. Effects of astragalus and saponins of *Panax notoginseng* on MMP-9 in patients with type 2 diabetic macroangiopathyl. *Zhongguo Zhong Yao Za Zhi* 29, no. 3 (2004): 264–66.

Liu, Z. G., et al. Effect of astragalus injection on immune function in patients with congestive heart failure. *Zhongguo Zhong Xi Yi Jie He Za Zhi* 23, no. 5 (2003): 351–53.

Lu, M.-C., et al. Effect of *Astragalus membranaceus* in rats on peripheral nerve regeneration: in vitro and in vivo studies. *J Trauma* 68, no. 2 (2010): 434–40.

Mao, S. P., et al. Modulatory effect of *Astragalus membranaceus* on Th1/Th2 cytokine in patients with herpes simplex keratitis. *Zhongguo Zhong Xi Yi Jie He Za Zhi* 24, no. 2 (2004): 121–23.

Mao, X. F., et al. Effects of ß-glucan obtained from the Chinese herb *Astragalus membranaceus* and lipopolysaccharide challenge on performance, immunological, adrenal, and somatotropic responses of weaning pigs. *J Anim Sci* 83 (2005): 2775–82.

Matkowski, A., et al. Flavonoids and phenol carboxylic acids in Oriental medicinal plant *Astragalus membranaceus* acclimated in Poland. *Z Naturforsch C* 58, no. 7–8 (2003): 602–4.

Peng, A., et al. Herbal treatment for renal diseases. *Ann Acad Med Singapore* 34 (2005): 44–51.

Schafer, P. *Astragalus membranaceus.* On the website of Chinese Medicinal Herb Farm. 2009. http://www.chinesemedicinalherbfarm.com/Astragalus%20membran3.pdf.

Shabbir, M. Z., et al. Immunomodulatory effect of polyimmune (*Astragalus membranaceus*) extract on humoral response of layer birds vaccinated against Newcastle disease virus. *Int J Agri Biol* 10 (2008): 585–87.

Shen, P., et al. Differential effects of isoflavones, from *Astragalus membranaceus* and *Pueraria thomsonii*, on the activation of PPARalpha, PPARgamma, and adipocyte differentiation in vitro. *J Nutr* 136 (2006): 899–905.

Sheng, B.-W., et al. *Astragalus membranaceus* reduces free radical-mediated injury to renal tubules in rabbits receiving high-energy shock waves. *Chin Med J* (English) 118, no. 1 (2005): 43–49.

Shi, F. S., et al. Effect of astragalus saponin on vascular endothelial cell and its function in burn patients. *Zhongguo Zhong Xi Yi Jie He Za Zhi* 21, no. 10 (2001): 750–51.

Su, L., et al. Effect of intravenous drip infusion of cyclophosphamide with high-dose astragalus injection in treating lupus nephritis. *Zhong Xi Yi Jie He Xue Bao* 5, no. 3 (2007): 272–75.

Sun, H., et al. Effect on exercise endurance capacity and antioxidant properties of *Astragalus membranaceus* polysaccharides (APS). *J Med Plant Res* 4, no. 10 (2010): 982–86.

Taixiang, W., et al. Chinese medical herbs for chemotherapy side effects in colorectal cancer patients. *Cochrane Database Syst Rev* 25, no. 1 (2005): CD0004540.

Tin, M. Y. Study of the anticarcinogenic mechanisms of *Astragalus Membranaceus* in colon cancer cells and tumor xenograft. Master's thesis, Hong Kong Baptist University, 2006. http://www.hkbu.edu.hk/~libimage/theses/abstracts/b20195643a.pdf.

Wang, F., et al. Effect of astragalus on cytokines in patients undergoing heart valve replacement. *Zhongguo Zhong Xi Yi Jie He Za Zhi* 28, no. 6 (2008): 495–98.

Wang, H. F., et al. Effects of *Astragalus membranaceus* on growth performance, carcass characteristics, and antioxidant status of broiler chickens. *Acta Agric Scand* 60, no. 3 (2010): 151–58.

Wang, M. S., et al. Clinical study on effect of astragalus injection and its immunoregulation action in treating chronic aplastic anemia. *Chin J Integr Med* 13, no. 2 (2007): 98–102.

Wojcikowski, K., et al. Effect of *Astragalus membranaceus* and *Angelica sinensis* combined with enalapril in rats with obstructive uropathy. *Phytotherapy Research* 24, no. 6 (2010): 875–84.

Wu, J., et al. Effect of astragalus injection on serious abdominal traumatic patients' cellular immunity. *Chin J Integr Med* 12, no. 1 (2006): 29–31.

Wu, Y., et al. Inhibition of *Astragalus membranaceus* polysaccharides against liver cancer cell HepG2. *African Journal of Microbiology Research* 4, no. 20 (2010): 2181–83.

Xian-qing, M., et al. Hypoglycemic effect of polysaccharide enriched extract of *Astragalus membranaceus* in diet induced insulin resistant C57BL/6J mice and its potential mechanism. *Phytomedicine* 16, no. 5 (2009): 416–25.

Xiaoyan, Z., et al. Effect of superfine pulverization on properties of *Astragalus membranaceus* powder. *Adv Powder Technol* 203, no. 3 (2010): 620–25.

Yang, W. J., et al. Synergistic antioxidant activities of eight traditional Chinese herb pairs. *Biol Pharm Bull* 32, no. 6 (2009): 1021–26.

Yao-Haur, K., et al. *Astragalus membranaceus* flavonoids (AMF) ameliorate chronic fatigue syndrome induced by food intake restriction plus forced swimming. *J Ethnopharmacol* 122, no. 1 (2009): 28–34.

Yu, D. H., et al. Studies of chemical constituents and their antioxidant activities from *Astragalus mongholicus* Bunge. *Biomedical and Environmental Sciences* 18 (2005): 297–301.

Zhang, J. G., et al. Clinical study on effect of astragalus injection on left ventricular remodeling and left ventricular function in patients with acute myocardial infarction. *Zhongguo Zhong Xi Yi Jie He Za Zhi* 22, no. 5 (2002): 346–48.

Zhang, J. G., et al. Effect of astragalus injection plasma levels of apoptosis-related factors in aged patients with chronic heart failure. *Chin J Integr Med* 11, no. 3 (2005): 187–90.

Zou, Y. H., et al. Effect of astragalus injection combined with chemotherapy on quality of life in patients with advanced non-small cell lung cancer. *Zhongguo Zhong Xi Yi Jie He Za Zhi* 23, no. 10 (2003): 733–35.

Zwickey, H., et al. The effect of *Echinacea purpurea*, *Astragalus membranaceus* and *Glycyrrhiza glabra* on CD25 expression in humans: a pilot study. *Phytother Res* 21, no. 11 (2007): 1109–12.

Berberine Plants

Abidi, P., et al. The medicinal plant goldenseal is a natural LDL-lowering agent with multiple bioactive components and new action mechanisms. *J Lipid Res* 47, no. 10 (2006): 2134–47.

Anonymous. Berberine monograph. *Altern Med Rev* 5, no. 2 (2000): 175–77.

Anonymous. *Mahonia bealei* (Fortune) Carrière. Entry in the U.S. Department of Agriculture Natural Resources Conservation Service PLANTS Database. http://plants.usda.gov/java/profile?symbol=MABE2 (accessed January 25, 2011).

Anonymous. Phellodendron. Wikipedia. http://en.wikipedia.org/wiki/Phellodendron (accessed January 25, 2010).

Anonymous. Phellodendron amurense. Wikipedia. http://en.wikipedia.org/wiki/Phellodendron_amurense (accessed January 25, 2010).

Anonymous. Tinospora cordifolia. Wikipedia. http://en.wikipedia.org/wiki/Tinospora_cordifolia (accessed January 25, 2011).

Anonymous. Weed of the week: Amur corktree. U.S. Department of Agriculture Forest Service, Forest Health Staff, Newtown Square, Penn., February 19, 2005. http://na.fs.fed.us/fhp/invasive_plants/weeds/amur-corktree.pdf.

Anonymous. Weed of the week: Japanese barberry. U.S. Department of Agriculture Forest Service, Forest Health Staff, Newtown Square, Penn., June 13, 2005. http://na.fs.fed.us/fhp/invasive_plants/weeds/japanese-barberry.pdf.

Arayne, M. S., et al. The berberis story: *Berberis vulgaris* in therapeutics, *Pak J Pharm Sci* 20, no. 1 (2007): 83–92.

Askri, H., et al. Effects of chloropromazine, berberine and verapamil on *Escherichia coli* heat-labile enterotoxin-induced intestinal hypersecretion in rabbit ileal loops. *J Med Microbiol* 27 (1988): 99–103.

Ball, A. R., et al. Conjugated berberine to a multidrug resistance pump inhibitor creates an effective antimicrobial. *ACS Chem Biol* 1, no. 9 (2006): 594–600.

Borysiewicz, J., et al. Determining the invasive capabilities of the exotic tree *Phellodendron amurense* Rupr. in northeastern North America. Presentation at the Botany 2010 conference, July 31 through August 4, 2010, Providence, Rhode Island. http://2010.botanyconference.org/engine/search/index.php?func=detail&aid=236; http://www.youtube.com/watch?v=C20tvFpBwUE.

Budzinski, J. W., et al. Modulation of human cytochrome P450 3A4 (CYP3A4) and P-glycoprotein (P-gp) in caco-2 cell monolayers by selected commercial-source milk thistle and goldenseal products. *Can J Physiol Pharmacol* 85, no. 9 (2007): 966–78.

Buhlmann, C., and G. Ross. *Quantitation of the alkaloids berberine, palmatine and jatrorrhizine in Mahonia stem by capillary electrophoresis.* Pub. no. 5990-3396EN. (Waldbronn, Germany: Agilent Technologies, March 1, 2009). http://chem.agilent.com/Library/applications/5990-3396EN.pdf.

Cao, X., et al. Why is it challenging to predict intestinal drug absorption and oral bioavailability in human using rat model. *Pharm Res* 23, no. 8 (2006): 1675–86.

Cernáková, M., et al. Antimicrobial activity of berberine—a constituent of *Mahonia aquifolium*. *Folia Microbiol* (Prague) 47, no. 4 (2002): 375–78.

Chen, C. M., et al. Determination of berberine in plasma, urine and bile by high-performance liquid chromatography. *J Chromatogr B Biomed Appl* 665, no. 1 (1995): 117–23.

Chen, F., et al. Optimization of a novel mucoadhesive drug deliver system with ion-exchange resin core loaded with berberine hydrochloride using central composite design methodology. *Yao Xue Xue Bao* 43, no. 9 (2008): 963–68.

Chen, M. L., et al. Chemical and biological differentiation of cortex phellodendri chinensis and cortex phellodendri amurensis. *Planta Med* 76, no. 14 (2010): 1530–35.

Chen, Y., et al. Characterization of the transportation of berberine in coptidis rhizoma extract through rat primary cultured cortical neurons. *Biomed Chromatogr* 22, no. 1 (2008): 28–33.

Chin, L. W., et al. Anti-herpes simplex virus effects of berberine from coptidis rhizoma, a major component of a Chinese herbal medicine, ching-wei-san. *Arch Virol* 155, no. 12 (2010): 1933–41.

Chiu, H. F., et al. The pharmacological and pathological studies on several hepatic protective crude drugs from Taiwan (I). *Am J Chin Med* 16, no. 3–4 (1988): 127–37.

Clement-Kruzel, S., et al. Immune modulation of macrophage pro-inflammatory response by goldenseal and astragalus extracts. *J Med Food* 11, no. 3 (2008): 493–98.

Cuéllar, M. J., et al. Topical anti-inflammatory activity of some Asian medicinal plants used in dermatological disorders. *Fitoterapia* 72, no. 3 (2001): 221–29.

Cui, W. S., et al. A new isocoumarin from bark of *Pellodendron chinense. Nat Prod Res* 17, no. 6 (2003): 427–29.

Deng, Y., et al. Simultaneous determination of berberine, palmatine and jatrorrhizine by liquid chromatography-tandem mass spectrometry in rat plasma and its application in a pharmacokinetic study after oral administration of coptis-evodia herb couple. *J Chromatogr B Analyt Technol Biomed Life Sci* 863, no. 2 (2008): 195–205.

Domadia, P. N., et al. Berberine targets assembly of *Escherichia coli* cell division protein FtsZ. *Biochemistry* 47, no. 10 (2008): 3225–34.

Dong, Y., et al. Absorption of extractive rhizoma coptidis in rat everted gut scas. *Zhongguo Zhong Yao Za Zhi* 33, no. 9 (2008): 1056–60.

Douglas, J. A., et al. Seasonal variation of biomass and bioactive alkaloid content of goldenseal, *Hydrastis canadensis. Fitoterapia* 81, no. 7 (2010): 925–28.

Draco Natural Products. Corydalis: when life is just a pain. *Extrax Fax* 2, no. 8 (1999): 1. http://www.dracoherbs.com/assets/Exfax%209908%20final%20-%20new%20addr.PDF.

Freile, M. L., et al. Antifungal activity of aqueous extracts and of berberine isolated from *Berberis heterophylla. Acta Farm Bonaerense* 25, no. 1 (2006): 83–88.

Freile, M. L., et al. Antimicrobial activity of aqueous extracts and of berberine isolated from *Berberis heterophylla. Fitoterapia* 74, no. 7–8 (2003): 702–5.

Garcia, G. E., et al. Akt- and CREB-mediated prostate cancer cell proliferation inhibition by nexrutine, a *Phellodendron amurense* extract. *Neoplasia* 8, no. 6 (2006): 523–33.

Garrison, R., et al. Effect of a proprietary *Magnolia* and *Phellodendron* extract on weight management: a pilot, double-blind, placebo-controlled clinical trial. *Altern Ther Health Med* 12, no. 1 (2006): 50–54.

Ghosh, R., et al. *Phellodendron amurense* bark extract prevents progression of prostate tumors in transgenic adenocarcinoma of mouse prostate: potential for prostate cancer management. *Anticancer Res* 30, no. 3 (2010): 857–66.

Ghosh, R., et al. Regulation of cox-2 by cyclic AMP response element binding protein in prostate cancer: potential role for nexrutine. *Neoplasia* 9, no. 11 (2007): 893–99.

Gilman, E. F., and D. Watson. Phellodendron amurense: *Amur corktree.* Florida Cooperative Extension Service, Institute of Food and Agricultural Sciences, University of Florida, May 2011. http://edis.ifas.ufl.edu/st437.

Giri, P., et al. Binding of protoberberine alkaloid coralyne with double stranded poly(A): a biophysical study. *Mol Biosyst* 4, no. 4 (2008): 341–48.

Grippa, E., et al. Inhibition of *Candida rugosa* lipase by berberine and structurally related alkaloids, evaluated by high-performance liquid chromatography. *Biosci Biotechnol Biochem* 63, no. 9 (1999): 1557–62.

Gui, S., et al. Study on preparation of berberine microemulsion and its absorption in intestine. *Zhongguo Zhong Yao Za Zhi* 34, no. 4 (2009): 398–401.

Gui, S. Y., et al. Preparation and evaluation of a microemulsion for oral delivery of berberine. *Pharmazie* 63, no. 7 (2008): 516–19.

Gupta, P. K., et al. Validation of a liquid chromatography-tandem mass spectrometric assay for the quantitative determination of hydrastine and berberine in human serum. *J Pharm Biomed Anal* 49, no. 4 (2009): 1021–26.

Gurley, B. J., et al. Effect of goldenseal (*Hydrastis canadensis*) and kava kava (*Piper methysticum*) supplementation on digoxin pharmacokinetics in humans. *Drug Metab Dispos* 35, no. 2 (2007): 240–5.

Gurley, B. J., et al. Supplementation with goldenseal (*Hydrastis canadensis*), but not kava kava (*Piper methysticum*), inhibits human CYP3A activity in vivo, *Clin Pharmacol Ther* 83, no. 1 (2008): 61–9.

Hajnická, V., et al. Effect of *Mahonia aquifolium* active compounds on interleukin-8 production in the human monocytic cell line THP-1. *Planta Med* 68, no. 3 (2002): 266–68.

Harikumar, K. B., et al. Inhibition of progression of erythroleukemia induced by Friend virus in BALB/c mice by natural products—berberine, curcumin and picroliv. *J Exp Ther Oncol* 7, no. 4 (2008): 275–84.

Hayashi, K., et al. Antiviral activity of berberine and related compounds against human cytomegalovirus. *Bioorg Med Chem Lett* 17, no. 6 (2007): 1562–64.

Head, Kathleen A. Natural approaches to prevention and treatment of infections of the lower urinary tract. *Altern Med Rev* 13, no. 3 (2008): 227–44.

Hua, W., et al. Determination of berberine in human plasma by liquid chromatography-electrospray ionization-mass spectrometry. *J Pharm Biomed Anal* 44, no. 4 (2007): 931–37.

Hwang, B. Y., et al. Antimicrobial constituents from goldenseal (the rhizomes of *Hydrastis canadensis*) against selected oral pathogens. *Planta Med* 69, no. 7 (2003): 623–27.

Imanshahidi, M., et al. Pharmacological and therapeutic effects of *Berberis vulgaris* and its active constituent, berberine. *Phytother Res* 22, no. 8 (2008): 999–1012.

Inbaraj, J. J., et al. Photochemistry and photocytotoxicity of alkaloids from goldenseal (*Hydrastis canadensis* L.). 2. Palmatine, hydrastine, canadine, and hydrastinine. *Chem Res Toxicol* 19, no. 6 (2006): 739–44.

Jahnke, G. D., et al. Developmental toxicity evaluation of berberine in rats and mice. *Birth Defects Res B Dev Reprod Toxicol* 77, no. 3 (2006): 195–206.

James, M. A., et al. Dietary administration of berberine or *Phellodendron amurense* extract inhibits cell cycle progression and lung tumorigenesis. *Mol Carcinog* 50, no. 1 (2011): 1–7.

Jia, F., et al. Identification of palmatine as an inhibitor of West Nile virus. *Arch Virol* 155, no. 8 (2010): 1325–29.

Kai-sum, M., et al. Coptis accumulation of active ingredients. Free Papers Download Center, May 17, 2008. http://eng.hi138.com/?i135909.

Kalman, D. S., et al. Effect of a proprietary *Magnolia* and *Phellodendron* extract on stress levels in healthy women: a pilot, double-blind, placebo-controlled clinical trial. *Nutr J* 21, no. 7 (2008): 11.

Karmakar, S. R., et al. Anti-carcinogenic potentials of a plant extract (*Hydrastis canadensis*): I. Evidence from in vivo studies in mice (*Mus musculus*). *Asian Pac J Cancer Prev* 11, no. 2 (2010): 545–51.

Kheir, M. M., et al. Acute toxicity of berberine and its correlation with the blood concentration in mice. *Food Chem Toxicol* 48, no. 4 (2010): 1105–10.

Khin-Maung-U, et al. Clinical trial of berberine in acute watery diarrhoea. *Br Med J (Clin Res Ed)* 291, no. 6509 (1985): 1061–65.

Khin-Maung-U, et al. Clinical trial of high-dose berberine and tetracycline in cholera. *J Diarrhoeal Dis Res* 5, no. 3 (1987): 184–87.

Kim, J. B., et al. The alkaloid berberine inhibits the growth of anoikis-resistant MCF-7 and MDA-MB-231 breast cancer cell lines by inducing cell cycle arrest. *Phytomedicine* 17, no. 6 (2009): 436–40.

Kim, J. H., et al. Effect of *Phellodendron amurense* in protecting human osteoarthritic cartilage and chondrocytes. *J Ethnopharmacol* 134, no. 2 (2011): 234–42. E-pub (preprint) December 21, 2010.

Kim, J. S., et al. Immunoquantitative analysis for berberine and its related compounds using monoclonal antibodies in herbal medicines. *Analyst* 129, no. 1 (2004): 87–91.

Kulkami, S. K., et al. Berberine: a plant alkaloid with therapeutic potential for central nervous system disorders. *Phytother Res* 24, no. 3 (2010): 317–24.

Kumar, A. P., et al. Akt/camp-responsive element binding protein/cyclin D1 network: a novel target for prostate cancer inhibition in transgenic adenocarcinoma of mouse prostate model mediated by nexrutine, a *Phellodendron amurense* bark extract. *Clin Cancer Res* 13, no. 9 (2007): 2784–94.

Kumar, A. P., et al. Natural products: potential for developing *Phellodendron amurense* bark extract for prostate cancer management. *Mini Rev Med Chem* 10, no. 5 (2010): 388–97.

Lau, C. W., et al. Cardiovascular actions of berberine. *Cardiovasc Drug Rev* 19, no. 3 (2001): 234–44.

Lauk, L., et al. Activity of *Berberis aetnensis* root extracts on *Candida* strains. *Fitoterapia* 78, no. 2 (2007): 159–61.

Lee, J. H., et al. Isolation and characterization of a novel glutathione S-transferase-activating peptide from the oriental medicinal plant *Phellodendron amurense*. *Peptides* 27, no. 9 (2006): 2069–74.

Lesnau, A., et al. Antiviral activity of berberine salts. *Pharmazie* 45, no. 8 (1990): 638–39.

Leu, C. H., et al. Constituents from the leaves of *Phellodendron amurense* and their antioxidant activity. *Chem Pharm Bull* (Tokyo), 54, no. 9 (2006): 1308–11.

408

Li, A., et al. Evaluation of antimicrobial activity of certain Chinese plants used in folkloric medicine. *World J Microbio Biotech* 24, no. 4 (2008): 569–72.

Li, A.-R., et al. Antimicrobial activity of four species of Berberidaceae. *Fitoterapia* 78, no. 5 (2007): 379–81.

Li, H. L., et al. Alkaloids from *Corydalis saxicola* and their anti-hepatitis B virus activity. *Chem Biodivers* 5, no. 5 (2008): 777–83.

Li, H. L., et al. Simultaneous determination of four active alkaloids from a traditional Chinese medicine *Corydalis saxicola* Bunting. (yanhuanglian) in plasma and urine samples by LC-MS-MS. *J Chromatogr B Analyst Technol Biomed Life Sci* 831, no. 1–2 (2006): 140–46.

Li, Y., et al. Effect of additives on absorption of *Coptis chinensis* total alkaloids and pharmacokinetics in mice. *Zhongguo Zhong Yao Za Zhi* 34, no. 3 (2009): 344–48.

Liepin, V. K., et al. Seasons, regions of procurement of Amur corktree bast (*Phellodendron amurense* Rupr.) and localization of berberine in it. *Farmatsiia* 17, no. 6 (1968): 65–69.

Lin, C. C., et al. Effects of oral administration of berberine on distribution and metabolism of 2-aminofluorene in Sprague-Dawley rats. *In Vivo* 21, no. 2 (2007): 321–28.

Lin, J. P., et al. Berberine induced down-regulation of matrix metalloproteinase-1, -2 and -9 in human gastric cancer cells (SNU-5) in vitro. *In Vivo* 22, no. 2 (2008): 223–30.

Liu, L., et al. Berberine suppresses intestinal disaccharidases with beneficial metabolic effects in diabetic states, evidences from in vivo and in vitro study. *Naunyn Schmiedebergs Arch Pharmacol* 381, no. 4 (2010): 371–81.

Liu, Y., et al. Simultaneous determination of seven alkaloids in *Phellodendron chinense* Schneid by high-performance liquid chromatography. *J AOAC Int* 93, no. 5 (2010): 1416–21.

Liu, Y. M., et al. A comparative study on commercial samples of phellodendri cortex. *Planta Med* 59, no. 6 (1993): 557–61.

Lu, S. S., et al. Berberine promotes glucagon-like peptide-1 (7-36) amide secretion in streptozotocin-induced diabetic rats. *J Endocrinol* 200, no. 2 (2009): 159–65.

Lu, T., et al. Simultaneous determination of berberine and palmatine in rat plasma by HPLC-ESI-MS after oral administration of traditional Chinese medicinal preparation huang-lian-jie-du decoction and the pharmacokinetic application of the method. *J Pharm Biomed Anal* 40, no. 5 (2006): 1218–24.

Lu, X. Y., et al. Enhancement of sodium caprate on intestine absorption and antidiabetic action of berberine. *AAPS Pharm Sci Tech* 11, no. 1 (2010): 372–82.

Ma, B. L., et al. Identification of the toxic constituents in rhizoma coptidis. *J Ethnopharmacol* 128, no. 2 (2010): 357–64.

Ma, L., et al. Absorption of coptisine chloride and berberrubine across human intestinal epithelial by using human Caco-2 cell monolayers. *Zhongguo Zhong Yao Za Zhi* 32, no. 23 (2007): 2523–27.

Maeng, H. J., et al. P-glycoprotein-mediated transport of berberine across Caco-2 cell monolayers. *J Pharm Sci* 91, no. 12 (2002): 2614–21.

Mahady, G. B., et al. In vitro susceptibility of *Helicobacter pylori* to isoquinoline alkaloids from *Sanguinaria canadensis* and *Hydrastis canadensis*. *Phytother Res* 17, no. 3 (2003): 217–21.

Min, Y. D., et al. Isolation of limonoids and alkaloids from *Phellodendron amurense* and their multidrug resistance (MDR) reversal activity. *Arch Pharm Res* 30, no. 1 (2007): 58–63.

Miyake, M., et al. Limonoids in *Phellodendron amurense* (Kihada). *Yakugaku Zasshi* 112, no. 5 (1992): 343–47.

Mori, H., et al. Principle of the bark of *Phellodendron amurense* to suppress the cellular immune response. *Planta Med* 60, no. 5 (1994): 445–49.

Mori, H., et al. Principle of the bark of *Phellodendron amurense* to suppress the cellular immune response: effect of phellodendrine on cellular and humoral immune responses. *Planta Med* 61, no. 1 (1995): 45–49.

Morisawa, TunyaLee. *Phellodendron amurense*. BugwoodWiki, updated March 23, 2009. http://wiki.bugwood.org/Phellodendron_amurense.

Musumeci, R., et al. *Berberis aetnensis* C. Presl. extracts: antimicrobial properties and interaction with ciprofloxacin. *Int J Antimicrob Agents* 22, no. 1 (2003): 48–53.

Oben, J., et al. *Phellodendron* and *Citrus* extracts benefit cardiovascular health in osteoarthritis patients: a double-blind, placebo-controlled pilot study. *Nutr J* 20, no. 7 (2008): 16.

Oben, J., et al. *Phellodendron* and *Citrus* extracts benefit joint health in osteoarthritis patients: a pilot, double-blind, placebo-controlled study. *Nutr J* 14, no. 8 (2009): 38.

Pan, G. Y., et al. The involvement of P-glycoprotein in berberine absorption. *Pharmacol Toxicol* 91, no. 4 (2002): 193–97.

Park, E. K. Antiinflammatory effects of a combined herbal preparation (RAH13) of *Phellodendron amurense* and *Coptis chinensis* in animal models of inflammation. *Phytother Res* 21, no. 8 (2007): 746–50.

Park, K. S., et al. Differential inhibitory effects of protoberberines on sterol and chitin biosyntheses in *Candida albicans*. *J Antimicrob Chemother* 43, no. 5 (1999): 667–74.

Park, K. S., et al. HWY-289, a novel semi-synthetic protoberberine derivative with multiple target sites in *Candida albicans*. *J Antimicrob Chemother* 47, no. 5 (2001): 513–19.

Ping, Yi., et al. Berberine reverses free-fatty-acid-induced insulin resistance in 3T3-L1 adipocytes through targeting IKK. *World J Gastroenterology* 14, no. 6 (2008): 876–83.

Pitta-Alvarez, S. I., et al. In vitro shoot culture and antimicrobial activity of *Berberis buxifolia* Lam. *In Vitro Cell Dev Biol Plant* 44, no. 6 (2008): 502–7.

Premkumar, J., et al. Activity and interactions of antibiotic and phytochemical combinations against *Pseudomonas aeruginosa* in vitro. *Int J Biol Sci* 6, no. 6 (2010): 556–68.

Quan, H., et al. Potent in vitro synergism of fluconazole and berberine chloride against clinical isolates of *Candida albicans* resistant to fluconazole. *Antimicrob Agents Chemother* 50, no. 3 (2006): 1096–99.

Qui, W., et al. Effect of berberine on the pharmacokinetics of substrates of CYP3A and P-gp. *Phytother Res* 23, no. 11 (2009): 1553–58.

Rabbani, G. H., et al. Mechanism and treatment of diarrhoea due to *Vibrio cholerae* and *Escherichia coli*: roles of drugs and prostaglandins. *Dan Med Bull* 43, no. 2 (1996): 173–85.

Rabbani, G. H., et al. Randomized controlled trial of berberine sulfate therapy for diarrhea due to enterotoxigenic *Escherichia coli* and *Vibrio cholerae*. *J Infect Dis* 155, no. 5 (1987): 979–84.

Rajaian, H., et al. *Berberis vulgaris* as growth promoter in broiler chickens. *Int J Poultry Sci* 5, no. 4 (2006): 395–97.

Read, R. A., and J. Zasada. *Phellodendron amurense* Rupr.: Amur corktree. In *Woody Plant Seed Manual*, by the U.S. Department of Agriculture Forest Service (USDAFS Agriculture Handbook 727), 783–85. Washington DC: U.S. Government Printing Office, 2008. http://www.nsl.fs.fed.us/O&P%20genera.pdf .

Rohrer, U., et al. Antimicrobial activity of *Mahonia aquifolium* and two of its alkaloids against oral bacteria. *Schweiz Monatsschr Zahnmed* 117 (2007): 1126–31.

Ropivia, J., et al. Isoquinolines from the roots of *Thalictrum flavum* L. and their evaluation as antiparasitic compounds. *Molecules* 15 (2010): 6476–84.

Sack, R. B., et al. Berberine inhibits intestinal secretory response of *Vibrio cholerae* and *Escherichia coli* enterotoxins. *Infect Immun* 35, no. 2 (1982): 471–75.

Sahelian, Ray. *Phellodendron*. Newsletter. http://raysahelian.com/phellodendron.html (accessed January 25, 2011).

Sato, I., et al. The study of dentifrice containing *Phellodendron amurense* extract on periodontal disease (II). The clinical effects of dentifrice containing *Phellodendron amurense* extract and anti-inflammatory agents. *Nihon Shishubyo Gakkai Kaishi* 30, no. 3 (1988): 887–900.

Scazzocchio, F. et al. Antibacterial activity of *Hydrastis canadensis* extract and its major isolated alkaloids. *Planta Med* 67, no. 6 (2001): 561–64.

Schinella, G. R., et al. Inhibition of *Trypanosoma cruzi* growth by medical plant extract. *Fitoterapia* 73, no. 7–8 (2002): 569–75.

Serafim, T. L., et al. Different concentrations of berberine result in distinct cellular localization patterns and cell cycle effects in a melanoma cell line. *Cancer Chemother Pharmacol* 61, no. 6 (2008): 1007–18.

Severina, I. I., et al. Transfer of cationic antibacterial agents berberine, palmatine, and benzalkonium through bimolecular planar phospholipid film and *Staphylococcus aureus* membrane. *IUBMB Life* 52, no. 6 (2001): 321–24.

Shahid, M., et al. Ethnobotanical studies on *Berberis aristata* DC. root extracts. *Afr J Biotechnol* 8, no. 4 (2009): 556–63.

Shi, R., et al. Influence of *Coptis chinensis* on pharmacokinetics of flavonoids after oral administration of radix scutellariae in rats. *Biopharm Drug Dispos* 30, no. 7 (2009): 398–410.

Shrya, K., et al. Significant differences in alkaloid content of *Coptis chinensis* (huanglian), from its related American species. *Chinese Med* 4 (2009): 17.

Singh, A., et al. Berberine: alkaloid with wide spectrum of pharmacological activities. *I J Nat Prod* 3 (2010): 64–75.

Slobodniková, L., et al. Antimicrobial activity of *Mahonia aquifolium* crude extract and its major isolated alkaloids. *Phytother Res* 18, no. 8 (2004): 674–76.

Stermitz, F. R., et al. 5'-methoxyhydnocarpin-D and pheophorbide A: *Berberis* species components that potentiate berberine growth inhibition of resistant *Staphylococcus aureus*. *J Nat Prod* 63, no. 8 (2000): 1146–49.

Stermitz, F. R., et al. Synergy in a medicinal plant: antimicrobial action of berberine potentiated by 5'-methoxyhydnocarpin, a multidrug pump inhibitor. *PNAS* 97, no. 4 (2000): 1433–37.

Subhuti, Dharmananda. New uses of berberine: a valuable alkaloid from herbs for "damp-heat" syndromes. Institute for Traditional Medicine (Portland, Ore.), April 2005. http://itmonline.org/articles/berberine/berberine.htm.

Sun, D., et al. Berberine sulfate blocks adherence of *Streptococcus pyogenes* to epithelial cells, fibronectin, and hexadecane. *Antimicrob Agents Chemother* 32, no. 9 (1988): 1370–74.

Suraj, Gupte. Use of berberine in treatment of giardiasis. *Am J Dis Child* 129, no. 7 (1975): 866.

Swearingen, Jil M. Plant Conservation Alliance's Alien Plant Working Group "Least Wanted": Japanese Barberry. U.S. National Park Service Plant Conservation Alliance, May 20, 2005. http://nps.gov/plants/alien/fact/beth1.htm.

Tan, X., et al. In situ intestinal absorption kinetics of berberine and jatrorrhizine from extractive rhizoma coptidis in rats. *Zhongguo Zhong Yao Za Zhi* 35, no. 6 (2010): 755–58.

Tanaka, Y., et al. A meningoencephalitic form of cerebral aspergillosis effectively treated with a derivative of berberine alkaloids (author's transl). *Rinsho Shinkeigaku* 18, no. 10 (1978): 635–40.

Taylor, C. E., et al. Control of diarrheal diseases. *Annu Rev Public Health* 10 (1989): 221–44.

410

Tegos, G., et al. Multidrug pump inhibitors uncover remarkable activity of plant antimicrobials. *Antimicrob Agents Chemother* 46, no. 10 (2002): 3133–41.

Tsai, P. L., et al. Hepatobiliary excretion of berberine. *Drug Metab Dispos* 32, no. 4 (2004): 405–12.

Turner, N., et al. Berberine and its more biologically available derivative, dihydroberberine, inhibit mitochondrial respiratory complex 1: a mechanism for the action of berberine to activate AMP-activated protein kinase and improve insulin action. *Diabetes* 57 (2008): 1414–18.

Uchiyama, T., et al. Anti-ulcer effect of extract from phellodendri cortex. *Yakugaku Zasshi* 109, no. 9 (1989): 672–76.

Van Berkel, G. J. Thin-layer chromatography/desorption electrospray ionization mass spectrometry: investigation of goldenseal alkaloids. *Anal Chem* 79, no. 7 (2007): 2778–89.

Vennerstrom, J. L., et al. Berberine derivatives as antileishmanial drugs. *Antimicro Agent Chemother* 34, no. 5 (1990): 918–21.

Villinski, J., et al. Antibacterial activity and alkaloid content of *Berberis thunbergii, Berberis vulgaris* and *Hydrastis canadensis*. *Pharma Biol* 41, no. 8 (2003): 551–57.

Volleková, A., et al. Antifungal activity of *Mahonia aquifolium* extract and its major protoberberine alkaloids. *Phytother Res* 17, no. 7 (2003): 834–37.

Volleková, A., et al. Isoquinoline alkaloids from *Mahonia aquifolium* stem bark are active against *Malassezia* spp. *Folia Microbiol* 46, no. 2 (2001): 107–11.

Wang, L., et al. Metabolism, transformation and distribution of *Coptis chinensis* total alkaloids in rat. *Zhongguo Zhong Yao Za Zhi* 35, no. 15 (2010): 2017–20.

Wang, M., et al. Studies on the chemical constituents of *Phellodendron chinense*. *Zhong Yao Cai* 32, no. 2 (2009): 208–10.

Wang, W., et al. In vitro antioxidant, antimicrobial and anti-herpes simplex virus type 1 activity of *Phellodendron amurense* Rupr. from China. *Am J Chin Med* 37, no. 1 (2009): 1–9.

Wang, X., et al. Berberine inhibits *Staphylococcus epidermidis* adhesion and biofilm formation on the surface of titanium alloy. *J Orthop Res* 27, no. 11 (2009): 1487–92.

Wang, X. Q., et al. Effect of rhizoma coptidis and radix rehmanniae with different ratio on pharmacokinetics of berberine in rats. *Zhongguo Zhong Yao Za Zhi* 32, no. 17 (2007): 1795–97.

Watanabe, Y., et al. The study of dentifrice containing *Phellodendron amurense* extracts on periodontal disease (I). The anti-inflammatory effects and clinical effects of *Phellodendron amurense* extract on periodontal disease. *Nihon Shishubyo Gakkai Kaishi* 30, no. 3 (1988): 875–86.

Weber, H. A., et al. Extraction and HPLC analysis of alkaloids in goldenseal. *Sheng Wu Gong Cheng Xue Bao* 20, no. 2 (2004): 306–8.

Wei, P. H., et al. Determination of alkaloids from *Coptis chinensis* Franch. and *Phellodendron amurense* Rupr. decocted together in baitouweng decocta by high performance capillary electrophoresis. *Se Pu* 20, no. 6 (2002): 554–56.

Wongbutdee, Jaruwan. Physiological effects of berberine. *Pharm Health Sci J* 4, no. 1 (2009): 78–83.

Wu, T. S., et al. Constituents from the leaves of *Phellodendron amurense* var. *wilsonii* and their bioactivity. *J Nat Prod* 66, no. 9 (2003): 1207–11.

Wu, W. N., et al. Alkaloids of *Thalictrum*. XXI. Isolation and characterization of alkaloids from the roots of *Thalictrum podocarpum*. *Lloydia* 40, no. 4 (1977): 384–94.

Wu, X., et al. Effects of berberine on the blood concentration of cyclosporine A in renal transplanted recipients: clinical and pharmacokinetic study. *Eur J Clin Pharmacol* 61, no. 8 (2005): 567–72.

Xin, H. W., et al. The effects of berberine on the pharmacokinetics of cyclosporine A in healthy volunteers. *Methods Find Exp Clin Pharmacol* 28, no. 1 (2006): 25–29.

Xu, Lihui., et al. Inhibitory effects of berberine on the activation and cell cycle progression of human peripheral lymphocytes. *Cell Mol Immun* 2, no. 4 (2005): 295–300.

Xu, Y., et al. Extracts of bark from the traditional Chinese herb *Phellodendron amurense* inhibit contractility of the isolated rat prostate gland. *J Ethnopharmacol* 127, no. 1 (2010): 196–99.

Yan, C., et al. Water-soluble chemical constituents from fruits of *Phellodendron chinense* var. *glabriusculum*. *Zhongguo Zhong Yao Za Zhi* 34, no. 22 (2009): 2895–97.

Yan, Q. N., et al. Study on the tissue distribution of berberine from rhizoma coptidis and compatibility with rhizoma coptidis and cortex cinnamomi in rats. *Zhong Yao Cai* 32, no. 4 (2009): 575–78.

Yang, C., et al. Effects of processing *Phellodendron amurense* with salt on anti-gout. *Zhongguo Zhong Yao Za Zhi* 30, no. 2 (2005): 145–48.

Yang, H. T., et al. Transport and uptake characteristics of a new derivative of berberine (CPU-86017) by human intestinal epithelial cell line: Caco-2. *Acta Pharmacol Sin* 24, no. 12 (2003): 1185–91.

Yao, M., et al. A reproductive screening test of goldenseal. *Birth Defects Res B Dev Reprod Toxicol* 74, no. 5 (2005): 399–404.

Ye, M., et al. Neuropharmacological and pharmacokinetic properties of berberine: a review of recent research. *J Pharm Pharmacol* 61, no. 7 (2009): 831–37.

Yi, L., et al. Simultaneous determination of baicalin, rhein and berberine in rat plasma by column-switching high-performance liquid chromatography. *J Chromatogr B Analyt Technol Biomed Life Sci* 838, no. 1 (2006): 50–55.

Yi, P., et al. Molecular mechanism of berberine in improving insulin resistance induced by free fatty acid through inhibiting nuclear transcription factor-kappaB p65 in 3T3-L1 adipocytes. *Zhongguo Zhong Xi Yi Jie He Za Zhi* 27, no. 12 (2007): 1099–104.

Yin, Jun., et al. Berberine improves glucose metabolism through induction of glycolysis. *Am J Physiol Endocrinol Metab* 294, no. 1 (2008): E148–156.

Yin, L., et al. Simultaneous determination of 11 active components in two well-known traditional Chinese medicines by HPLC coupled with diode array detection for quality control. *J Pharm Biomed Anal* 49, no. 4 (2009): 1101–8.

Yu, H. H., et al. Antimicrobial activity of berberine alone and in combination with ampicillin or oxacillin against methicillin-resistant *Staphylococcus aureus. J Med Food* 8, no. 4 (2005): 454–61.

Yu, Y., et al. Modulation of glucagon-like-peptide-1 release by berberine: in vivo and in vitro studies. *Biochem Pharmacol* 79, no. 7 (2010): 1000–1006.

Zhang, D., and T. Hartley. Phellodendron Ruprecht. In *Flora of China* 11, 75–76. St. Louis, MS: Missouri Botanical Garden Press; Beijing: Science Press, 2008.

Zhang, D. M., et al. Effect of baicalin and berberine on transport of nimodipine on primary-cultured, rat brain microvascular endothelial cells. *Acta Pharmacol Sin* 28, no. 4 (2007): 573–78.

Zhang, Q.-J., et al. Inhibitory activity of substance in seed and sarcocarp of *Phellodendron amurense*. In *Chinese Traditional and Herbal Drugs* 1 (2008) [in Chinese]. English abstract on Medicine & Hygiene website at http://medicine -hygiene.idnwhois.org/download. php?aid=32448 (accessed December 25, 2011).

Zhang, Y., et al. Studies on in vivo release of berberine hydrochloride from carboxymethyl konjac glucomannan pellets in rats. *Zhongguo Zhong Yao Za Zhi* 33, no. 13 (2008):1591–95.

Zhang, Y., et al. Study on release mechanism of berberine hydrochloride-loaded carboxymethyl konjac glucomannan pellets for colonic delivery. *Zhongguo Zhong Yao Za Zhi* 33, no. 1 (2008): 23–26.

Zheng, H., et al.. *Phellodendron amurense*: Amur corktree. In *Invasive Plants of Asian Origin Established in the United States and Their Natural Enemies* 1, 131–32. Morgantown, W.Va.: U.S. Department of Agriculture Forest Service, 2004. Online on the BugwoodWiki website: http://wiki.bugwood.org/uploads/ Phellodendron.pdf.

Zhou, H., et al. Determination of berberine in *Phellodendron chinense* Schneid and its processed products by TLC (thin layer chromatography) densitometry. *Zhongguo Zhong Yao Za Zhi* 20, no. 7 (1995): 405–7, 447.

Zhou, H. Y., et al. Ferulates, amurenlactone A and amurenamide A from traditional Chinese medicine cortex phellodendri amurensis. *J Asian Nat Prod Res* 19, no. 5–6 (2008): 409–13.

Zuo, Feng. Pharmacokinetics of berberine and its main metabolites in conventional and pseudo germ-free rats determined by liquid chromatography/ion trap mass spectrometry. *Drug Metab Dispos* 34, no. 12 (2006): 2064–71.

Bidens

Abajo, C., et al. In vitro study of the antioxidant and immunomodulatory activity of aqueous infusion of *Bidens pilosa. J Ethnopharmacol* 93, no. 2 (2004): 319–23.

Alarcon-Aguilar, F. J., et al. Investigation on the hypoglycemic effects of extracts of four Mexican medicinal plants in normal and alloxan-diabetic mice. *Phytother Res* 16, no. 4 (2002): 383–86.

Alvarez, A., et al. Gastric antisecretory and antiulcer activities of an ethanolic extract of *Bidens pilosa* L. var. *radiata* Schult. Bip. *J Ethnopharmacol* 67, no. 3 (1999): 333–40.

Alvarez, L., et al. Bioactive polyacetylenes from *Bidens pilosa. Planta Med* 62, no. 4 (1996): 355–57.

Andrade-Neto, V. F., et al. Antimalarial activity of *Bidens pilosa* L. (Asteraceae) ethanol extracts from wild plants collected in various localities or plants cultivated in human soil. *Phytother Res* 18, no. 8 (2004): 634–39.

Anonymous. Bidens pilosa. Wikipedia. http:// en.wikipedia.org/wiki/Bidens_pilosa (accessed January 14, 2011).

Anonymous. *Bidens pilosa* (herb). Entry in the Global Invasive Species Database, modified August 30, 2010. http:// issg.org/database/species/ecology. asp?si=1431&fr=1&sts=&lang=EN.

Anonymous. *Bidens pilosa* L., Asteraceae. Entry in the Pacific Island Ecosystems at Risk (PIER) database, updated March 5, 2010. http://hear. org/pier/species/bidens_pilosa.htm.

Anonymous. *Bidens pilosa* Linn. Newsodrome, September 28, 2011. http://newsodrome.com/ alternative_medicine_news/bidens-pilosa- linn-22584780.

Anonymous. *Presence of compounds in picao preto* (Bidens pilosa). Carson City, Nev.: Raintree Nutrition, 2004. http://rain-tree.com/picao- preto-chemicals.pdf.

Ashafa, A. O. T., et al. Screening the root extracts from *Bidens pilosa* L. var. *radiata* (Asteraceae) for antimicrobial potentials. *J Med Plant Res* 3, no. 8 (2009): 568–72.

Brandão, M. G. L., et al. Antimalarial activity of extracts and fractions from *Bidens pilosa* and other *Bidens* species (Asteraceae) correlated with the presence of acetylene and flavonoid compounds. *J Ethnopharmacol* 57 (1997): 131–38.

Chang, C. L., et al. Cytopiloyne, a polyacetylenic glucose, prevents type 1 diabetes in nonobese diabetic mice. *J Immunol* 178, no. 11 (2007): 6984–93.

Chang, C. L., et al. The distinct effects of a butanol fraction of *Bidens pilosa* plant extract on the development of Th1-mediated diabetes and Th2-mediated airway inflammation in mice. *J Biomed Sci* 12, no. 1 (2005): 79–89.

Chang, J. S., et al. Antileukemic activity of *Bidens pilosa* L. var. *minor* (Blume) Sherff and *Houttuynia cordata* Thunb. *Am J Chin Med* 29, no. 2 (2001): 303–12.

Chang, M.-H., et al. The low polar constituents from *Bidens pilosa* L. var. *minor* (Blume) Sherff. *J Chinese Chem Soc* 47 (2000): 1131–36.

Chang, S. L., et al. Flavonoids centaurein and centaureidin, from *Bidens pilosa*, stimulate IFN-gamma expression. *J Ethnopharmacol* 112, no. 2 (2007): 232–36.

Chang, S.-L., et al. Polyacetylenic compounds and butanol fraction from *Bidens pilosa* can modulate the differentiation of helper t cells and prevent autoimmune diabetes in non-obese diabetic mice. *Planta Med* 70, no. 11 (2004): 1045–51.

Chiang, L. C., et al. Anti-herpes simplex virus activity of *Bidens pilosa* and *Houttuynia cordata*. *Am J Chin Med* 31, no. 3 (2003): 355–62.

Chiang, Y. M., et al. Cytopiloyne, a novel polyacetylenic glucoside from *Bidens pilosa*, functions as a T helper cell modulator. *J Ethnopharmacol* 110, no. 3 (2007): 532–38.

Chiang, Y. M., et al. Metabolite profiling and chemopreventive bioactivity of plant extracts from *Bidens pilosa*. *J Ethnopharmacol* 95, no. 2–3 (2004): 409–19.

Chien, S. C., et al. Anti-diabetic properties of three common *Bidens pilosa* variants in Taiwan. *Phytochemistry* 70, no. 10 (2009): 1246–54.

Chih, H. W., et al. Anti-inflammatory activity of Taiwan folk medicine "ham-hong-chho" in rats. *Am J Chin Med* 23, no. 3–4 (1995): 273–78.

Chin, H. W., et al. The hepatoprotective effects of Taiwan folk medicine ham-hong-chho in rats. *Am J Chin Med* 24, no. 3–4 (1996): 231–40.

Chippaux, J. P., et al. Drug or plant substances which antagonize venoms or potentiate antivenins. *Bull Soc Pathol Exot* 90, no. 4 (1997): 282–85.

Corren, J., et al. Clinical and biochemical effects of a combination botanical product (ClearGuard) for allergy: a pilot randomized double-blind placebo-controlled trial. *Nutr J* 14, no. 7 (2008): 20.

Costa R. J., et al. In vitro study of mutagenic potential of *Bidens pilosa* Linné and *Mikania glomerata* Sprengel using the comet and micronucleus assays. *J Ethnopharmacol* 118, no. 1 (2008): 86–93.

Dimo, T., et al. Effects of leaf aqueous extract of *Bidens pilosa* (Asteraceae) on KCI- and norepinephrine-induced contractions of rat aorta. *J Ethnopharmacol* 60, no. 2 (1998): 179–82.

Dimo, T., et al. Effects of the aqueous and methylene chloride extracts of *Bidens pilosa* leaf on fructose-hypertensive rats. *J Ethnopharmacol* 76, no. 3 (2001): 215–21.

Dimo, T., et al. Hypotensive effects of a methanol extract of *Bidens pilosa* Linn on hypertensive rats. *C R Acad Sci III* 322, no. 4 (1999): 323–29.

Dimo, T., et al. Leaf methanol extract of *Bidens pilosa* prevents and attenuates the hypertension induced by high-fructose diet in Wistar rats. *J Ethnopharmacol* 83, no. 3 (2002): 183–91.

Dimo, T., et al. Possible mechanisms of action of the neutral extract from *Bidens pilosa* L. leaves on the cardiovascular system of anaesthetized rats. *Phytother Res* 17, no. 1 (2003): 1135–39.

Frida, L., et al. In vivo and in vitro effects of *Bidens pilosa* L. (Asteraceae) leaf aqueous and ethanol extracts on primed-oestrogenized rat uterine muscle. *Afr J Tradit Complement Altern Med* 5, no. 1 (2007): 79–91.

Garcia, M., et al. Screening of medicinal plants against *Leishmania amazonensis*. *Pharm Biol* 48, no. 9 (2010): 1053–58.

Gbedema, S. Y., et al. Modulation effect of herbal extracts on the antibacterial activity of tetracycline. *Int J Contemp Res Rev* 1, no. 4 (2010): 1–5.

Gbolade, A. A. Inventory of antidiabetic plants in selected districts of Lagos State, Nigeria. *J Ethnopharmacol* 121, no. 1 (2009): 135–39.

Geissberger, P., et al. Constituents of *Bidens pilosa* L.: do the components found so far explain the use of this plant in traditional medicine? *Acta Trop* 48, no. 4 (1991): 251–61.

Hoffmann, B., et al. Further acylated chalcones from *Bidens pilosa*. *Planta Med* 54, no. 5 (1988): 450–51.

Hoffmann, B., et al. New chalcones from *Bidens pilosa*. *Planta Med* 54, no. 1 (1988): 52–54.

Horiuchi, M., et al. Effects of *Bidens pilosa* L. var. *radiata* Scherff on experimental gastric lesion. *J Nat Med* 64, no. 4 (2010): 430–35.

Horiuchi, M., et al. Improvement of the antiiinflammatory and antiallerginic activity of *Bidens pilosa* L. var. *radiata* Scherff treated with enzyme (cellulosine). *J Health Sci* 54, no. 3 (2008): 294–301.

Hsu, H.-M., et al. Contrasting effects of aqueous tissue extracts from an invasive plant, *Bidens pilosa* L. var. *radiata*, on the performance of its sympatric plant species. *Taiwania* 54, no. 3 (2009): 255–60.

Hsu, Y. J., et al. Anti-hyperglycemic effects and mechanism of *Bidens pilosa* water extract. *J Ethnopharmacol* 122, no. 2 (2009): 379–83.

Hudson, J. B. Plant photosensitizers with antiviral properties. *Antiviral Res* 12, no. 2 (1989): 55–74.

Hudson, J. B., et al. Therapeutic potential of plant photosensitizers. *Pharmacol Ther* 49, no. 3 (1991): 181–222.

Jäger, A. K., et al. Screening of Zulu medicinal plants for prostaglandin-synthesis inhibitors. *J Ethnopharmacol* 52, no. 2 (1996): 95–100.

Khan, M. R., et al. Anti-microbial activity of *Bidens pilosa*, *Bischofia javanica*, *Elmerillia papuana* and *Sigesbekia orientalis*. *Fitoterapia* 72, no. 6 (2001): 662–65.

Krettli, A. U., et al. The search for new antimalarial drugs from plants used to treat fever and malaria or plants randomly selected: review. *Mem Inst Oswaldo Cruz* 96, no. 8 (2001): 1033–42.

Kumar, J. K., et al. A new disubstituted actylacetone from the leaves of *Bidens pilosa* Linn. *Nat Prod Res* 17, no. 1 (2003): 71–74.

Kumari, P., et al. A promising anticancer and antimalarial component from the leaves of *Bidens pilosa. Planta Med* 75, no. 1 (2009): 59–61.

Kviecinski, M. R., et al. Study of the antitumor potential of *Bidens pilosa* (Asteraceae) used in Brazilian folk medicine. *J Ethnopharmacol* 117, no. 1 (2008): 69–75.

Lans, Cheryl. Comparison of plants used for skin and stomach problems in Trinidad and Tobago with Asian ethnomedicine. *J Ethnobiol Ethnomed* 3 (2007): 1–25.

Leonard, D. B. Medicine at your feet: plants and food: *Bidens* spp. On the website of Medicine at Your Feet, produced by David Bruce Leonard, L.Ac. http://medicineatyourfeet.com/bidenspilosa.html (accessed January 14, 2011).

Makuzva, R., et al. Antimicrobial screening in *Bidens pilosa* and *Jatropha curcas*. Honors project publication, 1990, Department of Pharmacy, Faculty of Medicine, University of Zimbabwe. http://uz.ac.zw/medicine/pharmacy/pubs/1990.html.

Matsumoto, T., et al. Effects of *Bidens pilosa* L. var. *radiata* Scherff treated with enzyme on histamine-induced contraction of guinea pig ileum and on histamine release from mast cells. *J Smooth Muscle Res* 45, no. 2–3 (2009): 75–86.

Moundipa, P. F., et al. In vitro amoebicidal activity of some medicinal plants of the Bamun region (Cameroon). *Afr J Tradit Complement Altern Med* 2, no. 2 (2005): 113–21.

Mvere, B. *Bidens pilosa* L. Record in the Protabase database, ed. G. J. H. Grubben and O. A. Denton (PROTA: Plant Resources of Tropical Africa/Resources végétales de l'Afrique tropicale). Wageningen, Netherlands. http://database.prota.org/search.htm (accessed January 14, 2011).

Nguelefack, T. B., et al. Relaxant effects of the neutral extract of the leaves of *Bidens pilosa* Linn on isolated rat vascular smooth muscle. *Phytother Res* 19, no. 3 (2005): 207–10.

Ogunbinu, A. O., et al. Constituents of *Cajuns cajan* (L.) Millsp., *Moringa oleifera* Lam., *Heliotropium indicum* L. and *Bidens pilosa* L. from Nigeria. *Nat Prod Commun* 4, no. 4 (2009): 573–78.

Okoli, R. I., et al. Phytochemical and antimicrobial properties of four herbs from Edo State, Nigeria. *Report and Opinion* 1, no. 5 (2009): 67–73.

Oliviera, F. Q., et al. New evidences of antimalarial activity of *Bidens pilosa* roots extract correlated with polyacetylene and flavonoids. *J Ethnopharmacol* 93, no. 1 (2004): 39–42.

Ong, P. L., et al. The anticancer effect of protein-extract from *Bidens alba* in human colorectal carcinoma SW480 cells via the reactive oxidative species- and glutathione depletion-dependent apoptosis. *Food Chem Toxicol* 46, no. 5 (2008): 1535–47.

Parry, D. W., et al. Opaline silica deposits in the leaves of *Bidens pilosa* L. and their possible significance in cancer. *Annal Botany* 58 (1986): 641–47.

Pereira, R. L., et al. Immunosuppressive and anti-inflammatory effects of methanolic extract and the polyacetylene isolated from *Bidens pilosa* L. *Immunopharmacology* 43, no. 1 (1999): 31–37.

Priyanka, K., et al. A promising anticancer and antimalarial component from the leaves of *Bidens pilosa. Planta Med* 75, no. 1 (2009): 59–61.

Rabe, T., et al. Antibacterial activity of South African plants used for medicinal purposes. *J Ethnopharmacol* 56 (1997): 81–87.

Rojas, J. J., et al. Screening for antimicrobial activity of ten medicinal plants used in Colombian folkloric medicine: a possible alternative in the treatment of non-nosocomial infections. *BMC Complement Alt Med* 6 (2006): 2.

Sarg, T. M., et al. Constituents and biological activity of *Bidens pilosa* L. grown in Egypt. *Acta Pharm Hung* 61, no. 6 (1991): 317–23.

Sarker, S. D., et al. 5-O-methylhoslundin: an unusual flavonoid from *Bidens pilosa* (Asteraceae). *Biochem Syst Ecol* 28, no. 6 (2000): 591–93.

Sun, Y., et al. Cadmium tolerance and accumulation characteristics of *Bidens pilosa* L. as a potential Cd-hyperaccumulator. *J Hazard Mater* 161, no. 2–3 (2009): 808–14.

Sun, Y. B., et al. Characteristics of cadmium tolerance and bioaccumulation of *Bidens pilosa* L. seedlings. *Huan Jing Ke Xue* 30, no. 10 (2009): 3028–35.

Sun, Y. B., et al. Joint effects of arsenic and cadmium on plant growth and metal bioaccumulation: a potential Cd-hyperaccumulator and As-excluder *Bidens pilosa* L. *J Hazard Mater* 165, no. 1–3 (2009): 1023–28.

Sundararajan, P., et al. Studies of anticancer and antipyretic activity of *Bidens pilosa* whole plant. *Afr Health Sci* 6, no. 1 (2006): 27–30.

Suzigan, M. I., et al. An acqueous extract of *Bidens pilosa* L. protects liver from cholestatic disease: experimental study in young rats. *Acta Cir Bras* 24, no. 5 (2009): 347–52.

Tan, P. V., et al. Effects of methanol, cyclohexane and methylene chloride extracts of *Bidens pilosa* on various gastric ulcer models in rats. *J Ethnopharmacol* 73, no. 3 (2000): 415–21.

Tobinaga, S., et al. Isolation and identification of a potent antimalarial and antibacterial polyacetylene from *Bidens pilosa. Planta Med* 75, no. 6 (2009): 624–28.

Towers, G. H., et al. Potentially useful antimicrobial and antiviral phototoxins from plants. *Photochem Photobiol* 46, no. 1 (1987): 61–66.

Trivedi, P., et al. HPLC method development and validation of cytotoxic agent phenyl-heptatriyne in *Bidens pilosa* with ultrasonic-assisted cloud point extraction and preconcentration. *Biomed Chromatogr* 25, no. 6 (2011): 697–706. E-pub (preprint) September 1, 2010.

Ubillas, R. P., et al. Antihyperglycemic acetylenic glucosides from *Bidens pilosa. Planta Med* 66, no. 1 (2000): 82–83.

Usami, E., et al. Assessment of antioxidant activity of natural compound by water- and lipid-soluble antioxidant factor. *Yakugaku Zasshi* 124, no. 11 (2004): 847–50.

Valdés, H. A. L., et al. *Bidens pilosa* Linné. *Rev Cubana Plant Med* 1 (2001): 28–33.

Wang, R., et al. Polyacetylenes and flavonoids from the aerial parts of *Bidens pilosa*. *Planta Med* 76, no. 9 (2010): 893–96.

Wat, C. K., et al. Ultraviolet-mediated cytotoxic activity of phenylheptatriyne from *Bidens pilosa* L. *J Nat Prod* 42, no. 1 (1979): 103–11.

Waterhouse, D. F. *Bidens pilosa*. In *Biological Control of Weeds: Southeast Asian Prospects*, 26–33. Canberra: Australian Centre for International Agricultural Research, 1994. http://aciar.gov.au/files/node/2160/MN26%20Part%203.pdf.

Wei, S., et al. Screen of Chinese weed species for cadmium tolerance and accumulation characteristics. *Int J Phytoremediation* 10, no. 6 (2008): 584–97.

Wei, S. H., et al. Hyperaccumulative characteristics of 7 widely distributed weed species in composite family especially *Bidens pilosa* to heavy metals. *Huan Jing Ke Xue* 29, no. 10 (2008): 2912–18.

Wu, L. W., et al. A novel polyacetylene significantly inhibits angiogenesis and promotes apoptosis in human endothelial cells through activation of the CDK inhibitors and caspase-7. *Planta Med* 73, no. 7 (2007): 655–61.

Wu, L. W., et al. Polyacetylenes function as anti-angiogenic agents. *Pharm Res* 21, no. 11 (2004): 2112–19.

Wu, Y. S., et al. Season variations for metallic elements compositions study in plant *Bidens pilosa* L. var. *radiate* Sch. in central Taiwan. *Environ Monit Assess* 168, no. 1–4 (2010): 255–67.

Yang, H. L., et al. Protection from oxidative damage using *Bidens pilosa* extracts in normal human erythrocytes. *Food Chem Toxicol* 44, no. 9 (2006): 1513–21.

Yoshida, N., et al. *Bidens pilosa* suppresses interleukin-1beta-induced cyclooxygenase-2 expression through the inhibition of mitogen activated protein kinases phosphorylation in normal human dermal fibroblasts. *J Dermatol* 33, no. 10 (2006): 676–83.

Yuan, L. P., et al. Protective effects of total flavonoids of *Bidens pilosa* L. (TFB) on animal liver injury and liver fibrosis. *J Ethnopharmacol* 116, no. 3 (2008): 539–46.

Black Pepper/Piperine

Al-Fatimi, M., et al. Antimicrobial, cytotoxic and antioxidant activity of selected basidiomycetes from Yemen. *Pharmazie* 60, no. 10 (2005): 776–80.

Allameh, A., et al. Piperine, a plant alkaloid of the piper species, enhances the bioavailability of afloxin B1 in rat tissues. *Cancer Lett* 61, no. 3 (1992): 195–99.

Anonymous. Biological activities of piperine. Entry in Dr. Duke's Phytochemical and Ethnobotanical Databases. http://www.ars-grin.gov/duke (accessed February 27, 2011).

Anonymous. Chemicals in: *Piper nigrum* L. (Piperaceae). Entry in Dr. Duke's Phytochemical and Ethnobotanical Databases. http://www.ars-grin.gov/duke (accessed February 27, 2011).

Anonymous. Piperine. QuestHealthLibrary.com, a website of Quest Vitamins. http://www.questhealthlibrary.com/herbs/piperine (accessed January 30, 2010).

Atal, C. K. Biochemical basis of enhanced drug availability by piperine: evidence that piperine is a potent inhibitor of drug metabolism. *J Pharmacol Exp* 232, no. 1 (1985): 258–62.

Badmaev, V., et al. Piperine derived from black pepper increases the plasma levels of coenzyme Q10 following oral supplementation. *J Nutr Biochem* 11, no. 2 (2000): 109–13.

Bajad, S., et al. Antidiarrhoeal activity of piperine in mice. *Planta Med* 67, no. 3 (2001): 284–87.

Bang, J. S., et al. Anti-inflammatory and antiarthritic effects of piperine in human interleukin 1beta-stimulated fibroblast-like synoviocytes and in rat arthritis models. *Arthritis Res Ther* 11, no. 2 (2009): R49.

Bhardwaj, R. K., et al. Piperine, a major constituent of black pepper, inhibits human P-glycoprotein and CYP3A4. *J Pharmacol* 302, no. 2 (2002): 645–50.

Bishnoi, M., et al. Protective effect of curcumin and its combination with piperine (bioavailability enhancer) against haloperidol-associated neurotoxicity: cellular and neurochemical evidence. *Neurotox Res* 20, no. 3 (2011): 215–25. E-pub (preprint) November 13, 2010.

Chaudhry, N. M., et al. Bactericidal activity of black pepper, bay leaf, aniseed and coriander against oral isolates. *Pak J Pharm Sci* 19, no. 3 (2006): 214–18.

Chen, J., et al. The role of CYP3A4 and p-glycoprotein in food-drug and herb-drug interactions. *Pharmacist* 25, no. 9 (2006): 732–38.

Chonpathompikunlert, P., et al. Piperine, the main alkaloid of Thai black pepper, protects against neurodegeneration and cognitive impairment in animal model of cognitive deficit like condition of Alzheimer's disease. *Food Chem Toxicol* 48, no. 3 (2010): 798–802.

Chun, H., et al. Biochemical properties of polysaccharides from black pepper. *Biol Pharm Bull* 25, no. 9 (2002): 1203–8.

Dama, M. S., et al. Effect of trikatu pretreatment on the pharmacokinetics of pefloxacin administered orally in mountain Gaddi goats. *J Vet Sci* 9, no. 1 (2008): 25–29.

Fu, M., et al. Neuroprotective effect of piperine on primarily cultured hippocampal neurons. *Biol Pharm Bull* 33, no. 4 (2010): 598–603.

Gideon [pseud.]. Piperine multiplies the strength of many supplements and drugs. *Delano Report* (blog). http://Delano.com/blog/?tag=piperine (accessed 2/27/2011).

Gupta, S. K., et al. Comparative anti-nociceptive, anti-inflammatory and toxicity profile of nimesulide vs nimesulide and piperine combination. *Pharmacol Res* 41, no. 6 (2002): 657–62.

Horn, J. R., and P. D. Hansten. Get to know an enzyme: CYP3A4. *Pharmacy Times*, September 2008: 40–42.

Johri, R. K. Piperine-mediated changes in the permeability of rat intestinal epithelial cells. The status of gamma-glutamyl transpeptidase activity, uptake of amino acids and lipid peroxidation. *Biochem Pharmacol* 43, no. 7 (1992): 1401–7.

Lala, L. G., et al. Pharmacokinetic and pharmacodynamic studies on interaction of "trikatu" with diclofenac sodium. *J Ethnopharmacol* 91, no. 2–3 (2004): 277–80.

Lee, S. W., et al. Alkamides from the fruits of *Piper longum* and *Piper nigrum* displaying potent cell adhesion inhibition. *Bioorg Med Chem Lett* 18, no. 16 (2008): 4544–46.

Matheny, C., et al. Pharmacokinetic and pharmacodynamic implications of P-glycoprotein modulation. *Pharmacotherapy Publications* 21, no. 7 (2001): 1–2.

Mehmood, M. H., et al. Pharmacological basis for the medicinal use of black pepper and piperine in gastrointestinal disorders. *J Med Food* 13, no. 5 (2010): 1086–96.

Mujumdar, A. M., et al. Anti-inflammatory activity of piperine. *Jpn J Med Sci Biol* 43, no. 3 (1990): 95–100.

Mujumdar, A. M., et al. Effect of piperine on pentobarbitone induced hypnosis in rats. *Indian J Exp Biol* 28, no. 5 (1990): 486–87.

Najar, I. A., et al. Involvement of P-glycoprotein and CYP 3A4 in the enhancement of eteposide bioavailability by a piperine analogue. *Chem Biol Interact* 190, no. 2–3 (2011). E-pub (preprint) February 17, 2011.

Nakatani, N., et al. Chemical constituents of peppers (*Piper* spp.) and application to food preservation: naturally occurring antioxidative compounds. *Environ Health Perspect* 67 (1986): 135–42.

Oesterheld, Jessica. P-gp (ABCB1) Introduction. On the website of GeneMDRx. http://www.genemedrx.com/PGP_Introduction.php (accessed February 27, 2011).

Pathak, N., et al. Cytoprotective and immunomodulating properties of piperine on murine splenocytes: an in vitro study. *Eur J Pharmacol* 576, no. 1–3 (2007): 160–70.

Ramakrishnan, Pankajavalli. The role of P-glycoprotein in the blood-brain barrier. *Einstein Quart J Biol Med* 19 (2003): 160–65.

Rasheed, M., et al. Phytochemical studies on the seed extract of *Piper nigrum* Linn. *Nat Prod Res* 19, no. 7 (2005): 703–12.

Reddy, S. V., et al. Antibacterial constituents from the berries of *Piper nigrum*. *Phytomedicine* 11, no. 7–8 (2004): 697–700.

Rho, M. C., et al. ACAT inhibition of alkamides identified in the fruits of *Piper nigrum*. *Phytochemistry* 68, no. 6 (2007): 899–903.

Sabina, E. P., et al. A role of piperine on monosodium urate crystal-induced inflammation—an experimental model of gouty arthritis. *Inflammation* 34, no. 3 (2011). E-pub (preprint) 2010.

Sasidharan, I. Comparative chemical composition and antimicrobial activity of berry and leaf essential oils of *Piper nigrum* L. *IJBMR* 1, no. 4 (2010): 215–18.

Shingh, I. P., et al. Synthesis and antileishmanial activity of piperoyl-amino acid conjugates. *Eur J Med Chem* 45, no. 8 (2010): 3439–45.

Shoba, G., et al. Influence of piperine on the pharmacokinetics of curcumin in animals and human volunteers. *Planta Med* 64, no. 4 (1998): 353–56.

Suresh, D. V, et al. Binding of bioactive phyto-chemical piperine with human serum albumin: a spectrofluorometric study. *Biopolymers* 86, no. 4 (2007): 265–75.

Thummel, K. Gut instincts: CYP3A4 and intestinal drug metabolism. *J Clin Invest* 117, no. 11 (2007): 3173–76.

Volak, L. P., et al. Curcuminoids inhibit multiple human cytochromes P450, UDP-glucuronosyltransferase, and sulfotransferaseenzymes, whereas piperine is a relatively selective CYP3A4 inhibitor. *Drug Metab Dispos* 36, no. 8 (2008): 1594–605.

Zhang, W., et al. Dietary regulation of P-gp function and expression. *Expert Opin Drug Metab Toxicol* 5, no. 7 (2009): 789–801.

Zhou, S., et al. Herbal modulation of P-glycoprotein. *Drug Metab Rev* 36, no. 1 (2004): 57–104.

Boneset

Anonymous. Chemicals in: *Eupatorium perfoliatum* L. (Asteraceae). Entry in Dr. Duke's Phytochemical and Ethnobotanical Databases. http://ars-grin.gov/duke (accessed December 9, 2010).

Elsässer-Beile, U., et al. Cytokine production in leukocyte cultures during therapy with echinacea extract. *J Clin Lab Anal* 10, no. 6 (1996): 441–45.

Gassinger, C. A. A controlled clinical trial for testing of efficacy of the homeopathic drug *Eupatorium perfoliatum* D2 in the treatment of common cold (author's transl). *Arzneimittelforschung* 31, no. 4 (1981): 732–36.

Habtemariam, S., et al. Cytotoxicity and antibacterial activity of ethanol extract from leaves of a herbal drug, boneset (*Eupatorium perfoliatum*). *Phytother Res* 14, no. 7 (2000): 575–77.

Herz, W., et al. Sesquiterpene lactones of *Eupatorium perfoliatum*. *J Org Chem* 42, no. 13 (1977): 2264–71.

Lang, G., et al. Antiplasmodial activities of sesquiterpene lactones from *Eupatorium semialatum*, *Z Naturforsch C* 57, no. 3–4 (2002): 282–86.

Lira-Salazar, G., et al. Effects of homeopathic medications *Eupatorium perfoliatum* and *Arsenicum album* on parasitemia of *Plasmodium berghei*-infected mice. *Homeopathy* 95, no. 4 (2006): 223–28.

Maas, M., et al. Caffeic acid derivatives from *Eupatorium perfoliatum* L. *Molecules* 14, no. 1 (2008): 36–45.

Robinson, G., et al. Medical attributes of *Eupatorium perfoliatum*—boneset. Paper developed for a course in medical botany at Wilkes University, Wilkes-Barre, Penn., July 2007. http://klemow.wilkes.edu/Eupatorium.html.

Wagner, H., et al. Immunological studies of plant combination preparations. In-vitro and in-vivo studies on the stimulation of phagocytosis. *Arzneimittelforschung* 41, no. 10 (1991): 1072–76.

Woerdenbag, H. J. Enhanced cytostatic of the sesquiterpene lactone eupatoriopicrin by glutathione depletion. *Br J Cancer* 59, no. 1 (1989): 68–75.

Cryptolepis

Ameyaw, Y., et al. Quality and harvesting specifications of some herbalists in the eastern region of Ghana. *Ethnobotanical Leaflets* (2005). http://ethnoleaflets.com/leaflets/eghana.htm.

Ameyaw, Y., et al. The impact of pH and soil nutrients on the total alkaloid content of *Cryptolepis sanguinolenta* (Lindl.) Schtr. *Biosci Biotech Res Asia* 4, no. 2 (2007): 1.

Amponsah, K., et al. Manual for the propagation and cultivation of medicinal plants of Ghana. Accra, Ghana: Aburi Botanic Garden (University of Ghana), 2002. Available from CabDirect at http://cabdirect.org/abstracts/20073006217.html.

Anasah, C., et al. In vitro genotoxicity of the West African anti-malarial herbal *Cryptolepis sanguinolenta* and its major alkaloid cryptolepine. *Toxicology* 208, no. 1 (2005): 141–47.

Anonymous. Antimicrobial properties of some West African medicinal plants II. Antimicrobial activity of aqueous extracts of *Cryptolepis sanguinolenta* (Lindl.) Schlechter. *Quart. J. Crude Du Res* 17, no. 2 (1979): 78–80.

Anonymous. Cryptolepis: An African traditional medicine that provides hope for malaria victims. *Herbal Gram* 60 (2003): 54–59, 67.

Anonymous. *Cryptolepis buchanani*. Brief profile on the website of Ayurvedic Community at http://ayurvediccommunity.com/Botany.asp?Botname=Cryptolepis%20buchanani (accessed December 28, 2010).

Anonymous. Review of cryptoline. On the website of EurekaMag.com at http://eurekamag.com/review/c/427/cryptolepine.php (accessed November 20, 2010).

Anonymous. Selected African botanical remedies. http://academic.cengage.com/resource_uploads/downloads/049511541X_122179.pdf.

Anonymous. Shyamlata. On the website of AyurvedaConsultants.com at http://ayurvedaconsultants.com/images/doctor/ayurveda/ayurvedic-herb-shyamlata.aspx (accessed December 28, 2010).

Ansah, C., et al. Anxiogenic effects of an aqueous crude extract of *Cryptolepis sanguinolenta* (Periploceae) in mice. *Int J Pharmacol* 4, no. 1 (2008): 20–26.

Ansah, C., et al. Cryptolepine provokes changes in the expression of cell cycle proteins in growing cells. *Am J Pharmacol Tox* 4, no. 4 (2009): 177–85.

Ansah, C., et al. The popular herbal antimalarial, extract of *Cryptolepis sanguinolenta*, is potently cytotoxic. *Oxford J Life Sci Med Tox Sci* 70, no. 2 (2002): 245–51.

Ansah, C., et al. Reproductive and developmental toxicity of *Cryptolepis sanguinolenta* in mice. *Res J Pharmacol* 4, no. 1 (2010): 9–14.

Ansah, C., et al. Toxicological evaluation of the anti-malarial herb *Cryptolepis sanguinolenta* in rodents. *J Pharmacol Toxicol* 3 (2008): 335–43.

Appiah, Alfred A. The golden roots of *Cryptolepis sanguinolenta*. In *African natural plant products: new discoveries and challenges in chemistry and quality*, ed. H. R. Juliani, J. E. Simon, and C.-T. Ho, 231–39. ACS Symposium Series 1021. American Chemical Society, 2009.

Asase, A., et al. *Medicinal plants used for the treatment of malaria in Wechiau Community Hippopotamus Sanctuary in Ghana*. Abstract of an oral presentation made at the Society for Economic Botany's 48th annual meeting, June 4–7, 2007, at Lake Forest College, Chicago, Ill. http://econbot.org/_organization_/07_annual_meetings/meetings_by_year/2007/pdfs/abstracts/asase.pdf.

Bakhlet, A. O., et al. Therapeutic utility, constituents and toxicity of some medicinal plants: a review. *Vet Human Toxicol* 37, no. 3 (1995): 255–58.

Banerji, J., et al. A novel route to anticonvulsant imesatins and an approach to cryptolepine, the alkaloid from *Cryptolepis* sp. *Indian J Chem* 44B (2005): 426–29.

Bérangére, G., et al. Synthesis and evaluation of analogues of 10H-indol[3-2-b]-quinoline as G-quadruplex stabilizing ligands and potential inhibitors of the enzyme telomerase. *Org Biomol Chem* 2 (2004): 981–88.

Bierer, D. E., et al. Antihyperglycemic activities of crytolepine analogues: an ethnobotanical lead structure isolated from *Cryptolepis sanguinolenta*. *J Med Chem* 41, no. 15 (1998): 2754–64.

Bierer, D. E., et al. Ethnobotanical-directed discovery of the antihyperglycemic properties of cryptolepine: its isolation from *Cryptolepis sanguinolenta*, synthesis, and in vitro and in vivo activities. *J Med Chem* 41, no. 6 (1998): 894–901.

Bierer, D. E. Hypoglycemic agent from cryptolepis. U.S. Patent 5,917,052, filed September 28, 1994, and issued June 29, 1999.

Boakye-Yiadom, K., et al. Cryptolepine hydrochloride effect on *Staphylococcus aureus*. *J Pharm Sci* 68, no. 12 (1979): 1510–14.

Bugyei, K. A., et al. Clinical efficacy of a tea-bag formulation of *Cryptolepis sanguinolenta* root in the treatment of acute uncomplicated falciparum malaria. *Ghana Med J* 44, no. 1 (2010): 3–9.

Cimanga, K., et al. In vitro and in vivo antiplasmodial activity of cryptolepine and related alkaloids from *Cryptolepis sanguinolenta*. *J Nat Prod* 60, no. 7 (1997): 688–91.

Cimanga, K., et al. In vitro biological activities of alkaloids from *Cryptolepis sanguinolenta*. *Planta Med* 62, no. 1 (1996): 22–27.

Dankwa, Kwabena. Evaluation of antimalarial activity of four (4) *Cryptolepis sanguinolenta* based herbal preparations on *Plasmodium berghei* in mice. Thesis, Kwame Nkruma University of Science and Technology (Ghana), 2006. http://dspace.knust.edu.gh/dspace/handle/123456789/1590.

Dassonneville, L., et al. Cytotoxicity and cell cycle effects of the plant alkaloids cryptolepine and neocryptolepine: relation to drug-induced apoptosis. *Eur J Pharmacol* 409, no. 1 (2000): 9–18.

Gibbons, S., et al. Cryptolepine hydrochloride: a potent antimycobacterial alkaloid derived from *Cryptolepis sanguinolenta*. *Phytother Res* 17, no. 4 (2003): 434–36.

Grycová, Lenka. Applications of NMR to study structures of natural compounds. PhD thesis, Masaryk University, 2010. http://is.muni.cz/th/12679/prif_d/PhD_thesis_LG.pdf.

Guittat, L., et al. Interactions of cryptolepine and neocryptolepine with unusual DNA structures. *Biochemie* 85, no. 5 (2003): 535–47.

Hadden, C. E., et al. 11-isopropylcryptolepine: a novel alkaloid isolated from *Cryptolepis sanguinolenta* characterized using submicro NMR techniques. *J Nat Prod* 62, no. 2 (1999): 238–40.

Humenuik, R., et al. Cytotoxicity and cell cycle effects of novel indolo[2,3-b]quinoline derivatives. *Oncol Res* 13, no. 5 (2003): 269–77.

Iwu, Maurice M. The Associate Program on Ethnobiology, Socio-Economic Value Assessment and Community Based Conservation. Report DAMD17-99-2-9025, prepared for the U.S. Army Medical Research and Materiel Command, Fort Detrick, Md., October 2000. http://www.dtic.mil/cgi-bin/GetTRDoc?Location=U2&doc=GetTRDoc.pdf&AD=ADA406251.

Jansen, P. C. M., and Schmelzer, G. H. *Cryptolepis sanguinoleta* (Lindl.) Schltr. Record from Protabase database, ed. G. J. H. Grubben and O. A. Denton (PROTA: Plant Resources of Tropical Africa/Resources végétales de l'Afrique tropicale). Wageningen, Netherlands. http://database.prota.org/search.htm (accessed November 18, 2010).

Jaromin, A., et al. Liposomal formulation of DIMIQ, potential antitumor indolo[2,3-b] quinoline agent and its cytotoxicity on hepatoma Morris 5123 cells. *Drug Deliv* 15, no. 1 (2008): 49–56.

Jonckers, T. H., et al. Synthesis, cytotoxicity, and antiplasmodial and antitrypanosomal activity of new neocryptolepine derivatives. *J Med Chem* 45, no. 16 (2002): 3497–508.

Kaul, A., et al. Immunopotentiating properties of *Cryptolepis buchanani* root extract. *Phytother Res* 17, no. 10 (2003): 1140–44.

Laupattarakasem, P., et al. An evaluation of the activity related to inflammation of four plants used in Thailand to treat arthritis. *J Ethnopharmacol* 85, no. 2–3 (2003): 207–15.

Laupattarakasem, P., et al. In vitro and in vivo anti-inflammatory potential of *Cryptolepis buchanani*. *J Ethnopharmacol* 108, no. 3 (2006): 349–54.

Luo, J., et al. *Cryptolepis sanguinolenta*: an ethnobotanical approach to drug discovery and the isolation of a potentially useful new antihyperglycaemic agent. *Diabet Med* 15, no. 5 (1998): 367–74.

Luo, J., et al. Hypoglycemic agent from cryptolepis. U.S. Patent 5,629,319, filed June 6, 1995, and issued May 13, 1997.

Maurya, et al. Pharmaceutical composition comprising extract from plant *Cryptolepis buchanani* for tea. U.S. Patent 6,548,086, filed December 18, 2001, and issued April 15, 2003.

Mills-Robertson, F. C., et al. In vitro antimicrobial activity of *Cryptolepis sanguinolenta* (Periplocaceae). *Afr J Pharm Pharmacol* 3, no. 10 (2009): 476–80.

Mtshemla, Vathiswa. Synthesis of 2,3-diaryl-4-methoxyquinolines via palladium-catalyzed cross coupling reactions. Master's thesis, University of South Africa, May 2008. http://uir.unisa.ac.za/bitstream/handle/10500/2275/dissertation.pdf?sequence=1.

Noamesi, B. K., et al. Studies on cryptolepine. *Planta Med* 48, no. 5 (1983): 48–51.

Obua, C., et al. Antimalarial activity of some plants used in traditonal medicine in Uganda. *E C Afr J Pharma Sci* 5, no. 2 (2002): 1.

Olajide, O. A., et al. Anti-inflammatory properties of cryptolepine. *Phytother Res* 23, no. 10 (2009): 1421–25.

Olajide, O. A., et al. Synthetic cryptolepine inhibits DNA binding of NF-kappaB. *Bioorg Med Chem* 15, no. 1 (2007): 43–49.

Oluwafemi, A. J., et al. Evaluation of cryptolepine and huperzine derivatives as lead compounds towards new agents for the treatment of human African trypanosomiasis. *Nat Prod Commun* 4, no. 2 (2009): 193–98.

Otsyina, Hope R. Toxicological evaluation of *Cryptolepis sanguinolenta, Momordica charantia* and *Euphorbia hirta* in rats. Thesis, Kwame Nkruma University of Science and Technology (Ghana), 2008. http://dspace.knust.edu.gh:8080/jspui/handle/123456789/885.

Oyekan, A. O., et al. Cryptolepine inhibits platelet aggregation in vitro and in vivo and stimulates fibrinolysis ex vivo. *Gen Pharmacol* 19, no. 2 (1988): 233–37.

Pande, M., et al. Crystalization and preliminary X-ray analysis of cryptolepain, a novel glycosylated serine protease from *Cryptolepis buchanani*. *Acta Crystallogr Sect F Struct Biol Cryst Commun* 63, part 2 (2006): 74–80.

Paulo, A., et al. Antiplasmodial activity of *Cryptolepis sanguinolenta* alkaloids from leaves and roots. *Planta Med* 66, no. 1 (2000): 30–34.

Paulo, A., et al. Chemotaxonomic analysis of the genus *Cryptolepis. Biochem Syst Ecol* 31, no. 2 (2003): 155–66.

Paulo, A., et al. *Cryptolepis sanguinolenta* activity against diarrhoeal bacteria. *J Ethnopharmacol* 44, no. 2 (1994): 73–77.

Paulo, A., et al. In vitro antibacterial screening of *Cryptolepis sanguinolenta* alkaloids. *J Ethnopharmacol* 44, no. 2 (1994): 127–30.

Paulo, A., et al. Steroidal alkaloids from *Cryptolepis obtusa*. *Phytochemistry* 53, no. 3 (2000): 417–22.

Prasad, P. J. N., et al. Micropropagation of *Cryptolepis buchanani* Roem. & Schult. *Taiwania* 49, no. 1 (2004): 57–65.

Rao, V. R., et al. Interactions of cryptosin with mammalian cardiac beta-adrenoceptors. *Drug Chem Toxicol* 13, no. 2–3 (1990): 173–94.

Rauwald, H. W., et al. *Cryptolepis sanguinolenta*: antimuscarinic properties of cryptolepine and the alkaloid fraction at M1, M2 and M3 receptors. *Planta Med* 58, no. 6 (1992): 486–88.

Sawer, I. K., et al. The effect of cryptolepine on the morphology and survival of *Escherichia coli*, *Candida albicans* and *Saccharomyces cerevisiae*. *J Appl Bacteriol* 79, no. 3 (1995): 314–21.

Sawer, I. K., et al. The killing effect of cryptolepine on *Staphylococcus aureus*. *Lett Appl Microbiol* 40, no. 1 (2005): 24–29.

Silva, O., et al. Antimicrobial activity of Guinea-Bissau traditional remedies. *J Ethnopharmacol* 50, no. 1 (1996): 55–59.

Simon, J. E., et al. Medicinal crops of Africa. In *Issues in new crops and new uses*, ed. J. Janick and A. Whipkey, 322–31. Alexandria, Va.: ASHS Press, 2007. http://hort.purdue.edu/newcrop/ncnu07/pdfs/simon322-331.pdf.

Sittiwet, C., et al. Anti-bacterial activity of *Cryptolepis buchanani* aqueous extract. *Int J Biol Chem* 3 (2009): 90–94.

Soh, P. N., et al. Are West African plants a source of future antimalarial drugs? *J Ethnopharmacol* 114, no. 2 (2007): 130–40.

Tempesta, Michael S. The clinical efficacy of *Cryptolepis sanguinolenta* in the treatment of malaria. *Ghana Med J* 44, no. 1 (2010): 1–2.

Van Miert, S., et al. In vitro inhibition of beta-haematin formation, DNA interactions, neocryptolepine derivatives. *Exp Parasitol* 108, no. 3–4 (2004): 163–68.

Van Miert, S., et al. Isoneocryptolepine, a synthetic indoloquinoline alkaloid, as an antiplasmodial lead compound. *J Nat Prod* 68, no. 5 (2005): 674–77.

Venkateswara, R., et al. Cryptosin, a cardenolide from the leaves of *Cryptolepis buchanani*. *Phytochemistry* 28, no. 4 (1989): 1203–5.

Wright, C. W. Cryptolepine and development of new antimalarial agents. *Iran J Pharm Res (IJPR)* 3, suppl. 2 (2004): 17.

Wright, C. W. Recent developments in naturally derived antimalarials: cryptolepine analogues. *J Pharm Pharmacol* 59, no. 6 (2007): 899–904.

Yakubu, Clare Banoeng. "Nibima": a wonder plant for malaria treatment for Ghana. *Eyes on Malaria* 3 (online). http://eyesonmalaria.org/nibima.html.

Yeau, K. L., et al. The cardiotonic effect of a glycoside from *Cryptolepis buchanani*. *Yao Xue Xue Bao* 10 (1963): 561–65.

Zhu, H., et al. Chemical compound review: cymopol. Entry on WikiGenes website at http://wikigenes.org/e/chem/e/5386672.html (accessed November 18, 2010).

Zhu, H., et al. Mechanisms of induction of cell cycle arrest and cell death by cryptolepine in human lung adenocarcinoma A549 cells. *Oxford J Life Sci Med Tox Sci* 91, no. 1 (2006): 132–39.

Zhu, X. Y., et al. Synthesis and evaluation of isosteres of N-methyl indolo[3,2-b]-quinoline (cryptolepine) as new antinfective agents. *Bioorg Med Chem* 15, no. 2 (2007): 686–95.

Echinacea

Aboulella, A. M., et al. Phytotherapeutic effects of *Echinacea purpurea* in gamma-irradiated mice. *J Vet Sci* 8, no. 4 (2007): 341–51.

Anonymous. Echinacea: Monograph. *Altern Med Rev* 6, no. 4 (2001): 411–14.

Binns, S. E., et al. Light-mediated antifungal activity of echinacea extracts. *Planta Med* 66, no. 3 (2000): 241–14.

Birt, D. F. Echinacea in infection. *Am J Clin Nutr* 87, no. 2 (2008): 488S–92S.

Brush, J., et al. The effect of *Echinacea purpurea*, *Astragalus membranaceus* and *Glycyrrhiza glabra* on CD69 expression and immune cell activation in humans. *Phytother Res* 20, no. 8 (2006): 687–95.

Chaves, Fernando., et al. Effect of *Echinacea purpurea* (Asteraceae) aqueous extract on antibody response to *Bothrops asper* venom and immune cell response. *Rev Biol Trop Int J Trop Biol* 55, no. 1 (2007): 113–19.

Facino, R. M., et al. Echinacoside and caffeoyl conjugates protect collagen from free radical-induced degradation: a potential use of echinacea extracts in the prevention of skin photodamage. *Planta Med* 61, no. 6 (1995): 510–14.

Fuchikama, H., et al. Effects of herbal extracts on the function of human organic anion-transporting polypeptide OATP-B. *Drug Metab Dispos* 34, no. 4 (2006): 577–82.

Jurkstiene, V., et al. Compensatory reactions of immune sytem and action of purple coneflower (*Echinacea purpurea* (L.) Moench) preparations. *Medicina (Kaunas)* 40, no. 7 (2004): 657–62.

Kim, L. S., et al. Immunological activity of larch arabinogalactan and echinacea: a preliminary, randomized, double-blind, placebo-controlled trial. *Altern Med Rev* 7, no. 2 (2002): 138–49.

Kraus, G. A., et al. Synthesis and natural distribution of anti-inflammatory alkamides from echinacea. *Molecule* 11, no. 10 (2006): 758–67.

LaLone, C. A., et al. Echinacea species and alkamides inhibit prostaglandin E(2) production in RAW264.7 mouse macrophage cells. *J Agric Food Chem* 55, no. 18 (2007): 7314–22.

Lee, T.-T., et al. Flavonoid, phenol and polysaccharide content of *Echinacea purpurea* L. and its immunostimulant capacity in vitro. *Internl J Enviro Sci Dev* 1, no. 1 (2010): 5–9.

McCann, D. A., et al. Cytokine- and interferon-modulating properties of *Echinacea* spp. root tinctures stored at −20 degrees C for 2 years. *J Interferon Cytokine Res* 27, no. 5 (2007): 425–36.

Melchart, D., et al. Results of five randomized studies on the immunomodulatory activity of preparations of echinacea. *J Altern Complement Med* 1, no. 2 (1995): 145–60.

Miller, Sandra C. Echinacea: a miracle herb against aging and cancer? Evidence *in vivo* in mice. *Evid Based Complement Alternat Med* 2, no. 3 (2005): 309–14.

Mishima, S., et al. Antioxidant and immuno-enhancing effects of *Echinacea purpurea*. *Biol Pharm Bull* 27, no. 7 (2004): 1004–9.

Pleschka, S., et al. Anti-viral properties and mode of action of standardized *Echinacea purpurea* extract against highly pathogenic avian influenza virus (H5N1, H5N7) and swine-origin H1N1 (S-OIV). *Virol J* 13, no. 6 (2009): 197.

Raduner, S., et al. Alkylamides from echinacea are a new class of cannabinomimetics. Cannabinoid type 2 receptor-dependent and -independent immunomodulatory effects. *J Biol Chem* 281, no. 20 (2006): 14192–206.

Rininger, J. A., et al. Immunopharmacological activity of echinacea preparations following simulated digestion on murine macrophages and human peripheral blood mononuclear cells. *J Leukocyt Biol* 68 (2000): 503.

Roesler, J., et al. Application of purified polysaccharides from cell cultures of the plant *Echinacea purpurea* to mice mediates protection against systemic infections with *Listeria monocytogenes* and *Candida albicans*. *Int J Immunopharmacol* 13, no. 1 (1991): 27–37.

Romiti, N., et al. P-glycoprotein inhibitory activity of lipophilic constituents of *Echinacea pallida* roots in a human proximal tubular cell line. *Planta Med* 74, no. 3 (2008): 264–66.

Rousseau, B., et al. Investigation of anti-hyaluronidase treatment on vocal fold wound healing. *J Voice* 20, no. 3 (2006): 443–51.

Senchina, D. S., et al. Phenetic comparison of seven echinacea species based on immunomodulatory characteristics. *Econ Bot* 60, no. 3 (2006):205–11.

Senchina, D. S., et al. Year-and-a-half old, dried echinacea roots retain cytokine-modulating capabilities in an in vitro human older adult model of influenza vaccination. *Planta Med* 72, no. 13 (2006): 1207–15.

Sharma, M., et al. The potential use of echinacea in acne: control of *Propionibacterium acnes* growth and inflammation. *Phytother Res* 25, no. 4 (2011): 517–21. E-pub (preprint) September 9, 2010.

Sharma, S. M., et al. Bactericidal and anti-inflammatory properties of a standardized echinacea extract (Echinaforce): dual actions against respiratory bacteria. *Phytomedicine* 17, no. 8–9 (2010): 563–68.

Soudi, S., et al. Antileishmanial effect of *Echinacea purpurea* root extract cultivated in Iran. *Iran J Pharm Res* 6, no. 2 (2007): 147–49.

Spence, Katherine M. In vivo evaluation of immunomodulatory properties of crude extracts of *Echinacea* species and fractions isolated from *Echinacea purpurea*. Master's thesis, University of Southern Queensland (Toowoomba, Queensland), 1999. http://eprints.usq.edu.au/1512/.

Steinmüller, C., et al. Polysaccharides isolated from plant cell cultures of *Echinacea purpurea* enhance the resistance of immunosuppressed mice against systemic infections with *Candida albicans* and *Listeria monocytogenes*. *Int J Immunopharmacol* 15, no. 5 (1993): 605–14.

Stevenson, L. M., et al. Modulation of macrophage immune responses by echinacea. *Molecules* 10 (2005): 1279–85.

Tamta, H., et al. Variability in in vitro macrophage activation by commercially diverse bulk echinacea plant material is predominantly due to bacterial lipoproteins and lipopolysaccharides. *J Agric Food Chem* 56, no. 22 (2008): 10552–56.

Tunnerhoff, F. H., et al. Research in man and animal on the effect of echinacea extracts on artificial formation of connective tissues after fibrin implantations. *Arzneimittelforschung* 6, no. 6 (1956): 330–34.

Wagner, H., et al. Immunostimulant action of polysaccharides (heteroglycans) from higher plants. Preliminary communication. *Arzneimittelforschung* 34, no. 6 (1984): 659–61.

Wagner, H., et al. Immunostimulating action of polysaccharides (heteroglycans) from higher plants. *Arzneimittelforschung* 35, no. 7 (1985): 1069–75.

Wang, C. Y., et al. Genomics and proteomics of immune modulatory effects of a butanol fraction of *Echinacea purpurea* in human dendritic cells. *BMC Genomics* 13, no. 9 (2008): 479.

Zaporozhets, O. A., et al. Medicinal plants: spectrophotometric determination of hydroxycynnamic acid and related compounds in echinacea preparations. *Pharmaceutical Chem J* 37, no. 12 (2003): 632.

Zhai, Z., et al. Alcohol extract of *Echinacea pallida* reverses stress-delayed wound healing in mice. *Phytomedicine* 16, no. 6–7 (2009): 669–78.

Zhai, Z., et al. Alcohol extracts of echinacea inhibit production of nitric oxide and tumor necrosis factor-alpha by macrophages in vitro. *Food Agric Immunol* 18, no. 3–4 (2007): 221–36.

Zhai, Z., et al. Echinacea increases arginase activity and has anti-inflammatory properties in RAW 264.7 macrophage cells, indicative of alternative macrophage activation. *J Ethnopharmacol* 122, no. 1 (2009): 76–85.

Zhai, Z., et al. Enhancement of innate and adaptive immune functions by multiple *Echinacea* species. *J Med Food* 10, no. 3 (2007): 423–34.

Zwickey, H., et al. The effects of *Echinacea purpurea*, *Astragalus membranaceus* and *Glycyrrhiza glabra* on CD25 expression in humans: a pilot study. *Phytother Res* 21, no. 11 (2007): 1109–12.

Eleutherococcus

Anonymous. Eleutherococcus. Wikipedia. http://en.Wikipedia.org/wiki/Eleutherococcus (accessed December 9, 2010).

Anonymous. *Eleutherococcus pentaphyllus.* Entry in the U.S. Department of Agriculture Natural Resources Conservation Service PLANTS Database. http://plants.usda.gov/java/profile?symbol=ELPE6 (accessed 12/9/2010).

Anonymous. *Eleutherococcus senticosus.* Entry in the Plants for a Future database. http://pfaf.org/user/Plant.aspx?LatinName=Eleutherococcus+senticosus (accessed January 24, 2008).

Anonymous. *Eleutherococcus senticosus.* Wikipedia. http://en.Wikipedia.org/wiki/Eleutherococcus_senticosus (accessed December 9, 2010).

Anonymous. *Eleutherococcus senticosus*: monograph. *Altern Med Rev* 11, no. 2 (2006): 151–55.

Anonymous. Ginseng: *Eleutherococcus pentaphyllus.* State distribution map on the website of EDDMApS (Early Detection and Distribution Mapping System) at http://eddmaps.org/distribution/usstate.cfm?sub=21019 (accessed December 9, 2010).

Arushanian, E. B., et al. Effect of eleutherococcus on short-term memory and visual perception in healthy humans. *Eksp Klin Farmakol* 66, no. 5 (2003): 10–13.

Bączek, Katarzyna. Accumulation of biologically active compounds in eleuthero (*Eleutherococcus senticosus* /Rupr. Et Maxim./Maxim.) grown in Poland. *Herba Polonica* 55, no. 1 (2009): 7–13.

Barenboim, G. M. Part V: Eleutherococcus and adaptogens: generalizations and hypotheses. Eleutherococcus: application and the mechanism of action. Available online on the website of VitaOffice at http://vitaoffice.com/images/office/download/eleuthroandadaptogens.pdf (accessed December 19, 2011).

Barenboim, G. M., and N. B. Kozlova. Part III: Eleutherococcus extract as an agent increasing the biological resistance of man exposed to unfavorable factors. Use of eleutherococcus extract for increasing the biological resistance of man exposed to different unfavourable environmental factors (a review). Available online on the website of VitaOffice at http://vitaoffice.com/images/office/download/eleuthrobioresist.pdf (accessed December 19, 2011).

Barenboim, G. M., and L. A. Protozanova. Part IV: Eleutherococcus extract: prospective trends in application. General methodological principles of the use of eleutherococcus extract for decreasing the effects of embryotoxic factors. Available online on the website of VitaOffice at http://vitaoffice.com/images/office/download/eleuthrotrends.pdf (accessed December 19, 2011).

Bocharov, E. V., et al. Neuroprotective features of phytoadaptogens. *Vestn Ross Akad Med Nauk* 4 (2008): 47–50.

Cicero, A. F., et al. Effects of Siberian ginseng (*Eleutherococcus senticosus* Maxim.) on elderly quality of life: a randomized clinical trial. *Arch Gerentol Geriatr Suppl* 9 (2004): 69–73.

Dardymov, I. V. Part II: Study of the mechanism of action of eleutherococcus extract. Some aspects of the mechanism of action of eleutherococcus extract. Available online on the website of VitaOffice at http://vitaoffice.com/images/office/download/eleuthromechanism.pdf (accessed December 19, 2011).

Davydov, M., et al. *Eleutherococcus senticosus* (Rupr. & Maxim.) Maxim. (Araliaceae) as an adaptogen: a closer look. *J Ethnopharmacol* 72, no. 3 (2000): 345–93.

Deyama, T., et al. Constituents and pharmacological effects of *Eucommia* and Siberian ginseng, *Acta Pharmacol Sin* 22, no. 12 (2001): 1057–70.

Donovan, J. L., et al. Siberian ginseng (*Eleutherococcus senticosus*) effects on CYP2D6 and CYP3A4 activity in normal volunteers. *Drug Metab Dispos* 31, no. 5 (2003): 519–22.

Drozd, J., et al. Estimation of humoral activity of *Eleutherococcus senticosus*. *Acta Pol Pharm* 59, no. 9 (2002): 395–401.

Feng, S., et al. Determination of eleutheroside E and eleutheroside B in rat plasma and tissue by high-performance liquid chromatography using solid-phase extraction and photodiode array detection. *Eur J Pharm Biopharm* 62, no. 3 (2006): 315–20.

Gaffney, B. T., et al. The effects of *Eleutherococcus senticosus* and *Panax ginseng* on steroidal hormone indices of stress and lymphocyte subset numbers in endurance athletes. *Life Sci* 70, no. 4 (2001): 431–42.

Gaffney, B. T., et al. *Panax ginseng* and *Eleutherococcus senticosus* may exaggerate an already existing biphasic response to stress via inhibition of enzymes which limit the binding of stress hormones to their receptors. *Med Hypotheses* 56, no. 5 (2001): 567–72.

Glatthaar-Saalmüller, B., et al. Antiviral activity of an extract derived from roots of *Eleutherococcus senticosus*. *Antiviral Res* 50, no. 3 (2001): 223–28.

Hartz, A. J., et al. Randomized controlled trial of Siberian ginseng for chronic fatigue. *Psychol Med* 34, no. 1 (2004): 51–61.

Jeong, H. J., et al. Inhibitory effects of mast cell-mediated allergic reactions by cell cultured Siberian ginseng. *Immunopharmacol Immunotoxicol* 23, no. 1 (2001): 107–17.

Jung, C. H., et al. *Eleutherococcus senticosus* extract attenuates LPS-induced iNOS expression through the inhibition of Akt and JNK pathways in murine macrophage. *J Ethnopharmacol* 113, no. 1 (2007): 183–87.

Kang, J. S., et al. Quantitative determination of eleutheroside B and E from *Acanthopanax* species by high performance liquid chromatography. *Arch Pharm Res* 24, no. 5 (2001): 407–11.

Kaplan, E. Y., et al. Part I: Eleutherococcus extract. Action range study of the range of the adaptogenic action of *Eleutherococcus senticosus* Rupr. et Maxim. Available online on the website of VitaOffice at http://vitaoffice.com/images/office/download/eleuthroactionrange.pdf (accessed December 19, 2011).

Kimura, Y., et al. Effects of various *Eleutherococcus senticosus* cortex on swimming time, natural killer activity and corticosterone level in forced swimming stressed mice. *J Ethnopharmacol* 95, no. 2–3 (2004): 447–53.

Kuo, J., et al. The effect of eight weeks of supplementation with *Eleutherococcus senticosus* on endurance capacity and metabolism in human. *Chin J Physiol* 53 (2010): 1–7.

Lee, Jung J., et al. Extract of *Acanthopanax koreanum* for the treatment or prevention of hepatitis or the liver protective drug. U.S. Patent 7,309,504 B2, filed January 24, 2003, and issued December 18, 2007.

Lee, S., et al. Antiinflammatory activity of hyperin from *Acanthopanax chiisanensis* roots. *Arch Pharm Res* 27, no. 6 (2004): 628–32.

Li, W., et al. Acanthopanax for acute ischemic stroke. *Cochrane Database Syst Rev* 8, no. 3 (2009): CD007032.

Liu, Y, et al. Effects of *Acanthopanax giraldii* Harms var. *hispidus* Hoo polysaccharides on the human gastric cancer cell line SGC-7901 and its possible mechanism. *Chin Med J* 115, no. 5 (2002): 716–21.

Natural Products Research Institute at Seoul National University. *Eleutherococcus sessiliflorus*. In *Medicinal plants in the Republic of Korea*. WHO Regional Publications Western Pacific Series, no. 21. Manila: World Health Organization, 1998. http://wpro.who.int/internet/files/pub/97/105.pdf.

Panossian, A., et al. Stimulating effect of adaptogens: an overview with particular reference to their efficacy following single dose administration. *Phytother Res* 19, no. 10 (2005): 819–38.

Park, H. R., et al. Antioxidant activity of extracts from *Acanthopanax senticosus*. *Afr J Biotechnol* 5, no. 23 (2006): 2388–96.

Provalova, N. V., et al. Mechanisms underling the effects of adaptogens on erythropoiesis during paradoxical sleep deprivation. *Bull Exp Biol Med* 133, no. 5 (2002): 428–32.

Randall, R. P. *Eleutherococcus pentaphyllus* (Araliaceae). Entry in *A Global Compendium of Weeds*. Meredith, Victoria (Australia): R. G. and F. J. Richardson, 2002. Available on the website of the Hawaiian Ecosystems at Risk (HEAR) project at http://hear.org/gcw/species/eleutherococcus_pentaphyllus (accessed December 9, 2010).

Rogala, E., et al. The influence of *Eleutherococcus senticosus* on cellular and humoral immunological response of mice. *Pol J Vet Sci* 6, no. 3, suppl. (2003): 37–39.

Sang-Chul, J., et al. Chemical characteristics and immuno-stimulating properties of biopolymers extracted from *Acanthopanax sessiliflorus*. *J Biochem Mol Biol* 39, no. 1 (2006): 84–90.

Schmolz, M. W., et al. The synthesis of Rantes, G-CSF, IL-4, IL-5, IL-6, IL-12 and IL-13 in human whole-blood cultures is modulated by an extract from *Eleutherococcus senticosus* L. roots. *Phytother Res* 15, no. 3 (2001): 268–70.

Singh, N., et al. A comparative evaluation of some anti-stress agents of plant origin. *Ind J Pharmacol* 23, no. 2 (1991): 99–103.

Singh, N., et al. Effect of anti-stress plants on biochemical changes during stress reaction. *Ind J Pharmacol* 23, no. 3 (1991): 137–42.

Sithisarn, P., et al. Antioxidant activity of *Acanthopanax trifoliatus*. *Med Princ Pract* 18 (2009): 393–98.

Soya, H., et al. Extract from *Acanthopanax senticosus* Harms (Siberian ginseng) activates NTS and SON/PVN in the rat brain. *Biosci Biotechnol Biochem* 72, no. 9 (2008): 2467–80.

Steinmann, G. G., et al. Immunopharmacological in vitro effects of *Eleutherococcus senticosus* extracts. *Arzneimittelforschung* 51, no. 1 (2001): 76–83.

Szolomicki, J., et al. The influence of active components of *Eleutherococcus senticosus* on cellular defence and physical fitness in man. *Phytother Res* 14, no. 1 (2000): 30–35.

Tohda, C., et al. Inhibitory effects of *Eleutherococcus senticosus* extracts on amyloid beta(25-35)-induced neuritic atrophy and synaptic loss. *J Pharmacol Sci* 107, no. 3 (2008): 329–39.

Wang, Z., et al. Semipreparative separation and determination of eleutheroside E in *Acanthopanax giraldii* Harms by high-performance liquid chromatography. *J Chromatogr Sci* 43, no. 5 (2005): 249–52.

Weigant, F. A., et al. Plant adaptogens increase lifespan and stress resistance in *C. elegans*. *Biogerontology* 10, no. 1 (2009): 27–42.

Yi, J. M, et al. Effect of *Acanthopanax senticosus* stem on mast cell-dependent anaphylaxis. *J Ethnopharmacol* 79, no. 3 (2002): 347–52.

Yunfei, Deng. *Eleutherococcus humillimus*, a new combination in Chinese Araliaceae. *Novon* 13 (2003): 305–6.

Ginger

Ahui, M. L., et al. Ginger prevents Th2-mediated immune responses in a mouse model of airway inflammation. *Int Immunopharmacol* 8, no. 12 (2008): 1626–32.

Ajith, T. A., et al. *Zingiber officinale* Roscoe prevents acetaminophen-induced acute hepatotoxicity by enhancing hepatic antioxidant status. *Food Chem Toxicol* 45, no. 11 (2007): 2267–72.

Altman, R. D., et al. Effects of a ginger extract on knee pain in patients with osteoarthritis. *Arthritis Rheum* 44, no. 11 (2001): 2531–38.

Anonymous. Ginger. Herbs at a Glance fact sheet from the U.S. National Center for Complementary and Alternative Medicine, updated July 2010. http://nccam.nih.gov/health/ginger/.

Anonymous. Ginger. Profile on the website Herbs2000.com. http://herbs2000.com/herbs/herbs_ginger.htm (accessed February 9, 2011).

Anonymous. Ginger. Wikipedia. http://en.wikipedia.org/wiki/Ginger (accessed February 9, 2011).

Benchaluk, T., et al. Effects of *Zingiber officinale* Roscoe on methyl parathion intoxication in rats. *Chinag Mai Med J* 49, no. 3 (2010): 81–88.

Bensch, K., et al. Investigations into the antiadhesive activity of herbal extracts against *Campylobacter jejuni. Phytother Res* 25, no. 8 (2011): 1125–32. E-pub (preprint) January 31, 2011.

Betoni, J. E., et al. Synergism between plant extract and antimicrobial drugs used on *Staphylococcus aureus* diseases. *Mem Inst Oswaldo Cruz* 101, no. 4 (2006): 387–90.

Betz, O., et al. Is ginger a clinically relevant antiemetic? A systematic review of randomized controlled trials. *Forsch Komplementarmed Klass Naturheilkd* 12, no. 1 (2005): 14–23.

Bhat, J., et al. In vivo enhancement of natural killer cell activity through tea fortified with Ayurvedic herbs. *Phytother Res* 24, no. 1 (2010): 129–35.

Black, C. D., et al. Ginger (*Zingiber officinale*) reduces muscle pain caused by eccentric exercise. *J Pain* 11, no. 9 (2010): 894–903.

Borrelli, F., et al. Effectiveness and safety of ginger in the treatment of pregnancy-induced nausea and vomiting. *Obstet Gynecol* 105, no. 4 (2005): 849–56.

Carrasco, F. R., et al. Immunomodulatory activity of *Zingiber officinale* Roscoe, *Salvia officinalis* L. and *Syzygium aromaticum* L. essential oils: evidence for humor- and cell-mediated responses. *J Pharm Pharmacol* 61, no. 7 (2009): 961–67.

Chen, I. N., et al. Antioxidant and antimicrobial activity of Zingiberaceae plants in Taiwan. *Plant Foods Hum Nutr* 63, no. 1 (2008): 15–20.

Cwikla, C., et al. Investigations into the antibacterial activities of phytotherapeutics against *Helicobacter pylori* and *Campylobacter jejuni*. *Phytother Res* 24, no. 5 (2010): 649–56.

Daswani, P. G., et al. Antidiarrhoeal activity of *Zingiber officinale* (Rosc.). *Current Sci* 98, no. 2 (2010): 222–29,.

Datta, A., et al. Antifilarial effect of *Zingiber officinale* on *Dirofilaria immitis*. *J Helminthol* 61, no. 3 (1987): 268–70.

Demin, G., et al. Comparative antibacterial activities of crude polysaccharides and flavonoids from *Zingiber officinale* and their extraction. *Asian J Trad Med* 5, no. 6 (2010): 1.

Denyer, C. V., et al. Isolation of antirhinoviral sesquiterpenes from ginger (*Zingiber officinale*). *J Nat Prod* 57, no. 5 (1994): 658–62.

Dügenci, S. K., et al. Some medicinal plants as immunostimulant for fish. *J Ethnopharmacol* 88, no. 1 (2003): 99–106.

Egwurugwa, J. N., et al. Effects of ginger (*Zingiber officinale*) on cadmium toxicity. *Afr J Biotechnol* 6, no. 18 (2007): 2078–82.

Fischer-Rasmussen, W., et al. Ginger treatment of hyperemesis gravidarum. *Eur J Obstet Gynecol Reprod Biol* 38, no. 1 (1991): 19–24.

Foster, Steven. Ginger: *Zingiber officinale*—your food is your medicine. Monograph on the website of Steven Foster. http://stevenfoster.com/education/monograph/ginger2.html (accessed February 9, 2011).

Gato, C., et al. Lethal efficacy of extract from *Zingiber officinale* (traditional Chinese medicine) or [6]-shogaol and [6]-gingerol in *Anisakis* larvae in vitro. *Parasitol Res* 76, no. 8 (1990): 653–56.

Gaus, K., et al. Standardized ginger (*Zingiber officinale*) extract reduces bacterial load and suppresses acute and chronic inflammation in Mongolian gerbils infected with cagA *Helicobacter pylori*. *Pharm Biol* 47, no. 1 (2009): 92–98.

Ginger, C. D. Molecular/biochemical development of new drugs against macro- and microfilariae. *Acta Leiden* 59, no. 1–2 (1990): 315–28.

Haghighi, M., et al. Comparing the effects of ginger (*Zingiber officinale*) extract and ibuprofen on patients with osteoarthritis. *Arch Iran Med* 8, no. 4 (2005): 267–71.

Heeba, G. H., et al. Effect of combined administration of ginger (*Zingiber officinale* Roscoe) and atorvastatin on the liver of rats. *Phytomedicine* 17, no. 14 (2010): 1076–81.

Imanishi, N., et al. Macrophage-mediated inhibitory effect of *Zingiber officinale* Rosc, a traditional Oriental herbal medicine, on the growth of influenza A/Aichi/2/68 virus. *Am J Cin Med* 34, no. 1 (2006): 157–69.

Immanuel, G., et al. Dietary medicinal plant extracts improve growth, immune activity and survival of tilapia *Oreochromis mossambicus*. *J Fish Biol* 74, no. 7 (2009): 1462–75.

Iqbal, Z., et al. In vitro anthelmintic activity of *Allium sativum, Zingiber officinale, Cucurbita mexicana* and *Ficus religiosa. Int J Agr Biol* 3, no. 4 (2001).

Iqbal, Z., et al. In vivo anthelmintic activity of ginger against gastrointestinal nematodes of sheep. *J Ethnopharmacol* 106, no. 2 (2006): 285–87.

Iwami, M., et al. Inhibitory effects of zingerone, a pungent component of *Zingiber officinale* Roscoe, on colonic motility in rats. *J Nat Med* 65, no. 1 (2011): 89–94.

Jagetia, G. C., et al. Influence of ginger rhizome (*Zingiber officinale* Rosc) on survival, glutathione and lipid peroxidation in mice after whole-body exposure to gamma radiation. *Radiat Res* 160, no. 5 (2003): 584–92.

Khan, R., et al. Activity of solvent extracts of *Prosopis spicigera, Zingiber officinale* and *Trachyspermum ammi* against multidrug resistant bacterial and fungal. *J Infect Dev Ctries* 4, no. 5 (2010): 292–300.

Koh, E. M., et al. Modulation of macrophage functions by compounds isolated from *Zingiber officinale*. *Planta Med* 75, no. 2 (2009): 148–51.

Lakshmi, B. V., et al. Attenuation of acute and chronic restraint stress-induced perturbations in experimental animals by *Zingiber officinale* Roscoe. *Food Chem Toxicol* 48, no. 2 (2010): 530–35.

Lans, Cheryl. Ethnoveterinary medicines used to treat endoparasites and stomach problems in pigs and pets in British Columbia, Canada. *Vet Parasitol* 148, no. 3–4 (2007): 325–40.

Lee, S., et al. Liquid chromatographic determination of 6-, 8-, 10-gingerol and 6-shogaol in ginger (*Zingiber officinale*) as the raw herb and dried aqueous extract. *J AOAC Int* 90, no. 5 (2007): 1219–26.

Lin, R. J., et al. Larvicidal activities of ginger (*Zingiber officinale*) against *Angiostrongylus cantonensis*. *Acta Trop* 115, no. 1–2 (2010): 69–76.

Lin, R. J., et al. Larvicidal constituents of *Zingiber officinale* (ginger) against *Anisakis simplex*. *Plant Med* 76, no. 16 (2010): 1852–58.

Lopez, P., et al. Solid- and vapor-phase antimicrobial activities of six essential oils: susceptibility of selected foodborne bacterial and fungal strains. *J Agric Food Chem* 53, no. 17 (2005): 6939–46.

Maghsoudi, S., et al. Preventive effect of ginger (*Zingiber officinale*) pretreatment on renal ischemia-reperfusion in rats. *Eur Surg Res* 46, no. 1 (2011): 45–51.

Mahady, G. B., et al. Ginger (*Zingiber officinale* Roscoe) and the gingerols inhibit the growth of Cag A+ strains of *Helicobacter pylori*. *Anticancer Res* 23, no. 5A (2003): 3699–702.

Malu, S. P., et al. Antibacterial activity and medicinal properties of ginger (*Zingiber officinale*). *Global J Pure Applied Sci* 15, no. 3 (2009): 365–68.

Masoud, H., et al. Comparing the effects of ginger (*Zingiber officinale*) extract and ibuprofen on patients with osteoarthritis. *Arch Iran Med* 8, no. 4 (2005): 267–71.

Merawin, L. T., et al. Screening of microfilaricidal effects of plant extracts against *Dirofilaria immitis*. *Res Vet Sci* 88, no. 1 (2010): 142–47.

Nagoshi, C., et al. Synergistic effect of [10]-gingerol and aminoglycosides against vancomycin-resistant enterococci (VRE). *Biol Pharm Bull* 29, no. 3 (2006): 443–47.

Nanjundaiah, S. M., et al. Gastroprotective effect of ginger rhizome (*Zingiber officinale*) extract: role of gallic acid and cinnamic acid in H+, K+-ATPase/*H. pylori* inhibition and anti-oxidative mechanism. *Evid Based Complement Alternat Med*, no. 249487 (2011). E-pub (preprint) July 1, 2009. doi:10.1093/ecam/nep060.

Nogueira de Melo, G. A., et al. Inhibitory effects of ginger (*Zingiber officinale* Roscoe) essential oil on leukocyte migration in vivo and in vitro. *J Nat Med* 65, no. 1 (2011): 241–46.

Nya, E. J., et al. Use of dietary ginger, *Zingiber officinale* Roscoe, as an immunostimulant to control *Aeromonas hydrophila* infections in rainbow trout, *Oncorhynchus mykiss* (Walbaum). *J Fish Dis* 32, no. 11 (2009): 971–77.

Park, K. J. Evaluation of in vitro antiviral activity in methanol extracts against influenza virus type A from Korean medicinal plants. *Phytother Res* 17, no. 9 (2003): 1059–63.

Park, K. J., et al. In vitro antiviral activity of aqueous extracts from Korean medicinal plants against influenza virus type A. *J Microbiol Biotechnol* 15, no. 5 (2005): 924–29.

Park, M., et al. Antibacterial activity of [10]-gingerol and [12]-gingerol isolated from ginger rhizome against periodontal bacteria. *Phytother Res* 22, no. 11 (2008): 1446–49.

Presser, Art. Ginger. Fact sheet in the Smart Supplementation series. Knoxville, Tenn.: Huntington College of Health Sciences, 2001. http://hchs.edu/literature/Ginger.pdf.

Raji, Y., et al. Anti-inflammatory and analgesic properties of the rhizome extract of *Zingiber officinale*. *Afr J Biomed Res* 5 (2002): 121–24.

Reinhard, G., et al. Ginger—an herbal medicinal product with broad anti-inflammatory actions. *J Med Food* 8, no. 2 (2005): 125.

Sabul, B., et al. Caryophyllene-rich rhizome oil of *Zingiber nimmonii* from South India: chemical characterization and antimicrobial activity. *Phytochemistry* 67, no. 22 (2006): 2469–73.

Sasikumar, B., et al. *Ginger*. Extension pamphlet. Calicut, Kerala: Indian Institute of Spices Research, October 2008. http://spices.res.in/ pdf/package/ginger.pdf.

Sephavand, R., et al. Ginger (*Zingiber officinale* Roscoe) elicits antinociceptive properties and potentiates morphine-induced analgesia in the rat radiant heat tail-flick test. *J Med Food* 13, no. 6 (2010): 1397–401.

Sharma, A., et al. Antibacterial activity of medicinal plants against pathogens causing complicated urinary tract infections. *Indian J Pharm Sci* 71, no. 2 (2009): 136–39.

Shivanand, D. J., et al. Fresh organically grown ginger (*Zingiber officinale*): composition and effects on LPS-induced PGE2 production. *Phytochemistry* 65 (2004): 1937–54.

Shukla, Y., et al. Cancer preventive properties of ginger: a brief review. *Food Chem Toxicol* 45, no. 5 (2007): 683–90.

Singh, G., et al. Chemistry, antioxidant and antimicrobial investigations on essential oil and oleoresins of *Zingiber officinale*. *Food Chem Toxicol* 46, no. 10 (2008): 3295–302.

Sookkongwaree, K., et al. Inhibition of viral proteases by Zingiberaceae extracts and flavones isolated from *Kaempferia parviflora*. *Pharmazie* 61, no. 8 (2006): 717–21.

Srivastava, K. C., et al. Ginger (*Zingiber officinale*) in rheumatism and musculoskeletal disorders. *Med Hypotheses* 39, no. 4 (1992): 342–48.

Stephens, James M. *Ginger*—Zingiber officinale Roscoe. Publication HS600 from the Horticultural Sciences Department, Florida Cooperative Extension Service, Institute of Food and Agricultural Sciences, University of Florida, May 1994 (reviewed March 2009). http://edis. ifas.ufl.edu/pdffiles/MV/MV06700.pdf.

Tan, B. K., et al. Immunomodulatory and antimicrobial effects of some traditional Chinese medicinal herbs: a review. *Curr Med Chem* 11, no. 11 (2004): 1423–30.

Thongson, C., et al. Antimicrobial effect of Thai spices against *Listeria monocytogenes* and *Salmonella typhimurium* CT104. *J Food Prot* 68, no. 10 (2005): 2054–58.

Ueda, H., et al. Repeated oral administration of a squeezed ginger (*Zingiber officinale*) extract augmented the serum corticosterone level and had anti-inflammatory properties. *Biosci Biotechnol Biochem* 74, no. 11 (2010): 2248–52.

van Breemen, R. B., et al. Cyclooxygenase-2 inhibitors in ginger (*Zingiber officinale*). *Fitoterapia* 82, no. 1 (2011): 38–43.

Wang, H. M., et al. *Zingiber officinale* (ginger) compounds have tetracycline-resistance modifying effects against clinical extensively drug-resistant *Acinetobacter baumannii*. *Phytother Res* 24, no. 12 (2010): 1825–30.

Wang, X., et al. Anti-influenza agents from plants and traditional Chinese medicine. *Phytother Res* 20, no. 5 (2006): 335–41.

Wattanathorn, J., et al. *Zingiber officinale* mitigates brain damage and improves memory impairment in focal cerebral ischemic rat. *Evid Based Complement Alternat Med*, no. 429505 (2011). doi:10.1155/2011/429505.

Yip, Y. B., et al. An experimental study on the effectiveness of massage with aromatic ginger and orange essential oil for moderate-to-severe knee pain among the elderly in Hong Kong. *Complement Ther Med* 16, no. 3 (2008): 131–38.

Zhou, H. L., et al. The modulatory effects of the volatile oil of ginger on the cellular immune response in vitro and in vivo in mice. *J Ethnopharmacol* 105, no. 1–2 (2006): 301–5.

Zick, S. M., et al. Quantitation of 6-, 8- and 10-gingerols and 6-shogaol in human plasma by high-performance liquid chromatography with electrochemical detection. *Int J Biomed* 6, no. 3 (2010): 233–40.

Honey

Abdelatif, M., et al. Safety and efficacy of a new honey ointment on diabetic foot ulcers: a prospective pilot study. *J Wound Care* 17, no. 3 (2008): 108–10.

Acton, C. Medihoney: a complete wound bed preparation product. *Br J Nurs* 17, no. 11 (2008): S44, S46–48.

Adams, C. J., et al. Isolation by HPLC and characterization of the bioactive fraction of New Zealand manuka (*Leptospermum scoparium*) honey. *Carbohydr Res* 343, no. 4 (2008): 651–59.

Ahmed, A. K., et al. Honey-medicated dressing: transformation of an ancient remedy into modern therapy. *Ann Plast Surg* 50, no. 2 (2003): 143–47.

Alandejani, T., et al. Effectiveness of honey on *Staphylococcus aureus* and *Pseudomonas aeruginosa* biofilms. *Otolaryngol Head Neck Surg* 141, no. 1 (2009): 114–18.

Alvarez-Suarez, J. M., et al. Antioxidant and antimicrobial capacity of several monofloral Cuban honeys and their correlation with color, polyphenol content and other chemical compounds. *Food Chem Toxicol* 48, no. 8–9 (2010): 2490–99.

Alese, O. B., et al. Pyoderma gangrenosum and ulcerative colitis in the tropics. *Rev Soc Bras Med Trop* 41, no. 6 (2008): 664–67.

Al-Jabri, A. A., et al. Antibacterial activity of Omani honey alone and in combination with gentamicin. *Saudi Med J* 26, no. 5 (2005): 767–71.

Al-Jabri, A. A., et al. In vitro antibacterial activity of Omani and African honey. *Br J Biomed Sci* 60, no. 1 (2003): 1–4.

Al-Waili, N. S. The antimicrobial potential of honey from United Arab Emirates on some microbial isolates. *Med Sci Monit* 11, no. 12 (2005): BR433–38.

———. Identification of nitric oxide metabolites in various honeys: effect of intravenous honey on plasma and urinary nitric oxide metabolites concentrations. *J Med Food* 6, no. 4 (2003): 359–64.

———. Investigating the antimicrobial activity of natural honey and its effects on the pathogenic bacterial infections of surgical wounds and conjunctiva. *J Med Food* 7, no. 2 (2004): 210–22.

———. Mixture of honey, beeswax and olive oil inhibits growth of *Staphylococcus aureus* and *Candida albicans*. *Arch Med Res* 36, no. 1 (2005): 10–13.

———. Therapeutic and prophylactic effects of crude honey on chronic seborrheic dermatitis and dandruff. *Eur J Med Res* 6, no. 7 (2001): 306–8.

———. Topical honey application vs. acyclovir for the treatment of recurrent herpes simplex lesions. *Med Sci Monit* 10, no. 8 (2004): MT94–98.

Armstrong, D. G. Manuka honey improved wound healing in patients with sloughy venous leg ulcers. *Evid Based Med* 14, no. 5 (2009): 148.

Asadi-Pooya, A. A., et al. The antimycobacterial effect of honey: an in vitro study. *Riv Biol* 96, no. 3 (2003): 491–95.

Attia, W. Y., et al. The anti-tumor effect of bee honey in Ehrlich ascite tumor model of mice is coincided with stimulation of the immune cells. *Egypt J Immunol* 15, no. 2 (2008): 169–83.

Aysan, E., et al. The role of intra-peritoneal honey administration in preventing post-operative peritoneal adhesions. *Eur J Obstet Gynecol Reprod Biol* 104, no. 2 (2002): 152–55.

Ayyildiz, A., et al. Intraurethral honey application for urethral injury: an experimental study. *Int Urol Nephrol* 39, no. 3 (2007): 815–21.

Badawy, O. F., et al. Antibacterial activity of bee honey and its therapeutic usefulness against *Escherichia coli* O157:H7 and *Salmonella typhimurium* infection. *Rev Sci Tech* 23, no. 3 (2004): 1011–22.

Baghel, P. S., et al. A comparative study to evaluate the effect of honey dressing and silver sulfadiazine dressing on wound healing in burn patients. *Indian J Plast Surg* 42, no. 2 (2009): 176–81.

Bang, L. M., et al. The effect of dilution on the rate of hydrogen peroxide production in honey and its implications for wound healing. *J Altern Complement Med* 9, no. 2 (2003): 267–73.

Bansal, V., et al. Honey—a remedy rediscovered and its therapeutic utility. *Kathmandu Univ Med J (KUMJ)* 3, no. 3 (2005): 305–9.

Bardy, J., et al. A systematic review of honey uses and its potential value within oncology care. *J Clin Nurs* 17, no. 19 (2008): 2604–23.

Basson, N. J., et al. Antimicrobial activity of two South African honeys produced from indigenous *Leucospermum cordifolium* and *Erica* species on selected micro-organisms. *BMC Complement Altern Med* 15, no. 8 (2008): 41.

Basualdo, C., et al. Comparison of the antibacterial activity of honey from different provenance against bacteria usually isolated from skin wounds. *Vet Microbiol* 124, no. 3–4 (2007): 375–81.

Bell, S. G. The therapeutic use of honey. *Neonatal Netw* 26, no. 4 (2007): 247–51.

Beretta, G., et al. Quinoline alkaloids in honey: further analytical (HPLC-DAD-ESI-MS, multidimensional diffusion-ordered NMR spectroscopy), theoretical and chemometric studies. *J J Pharm Biomed Anal* 50, no. 3 (2009): 432–39.

Betts, J. The clinical application of honey in wound care. *Nurs Times* 104, no. 14 (2008): 43–44.

Bittman, S., et al. Does honey have a role in paediatric wound management? *Br J Nurs* 19, no. 15 (2010): S19–24 passim.

Blair, S. E., et al. The unusual antibacterial activity of medical-grade *Leptospermum* honey: antibacterial spectrum, resistance and transcriptome analysis. *Eur J Microbiol Infect Dis* 28, no. 10 (2009): 1199–208.

Blaser, G., et al. Effect of medical honey on wounds colonized or infected with MRSA. *J Wound Care* 16, no. 8 (2007): 325–28.

Boorn, K. L., et al. Antimicrobial activity of honey from the stingless bee *Trigona carbonaria* determined by agar diffusion, agar dilution, broth microdilution and time-kill methodology. *J Appl Microbial* 108, no. 5 (2010): 1534–43.

Boukraâ, L., et al. Additive action of honey and starch against *Candida albicans* and *Aspergillus niger*. *Rev Iberoam Micol* 24, no. 4 (2007): 309–11.

Boukraâ, L., et al. Additive activity of royal jelly and honey against *Pseudomonas aeruginosa*. *Altern Med Rev* 13, no. 4 (2008): 330–33.

Boukraâ, L., et al. Honey use in burn management: potentials and limitations. *Forsch Komplementmed* 17, no. 2 (2010): 74–80.

Boukraâ, L., et al. Rediscovering the antibiotics of the hive. *Recent Pat Antiinfect Drug Discov* 4, no. 3 (2009): 206–13.

Boukraâ, L., et al. Sahara honey shows higher potency against *Pseudomonas aeruginosa* compared to north Algerian types of honey. *J Med Food* 10, no. 4 (2007): 712–14.

Boukraâ, L., et al. Synergistic action of starch and honey against *Aspergillus niger* in correlation with diastase number. *Mycoses* 51, no. 6 (2008): 520–22.

Boukraâ, L., et al. Synergistic action of starch and honey against *Pseudomonas aeruginosa* in correlation with diastase number. *J Altern Complement Med* 14, no. 2 (2008): 181–84.

Chambers, J. Topical manuka honey for MRSA-contaminated skin ulcers. *Palliat Med* 20, no. 5 (2006): 557.

Chang, J., et al. The use of honey for wound care management: a traditional remedy revisited. *Home Healthc Nurse* 27, no. 5 (2009): 308–16.

Chernev, I., et al. Combined noncontact, low-frequency ultrasound and medical honey for the treatment of chronic wounds: a case series. *J Wound Ostomy Continence Nurs* 37, no. 4 (2010): 421–25. E-pub (preprint) 2010.

Cooper, R. Honey in wound care: antibacterial properties. *GMS Krankenhhyg Interdiszip* 2, no. 2 (2007): doc. 51.

Cooper, R. Using honey to inhibit wound pathogens. *Nurs Times* 104, no. 3 (2008): 46, 48–49.

Cooper, R. A., et al. Absence of bacterial resistance to medical-grade manuka honey. *Eur J Microbiol Infect Dis* 29, no. 10 (2010): 1237–41.

Cooper, R. A., et al. Antibacterial activity of honey against strains of *Staphylococcus aureus* from infected wounds. *J Royal Soc Med* 92 (1999): 283–85.

Cooper, R. A., et al. The efficacy of honey in inhibiting strains of *Pseudomonas aeruginosa* from infected burns. *J Burn Care Rehabil* 23, no. 6 (2002): 366–70.

Cooper, R. A., et al. Honey, health and longevity. *Curr Aging Sci* 3, no. 3 (2010): 239–41. E-pub (preprint) 2010.

Cooper, R. A., et al. The sensitivity to honey of Gram-positive cocci of clinical significance isolated from wounds. *J Appl Microbiol* 93, no. 5 (2002): 857–63.

Cutting, K. F. Honey and contemporary wound care: an overview. *Ostomy Wound Manage* 53, no. 11 (2007): 49–54.

Dai, T., et al. Topical antimicrobials for burn wound infections. *Recent Pat Antiinfect Drug Discov* 5, no. 2 (2010): 124–51.

Dunford, C. The use of honey-derived dressings to promote effective wound management. *Prof Nurse* 20, no. 8 (2005): 35–38.

Dunwoody, G., et al. The use of medical grade honey in clinical practice. *Br J Nurs* 17, no. 20 (2008): S38–44.

Eddy, J. J., et al. Practical consideration of using topical honey for neuropathic diabetic foot ulcers: a review. *WMJ* 107, no. 4 (2008): 187–90.

Emsen, M. A different and safe method of split thickness skin graft fixation: medical honey application. *Burns* 33, no. 6 (2007): 782–87.

English, H. K., et al. The effect of manuka honey on plaque and gingivitis: a pilot study. *J Int Acad Periodontol* 6, no. 2 (2004): 63–67.

Ergul, E., et al. The effect of honey on the intestinal anastomotic wound healing in rats with obstructive jaundice. *Bratisl Lek Listy* 111, no. 5 (2010): 265–70.

Estevinho, L., et al. Antioxidant and antimicrobial effects of phenolic compounds extracts of northeast Portugal honey. *Food Chem Toxicol* 46, no. 12 (2008): 3774–79.

Estrada, H., et al. Evaluation of the antimicrobial action of honey against *Staphyloccocus aureus, Staphylococcus epidermidis, Pseudomonas aeruginosa, Escherichia coli, Salmonella enteritidis, Listeria monocytogenes* and *Aspergillus niger*. Evaluation of its microbiological charge. *Arch Latinoam Nutr* 55, no. 2 (2005): 167–71.

Eyarefe, O. D., et al. Small bowel responses to enteral honey and glutamine administration following massive small bowel resection in rabbit. *Afr J Med Sci* 37, no. 4 (2008): 309–14.

Fangio, M. F., et al. Antimicrobial activity of honey the southeast of Buenos Aires Province against *Escherichia coli*. *Rev Argent Microbiol* 39, no. 2 (2007): 120–23.

French, V. M., et al. The antibacterial activity of honey against coagulase-negative staphylococci. *J Antimicrob Chemother* 56, no. 1 (2005): 228–31.

Genacias-Acuna, E. F. Active *Leptospermum* honey and negative pressure wound therapy for nonhealing postsurgical wounds. *Ostomy Wound Manage* 56, no. 3 (2010): 10–12.

Gethin, G., et al. Bacteriological changes in sloughy venous leg ulcers treated with manuka honey or hydrogel: an RCT. *J Wound Care* 17, no. 6 (2008): 241–44, 246–47.

Gethin, G., et al. Case series of use of manuka honey in leg ulceration. *Int Wound J* 2, no. 1 (2005): 10–15.

Gethin, G., et al. Manuka honey vs. hydrogel—a prospective, open label, multicentre, randomized controlled trial to compare desloughing efficacy and healing outcomes in venous ulcers. *J Clin Nurs* 18, no. 3 (2009): 466–74.

Gethin, G. T., et al. The impact of manuka honey dressings on the surface pH of chronic wounds. *Int Wound J* 5, no. 2 (2008): 185–94.

Gollu, A., et al. Effect of honey on intestinal morphology, intraabdominal adhesions and anastomotic healing. *Phytother Res* 22, no. 9 (2008): 1243–47.

Gottrup, F., et al. Current management of wound healing. *G Ital Dermatol Venereol* 144, no. 3 (2009): 217–28.

Gupta, A. K., et al. Role of antifungal agents in the treatment of seborrheic dermatitis. *Am J Clin Dermatol* 5, no. 6 (2004): 417–22.

Gurdal, M., et al. Predisposing factors and treatment outcome in Fournier's gangrene. Analysis of 28 cases. *Urol Int* 70, no. 4 (2003): 286–90.

Hashemi B., et al. Comparison between topical honey and mafenide acetate in treatment of auricular burn. *Am J Otolaryngol* 32, no. 1 (2011): 28–31. E-pub (preprint) November 24, 2009.

Hendrickson, M. A. Utilizing active *Leptospermum* honey dressings in the treatment of cutaneous small-vessel vasculitis. *Ostomy Wound Manage* 56, no. 4 (2010): 10–12.

Henriques A., et al. Free radical production and quenching in honeys with wound healing potential. *J Antimicrob Chemother* 58, no. 4 (2006): 773–77.

Henriques A. F., et al. The intracellular effects of manuka honey on *Staphylococcus aureus*. *Eur J Clin Microbiol Infect Dis* 29, no. 1 (2010): 45–50.

Heppermann, B. Towards evidence based emergency medicine: Best BETs from the Manchester Royal Infirmary. Bet 3. Honey for the symptomatic relief of cough in children with upper respiratory tract infections. *Emerg Med J* 26, no. 7 (2009): 522–23.

Holzgreve, H. Honey is better than aciclovir in herpes. *MMW Fortschr Med* 147, no. 3 (2005): 18.

Hon, J. Using honey to heal a chronic wound in a patient with epidermolysis bullosa. *Br J Nurs* 14, no. 19 (2005): S4–10 passim.

Iftikhar F., et al. Effects of acacia honey on wound healing in various rat models. *Phytother Res* 24, no. 4 (2010): 583–86.

Ingle, R., et al. Wound healing with honey – a randomised controlled trial. *S Afr Med J* 96, no. 9 (2006): 831–35.

Irish, J., et al. Antibacterial activity of honey from the Autralian stingless bee *Trigona carbonaria*. *Int J Antimicrob Agents* 32, no. 1 (2008): 89–90.

Irish, J., et al. Honey has an antifungal effect against *Candida* species. *Med Mycol* 44, no. 3 (2006): 289–91.

Johnson, D. W., et al. The honeypot study of protocol: a randomized controlled trial of exit-site application of Medihoney antibacterial wound gel for the prevention of catheter-associated infections in peritoneal dialysis patients. *Perit Dial Int* 29, no. 3 (2009): 303–9.

Jull, A., et al. Randomized clinical trial of honey-impregnated dressings for venous leg ulcers. *Br J Surg* 95, no. 2 (2008): 175–82.

Jull, A. B, et al. Honey as a topical treatment of wounds. *Cochrane Database Syst Rev* 8, no. 4 (2008): CD005083.

Khan, F. R., et al. Honey: nutritional and medicinal value. *Int J Clin Pract* 61, no. 10 (2007): 1705–7.

Khanal, B., et al. Effect of topical honey on limitation of radiation-induced oral mucositis: an intervention study. *Int J Oral Maxillofac Surg* 39, no. 12 (2010): 1181–85. E-pub (preprint) September 15, 2010.

Khoo, Y. T., et al. Wound contraction effects and antibacterial properties of tualang honey on full-thickness burn wounds in rats in comparison to hydrofibre. *BMC Complement Altern Med* 10 (2010): 48.

Kiefer, S., et al. (E,Z)-3-(3',5'-dimethoxy-4'-hydroxy-benzylidene)-2-indolinone blocks mast cell degranulation. *Eur J Pharm Sci* 40, no. 2 (2010): 143–47.

Koc, A. N., et al. Antifungal activity of Turkish honey against *Candida* spp. and *Trichosporon* spp: an in vitro evaluation. *Med Mycol* 47, no. 7 (2009): 707–12.

Kwakman, P. H., et al. How honey kills bacteria. *FASEB J* 24, no. 7 (2010): 2576–82.

Kwakman, P. H., et al. Medical-grade honey enriched with antimicrobial peptides has enhanced activity against antibiotic-resistant pathogens. *Eur J Clin Microbiol Infect Dis* 30, no. 2 (2011): 251–57. E-pub (preprint) October 7, 2010.

Kwakman, P. H., et al. Medical-grade honey kills antibiotic-resistant bacteria in vitro and eradicates skin colonization. *Clin Infect Dis* 46, no. 11 (2008): 1677–82.

Langemo, D. K., et al. Use of honey for wound healing. *Adv Skin Wound Care* 22, no. 3 (2009): 113–18.

Lay-flurrie, K. Honey in wound care: effects, clinical application and patient benefit. *Br J Nurs* 17, no. 11 (2008): S30, S32–36.

Lotfy, M., et al. Combined use of honey, bee propolis and myrrh in healing a deep, infected wound in a patient with diabetes mellitus. *Br J Biomed* 63, no. 4 (2006): 171–73.

Lusby, P. E., et al. Bactericidal activity of different honeys against pathogenic bacteria. *Arch Med Res* 36, no. 5 (2005): 464–67.

Lusby, P. E., et al. A comparison of wound healing following treatment with *Lavandula × allardii* honey or essential oil. *Phytother Res* 20, no. 9 (2006): 755–57.

Maeda, Y., et al. Antibacterial activity of honey against community-associated methicillin-resistant *Staphyloccocus aureus* (CA-MRSA). *Complement Ther Clin Pract* 14, no. 2 (2008): 77–82.

Majtán, J. Apitherapy—the role of honey in the chronic wound healing process. *Epidemiol Mikrobiol Imunol* 58, no. 3 (2009): 137–40.

Majtan, J., et al. Effect of honey and its major royal jelly protein 1 on cytokine and MMP-9 mRNA transcripts in human keratinocytes. *Exp Dermatol* 19, no. 8 (2010): e73–79.

Majtan, J., et al. Honeydew honey as a potent antibacterial agent in eradiation of multi-drug resistant *Stenotrophomonas maltophilia* isolates from cancer patients. *Phytother Res* 25, no. 4 (2011): 584–87. E-pub (preprint) September 29, 2010.

Majtan, J., et al. Is manuka honey the best type of honey for wound care? *J Hosp Infect* 74, no. 3 (2010): 305–6.

Makhdoom, A., et al. Management of diabetic foot by natural honey. *J Ayub Med Coll Abbottabad* 21, no. 1 (2009): 103–5.

Martos, I., et al. Flavonoids in monospecific eucalyptus honeys from Australia. *J Agric Food Chem* 48, no. 10 (2000): 4744–48.

Mavric, E., et al. Identification and quantification of methylglyoxal as the dominant antibacterial constituent of manuka (*Leptospermum scoparium*) honeys from New Zealand. *Mol Nutr Food Res* 52, no. 4 (2008): 483–89.

McIntosh, C. D., et al. Honey dressing versus paraffin tulle gras following toenail surgery. *J Wound Care* 15, no. 3 (2006): 133–36.

Mercan, N., et al. Antimicrobial activity and pollen composition of honey samples collected from different provinces in Turkey. *Nat Prod Res* 21, no. 3 (2007): 187–95.

Merckoll, P., et al. Bacteria, biofilm and honey: a study of the effects of honey on "planktonic" and biofilm-embedded chronic wound bacteria. *Scand J Infect Dis* 41, no. 5 (2009): 341–47.

Miorin, P. L., et al. Antibacterial activity of honey and propolis from *Apis mellifera* and *Tetragonisca angustula* against *Staphylococcus aureus*. *J Appl Microbiol* 95, no. 5 (2003): 913–20.

Misirlioglu, A., et al. Use of honey as an adjunct in the healing of split-thickness skin graft donor site. *Dermatol Surg* 29, no. 2 (2003): 168–72.

Moghazy, A. M., et al. The clinical and cost effectiveness of bee honey dressing in the treatment of diabetic foot ulcers. *Diabetes Res Clin Pract* 89, no. 3 (2010): 276–81.

Molan, P. C. The evidence supporting the use of honey as a wound dressing. *Int J Low Extrem Wounds* 5, no. 1 (2006): 40–54.

Molan, P. C., et al. Using honey to heal diabetic foot ulcers. *Adv Skin Wound Care* 21, no. 7 (2008): 313–16.

Moolanaar, M., et al. The effect of honey compared to conventional treatment on healing of radiotherapy-induced skin toxicity in breast cancer patients. *Acta Oncol* 45, no. 5 (2006): 623–24.

Motallebnejad, M., et al. The effect of topical application of pure honey on radiation-induced mucositis: a randomized clinical trial. *J Contemp Dent Pract* 9, no. 3 (2008): 40–47.

Mphande A. N., et al. Effects of honey and sugar dressings on wound healing. *J Wound Care* 16, no. 7 (2007): 317–19.

Mullai, V., et al. Bactericidal activity of different types of honey against clinical and environmental isolates of *Pseudomonas aeruginosa*. *J Altern Complement Med* 13, no. 4 (2007): 439–41.

Mundo, M. A., et al. Growth inhibition of foodborne pathogens and food spoilage organisms by select raw honeys. *Int J Food Microbiol* 97, no. 1 (2004): 1–8.

Namias, N. Honey in the management of infections. *Surg Infect* (Larchmont) 4, no. 2 (2003): 219–26.

Nasir, N. A., et al. Antibacterial properties of tualang honey and its effect in burn wound management: a comparative study. *BMC Complement Altern Med* 10 (2010): 31.

Natarajan, S., et al. Healing of an MRSA-colonized, hydroxyurea-induced leg ulcer with honey. *J Dermatolog Treat* 12, no. 1 (2001): 33–36.

Ndayisaba, G., et al. Treatment of wounds with honey. 40 cases. *Presse Med* 21, no. 32 (1992): 1516–18.

Oduwole, O., et al. Honey for acute cough in children. *Cochrane Database Syst Rev* 20, no. 1 (2010): CD007094.

Okeniyi, J. A., et al. Comparison of healing of incised abcess wounds with honey and EUSOL dressing. *J Altern Complement Med* 11, no. 3 (2005): 511–13.

Oladejo, O. W., et al. A comparative study of the wound healing properties of honey and *Ageratum conyzoides*. *Afr J Med Sci* 32, no. 2 (2003): 193–96.

Olaitan, P. B., et al. Honey: a reservoir for microorganisms and an inhibitory agent for microbes. *Afr Health Sci* 7, no. 3 (2007): 159–65.

Osuagwu, F. C., et al. Enhanced wound contraction in fresh wounds dressed with honey in Wistar rats (*Rattus novergicus*). *West Afr J Med* 23, no. 2 (2004): 114–18.

Ousey, K., et al. Topical antimicrobial agents for the treatment of chronic wounds. *Br J Community Nurs* 14, no. 9 (2009): S6–10 passim.

Panknin, H. T. Wound management with medicinal honey: an effective alternative to antiseptics especially in young children. *Kinderkrankenschwester* 28, no. 1 (2009): 29–30.

Patton, T., et al. Use of a spectrophotometric bioassay for determination of microbial sensitivity to manuka honey. *J Microbiol Methods* 64, no. 1 (2006): 84–95.

Paul, I. M., et al. Effect of honey, dextromethorphan, and no treatment on nocturnal cough and sleep quality for coughing children and their parents. *Arch Pediatr Adolesc Med* 161, no. 12 (2007): 1140–46.

Pieper, B. Honey-based dressings and wound care: an option for care in the United States. *J Wound Ostomy Continence Nurs* 36, no. 1 (2009): 60–66; quiz 67–68.

Rashad, U. M., et al. Honey as topical prophylaxis against radiochemotherapy-induced mucositis in head and neck cancer. *J Laryngol* 123, no. 2 (2009): 223–28.

Robson, V., et al. Standardized antibacterial honey (Medihoney) with standard therapy in wound care: randomized clinical trial. *J Adv Nurs* 65, no. 3 (2009): 565–75.

Robson, V., et al. Using leptospermum honey to manage wounds impaired by radiotherapy: a case series. *Ostomy Wound Manage* 55, no. 1 (2009): 38–47.

Rossiter, K., et al. Honey promotes angiogeneic activity in the rat aortic ring assay. *J Wound Care* 19, no. 10 (2010): 440, 442–46.

Rudzka-Nowak, A., et al. Application of manuka honey and GENADYNE A4 negative pressure wound therapy system in a 55-year old woman with extensive phlegmonous and necrotic lesions in the abdominal integuments and lumbar region after traumatic rupture of the colon. *Med Sci Monit* 16, no. 11 (2010): CS138–42.

Saber, A. Effect of honey versus intergel in intraperitoneal adhesion prevention and colonic anastomotic healing: a randomized controlled study in rats. *Int J Surg* 8, no. 2 (2010): 121–27.

Salomon, D., et al. Honey: from Noe to wound care. *Rev Med Suisse* 6, no. 246 (2010): 871–74.

Sare, J. L. Leg ulcer management with topical medical honey. *Br J Community Nurs* 13, no. 9 (2008): S22–26 passim.

Sayad, S. M., et al. Immune defense of rats immunized with fennel honey, propolis, and bee venom against staphylococcal infection. *J Med Food* 12, no. 3 (2009): 569–75.

Schumacher, H. H. Use of medical honey in patients with chronic venous leg ulcers after split-skin grafting. *J Wound Care* 13, no. 10 (2004): 451–52.

Shadkam, M. N., et al. A comparison of the effect of honey, dextromethorphan, and diphenhydramine on nightly cough and sleep quality in children and their parents. *J Altern Complement Med* 16, no. 7 (2010): 787–93.

Sharp, A. Beneficial effects of honey dressings in wound management. *Nurs Stand* 24, no. 7 (2009): 66–72 passim.

Shukrimi, A., et al. A comparative study between honey and povidone iodine as dressing solution for Wagner type II diabetic foot ulcers. *Med J Malaysia* 63, no. 1 (2008): 44–46.

Simon, A., et al. Antibacterial honey (Medihoney) for wound care of immunocompromised pediatric oncology patients. *GMS Krankenhhyg Interdiszip* 1, no. 1 (2006): doc. 18.

Simon, A., et al. Wound care with antibacterial honey (Medihoney) in pediatric hematology-oncology. *Support Care Cancer* 14, no. 1 (2006): 91–97.

Staunton, C. J., et al. The use of honey as a topical dressing to treat a large, devitalized wound in a stumptail macaque (*Macaca arctoides*). *Contemp Top Lab Anim Sci* 44, no. 4 (2005): 43–45.

Stephen-Haynes, J. Evaluation of a honey-impregnated tulle dressing in primary care. *Br J Community Nurs Suppl* (2004): S21–27.

Tan, H. T., et al. The antibacterial properties of Malaysian tualang honey against wound and enteric microorganisms in comparison to manuka honey. *BMC Complement Altern Med* 15, no. 9 (2009): 34.

Tanih, N. F., et al. An African perspective on *Helicobacter pylori*: prevalence of human infection, drug resistance, and alternative approaches to treatment. *Ann Trop Med Parasitol* 103, no. 3 (2009): 189–204.

Temaru, E., et al. Antibacterial activity of honey from stingless honeybees (Hymenoptera; Apidae; Meliponinae). *Pol J Microbiol* 56, no. 4 (2007): 281–85.

Timm, M., et al. Immunomodulatory effects of honey cannot be distinguished from endotoxin. *Cytokine* 42, no. 1 (2008): 113–20.

Tonks, A. J., et al. A 5.8-kDa component of manuka honey stimulates immune cells via TLR4. *J Leukoc Biol* 82, no. 5 (2007): 1147–55.

Tonks, A. J., et al. Honey stimulates inflammatory cytokine production from monocytes. *Cytokine* 21, no. 5 (2003): 242–47.

Tshukudu, G. M ., et al. Comparative in vitro study of honey based and silver based wound preparations on cell viability. *Burns* 36, no. 7 (2010): 1036–41.

Tushar, T., et al. Effect of honey on CYP3A4, CYP2D6 and CYP2C19 enzyme activity in healthy human volunteers. *Basic Clin Pharmacol Toxicol* 100, no. 4 (2007): 269–72.

van den Berg, A. J., et al. An in vitro examination of the antioxidant and anti-inflammatory properties of buckwheat honey. *J Wound Care* 17, no. 4 (2008): 172–74, 176–78.

Van der Weyden, E. A. Treatment of a venous leg ulcer with a honey alginate dressing. *Br J Community Nurs*, June 2005, suppl.: S21–27 passim.

———. The use of honey for the treatment of two patients with pressure ulcers. *Br J Community Nurs* 8, no. 12 (2003): S14–20.

Visavadia, B. G., et al. Manuka honey dressing: an effective treatment for chronic wound infections. *Br J Oral Maxillofac Surg* 46, no. 1 (2008): 55–56.

Visavadia, B. G., et al. Manuka honey dressing: an effective treatment for chronic wound infections. *Br J Oral Maxillofac Surg* 46, no. 8 (2008): 696–97.

Wang, X. H., et al. Antimutagenic effect of various honeys and sugars against Trp-p-1. *J Agric Food Chem* 50, no. 23 (2002): 6923–28.

White, R. The benefits of honey in wound management. *Nurs Stand* 20, no. 10 (2005): 57–64; quiz 66.

Wijesinghe, M., et al. Honey in the treatment of burns: a systematic review and meta-analysis of its efficacy. *N Z Med J* 122, no. 1295 (2009): 47–60.

Wilkinson, J. M., et al. Antibacterial activity of 13 honeys against *Escherichia coli* and *Pseudomonas aeruginosa*. *J Med Food* 8, no. 1 (2005): 100–103.

Wilson, V. Assessment and management of fungating wounds: a review. *Br J Community Nurs* 10, no. 3 (205): S28–34.

Yapucu, G., et al. Effectiveness of a honey dressing for healing pressure ulcers. *J Wound Ostomy Continence Nurs* 34, no. 2 (2007): 184–90.

Yuzbasioglu, M. F., et al. Administration of honey to prevent peritoneal adhesions in a rat peritonitis model. *Int J Surg* 7, no. 1 (2009): 54–57.

Zeiger, B. The use of active *Leptospermum* honey dressings to re-initiate the wound healing process. *Ostomy Wound Manage* 56, no. 1 (2010): 10.

Zeina, B., et al. Effect of honey versus thyme on rubella virus survival in vitro. *J Altern Complement Med* 2, no. 3 (1996): 345–48.

Zhao, Y. L., et al. Effects of different extracts from radix isatidis lymphocytes of mice by biothermodynamics. *Zhongguo Zhong Yao Za Zhi* 31, no. 7 (2006): 590–93.

Juniper Berry

Akkol, E. K., et al. A comparative study on the antinociceptive and anti-inflammatory activities of five *Juniperus* taxa. *J Ethnopharamacol* 125, no. 2 (2009): 330–36.

Ali, S. A., et al. Protective role of *Juniperus phoenicea* and *Cupressus sempervirens* against CCI4. *World J Gastrointest Pharmacol Ther* 1, no. 6 (2010): 123–31.

Almaarri, K., et al. Volatile compounds from leaf extracts *of Juniperus excelsa* growing in Syria via gas chromatography mass spectrometry±. *Anal Methods* 2 (2010): 673–77.

Al-Mustafa, A. H., et al. Antioxidant activity of some Jordanian medicinal plants used traditionally for the treatment of diabetes. *Pak J Biol Sci* 11, no. 3 (2008): 351–58.

Al-Qahtani, S. J., and M. Al-Shawaf. In vitro study effectiveness of Saudi plants' extracts against selected microorganisms. Abstract of a poster presentation at the preliminary program for the Saudi Dental Society Annual Scientific Meeting and IADR–Saudi Arabian Section General Assembly Meeting, Riyadh, Saudi Arabia, January 10–13, 2005. http://iadr.confex.com/iadr/saudi05/preliminaryprogram/abstract_71741.htm.

Angioni, A., et al. Chemical composition of the essential oils of *Juniperus* from ripe and unripe berries and leaves and their antimicrobial activity. *J Agric Food Chem* 51, no. 10 (2003): 3073–78.

Anonymous. Chinese medicine treatment of chronic obstructive pulmonary disease research. Free Papers Download Center, August 4, 2009. http://eng.hi138.com/?i120068.

Anonymous. Chinese medicine treatment of depression status. Free Papers Download Center, June 19, 2008. http://eng.hi138.com/?i123796.

Anonymous. Juniper berry. Brief monograph in the herb encyclopedia maintained by Flora Manufacturing and Distributing. http://florahealth.com/herbal_encyclopedia_int.cfm (accessed March 22, 2011).

Anonymous. Totarol. http://en.wikipedia.org/wiki/Totarol (accessed November 25, 2010).

Ateş, D. A., et al. Antimicrobial activities of various medicinal and commercial plant extracts. *Turk J Biol* 27 (2003): 157–62.

Barjaktarović, B., et al. Chemical composition of *Juniperus communis* L. fruits supercritical CO2 extracts: dependence on pressure and extraction time. *J Agric Food Chem* 53, no. 7 (2005): 2630–36.

Bergner, P. *Juniperus*: are juniper berries a kidney irritant? *Medical Herbalism* 6, no. 2 (1994): 12.

Butani, L., et al. Amelioration of tacrolimus-induced nephrotoxicity in rats using juniper oil. *Transplantation* 76, no. 2 (2003): 306–11.

Caldecott, T. Juniperus communis, Pinaceae. http://toddcaldecott.com/index.php/herbs/learning-herbs (accessed November 22, 2010).

Chavali, S. R., et al. Increased production of TNF-alpha and decreased levels of dienoic eicosanoids, IL-6 and IL-10 in mice fed menhaden oil and juniper oil diets in response to an intraperitoneal lethal dose of LPS. *Prostaglandins Leukot Essent Fatty Acids* 59, no. 2 (1998): 89–93.

Clark, A. M., et al. Antimicrobial properties of heartwood, bark/sapwood and leaves of *Juniperus* species. *Phytother Res* 4, no. 1 (1990): 15–19.

Committee on Herbal Medicinal Products (HMPC). List of references supporting the assessment of *Juniperus communis* L., pseudo-fructus. European Medicines Agency, November 12, 2009. http://www.ema.europa.eu/docs/en_GB/document_library/Herbal_-_List_of_references_supporting_the_assessment_report/2011/02/WC500102145.pdf.

Derwich, E., et al. Chemical composition of leaf essential oil of *Juniperus phoenicea* and evaluation of its antibacterial activity. *Int J Agric Biol* 12 (2010): 199–204.

Diğrak, M., et al. Antimicrobial activities of several parts of *Pinus brutia, Juniperus oxycedrus, Abies ciclicia, Cedrus libani* and *Pinus nigra. Phytother Res* 13, no. 7 (1999): 584–87.

El Sawi, S. A., and H. M. Motawe. Labdane, pimarane and abietane diterpenes from the fruits of *Juniperus phoenicea* L. grown in Egypt and their activities against human liver carcinoma. *Can J Pure Appl Sci* 2, no. 1 (2008): 115–22.

El Sawi, S. A., et al. Chemical composition, cytotoxic activity and antimicrobial activity of essential oils of leaves and berries of *Juniperus phoenicea* L. grown in Egypt. *Afr J Tradit Complement Altern Med* 4, no. 4 (2007): 417–26.

Ennajar, M., et al. The influence of organ, season and drying method on chemical composition and antioxidant and antimicrobial activities of *Juniperus phoenicea* L. essential oils. *J Sci Food Agric* 90, no. 3 (2010): 462–70.

Filipowicz, N., et al. Antibacterial and antifungal activity of juniper berry oil and its selected components. *Phytotherapy Research* 17 (2003): 227–31.

Filipowicz, N., et al. The phytochemical and genetic survey of common and dwarf juniper (*Juniperus communis* and *Juniperus nana*) identifies chemical races and close taxonomic identity of species. *Planta Med* 72, no. 9 (2006): 850–53.

Gavini, E., et al. Solid lipid microparticles (SLM) containing juniper oil anti-acne topical carriers: preliminary studies. *Pharm Dev Technol* 10, no. 4 (2005): 479–87.

Ghrabi, Zeineb. *Juniperus phoenicia* L. In *A Guide to Medicinal Plants in North Africa*, 161–63. Malaga, Spain: IUCN Center for Mediterranean Cooperation, 2005.

Gordien, A. Y., et al. Antimycobacterial terpenoids from *Juniperus communis* L. (Cuppressaceae). *J Ethnopharmacol* 126, no. 3 (2009): 500–505.

Jaiswal, R., et al. Totarol inhibits bacterial cytokinesis by perturbing the assembly dynamics of FtsZ. *Biochemistry* 46, no. 14 (2007): 4211–20.

Jimenez-Arellanes, A., et al. Activity against multidrug-resistant *Mycobacterium tuberculosis* in Mexican plants used to treat respiratory diseases. *Phytother Res* 17, no. 8 (2003): 903–8.

Johnston, W. H., et al. Antimicrobial activity of some Pacific Northwest woods against anaerobic bacteria and yeast. *Phytother Res* 15, no. 7 (2001): 586–88.

Jones, S. M., et al. Dietary juniper berry oil minimizes hepatic reperfusion injury in the rat. *Hepatology* 28, no. 4 (1998): 1042–50.

Karaman, F., et al. Antimicrobial activity of aqueous and methanol extracts of *Juniperus oxycedrus* L. *J Ethnopharmacol* 85, no. 2–3 (2003): 231–35.

Karchesy, J. *The literature of juniper utilization for oils and specialty products: a report to the Western Juniper Steering Committee*. Corvallis: Oregon State University Department of Forest Products, April 1, 1998. http://juniper.oregonstate.edu/bibliography/documents/php80YmFy_literature.pdf.

Kozan, E., et al. Evaluation of some plants used in Turkish folk medicine against parasitic infections for their in vivo anthelmintic activity. *J Ethnopharmacol* 108, no. 2 (2006): 211–16.

Lamnauer, D. *Juniperus oxycedrus* L. In *A Guide to Medicinal Plants in North Africa*, 157–160. Malaga, Spain: IUCN Center for Mediterranean Cooperation, 2005.

Lesjak, M. M., et al. *Juniperus sibirica* Burgsdorf as a novel source of antioxidant and anti-inflammatory agents. *Food Chemistry* 124, no. 3 (2010): 850–56.

Loizzo, M. R., et al. Phytochemical analysis and in vitro antiviral activities of the essential oils of seven Lebanon species. *Chem Biodivers* 5, no. 3 (2008): 461–70.

Mahady, G. B., et al. In vitro susceptibility of *Helicobacter pylori* to botanical extracts used traditionally for the treatment of gastrointestinal disorders. *Pytother Res* 19, no. 11 (2005): 988–91.

Marino, A., et al. In vitro effect of branch extracts of *Juniperus* species from Turkey on *Staphylococcus aureus* biofilm. *FEMS Immunol Med Microbiol* 59, no. 3 (2010): 470–76.

Martz, F., et al. Effect of latitude and altitude on the terpenoid and soluble phenolic composition of juniper (*Juniperus communis*) needles and evaluation of their antibacterial activity in the boreal zone. *J Agric Food Chem* 57, no. 20 (2009): 9575–84.

Miceli, N., et al. Comparative analysis of flavonoid profile, antioxidant and antimicrobial activity of the berries of *Juniperus communis* L. var. *communis* and *Juniperus communis* L. var. *saxatilis* Pall. from Turkey. *J Agric Food Chem* 57, no. 15 (2009): 6570–77.

Moein, M. R., et al. Analysis of antimicrobial, antifungal and anti-oxidant activities of *Juniperus excelsa* M. B subsp. *polycarpos* (K. Koch) Takhtajan essential oil. *Pharmacognosy Res* 2, no. 3 (2010): 128–31.

Mossa, J. S., et al. Antimycobacterial constituents from *Juniperus procera, Ferula communis* and *Plumbago zeylanica* and their in vitro synergistic activity with isonicotinic acid hydrazine. *Phytother Res* 18 (2004): 934–37.

Nixon, D., and D. Hobbs. The use of totarol to treat acne in an adolescent: a case study. *NZFP (New Zealand Family Physician)* 33, no. 4 (2006): 1–3, 2006.

Orhan, N., et al. Effects of *Juniperus oxycedrus* ssp. *oxycedrus* on tissue lipid peroxidation, trace elements (Cu, Zn, Fe) and blood glucose levels in experimental diabetes. *J Ethnopharmacol* 133, no. 2 (2011): 759–64.

Ottavioli, J., et al. Chemical variability of the needle oil of *Juniperus communis* ssp. *alpina* from Corsica. *Chem Biodivers* 6, no. 12 (2009): 2192–99.

Pankaj, K., et al. Identification of phytochemical content and antibacterial activity of *Juniperus communis* leaves. *Int J Biotechnol Biochem* 6, no. 1 (2004): 87–91.

Pepeljnjak, S., et al. Antimicrobial activity of juniper berry essential oil (*Juniperus communis* L., Cupressaceae). *Acta Pharm* 55, no. 4 (2005): 417–22.

Pubget. [Juniperus articles and abstracts.] http://pubget.com (search for "juniperus"; accessed November 22, 2010).

Rezvani, S., et al. Analysis and antimicrobial activity of the plant *Juniperus communis*. *Rasāyan J Chem* 2, no. 2 (2009): 257–60.

Sadeghi-aliabadi, H., et al. Evaluation of in vitro cytotoxic effects of *Juniperus foetidissima* and *Juniperus sabina* extracts against a panel of cancer cells. *Iran J Pharm Res* 8, no. 4 (2009): 281–86.

Salido, S., et al. Chemical studies of essential oils of *Juniperus oxycedrus* ssp. *badia*. *J Ethnopharmacol* 81, no. 1 (2002): 129–34.

Samoylenko, V., et al. Antiparasitic, nematicidal and antifouling constituents from *Juniperus* berries. *Phytother Res* 22, no. 12 (2008): 1570–76.

San Feliciano, A., et al. Antineoplastic and antiviral activities of some cyclolignans. *Planta Med* 59, no. 3 (1993): 246–49.

Sati, S. C., et al. Antibacterial potential of leaf extracts of *Juniperus communis* L. from Kumaun Himalaya. *Afr J Microbiol Res* 4, no. 12 (2010): 1291–94.

Schneider, I., et al. Inhibitory activity of *Juniperus communis* on 12(S)-HETE production in human platelets. *Planta Med* 70, no. 5 (2004): 471–74.

Smith, E. C., et al. The phenolic diterpene totarol inhibits multidrug efflux pump activity in *Staphylococcus aureus*. *Antimicrob Agents Chemother* 51, no. 12 (2007): 4480–83.

Van Slambrouck, S., et al. Effects of crude aqueous medicinal plant extracts on growth and invasion of breast cancer cells. *Oncol Rep* 17, no. 6 (2007): 1487–92.

Wanner, J., et al. Chemical composition and antibacterial activity of selected essential oils and some of their main compounds. *Nat Prod Commun* 5, no. 9 (2010): 1359–64.

Webster, D., et al. Antimycobacterial screening of traditional medicinal plants using the microplate resazurin assay. *Can J Microbiol* 56, no. 6 (2010): 487–94.

Licorice

Acharya, S. K., et al. A preliminary open trial on interferon stimulator (SNMC) derived from *Glycyrrhiza glabra* in the treatment of subacute hepatic failure. *Indian J Med Res* 98 (1993): 69–74.

Adams, L. S., et al. Analysis of the interactions of botanical extract combinations against the viability of prostate cancer cell lines. *Evid Based Complement Alternat Med* 3, no. 1 (2006): 117–24.

Agarwal, A., et al. An evolution of the efficacy of licorice gargle for attenuating postoperative sore throat: a prospective, randomized, single-blind study. *Anesth Analg* 109, no. 1 (2009): 77–81.

Aiyegoro, O. A., et al. Use of bioactive plant products in combination with standard antibiotics: implications in antimicrobial chemotherapy. *J Med Plants Res* 3, no. 13 (2009): 1147–52.

Aly, A. M. Licorice: a possible anti-inflammatory and anti-ulcer drug. *AAPS PharmSciTech* 6, no. 1 (2005): E74–82.

Ambawade, S. D., et al. Anticonvulsant activity of roots and rhizomes of *Glycyrrhiza glabra*. *Ind J Pharmacol* 34 (2002): 251–55.

Anonymous. Glycyrrhiza. Wikipedia. http://en.wikipedia.org/wiki/Glycyrrhiza (accessed February 7, 2011).

Anonymous. *Glycyrrhiza glabra*. *Altern Med Rev* 10, no. 3 (2005): 230–37.

Anonymous. *Glycyrrhiza* L. Entry in the U.S. Department of Agriculture Natural Resources Conservation Service PLANTS Database. http://plants.usda.gov/java/profile?symbol=GLYCY (accessed February 7, 2011).

Anonymous. *Glycyrrhiza lepidota*. Entry in the U.S. Department of Agriculture Natural Resources Conservation Service PLANTS Database. http://plants.usda.gov/java/profile?symbol=GLLE3 (accessed December 20, 2011).

Anonymous. *Glycyrrhiza uralensis*. Wikipedia. http://en.wikipedia.org/wiki/Glycyrrhiza_uralensis (accessed February 7, 2011).

Anonymous. Liquorice. Wikipedia. http://en.wikipedia.org/wiki/Liquorice (accessed February 7, 2011).

Aoki, F., et al. Clinical safety of licorice flavonoid oil (LFO) and pharmacokinetics of glabridin in healthy humans. *J Am Coll Nutr* 26, no. 3 (2007): 209–18.

Armanini, D., et al. Treatment of polycystic ovary syndrome with spironolactone plus licorice. *Eur J Obstet Gynecol Reprod Biol* 131, no. 1 (2007): 61–67.

Asl, M. N., et al. Review of pharmacological effects of *Glycyrrhiza* sp. and its bioactive compounds. *Phytother Res* 22, no. 6 (2008): 709–24.

Badam, L. In vitro antiviral activity of indigenous glycyrrhizin, licorice and glycyrrhizic acid (Sigma) on Japanese encephalitis virus. *J Commun Dis* 29, no. 2 (1997): 91–99.

Barthomeuf, C., et al. Conferone from *Ferula schtschurowskiana* enhances vinblastine cytotoxicity in MDCK-MDR1 cells by competitively inhibiting P-glycoprotein transport. *Planta Med* 72, no. 7 (2006): 634–39.

Belofsky, G., et al. Metabolites of the "smoke tree," *Dalea spinosa*, potentiate antibiotic activity against multidrug-resistant *Staphylococcus aureus*. *J Nat Prod* 69, no. 2 (2006): 261–64.

Belofsky, G., et al. Phenolic metabolites of *Dalea versicolor* that enhance antibiotic activity against model pathogenic bacteria. *J Nat Prod* 67, no. 3 (2004): 481–84.

Betoni, J. E. C., et al. Synergism between plant extract and antimicrobial drugs used on *Staphylococcus aureus* diseases. *Mem Inst Oswaldo Cruz* 101, no. 4 (2006): 387–90.

Biavatti, Maique W. Synergy: an old wisdom, a new paradigm for pharmacotherapy. *Braz J Pharm Sci* 45, no. 3 (2009): 371–78.

Biradar, Y. Evaluation of antimalarial activity of selected plants of Indian systems of medicine and study: the synergistic activity of the compounds present therein. PhD diss., Nirma University (India), December 9, 2010. http://ietd.inflibnet.ac.in/handle/10603/1379.

Bojian, B., et al. Glycyrrhiza Linnaeus. In *Flora of China* 10, 509–11. St. Louis, MS: Missouri Botanical Garden Press; Beijing: Science Press, 2010.

Burgess, J. A. Review of over-the-counter treatments for aphthous ulceration and results from use of a dissolving oral patch containing glycyrrhiza complex herbal extract. *J Contemp Dent Pract* 9, no. 3 (2008): 88–98.

Chérigo, L., et al. Bacterial resistance modifying tetrasaccharide agents from *Ipomoea murucoides*. *Phytochemistry* 70, no. 2 (2009): 222–27.

Chérigo, L., et al. Inhibitors of bacterial multidrug efflux pumps from the resin glycosides of *Ipomoea murucoides*. *J Nat Prod* 71, no. 6 (2008): 1037–45.

Chérigo, L., et al. Resin glycosides from the flowers of *Ipomoea murucoides*. *J Nat Prod* 69, no. 4 (2006): 595–99.

Cho, H. J., et al. Hexane/ethanol extract of *Glycyrrhiza uralensis* licorice exerts potent anti-inflammatory effects in murine macrophages and in mouse skin. *Food Chem* 121 (2010): 959–66.

Chung, S. Y., et al. Potent modulation of P-glycoprotein activity by naturally occurring phenylbutenoids from *Zingiber cassumunar*. *Phytother Res* 23, no. 4 (2009): 472–76.

Chung, S. Y., et al. Potent modulation of P-glycoprotein-mediated resistance by kaempferol derivatives isolated from *Zingiber zerumbet*. *Phytother Res* 21, no. 6 (2007): 565–69.

Cinatl, J., et al. Glycyrrhizin, an active component of liquorice roots, and replication of SARS-associated coronavirus. *Lancet* 361, no. 9374 (2003): 2045–46.

Cortés-Selva, F., et al. Dihydro-beta-agarofuran sesquiterpenes: a new class of reversal agents of the multidrug resistance phenotype mediated by P-glycoprotein in the protozoan parasite *Leishmania*. *Curr Pharm Des* 11, no. 24 (2005): 3125–39.

Dao, T. T., et al. Chalcones as novel influenza A (H1N1) neuraminidase inhibitors from *Glycyrrhiza inflata*. *Bioorg Med Chem Lett* 21, no. 1 (2011): 294–98. E-pub (preprint) November 5, 2010.

Dong, Y., et al. The anti-respiratory syncytial virus (RSV) effect of radix glycyrrhizae in vitro. *Zhong Yao Cai* 27, no. 6 (2004): 425–27.

Efferth, T., et al. Complex interactions between phytochemicals: the multi-target therapeutic concept of phytotherapy. *Curr Drug Targets* 12, no. 1 (2011): 122–32.

Elmadjian, F., et al. The action of mono-ammonium glycyrrhizinate on adrenalectomized subjects and its synergism with hydrocortisone. *J Clin Endocrinol Metab* 16, no. 3 (1956): 338–49.

Fiore, C., et al. Antiviral effects of *Glycyrrhiza* species. *Phytother Res* 22, no. 2 (2008): 141–48.

Follett, J., et al. Growing licorice (*Glycyrrhiza glabra* L.). New Zealand Center for Crop and Food Research broadsheet 121 (2000).

Foster, Steven. Licorice—Glycyrrhiza. Series of monographs on the website of Steven Foster. http://stevenfoster.com/education/monograph/licorice.html (accessed February 7, 2011).

Fuhrman, B., et al. Lycopene synergistically inhibits LDL oxidation in combination with vitamin E, glabridin, rosmarinic acid, carnosic acid, or garlic. *Antioxid Redox Signal* 2, no. 3 (2000): 491–506.

Gao, X., et al. Review of pharmacological effects of *Glycyrrhiza* radix and its bioactive compounds. *Zhongguo Zhong Yao Za Zhi* 34, no. 21 (2009): 2695–700.

Grankina, V. P., et al. Trace element composition of Ural licorice *Glycyrrhiza uralensis* Fisch. (Fabaceae family). *Contemp Probl Ecol* 2, no. 4 (2009): 396–99.

Grover, I. S., et al. Effect of liquorice [*Glycyrrhiza glabra* Linn.] as an adjuvant in newly diagnosed sputum smear-positive patients of pulmonary tuberculosis on directly observed treatment short course (DOTS) therapy. *Chest* 130, no. 4, suppl. (2006): 59S.

Hammouda, F. M., et al. *Glycyrrhiza glabra* L. In *A Guide to Medicinal Plants in North Africa*, 147–50. Malaga, Spain: IUCN Center for Mediterranean Cooperation, 2005. http://uicnmed.org/nabp/database/HTM/PDF/p94.pdf.

Hayashi, H., et al. Field survey of *Glycyrrhiza* plants in central Asia (2). Characterization of phenolics and their variation in the leaves of *Glycyrrhiza* plants collected in Kazakhstan. *Chem Pharm Bull* (Tokyo) 51, no. 11 (2003): 1147–52.

He, J., et al. Antibacterial compounds from *Glycyrrhiza uralensis*. *J Nat Prod* 69 (2006): 121–24.

Hirabayashi, K., et al. Antiviral activities of glycyrrhizin and its modified compounds against human immunodeficiency virus type 1 (HIV-1) and herpes simplex virus type 1 (HSV-1) in vitro. *Chem Pharm Bull* (Tokyo) 39, no. 1 (1991): 112–15.

Hoever, G., et al. Antiviral activity of glycyrrhizic acid derivatives against SARS-coronavirus. *J Med Chem* 48, no. 4 (2005): 1256–59.

Irani, M., et al. Leaves antimicrobial activity of *Glycyrrhiza glabra* L. *Iran J Pharm Res* 9, no. 4 (2010): 425–28.

Janke, R.. *Farming a few acres of herbs: licorice.* MF-2616. Kansas State University, May 2004. ksre.ksu.edu/library/hort2/mf2616.pdf.

Johns, C. Glycyrrhizic acid toxicity caused by consumption of licorice candy cigars. *CJEM* 11, no. 1 (2009): 94–96.

Ko, H. C., et al. The effect of medicinal plants used in Chinese folk medicine on RANTES secretion by virus-infected human epithelial cells. *J Ethnopharmacol* 107, no. 2 (2006): 205–10.

Kolbe, L., et al. Anti-inflammatory efficacy of licochalcone A: correlation of clinical potency and in vitro effects. *Arch Dermatol Res* 298, no. 1 (2006): 23–30.

Kondo, K., et al. Constituent properties of licorices derived from *Glycyrrhiza uralensis, G. glabra*, or *G. inflata* identified by genetic information. *Biol Pharm Bull* 30, no. 7 (2007): 1271–77.

Kuo, K., et al. Water extract of *Glycyrrhiza uralensis* inhibited enterovirus 71 in a human foreskin fibroblast cell line. *Am J Chin Med* 37, no. 2 (2009): 383–94.

Kusano, Eiji. How to diagnose and treat a licorice-induced syndrome with findings similar to that of primary hyperaldosteronism. *Intern Med* 43, no. 1 (2004): 5–6.

Kushiev, H., et al. Remediation of abandoned saline soils using *Glycyrrhiza glabra*: a study from the Hungry Steppes of central Asia. *Int J Agr Sust.* 3, no. 2): 102, 2005.

Lapi, F., et al. Myopathies associated with red yeast rice and liquorice: spontaneous reports from the Italian Surveillance System of Natural Health Products. *Br J Clin Pharmacol* 66, no. 4 (2008): 572–74.

León, I., et al. Pentasaccharide glycosides from the roots of *Ipomoea murucoides*. *J Nat Prod* 68, no. 8 (2005): 1141–46.

Li, X. L., et al. Antioxidant status and immune activity of glycyrrhiza in allergic rhinitis mice. *Int J Mol Sci* 12 (2011): 905–16.

Li, Y. S. Toxicity attenuation and efficacy potentiation effect of liquorice on treatment of rheumatoid arthritis with *Tripterygium wilfodii*. *Zhongguo Zhong Xi Yi Jie He Za Zhi* 26, no. 12 (2006): 1117–19.

Lin, J. C. Mechanism of action of glycyrrhizic acid in inhibition of Epstein-Barr virus replication in vitro. *Antiviral Res* 59, no. 1 (2003): 41–47.

Liu, X. R., et al. Treatment of intestinal metaplasia and atypical hyperplasia of gastric mucosa with xiao wei yan powder. *Zhongguo Zhong Xi Yi Jie He Za Zhi* 12, no. 10 (1992): 602–3, 580.

Martin, M. D., et al. A controlled trial of a dissolving oral patch concerning *glycyrrhiza* (licorice) herbal extract for the treatment of aphthous ulcers. *Gen Dent* 56, no. 2 (2008): 206–10.

Moghadamnia, A. A. The efficacy of the bioadhesive patches containing licorice extract in the management of recurrent aphthous stomatitis. *Phytother Res* 23, no. 2 (2009): 246–50.

Molnár, J., et al. Reversal of multidrug resistance by natural substances from plants. *Curr Top Med Chem* 10, no. 17 (2010): 1757–68.

Morel, C., et al. Isoflavones as potentiators of antibacterial activity. *J Agric Food Chem* 51, no. 19 (2003): 5677–79.

Muralidharan, P., et al. Cerebroprotective effect of *Glycyrrhiza glabra* Linn. root extract on hypoxic rats. *J Bangladesh Pharmacol Soc (BDPS)* 4 (2009): 60–64.

Nagoshi, Chihiro. Synergistic effect of [10]-gingerol and aminoglycosides against vancomycin-resistant enterococci (VRE). *Biol Pharm Bull* 29, no. 3 (2006): 443–47.

Nomura, T., et al. Chemistry of phenolic compounds of licorice (*Glycyrrhiza* species) and their estrogenic and cytotoxic activities. *Pure Appl Chem* 74, no. 7 (2002): 1199–206.

Parsaeimehr, A., et al. Producing friable callus for suspension of culture in *Glycyrrhiza glabra*. *Adv Enviro Biol* 3, no. 2 (2009): 125–28.

Pati, A. K. Licorice (*Glycyrrhiza glabra, G. uralensis*). Press release from Best Nutrition Products, Inc., Hayward, Calif., July 10, 2010. On the website of PRLog at http://prlog.org/10780323-licorice-glycyrrhiza-glabra-uralensis-dr-abhay-kumar-pati-best-nutrition-hayward-ca-usa.html.

Pompei, R., et al. Antiviral activity of glycyrrhizic acid. *Experientia* 36, no. 3 (1980): 304.

Pompei, R., et al. Glycyrrhizic acid inhibits virus growth and inactivates virus particles. *Nature* 281, no. 5733 (1979): 689–90.

Pompei, R., et al. Glycyrrhizic acid inhibits virus growth in embryonated eggs. *Microbiologica* 6, no. 3 (1983): 247–50.

Räikkönen, K., et al. Maternal licorice consumption and detrimental cognitive and psychiatric outcomes in children. *Am J Epidemiol* 170, no. 9 (2009): 1137–46.

Renjie, L., et al. Protective effect of *Glycyrrhiza glabra* polysaccharides against carbon tetrachloride-induced liver injury in rats. *Afr J Microbiol Res* 4, no. 16 (2010): 1784–87.

Saeedi, M., et al. The treatment of atopic dermatitis with licorice gel. *J Dermatolog Treat* 14, no. 3 (2003): 153–57.

Saif, M. W., et al. Phase I study of the botanical formulation PHY906 with capecitabine in advanced pancreatic and other gastrointestinal malignancies. *Phytomedicine* 17, no. 3–4 (2010): 161–69.

Sancar, M., et al. Comparative effectiveness of *Glycyrrhiza glabra* vs. omeprazole and misoprostol for the treatment of aspirin-induced gastric ulcers. *Afr J Pharm Pharmacol* 3, no. 12 (2009): 615–20.

Sato, J., et al. Antifungal activity of plant extracts against *Arthrinium sacchari* and *Chaetomium funicola*. *J Biosci Bioeng* 90, no. 4 (2000): 442–46.

Sato, Y., et al. Isoliquiritigenin, one of the antispasmodic principles of *Glycyrrhiza uralensis* roots, acts in the lower part of intestine. *Biol Pharm Bull* 30, no. 1 (2007): 145–49.

Schröfelbauer, B., et al. Glycyrrhizin, the main active compound in liquorice, attenuates pro-inflammatory responses by interfering with membrane-dependent receptor signaling. *Biochem J* 421, no. 3 (2009): 473–82.

Shibata, S. A drug over the millennia: pharmacognosy, chemistry, and pharmacology of licorice. *Yakugaku Zasshi* 120, no. 10 (2000): 849–62.

Shirazi, M., et al. An evaluation of antibacterial activity of *Glycyrrhiza glabra* extract on the growth of salmonella, shigella and ETEC *E. coli*. *J Biol Sci* 7 (2007): 827–29.

Simões, M., et al. Understanding antimicrobial activities of phytochemicals against multidrug resistant bacteria and biofilms. *J Nat Prod* 26 (2009): 746–57.

Sofia, H. N., and T. M. Walter. Review of *Glycyrrhiza glabra*, Linn. Siddha Papers 02 (01) (LR). ISSN 0974-2522. January 12, 2009. http://openmed. nic.in/3195/01/Glycyrrhiza_final.pdf.

Stavri, M., et al. Bacterial efflux pump inhibitors from natural sources. *J Antimicrob Chemo* 59 (2007): 1247–60.

Strandberg, T. E., et al. Birth outcome in relation to licorice consumption during pregnancy. *Am J Epidemiol* 153, no. 11 (2001): 1085–88.

Strandberg, T. E., et al. Preterm birth and licorice consumption during pregnancy. *Am J Epidemiol* 156, no. 9 (2002): 803–5.

Sui, X., et al. Antiviral effect of diammonium glycyrrhizinate and lithium chloride on cell infection by pseudorabies herpesvirus. *Antiviral Res* 85, no. 2 (2010): 346–53.

Sultana, S., et al. Antimicrobial, cytotoxic and antioxidant activity of methanolic extract of *Glycyrrhiza glabra*. *Agr Biol J N America* 1, no. 5 (2010): 957–60.

Tancevski, I., et al. Images in cardiovascular medicine. Malicious licorice. *Circulation* 117 (2008): e299.

Teelucksingh, S., et al. Potentiation of hydrocortisone activity in skin by glycyrrhetinic. *Lancet* 335, no. 8697 (1990): 1060–63.

Utsunomiya, T., et al. Glycyrrizin, an active component of licorice roots, reduces morbidity and mortality of mice infected with lethal doses of influenza virus. *Antimicrob Agents Chemother* 41, no. 3 (1997): 551–56.

Wagner, H., et al. Natural products chemistry and phytomedicine research in the new millennium: new developments and challenges. *ARKIVOC* 7 (2004): 277–84.

Wang, X. Q., et al. The anti-respiratory syncytial virus effect of active compound of *Glycyrrhiza* GD4 in vitro. *Zhong Yao Cai* 29, no. 7 (2006): 692–94.

Williamson, E. M., et al. Synergy: interactions within herbal medicines. *Eur Phyto J* 8, no. 5 (2001): 401–9.

Wolkerstoerfer, A., et al. Glycyrrhizin inhibits influenza A virus uptake into the cell. *Antiviral Res* 83, no. 2 (2009): 171–78.

Wu, T. H., et al. Hypouricemic effect and regulatory effects on autonomic function of shao-yao gan-cao tang, a Chinese herbal prescription, in asymptomatic hyperuricemic vegetarians. *Rheumatol Int* 28, no. 1 (2007): 27–31.

Yamashiki, M., et al. Effects of the Japanese herbal medicine "sho-saiko-to" (TJ-9) on interleukin-12 production in patients with HCV-positive liver cirrhosis. *Dev Immunology* 7, no. 1 (1999): 17–22.

Yasue, H., et al. Severe hypokalemia, rhabdomyolysis, muscle paralysis, and respiratory impairment in a hypertensive patient taking herbal medicines containing licorice. *Intern Med* 46, no. 9 (2007): 575–78.

Yim, S. B., et al. Protective effect of glycyrrhizin on 1-methyl-4-phenylpyridinium-induced mitochondrial damage and cell death in differentiated PC12 cells. *J Pharmacol Exper Therap* 321, no. 2 (2007): 816.

Yuan, H. N., et al. A randomized, crossover comparison of herbal medicine and bromocriptine against risperidone-induced hyperprolactinemia in patients with schizophrenia. *J Clin Psychopharmacol* 28, no. 3 (2008): 264–370.

Zhang, L., et al. Study on adscription of plasma effective constituents of rat after administrated with *Paeonia lacliflora* and *Glycyrrhiza uralensis*. *Zhongguo Zhong Yao Za Zhi* 32, no. 17 (2007): 1789–91.

Red Root

Alakurtti, S., et al. Pharmacological properties of the ubiquitous natural product betulin. *Eur J Pharm Sci* 1 (2006): 1–13.

Berry, A. M., et al. Bacteriohopanetetrol: abundant lipid in frankia cells and in nitrogen-fixing nodule tissue. *Plant Physiol* 95, no. 1 (1991): 111–15.

Bishop, J. G., et al. The effect of ceanothyn on blood coagulation time. *J Am Pharm Ass* 46, no. 7 (1957): 396–98.

Cichewicz, R. H. Chemistry, biological activity, and chemotherapeutic potential of betulinic acid for the prevention and treatment of cancer and HIV infection. *Med Res Rev* 24, no. 1 (2004): 90–114.

Cook, William. Ceanothus americanus. Entry in *The Physiomedical Dispensatory* (1869). Electronic version hosted on the website of *Medical Herbalism* journal. http://medherb.com/cook/home.htm.

de Sá, M. S., et al. Antimalarial activity of betulinic acid and derivatives in vitro against *Plasmodium falciparum* and in vivo in *P. berghei*-infected mice. *Parasitol Res* 105, no. 1 (2009): 275–79.

Delwiche, C. C., et al. Nitrogren fixation by *Ceanothus*. *Plant Physiol* 40, no. 6 (1965): 1045–47.

Eichenmüller, M., et al. Betulinic acid induces apoptosis and inhibits hedgehog signaling in rhabdomyosarcoma. *Br J Cancer* 103, no. 1 (2010): 43–51.

Emile, A., et al. Bioassay-guided isolation of antifungal alkaloids from *Melochia odorata*. *Phytother Res* 21, no. 4 (2007): 398–400.

Fisher, J. B., et al. What the towers don't see at night: nocturnal sap flow in trees and shrubs at two AmeriFlux sites in California. *Tree Physiol* 27, no. 4 (2007): 597–610.

Fu, J. Y. Betulinic acid ameliorates impairment of endothelium-dependent relaxation induced by oxidative stress in rat aorta. *Zhejiang Da Xue Xue Bao Yi Xue Ban* 39, no. 5 (2010): 523–29.

Giordano, A. A. S., et al. *Ceanothus americanus*: its effect on the coagulation time of the blood. *Arch Otolaryngol* 7, no. 6 (1928): 618–22.

Groot, J. T., et al. The pharmacology of *Ceanothus americanus*. I. Preliminary studies: hemodynamics and the effects on coagulation. *J Pharm Exper Therap* 30, no. 4 (1926): 275–91.

Klein, F. K., et al. Ceanothus alkaloids. Americine. *J Am Chem Soc* 90, no. 9 (1968): 2398–404.

Kommera, H., et al. Synthesis and anticancer activity of novel betulinic acid and betulin derivatives. *Arch Pharm* (Weinheim) 343, no. 8 (2010): 449–57.

Laferriere, J. E., et al. Mineral composition of some traditional Mexican teas. *Plant Food Hum Nutr* 41 (1991): 277–82.

Lan, P., et al. Understanding the structure-activity relationship of betulinic acid derivatives as anti-HIV-1 agents by using 3D-QSAR and docking. *J Mol Model* 17, no. 7 (2011): 1643–59. E-pub (preprint) October 27, 2010.

Laszczyk, M. N. Pentacytic triterpenes of the lupane, oleanane and ursane group as tools in cancer therapy. *Planta Med* 75, no. 15 (2009): 1549–60.

Leal, I. C., et al. Ceanothane and lupane type triterpenes from *Zizyphus joazeiro*—an anti-staphylococcal evaluation. *Planta Med* 76, no. 1 (2010): 47–52.

Lee, S. M., et al. Anti-complementary activity of triterpenoides from fruit of *Zizyphus jujuba*. *Biol Pharm Bull* 27, no. 11 (2004): 1883–86.

Lee, S. S., et al. Preparation and cytotoxic effect of ceanothic acid derivatives. *J Nat Prod* 61, no. 11 (1998): 1343–47.

Li, X. C., et al. Antimicrobial compounds from *Ceanothus americanus* against oral pathogens. *Phytochemistry* 46, no. 1 (1997): 97–102.

Li, Y., et al. Betulin induces mitochondrial cytochrome c release associated apoptosis in human cancer cells. *Mol Carcinog* 49, no. 7 (2010): 630–40.

Lo, Y. C. Betulinic acid stimulates the differentiation and mineralization of osteoblastic MC3T3-E1 cells: involvement of BMP/Runx2 and beta-catenin signals. *J Agric Food Chem* 58, no. 11 (2010): 6643–49.

Lucas, Joy. Ceanothus—a nice cup of tea & a piece of ague cake. Updated August 30, 2003. On the Homeopathic Materia Medica website at http://web.mac.com/joylucas/iWeb/Site/Materia%20Medica%20(2)_files/Ceanothus.pdf.

Lucero, M. E., et al. Composition of *Ceanothus gregii* oil as determined by stream distillation and solid-phase microextraction. *J Essent Oil Res* 22 (2010): 104–42.

Lynch, T. A., et al. An investigation of the blood coagulation principles from *Ceanothus americanus*. *J Am Pharm Assoc Am Pharm Assoc* (Baltimore) 47, no. 11 (1958): 816–19.

Moore, M. *Ceanothus: red root*. Folio on the website of the Southwest School of Botanical Medicine. http://www.swsbm.com/FOLIOS/RedRtFol.pdf (accessed December 21, 2011).

Rooney, R. F., et al. A case of poisoning from *Ceanothus velutinus*, resembling *Rhus* poisoning. *Cal State J Med* 3, no. 9 (1905): 290–91.

Roscoe, C. W., et al. A preliminary study of the alkaloidal principles of *Ceanothus americanus* and *Ceanothus velutinus*. *J Am Pharm Assoc* 49, no. 2 (1960): 108–12.

Saaby, L., et al. Isolation of immunomodulatory triterpene acids from a standardized rose hip powder (*Rosa canina* L.). *Phytother Res* 25, no. 2 (2011): 195–201. E-pub (preprint) 2010.

Salazar-Aranda, R., et al. Antimicrobial and antioxidant activities of plants from northeast of Mexico. *Evid Based Complement Alternat Med* e-pub (preprint) September 21, 2009.

Spjut, R. W. *Ceanothus*: Rhamnacea. On the website of World Botanical Associates. http://worldbotanical.com/ceanothus.htm (accessed December 9, 2010).

Steele, J. C., et al. In vitro and in vivo evaluation of betulinic acid as an antimalarial. *Phytother Res* 13, no. 2 (1999): 115–19.

Suksamram, S., et al. Ceanothane- and lupane-type triterpenes with antiplasmodial and antimycobacterial activities from *Ziziphus cambodiana*. *Chem Pharm Bull* (Tokyo) 54, no. 4 (2006): 535–37.

Takada, Y., et al. Betulinic acid suppresses carcinogen-induced NF-kappa B activation through inhibition of I kappa B alpha kinase and p65 phosphorylation: abrogation of cyclooxygenase-2 and matrix metalloprotease-9. *J Immunol* 171, no. 6 (2003): 3278–86.

Theraldsen, C. E., et al. Notes on blood reactions of the alkaloids of *Ceanothus americanus*. *Am J Physiol* 79, no. 3 (1926): 545–52.

Tschesche, R., et al. Alkaloids from Rhamnaceae. IV. Integerrin, an additional peptide alkaloid from *Ceanothus integgerrimus* Hock and Arn. *Tetrahedron Lett* 11 (1968): 1311–15.

Tschesche, R., et al. Integeressin and integerrenin, two peptide alkaloids from *Ceanothus integerrimus* Hook. and Arn. *Chem Ber* 100, no. 12 (1967): 3924–36.

Vijayan, V., et al. Betulinic acid inhibits endotoxin stimulated phosphorylation cascade and pro-inflammatory prostaglandin E(2) production in human peripheral blood mononuclear cells. *Br J Pharmacol* 162, no. 6 (2011): 1291–303. E-pub (preprint) 2010.

Wastle, H. Influence of tea leaves from *Ceanothus americanus* on blood pressure of hypertensive rats. *Fed Proc* 7, no. 1, part 1 (1948): 131.

Wollenweber, E., et al. Exudate flavonoids of eight species of *Ceanothus* (Rhamnaceae). *Z Naturforsch C* 59, no. 7–8 (2004): 459–62.

Yi, J. E. Immunomodulatory effects of betulic acid from the bark of white birch on mice. *J Vet Sci* 11, no. 4 (2010): 305–13.

Yogeeswari, P., et al. Betulinic acid and its derivatives: a review on their biological properties. *Curr Med Chem* 12, no. 6 (2005): 657–66.

Yoon, J. J., et al. Betulinic acid inhibits high glucose-induced vascular smooth muscle cells proliferation and migration. *J Cell Biochem* 111, no. 6 (2010): 1501–11.

Yun, Y., et al. Immunomodulatory activity of betulinic acid by producing pro-inflammatory cytokines and activation of macrophages. *Arch Pharm Res* 26, no. 12 (2003): 1087–95.

Reishi

Ahmadi, K., et al. *Ganoderma lucidum* induces the expression of CD40/CD86 on peripheral blood monocytes. *Iran J Immunol* 6, no. 2 (2009): 87–91.

Babu, P. D., et al. The sacred mushroom "reishi"—a review. *Am Eurasian J Botany* 1, no. 3 (2008): 107–10.

Bao, X. F., et al. Structural features of immunologically active polysaccharides from *Ganoderma lucidum*. *Phytochemistry* 59, no. 2 (2002): 175–81.

Bhagwan, S. S., et al. *Ganoderma lucidum*: a potent pharmacological macrofungus. *Curr Pharm Biotechnol* 10 (2009): 717–42.

Chan, W. K., et al. *Ganoderma lucidum* mycelium and spore extracts as natural adjuvants for immunotherapy. *J Altern Complement Med* 11, no. 6 (2005): 1047–57.

Chan, W. K., et al. Response of human dendritic cells to different immunomodulatory polysaccharides derived from mushroom and barley. *Int Immunol* 19, no. 7 (2007): 891–99.

Chang, Y. H., et al. *Ganoderma lucidum* extract promotes immune responses in normal BALB/c mice in vivo. *In Vivo* 23, no. 5 (2009): 755–59.

Chang, Y. H., et al. *Ganoderma lucidum* extracts inhibited leukemia WEHI-3 cells in BALB/c mice and promoted an immune response in vivo. *Biosci Biotechnol Biochem* 73, no. 12 (2009): 2589–94.

Chen, S. D., et al. Effects of fermentation products of *Ganoderma lucidum* on growth performance and immunocompetence in weanling pigs. *Arch Anim Nutr* 62, no. 1 (2008): 22–32.

Chen, W. C., et al. Effects of *Ganoderma lucidum* and krestin on subset T-cell in spleen of gamma-irradiated mice. *Am J Chin Med* 23, no. 3–4 (1995): 289–98.

Chen, W. Y., et al. Effect of reishi polysaccharides on human stem/progenitor cells. *Bioorg Med Chem* 18, no. 24 (2010): 8583–91.

Chen, X., et al. Monitoring of immune responses to a herbal immune-modulator in patients with advanced colorectal cancer. *Int Immunopharmacol* 6, no. 3 (2006): 499–508.

Cheng, C. H., et al. The effects of two different *Ganoderma* species (lingzhi) on gene expression in human monocytic THP-1 cells. *Nutr Cancer* 62, no. 5 (2010): 648–58.

Cheuk, W., et al. Regression of gastric large B-cell lymphoma accompanied by a florid lymphoma-like T-cell reaction: immunomodulatory effect of *Ganoderma lucidum* (lingzhi)? *Int J Surg Pathol* 15, no. 2 (2007): 180–86.

Eo, S. K., et al. Antiviral activities of various water and methanol soluble substances isolated from *Ganoderma lucidum*. *J Ethnopharmacol* 68, no. 1–3 (1999): 129–36.

Eo, S. K., et al. Possible mode of antiviral activity of acidic protein bound polysaccharides isolated from *Ganoderma lucidum* on herpes simplex viruses. *J Ethnopharmacol* 72, no. 3 (2000): 475–81.

Gao, Y., et al. Antibacterial and antiviral value of the genus *Ganoderma* P. Karst. species (Aphyllophoromycetideae): a review. *Int J Med Mushrooms* 5, no. 3 (2003): 20.

Gao, Y., et al. Effects of ganopoly (a *Ganoderma lucidum* polysaccharide extract) on the immune functions in advanced-stage cancer patients. *Immunol Invest* 32, no. 3 (2003): 201–15.

Gao, Y., et al. Effects of water-soluble *Ganoderma lucidum* polysaccharides on the immune functions of patients with advanced lung cancer. *J Med Food* 8, no. 2 (2005): 159–68.

Gill, S. K., et al. Toxicity of a traditional Chinese medicine, *Ganoderma lucidum*, in children with cancer. *Can J Clin Pharmacol* 15, no. 2 (2008): e275–85.

Hijikata, Y., et al. Herbal mixtures containing the mushroom *Ganoderma lucidum* improve recovery time in patients with herpes genitalis and labialis. *J Altern Complement Med* 13, no. 9 (2007): 985–87.

Hsu, H. Y., et al. Reishi immune-modulation protein induces interleukin-2 expression via protein kinase-dependent signaling pathways within human T cells. *J Cell Physiol* 215, no. 1 (2008): 15–26.

Hsu, M. J., et al. Polysaccharide purified from *Ganoderma lucidum* inhibits spontaneous and Fas-mediated apoptosis in human neutrophils through activation of the phosphatidylinositol 3 kinase/Akt signaling pathway. *J Leukoc Biol* 72, no. 1 (2002): 207–16.

Hsu, M. J., et al. Signaling mechanisms of enhanced neutrophil phagocytosis and chemotaxis by the polysaccharide purified from *Ganoderma lucidum*. *Br J Pharmacol* 139, no. 2 (2003): 289–98.

Hsu, T. L., et al. Profiling carbohydrate-receptor interaction with recombinant innate immunity receptor-Fc fusion proteins. *J Biol Chem* 284, no. 5 (2009): 34479–89.

Huang, S. Q., et al. Extraction of polysaccharide from *Ganoderma lucidum* and its immune enhancement activity. *Int J Biol Macromol* 47, no. 3 (2010): 336–41.

Huang, S. Q., et al. Optimization of alkaline extraction of polysaccharides from *Ganoderma lucidum* and their effect on immune function of mice. *Molecules* 15, no. 5 (2010): 3694–708.

Jeurink, P. V., et al. Immunomodulatory capacity of fungal proteins on the cytokine production of human peripheral blood mononuclear cells. *Int Immunopharmacol* 8, no. 8 (2008): 1124–33.

Ji, Z., et al. Immunomodulation of RAW264.7 macrophages by GLIS, a proteopolysaccharide from *Ganoderma lucidum*. *J Ethnopharmacol* 112, no. 3 (2007): 445–50.

Kim, K. C., et al. *Ganoderma lucidum* extract protects DNA from strand breakage caused by hydroxyl radical and UV irradiation. *Int J Mol Med* 4, no. 3 (1999): 273–77.

Kim, Y. S., et al. Antiherpetic activities of acidic protein bound polysaccharides isolated from *Ganoderma lucidum* alone and in combinations with interferons. *J Ethnopharmacol* 72, no. 3 (2000): 451–58.

Kohguchi, M., et al. Immuno-potentiating effects of the antler-shaped fruiting body of *Ganoderma lucidum* (rokkaku-reishi). *Biosci Biotechnol Biochem* 68, no. 4 (2004): 881–87.

Kuo, M. C., et al. *Ganoderma lucidum* mycelia enhance innate immunity by activating NF-kappaB. *J Ethnopharmacol* 103, no. 2 (2006): 217–22.

Li, W. J., et al. *Ganoderma atrum* polysaccharide induces antitumor activity via the mitochondrial apoptotic pathway related to activation of host immune response. *J Cell Biochem* e-pub (preprint) December 7, 2010.

Li, Y. Q., et al. Anti-hepatitis B activities of ganoderic acid from *Ganoderma lucidum*. *Biotechnol Lett* 28, no. 11 (2006): 837–41.

Lin, J. Y., et al. *Ganoderma tsugae* in vivo modulates Th1/Th2 and macrophage responses in an allergic murine model. *Food Chem Toxicol* 44, no. 12 (2006): 2025–32.

Lin, K. L., et al. Reishi polysaccharides induce immunoglobulin production through the TLR4/TLR2-mediated induction of transcription factor Blimp-1. *J Biol Chem* 281, no. 34 (2006): 24111–23.

Lin, Y. L., et al. An immunomodulatory protein, ling zhi-8, induced activation and maturation of human monocyte-derived dendritic cells by the NF-kappaB and MAPK pathways. *J Leukoc Biol* 86, no. 4 (2009): 877–89.

Lin, Y. L., et al. Polysaccharide purified from *Ganoderma lucidum* induced activation and maturation of human monocyte-derived dendritic cells by the NF-kappaB and p38 mitogen-activated protein kinase pathways. *J Leukoc Biol* 78, no. 2 (2005): 533–43.

Lin, Y. L., et al. Polysaccharide purified from *Ganoderma lucidum* induces gene expression changes in human dendritic cells and promotes T helper 1 immune response in BALB/c mice. *Mol Pharmacol* 70, no. 2 (2006): 637–44.

Lin, Z. B. Cellular and molecular mechanisms of immune-modulation by *Ganoderma lucidum*. *J Pharmacol Sci* 99, no. 2 (2005): 144–53.

Lin, Z. B., et al. Anti-tumor and immunoregulatory activities of *Ganoderma lucidum* and its possible mechanisms. *Acta Pharmacol Sin* 25, no. 11 (2004): 1387–95.

Moradali, M. F., et al. Investigation of potential antibacterial properties of methanol extracts from fungus *Ganoderma applanatum*. *Chemotherapy* 52, no. 5 (2006): 241–44.

Mothana, R. A., et al. Antiviral lanostanoid triterpenes from the fungus *Ganoderma pfeifferi*. *Fitoterapia* 74, no. 1–2 (2003): 177–80.

Mothana, R. A., et al. Ganomycins A and B, new antimicrobial farnesyl hydroquinones from the basidiomycete *Ganoderma pfeifferi*. *J Nat Prod* 63, no. 3 (2000): 416–18.

Neidermeyer, T. H., et al. Antiviral terpenoid constituents of *Ganoderma pfeifferi*. *J Nat Prod* 68, no. 12 (2005): 1728–31.

Ofodile, L. N., et al. Antimicrobial activity of some *Ganoderma* species from Nigeria. *Phytother Res* 19, no. 4 (2005): 310–13.

Oh, K. W., et al. Antiherpetic activities of acidic protein bound polysaccharide isolated from *Ganoderma lucidum* alone and in combinations with acyclovir and vidarabine. *J Ethnopharmacol* 72, no. 1–2 (2000): 221–27.

Quereshi, S., et al. Evaluation of antibacterial activity of different *Ganoderma lucidum* extracts. *People's J Scientif Res* 3, no. 1 (2010): 9–13.

Russell, R., et al. *Ganoderma*—a therapeutic fungal biofactory. *Phytochemistry* 67, no. 18 (2006): 1985–2001.

Sanodiya, B. S., et al. *Ganoderma lucidum*: a potent pharmacological macrofungus. *Curr Pharm Biotechnol* 10, no. 8 (2009): 717–42.

Shao, B. M., et al. Immune receptors for polysaccharides from *Ganoderma lucidum*. *Biochem Biophys Res Commun* 323, no. 1 (2004): 133–41.

Sliva, Daniel. *Ganoderma lucidum* in cancer research, *Leukemia Res* 30 (2006): 767–68.

Sliva, D., et al. Biological activity of spores and dried powder from *Ganoderma lucidum* for the inhibition of highly invasive human breast and prostate cancer cells. *J Altern Complement Med* 9, no. 4 (2003): 491–97.

Smania, E. F., et al. Antifungal activity of sterols and triterpenes isolated from *Ganoderma annulare*. *Fitoterapia* 74, no. 4 (2003): 375–77.

Smania, J. A., et al. Derivation does not influence antimicrobial and antifungal activities of applanoxicide acids and sterols from *Ganoderma* spp. *Z Naturforsch C* 61, no. 1–2 (2006): 31–34.

Spelman, K., et al. Traditional herbal remedies that influence cell adhesion molecule activity. *Phytother Res* 25, no. 4 (2011): 473–83. E-pub (preprint) November 23, 2010.

Stamets, P. Products for log and stump cultivation. On the website of Fungi Perfecti. http://www.fungi.com/plus/index.html (accessed January 30, 2012).

Sun, L. X., et al. Promoting effects of *Ganoderma lucidum* polysaccharides on B16F10 cells to activate lymphocytes. *Basic Clin Pharmacol Toxicol* 108, no. 3 (2011): 149–54. E-pub (preprint) October 22, 2010.

Volman, J. J., et al. Effects of mushroom-derived beta-glucan-rich polysaccharide extracts on nitric oxide production by bone marrow-derived macrophages and nuclear factor-kappaB transactivation in Caco-2 reporter cells: can effects be explained by structure? *Mol Nutr Food Res* 54, no. 2 (2010): 268–76.

Wachtel-Galor, S., et al. *Ganoderma lucidum* ("lingzhi"), a Chinese medicinal mushroom: biomarker responses in a controlled human supplementation study. *Br J Nutr* 91, no. 2 (2004): 263–69.

Wang, G., et al. Enhancement of IL-2 and IFN-gamma expression and NK cells activity involved in the anti-tumor effect of ganoderic acid Me in vivo. *Int Immunopharmacol* 7, no. 6 (2007): 864–70.

Wang, X., et al. Effects of *Ganoderma lucidum* polysaccharides on CYP2E1, CYP1A2 and CYP3A activities in BCG-immune hepatic injury in rats. *Biol Pharm Bull* 30, no. 9 (2007): 1702–6.

Wang, X., et al. HPLC method for the determination and pharmacokinetic studies of four triterpenoids in rat plasma after oral administration of *Ganoderma lucidum* extract. *Biomed Chromatogr* 21, no. 4 (2007): 389–96.

Wasser, S. P. Reishi or ling zhi (*Ganoderma lucidum*). In *Encyclopedia of Dietary Supplements*, ed. P. M. Coates et al., 603–22. New York: Marcel Dekker, 2005. Reproduced online at http://alohamedicinals.com/reishi.pdf.

Xie, J. T., et al. *Ganoderma lucidum* extract inhibits proliferation of SW 480 human colorectal cancer cells. *Exp Oncol* 28, no. 1 (2006): 25–29.

Yeh, C. H., et al. Polysaccharides PS-G and protein LZ-8 from reishi (*Ganoderma lucidum*) exhibit diverse functions in regulating murine macrophages and T lymphocytes. *J Agric Food Chem* 58, no. 15 (2010): 8535–44.

Yin, G., et al. Chinese herbs (astragalus radix and *Ganoderma lucidum*) enhance immune response of carp, *Cyprinos carpio*, and protection against *Aeromonas hydrophila*. *Fish Shellfish Immunol* 26, no. 1 (2009): 140–45.

Yoon, S. Y., et al. Antimicrobial activity of *Ganoderma lucidum* extract alone and in combination with some antibiotics. *Arch Pharm Res* 17, no. 6 (1994): 438–42.

Yue, G. G., et al. Comparative studies of various *Ganoderma* species and their different parts with regard to their antitumor and immunomodulating activities in vitro. *J Altern Complement Med* 12, no. 8 (2006): 777–89.

Yuen, J. W., et al. Anticancer effects of *Ganoderma lucidum*: a review of scientific evidence. *Nutr Cancer* 53, no. 1 (2005): 11–17.

Zhang, G. L., et al. Hepatoprotective role of *Ganoderma lucidum* polysaccharide against BCG-induced immune liver injury in mice. *World J Gastroenterol* 8, no. 4 (2002): 728–33.

Zhang, J., et al. GLIS, a bioactive proteoglycan fraction from *Ganoderma lucidum*, displays anti-tumour activity by increasing both humoral and cellular immune response. *Life Sci* 87, no. 19–22 (2010): 628–37.

Zhang, J. P., et al. Lipid extract from completely sporoderm-broken germinating *Ganoderma sinensis* spores elicits potent antitumor immune responses in human macrophages. *Phytother Res* 23, no. 6 (2009): 844–50.

Zhang, Y., et al. Effects of *Ganoderma lucidum* capsules on T lymphocytes subsets in football players on "living high-training low." *Br J Sports Med* 42, no. 10 (2008): 819–22.

Zhao, H., et al. Enteric mucosal immune response might trigger the immunomodulation activity of *Ganoderma lucidum* polysaccharide in mice. *Planta Med* 76, no. 3 (2010): 223–27.

Zhou, G. Q., et al. Effect of *Ganoderma lucidum* polysaccharides on intestinal mucosal immune system in H22 liver cancer bearing mice. *Zhongguo Zhong Xi Yi Jie He Za Zhi* 29, no. 4 (2009): 335–39.

Zhou, X., et al. Ganodermataceae: natural products and their related pharmacological functions. *Am J Chin Med* 35, no. 4 (2007): 559–74.

Zhu, X. L., et al. Effects of *Ganoderma lucidum* polysaccharides on proliferation and cytotoxicity of cytokine-induced killer cells. *Acta Pharmacol Sin* 26, no. 9 (2005): 1130–37.

Rhodiola

Abidoff, M., and Z. Ramazanov. *Rhodiola rosea*: the herbal heavyweight from Russia. *Muscle Development* (January 2003). http://vitalityplus.com.au/articles/RhodiolaPDF%20on%20Physical%20Performance.pdf.

Abidov, M., et al. Effect of extracts from *Rhodiola rosea* and *Rhodiola crenulata* (Crassulaceae) roots on ATP content in mitochondria of skeletal muscles. *Bull Exp Biol Med* 136, no. 6 (2003): 585–87.

Abidov, M., et al. Extract of *Rhodiola rosea* radix reduces the level of C-reactive protein and creatinine kinase in the blood. *Bull Exp Biol Med* 138, no. 1 (2004): 63–64.

Akgul, Y., et al. Lotaustralin from *Rhodiola rosea* roots. *Fitoterapia* 75, no. 6 (2004): 612–14.

An, F., et al. Determination of salidroside in eight *Rhodiola* species by TLC-UV spectrometry. *Zhongguo Zhong Yao Za Zhi* 23, no. 1 (1998): 43–44, 64.

Anonymous. Rhodiola. On the website of Paradise Herbs. http://paradiseherbs.com/media/uploads/research/Rhodiola.pdf (accessed February 8, 2012).

Anonymous. *Rhodiola integrifolia* Raf. Entry in the U.S. Department of Agriculture Natural Resources Conservation Service PLANTS Database. http://plants.usda.gov/java/profile?symbol=RHINI (accessed December 10, 2010).

Anonymous. *Rhodiola rhodantha.* Entry in Plants for a Future database. http://www.pfaf.org/user/Plant.aspx?LatinName=Rhodiola+rhodantha (accessed December 21, 2011).

Anonymous. *Rhodiola rhodantha.* Entry in the U.S. Department of Agriculture Natural Resources Conservation Service PLANTS Database. http://plants.usda.gov/java/profile?symbol=RHRH4 (accessed December 10, 2010).

Anonymous. *Rhodiola rosea.* Monograph. *Altern Med Rev* 7, no. 5 (2002): 421–23.

Anonymous. *Rhodiola rosea.* Wikipedia. http://en.Wikipedia.org/wiki/Rhodiola_rosea (accessed February 12, 2011).

Anonymous. *Rhodiola rosea* L. Entry in the Global Biodiversity Information Facility database. http://data.gbif.org/search/taxa/Rhodiola%20rosea (accessed December 10, 2010).

Anonymous. *Rhodiola rosea* L. Entry in the U.S. Department of Agriculture Natural Resources Conservation Service PLANTS Database. http://plants.usda.gov/java/profile?symbol=RHRO3 (accessed December 10, 2010).

Anonymous. Study on the chemical constituents from *Rhodiola bupleuroldes.* Magazine abstract, October 10, 2008. http://jokefans.com/read.php/4735.htm.

Arora, R., et al. Evaluation of radioprotective activities *Rhodiola imbricata* Edgew—a high altitude plant. *Mol Cell Biochem* 273, no. 1–2 (2005): 209–23.

Aslanyan, G., et al. Double-blind, placebo-controlled, randomized study of single dose effects of ADAPT-232 on cognitive functions. *Phytomedicine* 17, no. 7 (2010): 494–99.

Battistelli, M., et al. *Rhodiola rosea* as antioxidant in red blood cells: ultrastructural and hemolytic behaviour. *Eur J Histochem* 49, no. 3 (2005): 243–54.

Bocharova, O. A., et al. The effect of a *Rhodiola rosea* extract on the incidence of recurrences of a superficial bladder cancer (experimental clinical research). *Urol Nefrol* (Moscow) 2 (1995): 46–47.

Brown, R. P., et al. *Rhodiola rosea:* a phytomedicinal overview. *HerbalGram* 56 (2002): 40–52.

Bystritsky, A., et al. A pilot study of *Rhodiola rosea* (Rhodax) for generalized anxiety disorder (GAD). *J Altern Complement Med* 14, no. 2 (2008): 175–80.

Calcabrini, C., et al. *Rhodiola rosea* ability to enrich cellular antioxidant defences of cultured human keratinocytes. *Arch Dermatol Res* 302, no. 3 (2010): 191–200.

Cao, L. L., et al. The effect of salidroside on cell damage induced by glutamate and intracellular free calcium in PC12 cells. *J Asian Nat Prod Res* 8, no. 1–2 (2006): 159–65.

Chem, X., et al. Hypoglycemic effect of *Rhodiola sachalinensis* A. Bor. polysaccharides: comparison of administration in different ways. *Zhongguo Zhong Yao Za Zhi* 21, no. 11 (1996): 685–87.

Chen, C. H., et al. Antioxidant activity of some plant extracts towards xanthine oxidase, lipoxygenase and tyrosinase. *Molecules* 14, no. 8 (2009): 2947–58.

Chen, Q. G., et al. The effects of *Rhodiola rosea* extract on 5-HT level, cell proliferation and quantity of neurons at cerebral hippocampus of depressive rats. *Phytomedicine* 16, no. 9 (2009): 830–38.

Chen, T. S., et al. Antioxidant evaluation of three adaptogen extracts. *Am J Chin Med* 36, no. 6 (2008): 1209–17.

Chen, X., et al. Protective effect of salidroside against H2O2-induced cell apoptosis in primary culture of rat hippocampal neurons. *Mol Cell Biochem* 332, no. 1–2 (2009): 85–93.

Cui, S., et al. Determination of p-tyrosol and salidroside in three samples of *Rhodiola crenulata* and one of *Rhodiola kirilowii* by capillary zone electrophoresis. *Anal Bioanal Chem* 377, no. 2 (2003): 370–74.

Darbinyan, V., et al. Clinical trial of *Rhodiola rosea* L. extract SHR-5 in the treatment of mild to moderate depression. *Nord J Psychiatry* 61, no. 5 (2007): 343–48.

Darbinyan, V., et al. *Rhodiola rosea* in stress induced fatigue—a double blind cross-over study of a standardized extract SHR-5 with a repeated low-dose regimen on the mental performance of healthy physicians during night duty. *Phytomedicine* 7, no. 5 (2000): 365–71.

De Bock, K., et al. Acute *Rhodiola rosea* intake can improve endurance exercise performance. *Int J Sport Nutr Exerc Metab* 14, no. 3 (2004): 298–307.

De Sanctis, R., et al. In vitro protective effect of *Rhodiola rosea* extract against hypochlorous acid-induced oxidative damage in human erythrocytes. *Biofactors* 20, no. 3 (2004): 147–59.

Dieamant, G. C., et al. Neuroimmunomodulatory compound for sensitive skin care: in vitro and clinical assessment. *J Cosmet Dermatol* 7, no. 2 (2008): 112–19.

Evdokimov, V. G., et al. Effect of cryopowder *Rhodiola rosea* L. on cardiorespiratory parameters and physical performance of humans. *Aviakosm Ekolog Med* 43, no. 6 (2009): 52–56.

Evstatieva, L., et al. Chemical composition of the essential oils of *Rhodiola rosea* L. of three different origins. *Pharmacogn Mag* 6, no. 24 (2010): 256–58.

Fan, W., et al. Prolyl endopeptidase inhibitors from the underground part of *Rhodiola sachalinensis. Chem Pharm Bull* (Tokyo) 49, no. 4 (2001): 396–401.

Fintelmann, V., et al. Efficacy and tolerability of a *Rhodiola rosea* extract in adults with physical and cognitive deficiencies. *Adv Ther* 24, no. 4 (2007): 929–39.

Galambosi, B. Demand and availability of *Rhodiola rosea* L. raw material. Chapter 16 in *Medicinal and Aromatic Plants*, ed. R. J. Bogers et al., 223–36. Wageningen UR Frontis series, vol. 17. Springer, 2006.

Gao, D., et al. Antidiabetic potential of *Rhodiola sachalinensis* root extract in streptozotocin-induced diabetic rats. *Methods Find Exp Clin Pharmacol* 31, no. 6 (2009): 375–81.

Gauger, K. J., et al. *Rhodiola crenulata* inhibits the tumorigenic properties of invasive mammary epithelial cells with stem cell characteristics. *J Med Plants Res* 4, no. 6 (2010): 446–54.

Goel, H. C., et al. Radioprotection by *Rhodiola imbricata* in mice against whole-body lethal irradiation. *J Med Food* 9, no. 2 (2006): 154–60.

Grace, M. H., et al. Phytochemical characterization of an adaptogenic preparation from *Rhodiola heterodonta*. *Nat Prod Commun* 4, no. 8 (2009): 1053–58.

Guest, H. J. Molecular phylogeography of *Rhodiola integrifolia* (Crassulaceae) and its postglacial recolonization of north-western North America. Poster presented at the Botany 2006 conference at California State University at Chico, July 28–August 2, 2006. http://2006.botanyconference.org/engine/search/index.php?func=detail&aid=668.

Guest, H. J. Systematic and phylogeographic implications of molecular variation in the western North American roseroot, *Rhodiola integrifolia* (Crassulaceae). Master's thesis, University of Victoria (British Columbia), 2001. http://hdl.handle.net/1828/2812.

Guo, Y. Synthesis, biological activity of salidroside and its analogues. *Chem Pharm Bull* (Tokyo) 58, no. 12 (2010): 1627–29.

Gupta, A., et al. Effects of *Rhodiola imbricata* on dermal wound healing. *Planta Med* 73, no. 8 (2007): 774–77.

Gupta, V., et al. Anti-oxidative effect of *Rhodiola imbricata* root extract in rats during cold, hypoxia and restraint (C-H-R) exposure and post-stress recovery. *Food Chem Toxicol* 48, no. 4 (2010): 1019–25.

Gupta, V., et al. A dose dependent adaptogenic and safety evaluation of *Rhodiola imbricata* Edgew, a high altitude rhizome. *Food Chem Toxicol* 46, no. 5 (2008): 1645–52.

Gupta, V., et al. Mechanism of action of *Rhodiola imbricata* Edgew during exposure to cold, hypoxia and restraint (C-H-R) stress induced hypothermia and post stress recovery in rats. *Food Chem Toxicol* 47, no. 6 (2009): 1239–45.

Ha, Z., et al. The effect of rhodiola and acetazolamide on the sleep architecture and blood oxygen saturation in men living at high altitude. *Zhonghua Jie He He Hu Xi Za Zhi* 25, no. 9 (2002): 527–30.

Hellum, B. H., et al. Potent in vitro inhibition of CYP3A4 and P-glycoprotein by *Rhodiola rosea*. *Planta Med* 76, no. 4 (2010): 331–38.

Huang, S. C., et al. Attenuation of long-term *Rhodiola rosea* supplementation on exhaustive swimming-evoked oxidative stress in the rat. *Chin J Physiol* 52, no. 5 (2009): 316–24.

Hung, S. K., et al. The effectiveness and efficacy of *Rhodiola rosea* L.: a systematic review of randomized clinical trials. *Phytomedicine* 18, no. 4 (2011): 235–44. E-pub (preprint) October 30, 2010.

Iaremiĭ, I. N., et al. Hepatoprotective properties of liquid extract of *Rhodiola rosea*. *Eksp Klin Farmakol* 65, no. 6 (2002): 57–59.

Jafari, M., et al. *Rhodiola*: a promising anti-aging Chinese herb. *Rejuvenation Res* 10, no. 4 (2007): 587–602.

Jang, S. L. Salidroside from *Rhodiola sachalinensis* protects neuronal PC12 cells against cytotoxicity induced by amyloid-beta. *Immunopharmacol Immunotoxicol* 25, no. 3 (2003): 295–304.

Jeong, H. J., et al. Neuraminidase inhibitory activities of flavonoids isolated from *Rhodiola rosea* roots and their in vitro anti-influenza viral activities. *Bioorg Med Chem* 17, no. 19 (2009): 6816–23.

Kang, S., et al. Comparative study of the constituents from 10 *Rhodiola* plants. *Zhong Yao Cai* 20, no. 12 (1997): 616–18.

Kanupriya., et al. Cytoprotective and antioxidant activity of *Rhodiola imbricata* against tert-butyl hydroperoxide induced oxidative injury in U-937 human macrophages. *Mol Cell Biochem* 275, no. 1–2 (2005): 1–6.

Kelly, G. S. *Rhodiola rosea*: a possible plant adaptogen. *Altern Med Rev* 6, no. 3 (2001): 293–302.

Khanum, F., et al. *Rhodiola rosea*: a versatile adaptogen. *Inst Food Tech* 4 (2005): 55–62.

Kobayashi, K., et al. Constituents of *Rhodiola rosea* showing inhibitory effect on lipase activity in mouse plasma and alimentary canal. *Planta Med* 74, no. 14 (2008): 1716–19.

Kormosh, N., et al. Effect of a combination of extract from several plants on cell-mediated and humoral immunity of patients with advanced ovarian cancer. *Phytother Res* 20, no. 5 (2006): 424–25.

Kucinskaite, A., et al. Evaluation of biologically active compounds in roots and rhizomes of *Rhodiola rosea* L. cultivated in Lithuania. *Medicina* (Kaunas) 43, no. 6 (2007): 487–494, 2007.

Kucinskaite, A., et al. Experimental analysis of therapeutic properties of *Rhodiola rosea* L. and its possible application in medicine. *Medicina* (Kaunas) 40, no. 7 (2004): 614–19.

Kwon, Y. I., et al. Evaluation of *Rhodiola crenulata* and *Rhodiola rosea* for management of type II diabetes and hypertension. *Asia Pac J Clin Nutr* 15, no. 3 (2006): 425–32.

Lee, F. T., et al. Chronic *Rhodiola rosea* extract supplementation enforces exhaustive swimming tolerance. *Am J Chin Med* 37, no. 3 (2009): 557–72.

Lee, M. W., et al. Antioxidative phenolic compounds from the roots of *Rhodiola sachalinensis* A. Bor. *Arch Pharm Res* 23, no. 5 (2000): 455–58.

Lei, Y., et al. Chemical composition of the essential oils of two *Rhodiola* species from Tibet. *Z Naturforsch C* 58, no. 3–4 (2003): 161–64.

441

Li, C., et al. Study on the extraction process for saldroside and p-tyrosol in *Rhodiola crenulata*. *Zhong Yao Cai* 29, no. 11 (2006): 1239–41.

Li, H. B., et al. Salidroside stimulated glucose uptake in skeletal muscle cells by activating AMP-activated protein kinase. *Eur J Pharmacol* 588, no. 2–3 (2008): 165–69.

Li, H. X., et al. Production of Th1- and Th2-dependent cytokines induced by the Chinese medicine herb, *Rhodiola algida*, on human peripheral blood monocytes. *J Ethnopharmacol* 123, no. 2 (2009): 257–66.

Li, J., et al. Effect of rhodiola on expressions of Flt-1, KDR and Tie-2 in rats with ischemic myocardium. *Zhongguo Zhong Xi Yi Jie He Za Zhi* 25, no. 5 (2005): 445–48.

Li, T., et al. Identification and comparative determination of rhodionin in traditional Tibetan medicinal plants of fourteen *Rhodiola* species by high-performance liquid chromatography-photodiode array detection and electrospray ionization-mass spectrometry. *Chem Pharm Bull* (Tokyo) 56, no. 6 (2008): 807–14.

Li, T., et al. Pharmacological studies on the sedative and hypnotic effect of salidroside from the Chinese medicinal plant *Rhodiola sachalinensis*. *Phytomedicine* 14, no. 9 (2007): 601–4.

Li, X., et al. Bioactive constituents from Chinese natural medicines. XXIX. Monoterpene and monoterpene glycosides from the roots of *Rhodiola sachalinensis*. *Chem Pharm Bull* (Tokyo) 56, no. 4 (2008): 612–15.

Liu, Q., et al. Phenolic components from *Rhodiola dumulosa*. *Zhongguo Zhong Yao Za Zhi* 33, no. 4 (2008): 411–13.

Lovieno, N., et al. Second-tier natural antidepressants: review and critique, *J Affect Disord* 130, no. 3 (2011): 343–57. E-pub (preprint) June 26, 2010.

Luo, D., et al. Studies on the chemical constituents from *Rhodiola dumulosa* (I). *Zhong Yao Cai* 28, no. 2 (2005): 98–99.

Ma, G., et al. Rhodiolosides A–E, monoterpene glycosides from *Rhodiola rosea*. *Chem Pharm Bull* (Tokyo) 54, no. 8 (2006): 1229–33.

Majewska, A., et al. Antiproliferative and antimitotic effect, S phase accumulation and induction of apoptosis and necrosis after treatment of extract from *Rhodiola rosea* rhizomes on HL-60 cells. *J Ethnopharmacol* 103, no. 1 (2006): 43–52.

Maslov, L. N., et al. Antiarrhythmic activity of phytoadaptogens in short-term ischemia-reperfusion of the heart and postinfarction cardiosclerosis. *Bull Exp Biol Med* 147, no. 3 (2009): 331–34.

Maslova, L. V., et al. The cardioprotective and antiadrenergic activity of an extract of *Rhodiola rosea* in stress. *Eksp Klin Farmakol* 57, no. 6 (1994): 61–63.

Mattioli, L., et al. Effects of *Rhodiola rosea* L. extract on behavioural and physiological alterations induced by chronic mild stress in female rats. *J Psychopharmacol* 23, no. 2 (2009): 130–42.

Mattioli, L., et al. *Rhodiola rosea* L. extract reduces stress- and CRF-induced anorexia in rats. *J Psychopharmacol* 21, no. 7 (2007): 742–50.

Meng, L. Q., et al. Effection of observation Xinnaoxin capsules in treatment of chronic cerebral circulatory insufficiency. *Zhongguo Zhong Yao Za Zhi* 32, no. 17 (2007): 1798–800.

Ming, D. S., et al. Bioactive compounds from *Rhodiola rosea* (Crassulaceae). *Phytother Res* 19, no. 9 (2005): 740–43.

Mishra, K. P., et al. Adjuvant effect of aqueous extract of *Rhodiola imbricata* rhizome on the immune responses to tetanus toxoid and ovalbumin in rats. *Immunopharmacol Immunotoxicol* 32, no. 1 (2010): 141–46.

Mishra, K. P., et al. Aqueous extract of *Rhodiola imbricata* rhizome inhibits proliferation of an erythroleukemic cell line K-562 by inducing apoptosis and cell cycle arrest at G2/M phase. *Immunobiology* 213, no. 2 (2008): 125–31.

Mishra, K. P., et al. Aqueous extract of *Rhodiola imbricata* rhizome stimulates proinflammatory mediators via phosphorylated IkappaB and transcription factor nuclear factor-kappaB. *Immunopharmacol Immunotoxicol* 28, no. 2 (2006): 201–12.

Mishra, K. P., et al. Aqueous extract of *Rhodiola imbricata* rhizome stimulates Toll-like receptor 4, granzyme-B and Th1 cytokines in vitro. *Immunobiology* 214, no. 1 (2009): 27–31.

Mook-Jung, I., et al. Neuroprotective effects of constituents of the Oriental crude drugs, *Rhodiola sacra, R. sachalinensis* and tokaku-joki-to, against beta-amyloid toxicity, oxidative stress and apoptosis. *Biol Pharm Bull* 25, no. 8 (2002): 1101–4.

Moran, R. V. *Rhodiola integrifolia*. In *Flora of North America* 8, ed. Flora of North America Steering Committee, 164–66. New York and Oxford, 2009. http://efloras.org/florataxon.aspx?flora_id=1&taxon_id=250092043.

Morgan, M., et al. *Rhodiola rosea*—rhodiola. *Chem Pharm Bull* (Tokyo) 47 (2005): 1–4.

Nakamura, S., et al. Bioactive constituents from Chinese natural medicines. XXXVI. Chemical structures and hepatoprotective effects of constituents from roots of *Rhodiola sachalinensis*. *Chem Pharm Bull* (Tokyo) 55, no. 10 (2007): 1505–11.

Nakamura, S., et al. Bioactive constituents from Chinese natural medicines. XXXVIII. Chemical structures of acyclic glycosides from the roots of *Rhodiola crenulata*. *Chem Pharm Bull* (Tokyo) 56, no. 4 (2008): 536–40.

Narimanian, M., et al. Impact of Chisan (ADAPT-232) on the quality-of-life and its efficacy as an adjuvant in the treatment of acute non-specific pneumonia. *Phytomedicine* 12, no. 10 (2005): 723–29.

Olsson, E. M., et al. A randomized, double-blind, placebo-controlled, parallel-group study of the standardized extract SHR-5 of the roots of *Rhodiola rosea* in the treatment of subjects with stress-related fatigue. *Planta Med* 75, no. 2 (2009): 105–12.

Pae, H. O., et al. *Rhodiola sachalinesis* induces the expression of inducible nitric oxide synthase gene by murine fetal hepatocytes (BNL CL. 2). *Immunopharmacol Immunotoxicol* 23, no. 1 (2001): 25–33.

Panossian, A., et al. Comparative study of *Rhodiola* preparations on behavioral despair of rats. *Phytomedicine* 15, no. 1–2 (2008): 84–91.

Panossian, A., et al. Evidence-based efficacy of adaptogens in fatigue, and molecular mechanisms related to their stress-protective activity. *Curr Clin Pharmacol* 4, no. 3 (2009): 198–219.

Panossian, A., et al. Rosenroot (*Rhodiola rosea*): traditional use, chemical composition, pharmacology and clinical efficacy. *Phytomedicine* 17, no. 7 (2010): 481–93.

Parisi, A., et al. Effects of chronic *Rhodiola rosea* supplementation on sport performance and antioxidant capacity in trained male: preliminary results. *J Sports Med Phys Fitness* 50, no. 1 (2010): 57–63.

Pashkevich, I. A., et al. Comparative evaluation of effects of p-tyrosol and *Rhodiola rosea* extract on bone marrow cells in vivo. *Eksp Klin Farmakol* 66, no. 4 (2003): 50–52.

Peng, J. N., et al. Chemical constituents of *Rhodiola kirilowii* (Regel) Regel. *Zhongguo Zhong Yao Za Zhi* 19, no. 11 (1994): 676–77, 702.

Peng, J. N., et al. Studies on the chemical constituents of *Rhodiola fastigita*. *Yao Xue Xue Bao* 31, no. 10 (1996): 798–800.

Pererva, T. P., et al. Interaction of *Ungernia victoris*, *Rhodiola rosea* and *Polyscias filicifolia* plant extracts with bacterial cells. *Tsitol Genet* 44, no. 4 (2010): 34–40.

Perfumi, M., et al. Adaptogenic and central nervous sytem effects of single doses of 3% rosavin and 1% salidroside *Rhodiola rosea* L. extract in mice. *Phytother Res* 21, no. 1 (2007): 37–43.

Pickut, W. The uses of the *Rhodiola integrifolia* herb. LIVESTRONG.com, July 13, 2010. http://livestrong.com/article/173782-the-uses-of-the-rhodiola-integrifolia-herb/.

Platikanov, S., et al. Introduction of wild golden root (*Rhodiola rosea* L.) as a potential economic crop in Bulgaria. *Econ Bot* 20, no. 10 (2008): 1–7.

Pooja., et al. Anti-inflammatory activity of *Rhodiola rosea*—"a second-generation adaptogen." *Phytother Res* 23, no. 8 (2009): 1099–102.

Qin, Y. J., et al. Effects of *Rhodiola rosea* on level of 5-hydroxytryptamine, cell proliferation and differentiation, and number of neuron in cerebral hippocampus of rats with depression induced by chronic mild stress. *Zhongguo Zhong Yao Za Zhi* 33, no. 23 (2008): 2842–46.

Qu, Z. Q., et al. Pretreatment with *Rhodiola rosea* extract reduces cognitive impairment induced by intracerebroventricular streptozotocin in rats: implications of anti-oxidative and neuroprotective effects. *Biomed Environ Sci* 22, no. 4 (2009): 318–26.

Rohloff, J., et al. Volatiles from rhizomes of *Rhodiola rosea* L. *Phytochemistry* 59, no. 6 (2002): 655–61.

Ruan, X., et al. Analysis on the trace element and amino acid content in xinjiang 6 series *Rhodiola* L. plant. *Guang Pu Xue Yu Guang Pu Fen Xi* 21, no. 4 (2001): 542–44.

Schittko, U., and J. Grann. *Rhodiola integrifolia*: hybrid origin and medicinal ancestry. In *Proceedings of the North Dakota Academy of Science*, April 2008. Available online on the CBS Interactive website at http://findarticles.com/p/articles/mi_hb253/is_62/ai_n29437249/.

Schriner, S. E., et al. Decreased mitochondrial superoxide levels and enhanced protection against paraquat in *Drosophila melanogaster* supplemented with *Rhodiola rosea*. *Free Radic Res* 43, no. 9 (2009): 836–43.

Schriner, S. E., et al. Protection of human cultured cells against oxidative stress by *Rhodiola rosea* without activation of antioxidant defenses. *Free Radic Biol Med* 47, no. 5 (20009): 577–84.

Schutgens, F. W., et al. The influence of adaptogens on ultraweak biophoton emission: a pilot-experiment. *Phytother Res* 23, no. 8 (2009): 1103–8.

Seikou, N., et al. Bioactive constituents from Chinese natural medicines. XXVI. Chemical structures and hepatoprotective effects of constituents from roots of *Rhodiola sachalinensis*. *Chem Pharm Bull* (Tokyo) 55, no. 10 (2007): 1505–11.

Seo, W. G., et al. The aqueous extract of *Rhodiola sachalinensis* root enhances the expression of inducible nitric oxide synthase gene in RAW264.7 macrophages. *J Ethnopharmacol* 76, no. 1 (2001): 119–23.

Shen, W., et al. Effects of rhodiola on expression of vascular endothelial cell growth factor and angiogenesis in aortic atherosclerotic plaque of rabbits. *Zhongguo Zhong XI Yi Jie He Za Zhi* 28, no. 11 (2008): 1022–5.

Shevtsov, V. A., et al. A randomized trial of two different doses of a SHR-5 *Rhodiola rosea* extract versus placebo and control of capacity for mental work. *Phytomedicine* 19, no. 2–3 (2003): 95–105.

Shi, C. D., et al. Automatic nervous system mediates the cardiovascular effects of *Rhodiola sacra* radix in rats. *J Ethnopharmacol* 119, no. 2 (2008): 284–90.

Sio-Po, I., et al. Association of free radicals and the tissue renin-angiotensin system: prospective effects of *Rhodiola*, a genus of Chinese herb, on hypoxia-induced pancreatic injury, *JOP* 2, no. 1 (2001): 16–25.

Skopinska-Rózewska, E., et al. The effect of *Rhodiola quadrafida* extracts on cellular immunity in mice and rats. *Pol J Vet Sci* 11, no. 2 (2008): 105–11.

Skopinska-Rózewska, E., et al. The influence of *Rhodiola quadrifida* 50% hydro-alcoholic extract and salidroside on tumor-induced angiogenesis in mice. *Pol J Vet Sci* 11, no. 2 (2008): 97–104.

Smith, H. I. Materia medica of the Bella Coola and neighboring tribes of British Columbia. In *Annual report for 1927*, bulletin no. 56 of the Canada Department of Mines and the National Museum of Canada, 47–68. Ottawa: F. A. Acland, 1929. Reproduced online at http://wolf.mind. net/swsbm/Ethnobotany/Bella_Coola_Materia_Medica.pdf.

Spasov, A. A., et al. A double-blind, placebo-controlled pilot study of the stimulating and adaptogenic effect of *Rhodiola rosea* SHR-5 extract on the fatigue of students caused by stress during an examination period with a repeated low-dose regimen. *Phytomedicine* 7, no. 2 (2000): 85–89.

Spasov, A. A., et al. The effect and preparation rodakson on the psychophysiological and physical adaptation of students to an academic load. *Eksp Klin Farmakol* 63, no. 1 (2000): 76–78.

Tan, C. B., et al. Protective effect of salidroside on endothelial cell apoptosis induced by cobalt chloride. *Biol Pharm Bull* 32, no. 8 (2009): 1359–63.

Tolonen, A., et al. Phenylpropanoid glycosides from *Rhodiola rosea*. *Chem Pharm Bull* (Tokyo) 51, no. 4 (2003): 467–70.

Tu, Y., et al. *Rhodiola crenulata* induces death and inhibits growth of breast cancer cell lines. *J Med Food* 11, no. 3 (2008): 413–23.

van Diermen, D., et al. Monoamine oxidase inhibition by *Rhodiola rosea* L. roots. *J Ethnopharmacol* 122, no. 2 (2009): 397–401.

Walker, T. B., et al. Does *Rhodiola rosea* possess ergogenic properties? *Int J Sport Nutr Exerc Metab* 16, no. 3 (2006): 305–15.

Wang, H., et al. The in vitro and in vivo antiviral effects of salidroside from *Rhodiola rosea* L. against Coxsackievirus B3. *Phytomedicine* 16, no. 2–3 (2009): 146–55.

Wang, Q., et al. Salidroside protects the hypothalamic-pituitary-gonad axis of male rats undergoing negative psychological stress in experimental navigation and weight exercise. *Zhongua Nan Ke Xue* 15, no. 4 (2009): 331–36.

Wiedenfeld, H., et al. Phytochemical and analytical studies of extracts from *Rhodiola rosea* and *Rhodiola quadrifida*. *Pharmazie* 62, no. 4 (2007): 308–11.

Wójcik, R., et al. The effect of Chinese medicinal herb *Rhodiola kirilowii* extracts on cellular immunity in mice and rats. *Pol J Vet Sci* 12, no. 3 (2009): 399–405.

Wong, Y. C., et al. Chemical constituents and anti-tuberculosis activity of root of *Rhodiola kirilowii*. *Zhongguo Zhong Yao Za Zhi* 33, no. 13 (2008): 1561–65.

Wu, T., et al. Cardioprotection of salidroside from ischemia/reperfusion injury by increasing N-acetylglucosamine linkage to cellular proteins. *Eur J Pharmacol* 613, no. 1–3 (2009): 93–99.

Wu, Y. L., et al. Hepatoprotective effects of salidroside on fulminant hepatic failure induced by D-galactosamine and lipopolysaccharide in mice. *J Pharm Pharmacol* 61, no. 10 (2009): 1375–82.

Xu, K. J., et al. Preventive and treatment effect of composite rhodiolae on acute lung injury in patients with severe pulmonary hypertension during extracorporeal circulation. *Zhongguo Zhong Xi Yi Jie He Za Zhi* 23, no. 9 (2003): 648–50.

Yan, X., et al. Seasonal variations in biomass and salidroside content in roots of *Rhodiola sachalinensis* as affected by gauze and red film shading. *Ying Yong Sheng Tai Xue Bao* 15, no. 3 (2004): 382–86.

Yoshikawa, M., et al. Bioactive constituents of Chinese natural medicines. II. Rhodiolae radix. (1). Chemical structures and antiallergic activity of rhodiocyanosides A and B from the underground part of *Rhodiola quadrifida* (Pall.) Fisch. et May. (Crassulaceae). *Chem Pharm Bull* (Tokyo) 44, no. 11 (1996): 2086–91.

Yoshikawa, M., et al. Bioactive constituents of Chinese natural medicines. IV. Rhodiolae radix. (2). On the histamine release inhibitors from the underground part of *Rhodiola sacra* (Prain ex Hamet) S. H. Fu (Crassulaceae): chemical structures of rhodiocyanoside D and sacranosides A and B. *Chem Pharm Bull* (Tokyo) 45, no. 9 (1997): 1498–503.

Yoshikawa, M., et al. Rhodiocyanosides A and B, new antiallergic cyanoglycosides from Chinese natural medicine "si lie hong jing tain," the underground part of *Rhodiola quadrifida* (Pall.) Fisch. et Mey. *Chem Pharm Bull* (Tokyo) 43, no. 7 (1995): 1245–47.

Yousef, G. G., et al. Comparative phytochemical characterization of three *Rhodiola* species. *Phytochemistry* 67 (2006): 2380–91.

Yu, S., et al. Involvement of ERK1/2 pathway in neuroprotection by salidroside against hydrogen peroxide-induced apoptotic cell death. *J Mol Neurosci* 40, no. 3 (2010): 321–31.

Yu, S., et al. Neuroprotective effects of salidroside in the PC12 cell model exposed to hypoglycemia and serum limitation. *Cell Mol Neurobiol* 28, no. 8 (2008): 1067–78.

Zhang, J., et al. Salidroside protects cardiomyocyte against hypoxia-induced death: a HIF-1alpha-activated and VEGF-mediated pathway. *Eur J Pharmacol* 607, no. 1–3 (2009): 6–14.

Zhang, L., et al. Neuroprotective effects of salidroside against beta-amyloid-induced oxidative stress in SH-SY5Y human neuroblastoma cells. *Neurochem Int* 57, no. 5 (2010): 547–55.

Zhang, L., et al. Protective effects of salidroside on hydrogen peroxide-induced apoptosis in SH-SY5Y human neuroblastoma cells. *Eur J Pharmacol* 564, no. 1–3 (2007): 18–25.

Zhang, S., et al. Early use of Chinese drug rhodiola compound for patients with post-trauma and inflammation in prevention of ALI/ARDS. *Zhonghua Wai Ke Za Zhi* 37, no. 4 (1999): 238–40.

Zhang, S., et al. Extraction of flavonoids from *Rhodiola sachlinesis* A. Bor by UPE and the antioxidant activity of its extract. *Nat Prod Res* 22, no. 2 (2008): 178–87.

Zhang, W. S., et al. Protective effects of salidroside on injury induced by hypoxia/hypoglycemia in cultured neurons. *Zhongguo Zhong Yao Za Zhi* 29, no. 5 (2004): 459–62.

Zhang, Z., et al. The effect of rhodiola capsules on oxygen consumption of myocardium and coronary artery blood flow in dogs. *Zhongguo Zhong Yao Za Zhi* 23, no. 2 (1998): 104–6.

Zhao, H. W., et al. *Rhodiola sacra* aqueous extract (RSAE) improves biochemical and sperm characteristics in cryopreserved boar semen. *Theriogenology* 71, no. 5 (2009): 849–57.

Zhou, X., et al. *Rhodiola sachalinensis* suppresses T241 fibrosarcoma tumor cells proliferation in vitro and growth in vivo. *Zhong Yao Cai* 31, no. 9 (2008): 1377–80.

Zhou, X., et al. Salidroside production by hairy roots of *Rhodiola sachalinensis* obtained after transformation with *Agrobacterium rhizogenes*. *Biol Pharm Bull* 30, no. 3 (2007): 439–42.

Zhu, B. W., et al. Reduction of noise-stress-induced physiological damage by radices of astragali and rhodiolae: glycogen, lactic acid and cholesterol contents in liver of the rat. *Biosci Biotechnol Biochem* 67, no. 9 (2003): 1930–36.

Zhu, B. W., et al. Resistance imparted by traditional Chinese medicines to the acute change of glutamic pyruvic transaminase, alkaline phosphatase and creatine kinase activities in rat blood caused by noise. *Biosci Biotechnol Biochem* 68, no. 5 (2004): 1160–63.

Zhu, L., et al. Prevention of *Rhodiola–Astragalus membranaceus* compounds against simulated plateau hypoxia brain injury in rat. *Space Med Med Eng* (Beijing) 18, no. 4 (2005): 303–5.

Zhuravlev, Y. N., et al. Medicinal plants of the Kurile Islands. *Botanical News from the Russian Far East* 2 (2005): 1–2.

Zubeldia, J. M., et al. Exploring new applications for *Rhodiola rosea*: can we improve the quality of life of patients with short-term hypothyroidism induced by hormone withdrawal? *J Med Food* 13, no. 6 (2010): 1287–92.

Zuo, G., et al. Activity of compounds from Chinese herbal medicine *Rhodiola kirilowii* (Regel) Maxim against HCV NS3 serine protease. *Antiviral Res* 76, no. 1 (2007): 86–92.

Sida

Adeniyi, S. A., et al. Preliminary phytochemical analysis and insecticidal activity of ethanolic extracts of four tropical plants (*Vernonia amygdalina, Sida acuta, Ocimum gratissimum* and *Telfaria occidentalis*) against beans weevil (*Acanthscelides obtectus*). *Int J Phys Sci* 5, no. 6 (2010): 753–62.

Agyarko, K., et al. Metal levels in some refuse dump soils and plants in Ghana. *Plant Soil Environ* 56, no. 5 (2010): 244–51.

Ahmed, F., et al. Cryptolepine, isolated from *Sida acuta*, sensitizes human gastric adenocarcinoma cells to TRAIL-induced apoptosis. *Phytother Res* 25, no. 1 (2011): 147–50. E-pub (preprint) 2010.

Ahmed, M. U. Cyclopropenoid fatty acids in seed oils of *Sida acuta* and *Sida rhombifolia* (Malvaceae). *J Am Oil Chem Sci* 53, no. 11 (1976): 698–99.

Alesiani, D., et al. Identification of phenolic compounds from medicinal and melliferous plants and their cytotoxic activity in cancer cells. *Caryologia* 60, no. 1–2 (2007): 90–95.

Ananil, K., et al. Investigation of medicinal plants of Togo for antiviral and antimicrobial activities. *Pharm Biol* 38, no. 1 (2000): 40–45.

Anonymous. Country mallow. Brief profile on the HolisticOnLine.com website. http://holistic-online.com/herbal-med/_Herbs/h129.htm (accessed January 9, 2011).

Anonymous. Country mallow. Entry in the Oshims. com herb directory. http://oshims.com/herb-directory/c/country-mallow (accessed January 9, 2011).

Anonymous. Ethnobotanical uses: *Sida acuta*. Dr. Duke's Phytochemical and Ethnobotanical Databases, online at http://ars-grin.gov/duke (accessed November 20, 2010).

Anonymous. Gulipas: *Sida cordifolia* Linn. Brief profile in Philippine Medicinal Plants database hosted on the StuartXchange.org website, updated November 2011. http://stuartxchange.org/Gulipas.html.

Anonymous. Nagabala. Brief profile on the HolisticOnLine.com website. http://holistic-online.com/herbal-med/_Herbs/h_sida-spinosa.htm (accessed January 9, 2011).

Anonymous. *Sida acuta*. Entry in the Listing of Interesting Plants of the World, on the Australian New Crops website. http://newcrops.uq.edu.au/listing/species_pages_S/Sida_acuta.htm (accessed November 15, 2010).

Anonymous. *Sida acuta*. Entry in the Pacific Island Ecosystems at Risk (PIER) database, updated December 27, 2010. http://hear.org/pier/species/sida_acuta.htm.

Anonymous. *Sida acuta*. Ethnobotanical Garden forum on the Shroomery Message Board. http://shroomery.org/forums/showflat.php/Number/945022 (accessed January 9, 2011).

Anonymous. *Sida acuta* Burm. f. Brief profile on website of Globinmed (Global Information Hub on Integrated Medicine). http://globinmed.com/index.php?option=com_content&view=article&id=79111:sida-acuta-burm-f&catid=721:s (accessed November 15, 2010).

Anonymous. *Sida* L. Entry in the U.S. Department of Agriculture Natural Resources Conservation Service PLANTS Database. http://plants.usda.gov/java/profile?symbol=SIDA (accessed November 15, 2010).

Anonymous. *Sida rhombifolia*. Brief profile on the website of Shaman Australis Botanicals. http://shaman-australis.com.au/shop/index.php?cPath=21_35_108 (accessed November 20, 2010).

Anonymous. *Sida rhombifolia* L.—Malvaceae. Chemicals and activities of the plant as given in Dr. Duke's Phytochemical and Ethnobotanical Databases, online at http://ars-grin.gov/duke (accessed November 20, 2010).

Anonymous. Taxon: *Sida acuta* Burm. f. Entry in the USDA Germplasm Resources Information Network (GRIN) database. http://www.ars-grin.gov/cgi-bin/npgs/html/taxon.pl?33885 (accessed November 20, 2010).

Assam, J. P., et al. In vitro antibacterial activity and acute toxicity studies of aqueous-methanol extract of *Sida rhombifolia* Linn. (Malvaceae). *BMC Complement Alt Med* 10, no. 40 (2010): 1–7.

Balakrishnan, V., et al. Ethanoveterinary studies amoung farmers in Dindigul District Tamil Nadu, India. *Global J Pharm* 3, no. 1 (2009): 15–23.

Banzouzi, J.-T., et al. Studies on medicinal plants of Ivory Coast: investigation of *Sida acuta* for in vitro antiplasmodial activities and identification of an active constituent. *Phytomed Int J Phytother Phytopharm* 11, no. 4 (2004): 338–41.

Bhawani, S. A., et al. Thin-layer chromatographic analysis of steroids: a review. *Trop J Pharm Res* 9, no. 3 (2010): 301–13.

Bonjean, K., et al. The DNA intercalating alkaloid cryptolepine interferes with topoisomerase II and inhibits primarily DNA synthesis in B16 melanoma. *Biochemistry* 37, no. 15 (1998): 5136–46.

Cao, J. H., et al. Studies of the chemical constituents of the herb huanghuaren (*Sida acutá* Burm. f.). *Zhongguo Zhong Yao Za Zhi* 18, no. 11 (1993): 681–703.

Chowdhury, A., et al. Phytochemical and biological investigations of *Sida rhomboidea* Linn. *Internet J Alt Med* 7, no. 2 (2009): 1–10.

Darwish, F. M. M., et al. Ecdysteroids and other constituents from *Sida spinosa*. *Phytochemistry* 62, no. 8 (2003): 1179–84.

Datusalia, A. K., et al. Antidepressant-like potential of *Sida tiagii* Bhandari fruits in mice. *J Health Sci* 55, no. 4 (2009): 641–48.

Datusalia, A. K., et al. Anxiolytic and antiseizure effects of *Sida tiagii* Bhandri. *J Health Sci* 54, no. 5 (2008): 544–50.

Dinan, L., et al. Phytoecdysteroid profiles in seeds of *Sida* spp. (Malvaceae). *Phytochem Anal* 12, no. 2 (2001): 110–19.

Edeoga, H. O., et al. Phytochemical constituents of some Nigerian medicinal plants. *Afr J Biotechnol* 4, no. 7 (2005): 685–88.

Ediriweera, E.R.H.S.S. A review of medicinal uses of weeds in Sri Lanka. *Tropical Agricultural Research & Extension* (Sri Lanka) 10 (2007): 11–16. http://sljol.info/index.php/TARE/article/viewFile/1865/1556.

Ekor, M., et al. Comparative evaluation of the protective effect of the ethanolic and methanolic leaf extracts of *Sida acuta* against hyperglycaemia and alterations of biochemical and haematological indices in alloxan diabetic rats. *J Pharmacol Toxicol* 5 (2010): 1–12.

Ekpo, M. A., et al. Antimicrobial activity of ethanolic and aqueous extracts of *Sida acuta* on microorganisms from skin infections. *J Med Plant Res* 3, no. 9 (2009): 621–24.

Flanagan, G. J., et al. The successful biological control of spinyhead sida, *Sida acuta* [Malvaceae], by *Calligrapha pantherina* (Col: Chrysomelidae) in Australia's Northern Territory. In *Proceedings of the X International Symposium on Biological Control of Weeds, July 4–14, 1999*, ed. Neal R. Spencer, 35–41. Bozeman: Montana State University, 2000.

Gupta, A. K., et al. Phytoextraction capacity of the plants growing on tannery sludge dumping sites. *Bioresour Technol* 98, no. 9 (2007): 1788–94.

Hudson, J. B., et al. Further investigations on the antiviral activities of medicinal plants of Togo. *Pharm Biol* 38, no. 1 (2000): 46–50.

Idu, M., et al. Ethnobotanical plants used for oral healthcare among the Esan tribe of Edo State, Nigeria. *Ethnobotanical Leaflets* 13 (2009): 548–63.

Idu, M., et al. Ethnobotanical uses of plants among the Binis in the treatment of ophthalmic and ENT (ear, nose and throat) ailments. *Ethnobotanical Leaflets* 13 (2009): 480–503.

Iroha, I. R., et al. Evaluation of the antibacterial activity of extracts of *Sida acuta* against clinical isolates of *Staphyloccocus aureus* isolated from human immunodeficiency virus/acquired immunodeficiency syndrome patients. *Res J Pharmacol* 3, no. 2 (2009): 22–25.

Jang, D. S., et al. Compounds obtained from *Sida acuta* with the potential to induce quinone reductase and to inhibit 7,12-dimethylbenz[a]anthracene-induced preneoplastic lesions in a mouse mammary organ culture model. *Arch Pharm Res* 26, no. 8 (2003): 585–90.

Karou, D., et al. Antibacterial activity of alkaloids from *Sida acuta*. *Afr J Biotechnol* 5, no. 2 (2006): 195–200.

Karou, D., et al. Antimalarial activity of *Sida acuta* Burm. f. (Malvaceae) and *Pterocarpus erinaceus* Poir. (Fabaceae). *J Ethnopharm* 89 (2003): 291–94.

Karou, S. D., et al. *Sida acuta* Burm. f.: a medicinal plant with numerous potencies. *Afr J Biotechnol* 6, no. 25 (2007): 2953–59.

Khan, M. H., et al. Herbal remedies of asthma in Thoubal District of Manipur in north east India. *Indian J Nat Prod Res* 1, no. 1 (2010): 80–84.

Khatoon, S., et al. HPTLC method for chemical standardization of *Sida* species and estimation of the alkaloid ephedrine. *J Planar Chromato* 18 (2005): 364–67.

Kiessoun, K., et al. Polyphenol contents, antioxidant and anti-inflammatory activities of six Malvaceae species traditionally used to treat hepatitis B in Burkina Faso. *Eur J Sci Res* 44, no. 4 (2010): 570–580, 2010.

Leonard, D. B. *Medicine at your feet: healing plants of the Hawaiian kingdom*. Sida rhombifolia *(huang hua mu)*. 2008. http://medicineatyourfeet.com/Sida_rhombifolia.pdf.

Londonkar, R. L., et al. Phytochemical and contraceptive property of *Sida acuta* Burm. f. Ind. in albino rats. *Int J PharmTech Res* 1, no. 4 (2009): 1260–66.

Malairajan, P., et al. Analgesic activity of some Indian medicinal plants *J Ethnopharmacol* 106, no. 3 (2006): 425–28.

Malairajan, P., et al. Antiulcer activity of *Sida acuta* Burm. *Nat Prod Sci* 12, no. 3 (2006): 150–52.

Matsut, T. A., et al. The plant alkaloid cryptolepine induces p21 and cell cycle arrest in a human osteosarcoma cell line. *Int J Oncol* 31 (2007): 915–22.

Mishra, M. P. Traditional-ethnoherbological and medicinal properties of *Sida* plant. On the website Ecosensorium.org, November 4, 2009. http://ecosensorium.org/2009/11/traditional-ethnoherbological-and.html.

Mott, J. J., et al. Germination and establishment of the weeds *Sida acuta* and *Pennisetum pedicellatum* in the Northern Territory. *Australian J Exper Agr Animal Husb* 20, no. 105 (1980): 463–69.

Nguyen-Pouplin, J., et al. Antimalarial and cytotoxic activities of ethnopharmacologically selected medicinal plants from south Vietnam. *J Ethnopharm* 109 (2007): 417–27.

Oboh, I. E., et al. Antimicrobial activity of the ethanol extract of the aerial parts of *Sida acuta* Burm. f. (Malvaceae). *Trop J Pharm Res* 6, no. 4 (2007): 809–13.

Ogie-Odia, E. A., et al. Assessment of some therapeutic plants of the Abbi People in Ndokwa West L.G.A. of Delta State, Nigeria. *Ethnobotanical Leaflets* 13 (2009): 989–1002.

Orech, F. O., et al. Potential toxicity of some traditional leafy vegetables consumed in Nyang'Oma Division, western Kenya. *Afr J Food Nutr Sci* 5, no. 1 (2005): 1–13.

Otero, R., et al. Snakebites and ethnobotany in the northwest region of Colombia. Part II. Neutralization of lethal and enzymatic effects of *Bothrops atrox* venom. *J Ethnopharmacol* 71, no. 3 (2000): 505–11.

Otero, R., et al. Snakebites and ethnobotany in the northwest region of Colombia. Part III. Neutralization of the haemorrhagic effect of *Bothrops atrox* venom. *J Ethnopharmacol* 73, no. 1–2 (2000): 233–41.

Oudhia, P. Khareti or bala (*Sida cordifolia* Linn.). Fact sheet on the website of the NewCROP program at Purdue University, 2004. http://www.hort.purdue.edu/newcrop/CropFactSheets/bala.html (accessed January 9, 2011).

———. Traditional medicinal knowledge about common herbs in Chattisgarh, India: interactions with the rice farmers of Tilda region. Research article on the website Botanical.com. http://botanical.com/site/column_poudhia/articles/_1130.html (accessed 11/20/2010).

———. Traditional medicinal uses of gangeran (*Sida spinosa*) in Chhattisgarh, India. Research article on the website Botanical.com. http://botanical.com/site/column_poudhia/articles/_1645.html (accessed November 20, 2010).

Prakash, A., et al. Alkaloid constituents of *Sida acuta, S. humilis, S. rhombifolia* and *S. spinosa. Planta Med* 43, no. 12 (1981): 384–88.

Rajakaruna, N., et al. Antimicrobial activity of plants collected from serpentine outcrops in Sri Lanka. *Pharm Biol* 40, no. 3 (2002): 235–44.

Rao, R. E., et al. Studies on fixed oil of seeds of *Sida acuta* Burm. *J Am Oil Chem Soc* 50, no. 5 (1973): 168–69.

Saganuwan, A. S., et al. Evaluation of *Sida acuta* subspecie *acuta* leaf/flower combination for antimicrobial activity and phytochemical constituents. *Afr J Clin Exper Microbiol* 7, no. 2 (2006): 83–88.

Sreedevi, C. D., et al. Hepatoprotective studies on *Sida acuta* Burm. f. *J Ethnopharmacol* 124, no. 2 (2009): 171–75.

Sutradhar, R. K., et al. Bioactive alkaloid from *Sida cordifolia* Linn. with analgesic and anti-inflammatory activities. *Iran J Pharm Ther* 5, no. 2 (2006): 175–78.

Williams, R., et al. *A native growing season forage for wildlife—teaweed,* Sida acuta Burm. f. Publication FOR 114, one of a series of the School of Forest Resources and Conservation, Florida Cooperative Extension Service, Institute of Food and Agricultural Sciences, University of Florida. First published December 2006; revised March 2011. http://edis.ifas.ufl.edu/pdffiles/FR/FR16800.pdf.

Usnea

Chifiriuc, M. C., et al. In vitro study of the inhibitory activity of usnic acid on dental plaque biofilm. *Roum Arch Microbiol Immunol* 68, no. 4 (2009): 215–22.

Cocchietto, M., et al. A review of usnic acid, an interesting natural compound. *Naturwissenschaften* 89, no. 4 (2002): 137–46.

Doell, Janet. The saga of *Usnea longissima* in California. *Bull Cal Lichen Soc* 11, no. 2 (2004): 37–44.

Elo, H., et al. Potent activity of the lichen antibiotic (+)-usnic acid against clinical isolates of vancomycin-resistant enterococci and methicillin-resistant *Staphylococcus aureus. Naturwissenschaften* 94, no. 6 (2007): 465–68.

Esme, H., et al. Investigation of the germicidal effect of usnic acid, betadine, savlosol, and desderman on the protoscolexes of lung hydatid cysts. *Tukiye Parazitol Derg* 31, no. 2 (2007): 101–4.

Fazio, A. T., et al. Lichen secondary metabolites from the cultured lichen mycobionts of *Teloschistes chryophthamus* and *Ramalina celastri* and their antiviral activities. *Z Naturforsch C* 62, no. 7–8 (2007): 543–49.

Hariharan, G. N., et al. Checklist of lichens and lichenicolous fungi of Tamil Nadu (India). On the website of the Environmental Information System Centre, September 1, 2007. http://tnenvis.nic.in/Lichens/tamil-nadu.htm.

Ingólfsdóttir, K. Usnic acid. *Phytochemistry* 61, no. 7 (2002): 729–36.

Kim, M. S., et al. Melanogenesis inhibitory effects of methanolic extracts of *Umbilicaria esculenta* and *Usnea longissima. J Microbiol* 45, no. 6 (2007): 578–82.

Kreander, K., et al. A rapid screening method for detecting active compounds against erythromycin-resistant bacterial strains of Finnish origin. *Folia Micobiol* 50, no. 6 (2005): 487–93.

Lans, C., et al. Ethnoveterinary medicines used for ruminants in British Columbia, Canada. *J Ethnobiol Ethnomed* 26, no. 3 (2007): 11.

Lauterwein, M., et al. In vitro activities of the lichen secondary metabolites vulpinic acid, (+)-usnic acid, and (-)-usnic acid against aerobic and anaerobic microorganisms. *Antimicrob Agents Chemother* 39, no. 11 (1995): 2541–43.

Lira, M. C., et al. In vitro uptake and antimycobacterial activity of liposomal usnic acid formulation. *J Liposome Res* 19, no. 1 (2009): 49–58.

Molnár, K., et al. Current results on biological activities of lichen secondary metabolites: a review. *Z Naturforsch C* 65, no. 3–4 (2010): 157–73.

Paranagama, P. A., et al. Heptaketides from *Corynespora* sp. inhibiting the cavern beard lichen, *Usnea cavernosa*: first report of metabolites of an endolichenic fungus. *J Nat Prod* 70 (2007): 1700–1705.

Paudel, B., et al. Antibacterial activities of ramlin, usnic acid and its three derivatives isolated from the Antarctic lichen *Ramalina terebrata*. *Z Naturforsch C* 65, no. 1–2 (2010)): 34–38.

Ramos, D. F., et al. Antimycobacterial activity of usnic acid against resistant and susceptible strains of *Mycobacterium tuberculosis* and non-tuberculous mycobacteria. *Pharm Biol* 48, no. 3 (2010): 260–63.

Rawat, M. S. M., et al. Chemical study on Garhwal Himalayan lichen: *Usnea emidotteries*. *Ind J Chem* 45B (2006): 2566–70.

Rowe, J. G., et al. Antibacterial activity of some lichens from southern Spain. *Ann Pharm Fr* 47, no. 2 (1989): 89–94.

Storaunet, K. O., et al. Effect of logging on the threatened epiphytic lichen *Usnea longissima*: a comparative and retrospective approach. *Silva Fennica* 42, no. 5 (2008): 685.

Verma, N., et al. Antioxidant and hepatoprotective activity of a lichen *Usnea ghattensis* in vitro. *Appl Biochem Biotechnol* 152, no. 2–3 (2008): 167–81.

Vijayan, P., et al. Antiviral activity of medicinal plants of Nilgiris. *Indian J Med Res* 120, no. 1 (2004): 24–29.

Wang, X. P., et al. Plasmid elimination effect of usnic acid on the antibiotic-resistant *Staphylococcus aureus*. *Zhong Yao Cai* 29, no. 1 (2006): 36–39.

Weckesser, S., et al. Screening of plant extracts for antimicrobial activity against bacteria and yeasts with dermatological relevance. *Phytomedicine* 14, no. 7–8 (2007): 508–16.

Wei, L. L., et al. In vitro effect of (+)-usnic acid on *Toxoplasma gondii* tachyzoites. *Zhongguo Ji Sheng Chong Xue Yu Ji Sheng Chong Bing Za Zhi* 26, no. 6 (2008): 438–41.

Yamamoto, Y., et al. Screening of tissue cultures and thalli of lichens and some of their active constituents for inhabitation of tumor promoter-induced Epstein-Barr virus activation. *Chem Pharm Bull* (Tokyo) 43, no. 8 (1995): 1388–90.

INDEX

A

By the Same Author

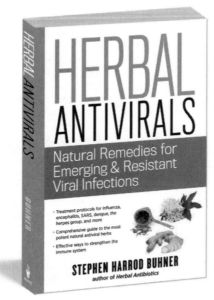

416 pages. Paper. ISBN 978-1-61212-160-4.

Praise for Stephen Harrod Buhner's *Herbal Antivirals*

"This book is a must for every herbalist and every health-care worker's office — full of plants and ideas that can make a difference!"
— **Kate Gilday, herbalist and Ayurvedic lifestyle consultant, Woodland Essence**

"Elegant, articulate and brilliantly researched. Given the critical nature of our ecological fragility, this book is a must for every practitioner's library."
— **Kathleen Maier, RH (AHG), Sacred Plant Traditions, LLC**

"Provides an alternative — and life-saving — solution."
— **Laurie Regan, PhD, ND, Dean of Classical Chinese Medicine, National College of Natural Medicine, and cohost of *True Nature Radio***

Herbs for Hepatitis C and the Liver

Important information and practical guidance for protecting the liver and strengthening the immune system.

Join the conversation. Share your experience with this book, learn more about Storey Publishing's authors, and read original essays and book excerpts at storey.com. Look for our books wherever quality books are sold or by calling 800-441-5700.